The Pharmacy Technician:

A Comprehensive Approach

Jahangir Moini, M.D., M.P.H.

Director of Pharmacy Technician Programs
Florida Metropolitan University
Melbourne, Florida

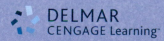
DELMAR
CENGAGE Learning

Australia • Brazil • Japan • Korea • Mexico • Singapore • Spain • United Kingdom • United States

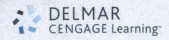

The Pharmacy Technician: A Comprehensive Approach
Jahangir Moini

Vice President, Health Care Business Unit:
  William Brottmiller

Editorial Director: Cathy L. Esperti

Acquisitions Editors: Maureen Rosener

Developmental Editor: Darcy M. Scelsi

Editorial Assistant: Elizabeth Howe

Marketing Director: Jennifer McAvey

Marketing Coordinator: Chris Manion

Art and Design Specialist: Alex Vasilakos

Production Coordinator: Jessica McNavich

Project Editor: Daniel Branagh

For product information and technology assistance, contact us at
Cengage Learning Customer & Sales Support, 1-800-354-9706

For permission to use material from this text or product,
submit all requests online at **www.cengage.com/permissions**
Further permissions questions can be emailed to
permissionrequest@cengage.com

Library of Congress Control Number: 2004058805

ISBN-13: 978-1-4018-5791-2

ISBN-10: 1-4018-5791-4

Delmar
Executive Woods
5 Maxwell Drive
Clifton Park, NY 12065
USA

Cengage Learning is a leading provider of customized learning solutions with office locations around the globe, including Singapore, the United Kingdom, Australia, Mexico, Brazil, and Japan. Locate your local office at **international.cengage.com/region**

Cengage Learning products are represented in Canada by Nelson Education, Ltd.

For your lifelong learning solutions, visit **delmar.cengage.com**

Visit our corporate website at **cengage.com**

Notice to the Reader

Publisher does not warrant or guarantee any of the products described herein or perform any independent analysis in connection with any of the product information contained herein. Publisher does not assume, and expressly disclaims, any obligation to obtain and include information other than that provided to it by the manufacturer. The reader is expressly warned to consider and adopt all safety precautions that might be indicated by the activities herein and to avoid all potential hazards. By following the instructions contained herein, the reader willingly assumes all risks in connection with such instructions. The publisher makes no representations or warranties of any kind, including but not limited to, the warranties of fitness for particular purpose or merchantability, nor are any such representations implied with respect to the material set forth herein, and the publisher takes no responsibility with respect to such material. The publisher shall not be liable for any special, consequential, or exemplary damages resulting, in whole or part, from the readers' use of, or reliance upon, this material.

Printed in China by China Translation & Printing Services Limited
7 8 9 10 12 11 10 09

Dedication

This book is dedicated to:

The living memory of my father, and my sister Pari,

My loving and caring family:
Mother, wife, and daughters

My colleagues, staff,
past and present Pharmacy Technician students
at Florida Metropolitan University

This book is also dedicated to:
Sharlee Brittingham,
Former President of FMU, Melbourne Campus,
who established
the first associate-degree program for Pharmacy Technicians.

Table of Contents

13 Safety in the Workplace ▪ 144

14 Computer Applications in Drug-Use Control ▪ 156

15

Communications ▪ 168

SECTION IV

MATHEMATICS REVIEW ▪ 181

16 Basic Mathematics ▪ 183

SECTION V

DRUG CLASSIFICATIONS ▪ 229

19 Biopharmaceutics ▪ 231

20 Antimicrobial Agents ▪ 240

SECTION VI

SPECIAL POPULATIONS ▪ 419

Contributors

Maggie Carpenter, PharmD
Adjunct Professor
Florida Metropolitan University
Director of Pharmacy Department
Sea Pines Hospital
Melbourne, Florida

Joseph Infantino, MD
Retired Gynecologist
Adjunct Professor
Florida Metropolitan University
Melbourne, Florida

Patricia A. Lawton, RN
Retired Nurse
Adjunct Professor
Florida Metropolitan University
Melbourne, Florida

Mahkameh Moini
Nova-Southeastern University
School of Dental Medicine
Fort Lauderdale, Florida

Stephanie K. Mullin, RN, MSN, CPNP
Pediatric Nurse Practitioner
Medical College of Wisconsin
Children's Hospital of Wisconsin
Milwaukee, Wisconsin

Susan Neil, MBA, RNP, LMIF
Chief Operating Officer
Alternate Family Care Inc.
West Palm Beach, Florida

Nicole Ostroff-Bologna, CMA, BS
Academic Advisor
Adjunct Professor
Florida Metropolitan University
Melbourne, Florida

Jeanette Pham, ARNP, BC
Adjunct Professor
Florida Metropolitan University
Melbourne, Florida

Vincent E. Trunzo, RPh, MSM
Adjunct Professor
Florida Metropolitan University
Director of Pharmacy, Health First Inc.
Holmes Regional Medical Center
Melbourne, Florida

Greg Vadimsky, PharmTech
Pharmacy Technician in Training
Florida Metropolitan University
Melbourne, Florida

Contributors

Reviewers

Renee Acosta, RPh, MS
Pharmacy Technician Department Chair
Austin Community College
Austin, Texas

Jeanie Barkett, B.S. Pharm
Professor
Clark College
Vancouver, Washington

Nora Chan, PharmD
Pharmacy Technician Program Coordinator
San Francisco Community College
San Francisco, California

Christopher W. Miller, PharmD, BCPP
Director of Pharmacy Services
Circles of Care, Inc.
Melbourne, Florida

James Mizner, RPh, MBA
Pharmacy Technician Program Coordinator
Applied Career Training
Rosslyn, Virginia

Stephanie Mullen, RN, MSN, CPNP
Pediatric Nurse Practitioner
Medical College of Wisconsin
Children's Hospital of Wisconsin
Milwaukee, Wisconsin

Agnes Pucillo, BSN, ACHI, RHE
Educational Supervisor for Allied Health
The Cittone Institute
Edison, New Jersey

Karen Snipe, CPhT, AS, BA, MAEd
Pharmacy Technician Program Coordinator
Trident Technical College
Charleston, South Carolina

Preface

The profession and practice of pharmacy have been revolutionized during the past decade. The reasons for this revolution include technology, research, new diseases, new drugs, new treatments, and new health care systems in the United States. Today, pharmacists and technicians have greater responsibilities in the field of medicine. Because of changing health care systems and costs of patient care, management of insurance policies and operation of pharmacies have shifted into a new era of responsibility. The duties of both pharmacists and technicians have been increased and changed by this revolution.

Pharmacy technicians must be more knowledgeable and skillful about preparing and dispensing medications in both the institutional and community pharmacy settings. Preparing medications involves using sterile and nonsterile techniques, compounding drugs, packaging, and labeling. These duties are challenging for pharmacy technicians. However, the most important role for pharmacy technicians is to be able to assist pharmacists in preventing medication errors.

This text is designed to give a comprehensive body of information and tools to pharmacy technicians and their educators. It contains 32 chapters and many questions and exercises that will help ensure better understanding of the text. Each chapter in this book begins with an outline, a list of objectives, and a glossary of terms. At the end of each chapter is a set of review questions. The book is printed in full color, which helps to better illustrate important concepts in the text.

My intention in writing this book was to provide an excellent source for pharmacy technicians that they could rely on to understand the art of pharmacy as well as its profession and practice.

Supplements

Electronic Classroom Manager to accompany The Pharmacy Technician: A Comprehensive Approach ISBN: 1-4018-5792-2

- The Electronic Classroom manager provides all the tools an instructor will need to plan and implement course work on an easy-to-use CD-ROM. Included on the CD are the Instructor's Manual, the testbank, and Microsoft® PowerPoint® Presentations.
- The Instructor's Manual includes lecture outlines, teaching strategies, and the answers to the end of chapter questions for each chapter.

- The testbank includes more than 1400 questions. Question types include multiple choice, completion, problem, and matching.
- The PowerPoint® presentations correlate to the chapters in the book.

Additional Products

Comprehensive Exam Review for the Pharmacy Technician, by Jahangir Moini (ISBN: 1-4018-4131-7)

Comprehensive Exam Review for the Pharmacy Technician provides a review of the material covered in a two-year pharmacy technician program and prepares individuals to pass the national certification exam (PTCE).

Essential material summaries provide a concentrated review of the topics covered on the national certification exam. Each chapter ends with a multiple choice quiz to reinforce the chapter material. An additional 400 questions and answers for self-evaluation are included at the end of the book to reinforce knowledge on a specific subject or assess overall knowledge of all topics covered in the book. An appendix containing a 150-item test with questions written in the style of the National Certification exam is included along with 30 examples of case studies. Answers for all of the quizzes and tests in the book are provided. Also provided with the book is a CD-ROM containing an additional 600 multiple choice questions and answers.

CourseForward for the Pharmacy Technician (ISBN: 1-4018-3959-2 [Faculty Guides]; 1-4018-3960-6 [Learning Guides])

CourseForward is a complete modular curriculum solution that breaks down content into topics for ease of learning and serves as a road map for course material. CourseForward provides PowerPoint® presentations, Faculty Teaching Guides, and Student Learning Guides that lead both the instructor and student step-by-step through each course. It also delivers tools that add extra support for students who need them, and more challenging materials for those who want to explore topics in depth. CourseForward is designed for instructors to enable them to spend less time planning and more time teaching.

About the Author

Dr. Moini is a/an:
Husband
Father
Author
Physician
Professor
Director
Chairman
Chief Proctor
Biological Scientist III
Epidemiologist
Health Educator Consultant
Physician Liaison of the Florida Society of Medical Assistants

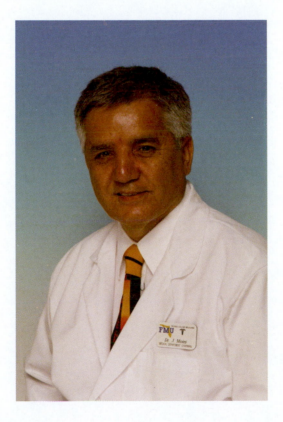

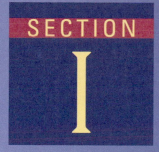

SECTION

I

Introduction

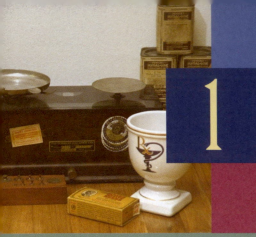

1 History of Pharmacy

OBJECTIVES

Upon completion of this chapter, the reader should be able to

1. Describe the historical evolution of the profession of pharmacy.
2. Discuss Hippocrates, the "father of medicine," and his role in the history of medicine.
3. Name the "father of botany" and the "father of toxicology."
4. Explain the establishment of the "pharmacy shop" operated by a pharmacist.
5. Describe the first attempts to regulate pharmacy.
6. Discuss the period of the Renaissance as it relates to the field of pharmacy.
7. Describe the Empiric Era and its impact on the field of pharmacy.
8. Explain the Industrialization Era and its impact on the field of pharmacy.
9. Describe the Patient Care Era.
10. Discuss the future of the field of pharmacy.

GLOSSARY

dosage form The make up of a particular type of drug; the form in which it is given.

formulary A document that specifies particular drug forms and compositions.

pharmaceutical care Term used to describe the care provided to a patient by the pharmacy, which encompasses all aspects of drug therapy from dispensing to drug monitoring.

pharmacy shop Term used to describe the first stand-alone pharmacies.

OVERVIEW

Pharmacy is an old and intriguing profession that was once filled with mystery and unknown methods. These have evolved into the art and science of preparing, preserving, compounding, and dispensing medicines. The field of pharmacy is as old as mankind yet as new as present-day medicines. We study the history of pharmacy because its evolution parallels the evolution of mankind. Its history also reflects the evolution of societies based on their people and cultural level, religious beliefs, scientific abilities, geographical location, and participation in the events of war. The evolution of the profession of pharmacy can be divided into five historical periods:

- Ancient Era—The beginning of time to 1600 AD
- Empiric Era—1600 to 1940
- Industrialization Era—1940 to 1970
- Patient Care Era—1970 to Present
- Biotechnology and Genetic Engineering — The new horizon

During these times pharmacy evolved to meet the changing needs of the world's societies in their quest to treat and prevent disease.

ANCIENT ERA

One can argue that the first ancient man was the first pharmacist. Acting through his natural instinct, he sought remedies for injuries and illness. He had to use the materials that were available in his surroundings. Through trial, error, and observation early man learned which items were effective. Leaves, mud, and cool water were used to stop bleeding and heal wounds. Clay was dried to splint broken bones. Many of these uses of natural products were discovered by observing injured animals. The methods the animals used to treat their injuries became the methods of early man as well, such as using mud to pack wounds.

As early man began to associate with others and form tribes in geographical locations, he applied his knowledge to help the members of his tribe. Generally one member of the tribe gained a reputation for possessing a greater knowledge of the techniques of healing. This person became a valuable member of the tribe because culturally the desire was to preserve the existence of the tribe. Knowledge of the healing properties of plants and mud that had been originally gained through experience was then passed down to younger members of the tribe.

At some point during this period early man developed the ability to document his experiences with healing materials. This information was documented on clay tablets, which provided the earliest know record written around 2600 BC. Documentation assisted in the preservation of experiences for future use. Concurrently, the use of natural substances was evolving in Egypt, Mesopotamia, and China. In 1875 in Egypt, George Ebers found one of the earliest written records, the Ebers Papyrus, written around 1500 BC. It contained formulas for more than 800 remedies. The belief was that bad spirits caused diseases and that the cure for disease was to drive off the bad spirit from the sick person. Each tribe had a designated member who could understand and control the spirits through spiritual rituals and the use of concoctions of plants and other natural materials. This person was the equivalent of a priest, pharmacist, and physician all in one. This position within society was held in high regard.

In the region of ancient Mesopotamia in the city of Babylonia the earliest known record of the practice of pharmacy by the priest, pharmacist, and physician was kept (around 2600 BC). From this Babylonian city, the science of drugs, organized pharmacy, and medicine had its beginnings.

In this same time period (about 2000 BC), the Chinese were developing an interest in herbs as having value in the cure of diseases. Shen Nung is reported (although not confirmed) to have written the first Pen T'sao, a native herbal treatise recording 365 drugs.

Around 600 BC the first attempts to approach medicine and medicines scientifically were being made in Greece. The Greeks began thinking logically about diseases rather than relying on spiritual explanations for physical phenomena. Hippocrates (about 400 to 361 BC), the "father of medicine," was a philosopher, physician, and pharmacist. He liberated medicine from the mystic and bad spirits. He is also known for authoring the Oath of Hypocrites; however some feel that it was actually written after his death. This code of ethics is still used today. Theophrastus, called the "father of botany," was an early (about 300 BC) Greek philosopher and scientist. He wrote about observations on the classification of plants by their various parts. Aristotle followed Theophrastus and wrote on the composition of matter. He produced the foundation for the later discovery of atoms and atomic theory. As the use of plants increased, some were found to be poisons that could be used for murders and other plants produced adverse effects. Mithridates (120 to 63 BC) studied the adverse effects of plants and later became know as the "father of toxicology."

As the world began to expand its horizons, men began to fight in wars. The Romans conquered the Greeks. Because the Romans drew much of their culture from the Greeks, this era became know as the Greco-Roman era. This adoption of Greek culture was especially true in medicine. The practice of the healing arts began in the Roman culture with the arrival of the Greek physicians. What the Romans added to the Greek system of knowledge was the organization of medical and pharmaceutical knowledge and the conversion of theory into rules and dogma. Sometime during the first century AD Dioscorides began this transition of the Greek system of knowledge to the Roman system of science. His written herbal treatise is known as *De Materia Medica* and was considered a major authority on drugs for 16 centuries.

For this reason some have considered him to be the "father of pharmacology." After Dioscorides, Galen (about 129 or 130 to 199 or 200 AD), a Greek physician, followed and had a greater impact on medicine and pharmacy than Dioscorides. His great work was *Methodo medendi* (*On the Art of Healing*). Galen was a highly revered figure in the history of medicine and pharmacy. His works greatly overshadowed those of Celsus, Scribonius Largus, Pliny, Aretaeus, and Oribasius. Galen was a physician who was especially critical of those physicians who did not prepare their own remedies. Both the Greek and the Roman physicians were responsible for preparing their own prescriptions. The twin brothers, Cosmos and Damien, the patron saints of pharmacy and medicine, represent the close relationship of pharmacy and medicine. Both were Christians who practiced pharmacy and medicine in about 300 AD. Some physicians, however, used preparers of remedies. Over a period of time the Romans produced a group of functionaries concerned with the preparation of prescriptions:

- pharmacopoei—makers of remedies
- pharmacotritae—drug grinders
- unguentarii—makers of ointments
- pigmentarii—makers of cosmetics (eventually became preparers of and dealers in drugs)
- pharmacopolae—sellers of drugs
- pharmacopolae circumforaneae—itinerant vendors of drugs
- sellulari—sellers of drugs who kept shops or stalls
- aromatarii—dealers in spices

The pharmacist as known today had not yet evolved when the Western Roman Empire came to an end in 476 AD. After the fall of the Roman Empire little progress was made in advancing pharmacy and medicine in the Western world. One has to turn to the Arab world to see any major advances. With these advances in medicine others were required to perform the pharmacy tasks; thus, the division of pharmacy and medicine evolved. Three major advances occurred in pharmacy at this time: formularies, dosage forms, and pharmacy shops. The **formulary** was a continuation of the documentation of the knowledge of specific drug information intended for use by pharmacists and other preparers of medicine. The **dosage form** was introduced to the Western world. No longer were drugs harvested from the herb garden. They were now incorporated into sweetened dosage forms, such as syrups, conserves, confections, and juleps, all of which were mixed with sugar and honey. Thus, the myth that only bitter medicines were efficacious was disproved. The most significant advance was the establishment of the pharmacy shop operated by a pharmacist. The first **pharmacy shop** appeared in Baghdad in about 762 AD. This is the earliest documentation of the existence and operation of a privately owned pharmacy shop. The development of hospitals also played a role in the separation of pharmacy from medicine. In about 1190, a hospital in Marrakech had a room designated as a pharmacy. In the Arab world, once pharmacies were established, the duties, character, and responsibilities of a pharmacist were delineated.

A great change in attitudes occurred in the Western world with the greater interest in pharmacy and drug therapy. The advances and knowledge of the Greek and the Arabic worlds had to be transferred and preserved for the Western world to advance. The monasteries of the Christian world were repositories of learning, and the monks worked to acquire and preserve ancient knowledge. The change in attitude also resulted in the establishment of two centers of learning, one at Salerno, in southern Italy, and a second in Toledo, Spain. Salerno had a medical center that attracted students and patients. The school at Salerno, thought to be Europe's first university, was responsible for major contributions to pharmacy and medicine.

The first attempts to regulate pharmacy appear to have occurred in southern Italy around the school in Salerno. In about the twelfth century, guilds of pharmacists came into existence. Through the guilds, pharmacists found an organization of their own in local towns. A very important event occurred between 1231 and 1240 AD when the Holy Roman Emperor Frederick II issued an edict regulating medicine. It contained the Magna Carta of Pharmacy, and it separated pharmacy from medicine. For the first time, an edict legally recognized pharmacy as a separate profession in Western Europe.

The period from 1350 to 1650 AD, the later stages of the Middle Ages, is known as the Renaissance. It was a period of rebirth of interest in the classical world, art, literature, philosophy, education, religion, and science and was dominated by secularism, individualism, and humanism. Theophrastus Phillippus Aureolus Bombastus von Hohenheim, also know as Paracelsus, stimulated a revolution in pharmacy. He was a Swiss-born physician who emphasized a chemical rather than botanical orientation to medicine and contradicted the Galenic theories of the past. He believed that disease was a chemical manifestation and should be treated chemically. During this time, monasteries remained important centers of learning for pharmacy. The monasteries maintained their own pharmacies to treat the poor. As a political unit the city/state structure began to decline in power and the larger political unit, the country/nation/state, evolved and its governing power increased. The practice of pharmacy began to vary from country to country. The structural governing body of the profession of pharmacy became the guilds in a form of self-regulation. The guilds gained in strength over time and set educational standards and experiential requirements that had to be met before an individual could practice pharmacy.

In many cases the pharmacist did not have a friendly relationship with physicians. The pharmacist was often associated with "spicers" (those associated with dealing in spices). In small towns the pharmacist was forced into the same guild as the spicers. Physicians contended that pharmacists were ignorant of the medical profession, diagnosed and prescribed when they were unqualified, and were constantly making errors in compounding and dispensing. This conflict continued well into the eighteenth century. The Germans more tightly controlled the practice of pharmacy. While the rest of the world controlled the practice of pharmacy through the self-governing of the guilds, Germany used governmental controls to regulate the profession of pharmacy.

The royalty of various countries created another role for the pharmacist, known as the Court Apothecary or the Royal Apothecary, who provided pharmacy and other services to the royal family. This was a very prestigious and honored position that paid well. These pharmacists lived a very rich lifestyle.

The Renaissance was also a period in which new areas of the world were explored. During this exploration new medicinal herbal substances such as plants, trees, and seeds were sought. With the new findings came the desire to document and preserve this new knowledge in herbal treatises, pharmacopeias, and handbooks. In summary, during the Renaissance period of the Middle Ages, pharmacy went through many changes:

- Pharmacy became an independent profession separated from the physician.
- The profession of pharmacy achieved status and became socially accepted.
- Regulations increased the integrity and performance of the profession.
- An extensive pharmaceutical literature was created.
- University education of pharmacists was required.
- Importation of larger quantities of known drugs occurred.
- Importation of new drugs from the New World and the Orient occurred.
- New chemical medicines were introduced that gave pharmacists broader expertise.

EMPIRIC ERA

During the Renaissance, pharmacists in Continental Europe had attained impressive social status and recognition as health care providers. Their actions were, however, still tightly controlled through self-regulation, quasi-government control, and government control. The medical profession also carefully watched them. The pharmacopeia became a regulatory tool used by the government to protect public health through standardization of medicines. Governmental control also guaranteed that pharmacists compounded and dispensed the medicine. Scientific knowledge had not yet become highly developed during this time. Knowledge of anatomy, physiology, and biochemistry was extremely limited or nonexistent. There was, however, a questioning of the effectiveness of many of the medicines listed in the popular pharmacopeia. A typical pharmacopeia contained three sections as listed in Table 1-1.

TABLE 1-1.   A Typical Pharmacopeia

SECTION I	SECTION II	SECTION III
Vegetable simples	Composita galencia (galenicals)	Chemical compositions
Roots	Distilled waters	Mercury
Barks	Spirits	Antimony
Herbs	Distilled vinegars	Sulfur
Leaves	Tinctures	
Flowers	Elixirs	
Fruits	Decoctions	
Seeds	Simple syrups	
Gums	Compound syrups	
Resins	Purging compound syrups	
Balsams	Aromatic powders	
Tears	Pills	
Fungi	Extracts	
	Troches	
Animalia	Expressed oils	
	Distilled oils	
Mineralia	Balsams	
	Unguents	
Metalla	Plasters	
	Cerates	
Lapides et salia terrae		
Marina		

Many medicines of questionable benefit were purged from these texts. This questioning also created an interest in testing of drugs and especially an interest in the toxicological effects of drugs and how medicines worked in the human body.

Pharmacy in the New World was a reflection of pharmacy in Europe (e.g., France, Spain, Italy, and England). Pharmacists did not participate in the colonization of the New World, and, thus, physicians prepared their own remedies. The practice of pharmacy did not begin to develop in the colonies until the eighteenth century. Benjamin Franklin started the first hospital in 1751. It had a pharmacy and the first hospital pharmacist was Jonathan Roberts. During the early years of America, there was little control over the practice of pharmacy. William Proctor (1817 to 1874), who later became known, as the "father of American pharmacy" was the greatest influence on the practice of pharmacy during his time. He devoted his time and attention to the advancement of pharmacy. He was the owner of an apothecary shop, an editor, a leader in organizing the profession of pharmacy, a teacher, and scientist. His performance in each of the facets of his career was, as stated by his son, "incredible." As a leader in organizing the profession of pharmacy, William Proctor introduced "control" into the practice of pharmacy in America.

Monastic pharmacies began to disappear toward the end of the eighteenth century. This was due to the competition between cloistered and secular pharmacists. Continuing conflict between religion and political systems caused monarchs to close pharmacies in the monasteries.

The major contribution of pharmacists to science was in the area of chemistry. Ironically, although pharmacists worked with plants as medicines for centuries, little contribution to the science of botany was made by pharmacists. During the seventeenth and eighteenth centuries the following chemicals were identified: sodium sulfate, ammonium sulfate, zinc chloride, oxygen, nitrogen, chlorine, glycerin, manganese, ammonia, some organic and inorganic acids, calomel, phosphorus, and ether. During the eighteenth century, the following medicines were identified: quinine, caffeine, morphine, hyoscyamine, codeine, atropine, niacin, diphtheria antitoxin, prontosil, adrenalin, penicillin, arsphenamine, phenobarbital, thyroxine, estrone, and testosterone. In the nineteenth century developments in the field of chemistry continued. The beginnings of the field of organic chemistry occurred during this time. No major changes in pharmacy practice occurred in this period; however, many of the advances in chemistry during this period laid the foundation for the next period, the Industrialization Era (1940 to 1970).

INDUSTRIALIZATION ERA

In an article presented to the American Pharmacy Association at its annual convention in Detroit in 1914, Dr. Frank O. Taylor stated that, "Up to the time of the early sixties (1860) it had been the almost universal custom for each pharmacist to prepare for himself such galenical preparations as he needed, but about this time several firms began manufacturing work on a small scale, developing this in most cases in retail drugstores that had been established for some years. The idea of centralized manufacture of medicinal preparations was just in its infancy and was probably not recognized as such at that time. . . ." He then described four periods of development of manufacturing pharmacy, which were later increased to eight periods (see Table 1-2).

The impetus for industrialization becoming a factor in the practice of pharmacy in America was the occurrence of major wars: the Civil War, World War I, and World War II. These major conflicts led to the development of weapons capable of causing increasingly serious injuries. This, in turn, led to greater demand for medicines and medical procedures to treat these injuries. The demand was so great that the processes for producing medications in place at the time were not adequate for producing the quantities required during a major war. Industrial manufacturing processes had to be developed to meet this need. The most important manufacturing advance in the industrialization

TABLE 1-2.	Periods of Development of Manufacturing Pharmacy
Original four	Formative Period (1867–1874)
	Botanical Research Period (1875–1882)
	Standardization Period (1882–1894)
	Biological Period (1895–present time)
Added at later date	Organic Chemical Synthesis, beginning 1883
	Hormones, beginning 1901
	Vitamins, beginning 1909
	Antibiotics, beginning 1940

of the practice of pharmacy was the development of new machines for rapid mass production of medicines.

Even though the roots of the industrial pharmacy were in the retail pharmacy, its development did not proceed without opposition. Many retail pharmacists protested against what they call an encroachment upon their professional practice. Ironically both types of pharmacy practice survived and still have a role in the profession of pharmacy. The new scientific discoveries of the Industrialization Era provided the following advancements to the practice of pharmacy: standardization, biologically prepared products, complex chemical synthesis, and the increasing use of parenteral medications. There was also a greater acceptance by the public of the attractive products that were mass-produced. The retail pharmacists became more accepting of the ease and convenience of dispensing the products of mass production. They also realized that industry-prepared products were new creations or specialties and that preparation of these products was not within the means of the average retail pharmacy. Retail pharmacy survived the growth of the pharmaceutical industry and also experienced increased volumes. This was due to two facts:

1. The pharmaceutical industry created new needs that were advantageous to the retail pharmacy.
2. The retail pharmacy has proved to be indispensable and irreplaceable as the fitting and distributing agency of medicinal products. There is a limit to the centralization, mechanization, and standardization that is possible in medicine and pharmacy.

Research, another focus of industry, began to proliferate during this period. Investigation into medicines and their effects in some form occurred through the ages of pharmaceutical development. Not until the development of the basic sciences—biology, chemistry, and physics—did systematic research of medicines realize substantial success. The phenomenal growth of research resulted from the financial support of the pharmaceutical industry.

PATIENT CARE ERA

The beginning of the Patient Care Era was marked by an increasing concentration on research to develop new medicines, especially by pharmaceutical manufacturers. This focus produced an increasing number of medicines with a greater number of pharmacological activities. Well-coordinated teams of scientists (biologists, chemists, engineers, physicians, pharmacists, and toxicologists) and other professionals (statisticians and financial managers) now performed research. Pharmaceutical research moved from the empirical, intuitive, and serendipitous to a rational, targeted approach. This new approach facilitated development of ideal drugs to meet specific needs through the use of a computer. Thus, many new drugs have been developed, making major contributions to the health and well-being of mankind.

With the plethora of new drugs came many complications. Multiple drug therapy led to adverse drug reactions, drug interactions (with other drugs, foods, and laboratory tests), and different outcomes with sub- or supertherapeutic doses. As a result of these complications, a more demanding and educated public had higher expectations of the profession of pharmacy. The pharmacist was expected to be a therapeutic advisor and patient advocate when pharmaceutical services were provided. The patient advocacy role creates an expectation for patients that the pharmacist will ensure achievement of the maximal outcome with minimal harmful effects from their drug therapy. This patient-focused approach to drug therapy concentrated on the drug and was thought of as "drug control" or "drug monitoring." This new role did not relieve the pharmacist from the responsibility of dispensing medications. To incorporate the dispensing role with the patient care role, C. D. Hepler established the concept of **pharmaceutical care** in the late 1980s. This concept expands the role of the profession from dispensing to include all aspects of drug therapy. The education of the pharmacist, as this role evolves, will not only be scientific based but will also now have to focus on human behavior as it relates to providing patient-focused care. Education in human behavior, communication management, and problem-solving skills must be provided for pharmacists to practice in the new environment.

BIOTECHNOLOGY AND GENETIC ENGINEERING—THE NEW HORIZON

We are at the beginning of a new era in the field of pharmacy. Much research in the area of gene therapy is being conducted. Some diseases have been related to genetic defects. It is hoped that by modifying the genetic make-up of a patient with a disease, the disease may be cured totally or at least partially. Currently, limited numbers of medications are being produced through recombinant DNA technology. Some of today's medications are available from natural sources but these are prone to producing allergic reactions due to naturally occurring proteins. An early product produced by this method was insulin. Some other products produced by this method are used as therapies for cancer, anemia, and hepatitis.

SUMMARY

Pharmacy is a profession as old as time itself. It has evolved in parallel with the evolution of man. The earliest "drugs" were products taken from nature. Man's curiosity sparked a basic desire to determine why and how these drugs worked and to develop more drugs to treat more illnesses. Thus, in the evolution of research the focus was first on botanical drugs and then on chemicals. Future therapies may come from the biotechnological processes or from the gene modification process. There may even be chemicals yet to be discovered and synthesized that may change the way a disease is treated or even produce a cure for cancer or the common cold. The future of pharmacy lies in the research of the future.

CRITICAL THINKING

1. Create a timeline establishing the history of pharmacy through each era. Be sure to name the key events that shaped the profession as well as the key individuals who contributed to the profession.
2. Research the early attempts to regulate pharmacy. What were the reasons for establishing such regulations? What were the advantages and disadvantages of this regulation to pharmacy as a profession?
3. What are the goals of biotechnology and gene research? How do you think this will change pharmacy as it is known today?

REFERENCES

Bender, G. A. (1996). *Great moments in pharmacy.* Detroit, MI: Northwood Institute Press.

Brown, T. R. (1992). *Handbook of institutional pharmacy practice,* 3rd ed. Bethesda, MD: American Society of Hospital Pharmacists.

Cowan, D. L., & Helfand, W. H. (1990). *Pharmacy: An illustrated history.* New York: Harry N. Abrams.

REVIEW QUESTIONS

1. Jonathan Roberts is known as the
   A. father of pharmacology.
   B. father of toxicology.
   C. first American hospital pharmacist.
   D. father of botany.

2. Benjamin Franklin is known as the
   A. father of American pharmacy.
   B. patron saint of pharmacy.
   C. father of medicine.
   D. founder of the first American hospital.

3. Hippocrates is known as the
   A. father of American pharmacy.
   B. patron saint of pharmacy.
   C. father of medicine.
   D. founder of the first American hospital.

4. Cosmos and Damien are known as the
   A. fathers of American pharmacy.
   B. patron saints of pharmacy.
   C. fathers of medicine.
   D. founders of the first American hospital.

5. Who was the "father of toxicology"?
   A. Mithridates
   B. Cosmos
   C. Benjamin Franklin
   D. William Proctor

6. William Proctor is known as the
   A. father of pharmacology.
   B. father of toxicology.
   C. father of American pharmacy.
   D. father of botany.

7. Who followed Theophrastus and wrote on the composition of matter?
   A. Mithridates
   B. Hippocrates
   C. Aristotle
   D. Benjamin Franklin

8. The establishment of the "pharmacy shop," operated by a pharmacist, first occurred in
   A. Baghdad.
   B. Rome.
   C. Salerno.
   D. Spain.

9. The "father of pharmacology" was
   A. Benjamin Franklin.
   B. Mithridates.
   C. Dioscorides.
   D. William Proctor.

10. Industrial pharmacy found its roots in
    A. medicine.
    B. biology.
    C. the monastery.
    D. retail pharmacy.

The Foundation of Pharmaceutical Care

OUTLINE

OBJECTIVES

Upon completion of this chapter, the reader should be able to

1. Discuss the characteristics that make the practice of the pharmacy technician a profession.
2. Identify the three general areas in which skills will be measured on the Pharmacy Technician Certification Exam.
3. Explain why continuing education is important for the pharmacy technician.
4. Explain control of the drug use process.
5. Name five professional organizations related to the field of pharmacy.
6. Explain the United States Pharmacopeia (USP).
7. Describe job opportunities for pharmacy technicians.

GLOSSARY

American Association of Colleges of Pharmacy (AACP) A national organization that includes all 88 pharmacy colleges and schools in the United States, representing the interests of pharmaceutical education and educators; http://www.aacp.org.

American Association of Pharmaceutical Scientists (AAPS) An organization that represents pharmaceutical scientists employed in academia, industry, government, and other research institutions; http://www.aaps.org.

American Association of Pharmacy Technicians (AAPT) An organization that represents pharmacy technicians and promotes certification of technicians; http://www.pharmacytechnician.com.

American College of Clinical Pharmacy (ACCP) A professional and scientific society that provides leadership, education, advocacy, and resources for clinical pharmacists; http://www.accp.com.

American Council on Pharmaceutical Education (ACPE) A national accrediting agency for pharmacy education programs.

American Pharmacists Association (APhA) The largest of the national pharmacy organizations, consisting of three academies: the Academy of Pharmacy Practice and Management (APhA-APPM), the Academy of Pharmaceutical Research and Science (APhA-APRS), and the Academy of Students of Pharmacy (APhA-APS); http://www.aphanet.org.

American Society of Health-System Pharmacists (ASHP) A large organization that represents pharmacists who practice in hospitals, health maintenance organizations (HMOs), long-term care facilities, home care agencies, and other institutions; http://www.ashp.org.

assay and control A group with the responsibility for auditing the control system and evaluating product quality.

drug control A method used to eliminate or reduce the potential harm of the drug distributed.

pharmacy The art and science of dispensing and preparing medication and providing of drug-related information to the public.

GLOSSARY continued

Pharmacy Technician Certification Board (PTCB) An organization that prepares and administers the standard national exam for certification as a pharmacy technician; http://www.ptcb.org.

Pharmacy Technician Certification Exam (PTCE) A standardized national exam for certification to become a pharmacy technician.

Pharmacy Technician Educators Council (PTEC) An association of educators who prepare people for careers as pharmacy technicians; http://www.rxptec.org.

profession A group that requires specialized education and intellectual knowledge.

quality control An organized effort of all individuals directly or indirectly involved in the production, packaging, and distribution of quality medications, which are safe, effective, and acceptable.

quality control unit A group with the responsibility for auditing the control system and evaluating product quality.

United States Pharmacopeia (USP) A nonprofit organization that sets standards for the identity, strength, quality, purity, packaging, and labeling of drug products.

OVERVIEW

A **profession** is a group that requires specialized education and intellectual knowledge. Professionals have a knowledge base that others do not possess but which others need the services of. Therefore, professionals have certain social and societal obligations to apply their knowledge for the good of the community they work in. There are several characteristics that classify particular fields as professions. A profession is characterized by the following:

- A specialized body of knowledge based upon advanced education that continues to expand throughout a person's career
- Provision of a unique service to society
- Responsibility to those being provided the service
- Membership that shares a common identity, values, and belief system
- A code of ethics

Pharmacy professionals are concerned with matters that are vital to the health or well-being of their patients. Working in the field of pharmacy is typically considered to be a more socially useful profession than many other occupations, but social utility alone does not make an occupation a profession. Throughout this chapter, we will examine the characteristics of the field of pharmacy that make it a profession.

THE PROFESSION OF PHARMACY

Pharmacy is the art and science of dispensing and preparing medication and providing drug-related information to the public. It involves interpreting prescription orders; compounding, labeling, and dispensing drugs and devices; selecting drug products and conducting drug utilization reviews; monitoring patients; and providing cognitive services related to use of medications and devices. Today, pharmaceutical care is a necessary element of total health care. Practitioners perform highly useful social and health care–related functions. They improve the quality of life of patients by assisting in the curing and prevention of diseases and disease processes. They share common identities, values, and belief systems with the other members of the medical community with whom they interact. This cohesiveness aids in helping to eliminate or reduce symptoms of and correctly diagnose conditions and in altering physiological processes so that desired outcomes are achieved. The practitioner should value the provision of truthful, accurate, understandable information to ensure minimal patient risk and take care to treat everyone equally, without prejudice toward race, religion, social or marital status, sex, sexual orientation, age, or health. The wishes of competent patients who refuse medication, treatments, or services should be observed, and the dignity of patients with diminished competence should be respected as well.

Educational Requirements

As stated earlier, one of the characteristics of a profession is a specialized body of knowledge. This begins with furthering one's education beyond high school. There are two career paths in the field of pharmacy: pharmacist and pharmacy technician. Each of these careers has specific educational requirements and skill sets. In the Fall 1994, more than 33,000 students were enrolled in U.S. colleges of pharmacy in the pursuit of their initial degree in professional pharmacy practice. Of these, 63% were women. Enrollment in colleges of pharmacy has been increasing steadily since 1984. As of 1992, a majority of pharmacy colleges voted to change the type of professional degree awarded to the doctor of pharmacy (Pharm D) degree. Some schools will continue to offer the bachelor of science in pharmacy (BS Pharm) degree for the foreseeable future. Either degree fulfills the requirements for taking the licensure examination of a state board of pharmacy to practice pharmacy. A Pharm D degree requires 4 years of professional study after a minimum of 2 years of prepharmacy study, for a total of 6 academic years after high school. Including prepharmacy study, the minimum education program for a BS in Pharm is 5 academic years.

The Pharmacist

Like the profession of medicine, pharmacy practice has become much more specialized during the past 25 years. Specialties in pharmacy may include ambulatory care, pharmacy administration, drug information, community practice, geriatrics, industry, managed care, long-term care, home health care, oncology, and nutritional support. Table 2-1 shows the basic duties of the pharmacist.

The Pharmacy Technician

The role of the pharmacy technician has been expanding in recent years, and the number of pharmacy technicians is increasing. Many clerical and technical tasks that were previously performed by pharmacists are now performed by pharmacy technicians. The training and certification of pharmacy technicians expands their role within the profession, which ultimately allows the pharmacist to spend more time delivering pharmaceutical care services. Recent studies indicate that pharmacy technicians are now involved in wider areas of pharmacy practice. These studies show that in addition to assisting with outpatient prescription dispensing, many community pharmacy technicians participate in purchasing, inventory control, billing, and repackaging products. Educational requirements for pharmacy technicians include preparation for work in any number of health care facilities and retail establishments. These include hospitals, medical centers, teaching facilities, outpatient clinics, urgent care centers, and retail and wholesale pharmacies. The core requirements included in the 2-year associate degree program are the following: administrative and professional aspects of pharmacy, terminology, calculations, anatomy, pathophysiology, pharmacology, medical mathematics, customer relations, and study of health care delivery systems and current issues in the practice of pharmacy. Most hospital pharmacy technicians assist with inpatient medication dispensing and may also prepare intravenous admixtures and engage in compounding of nonsterile preparations, repackaging, purchasing, and billing. The basic duties of the pharmacy technician will be discussed in detail in Chapters 7 and 8.

Obtaining Certification as a Pharmacy Technician

Pharmacy technicians can choose to become certified in their profession. Certification is obtained by taking and passing a standardized national exam, the **Pharmacy Technician Certification Exam (PTCE).** Certification is a valuable component for the pharmacy technician's career. The certification exam is prepared by the **Pharmacy Technician Certification Board (PTCB)** and tests competency in basic functions of the pharmacy and its activity. Skills are measured in three general areas:

1. Assisting the pharmacist in serving patients
2. Maintaining medication and inventory control systems
3. Participating in the administration and management of pharmacy

The exam, which lasts for 3 hours, contains 140 multiple-choice questions, 15 of which are not actually scored. The nonscored questions are used for statistical purposes only. A score of at least 650 (of a possible 300 to 900) is required to pass. Certification is valid for 2 years and must then be renewed.

Assisting the Pharmacist in Serving Patients

The questions that address assisting the pharmacist in serving patients account for 64% of the exam. This portion includes approximately 70 to 80 questions and covers both retail and hospital settings. Technicians must prepare themselves for questions about how to interpret the prescription order; the structure and use of the patient profile; and the dispensing, labeling, storage, and delivery of medications. Questions about drug calculations are also included. Overall, pharmacy technicians should have the ability to work with people because of the large amount of personal contact they will have in their day-to-day duties, both with the public and with professionals in other medical disciplines. Having a solid interest in science and medicine is also helpful. Another requirement is that pharmacy technicians need to be flexible about work schedules.

Maintaining Medication and Inventory Control Systems

The portion of the exam that addresses maintaining medication and inventory control systems includes questions about storage of medications in the pharmacy, the ordering and inventory process, prepackaging and unit-dose distribution, labeling, and record-keeping. These questions account for 25% of the exam (30 to 40 questions).

TABLE 2-1. Roles of the Pharmacist

- Initiating, adjusting, or renewing medication orders/prescriptions based on knowledge and expertise
- Using a drug list recommended by the pharmacy and therapeutics committee
- Monitoring dosages for continuing clientele
- Dispensing nonprescription medications as requested
- If required, assisting in administration of oral and parenteral medications, performing venipunctures, and administering intravenous fluids
- Signing all entries in the medical records
- Ordering tests and laboratory studies appropriate for the medications they are approved to initiate, adjust, or renew
- Offering consultation as required on the substances that they control

Participating in the Administration and Management of Pharmacy

The questions that test knowledge about participating in the administration and management of pharmacy deal with issues of safety, cleanliness, infection control, pharmacy law, communications, and computers. These questions account for 11% of the exam (15 to 25 questions).

Continuing Education

The practicing pharmacy technician must keep up with the changes that are occurring rapidly within the profession. Education does not end with the completion of formal training. The traditional roles of the pharmacist and pharmacy technician are changing, and new services are being identified as functions for both. Therefore, a personal commitment to continue education is essential. Pharmacy technicians need to have a specialized body of knowledge about aspects of their job, including the various types of pharmacy practices they may work in (i.e., community or hospital settings), the constantly changing medications they may work with, and recognition of adverse effects and interactions of drugs. They will regularly assist the pharmacist in providing patient support, giving information to patients, attending to special needs of patients (especially of geriatric patients), and overseeing the use of nutritional supplements, in addition to being involved in packaging control, pharmacoeconomics, and even poison control. Lifelong learning is becoming part of the philosophy of professional education, and, through it, a sustaining influence for nurturing of the profession is being supplied. The amount of medical knowledge is said to double every 5 years. Much can be learned by reading or reviewing the pharmacy literature that arrives in the daily mail and articles that appear in professional magazines and related newsletters. Continuing education classes, seminars, and workshops are available to enhance the professional's knowledge of pharmacy and pharmacy affairs. Continuing education units (CEUs) may be required to maintain certification as a pharmacy technician. To become eligible for recertification every 2 years, certified pharmacy technicians must meet the requirements of obtaining 20 contact hours of pharmacy-related continuing education. At least 1 contact hour must be in pharmacy law, which can be accomplished through various means, such as an educational meeting. Continuing education credits can be obtained through many sources, including the American Association of Pharmacy Technicians (AAPT) and various other agencies and educational institutions. CEUs are often awarded for participation in professional seminars and workshops.

Providing Services to the Community

A pharmacy practice should maintain high standards of medication dispensing in serving the needs of its customers. Giving out proper information and offering fair prices are also important parts of the daily business in a pharmacy. To a lesser degree today than previously because of the availability of prepackaged medications, specialized compounding (inside the pharmacy) is occasionally required. Accessible, quality pharmaceutical care, given with compassion and concern for patients, is essential to the success of the pharmacy. The pharmacy staff should continually strive to improve, regularly treating all customers with the dignity and respect they deserve. Other activities that are extensions of regular pharmacy practice include health fairs and fundraisers that serve to heighten community awareness of support groups and available assistance for specific diseases and conditions and educational programs for future practitioners of pharmacy.

Responsibility to Those Being Served

Developing methods for standardization and control of medicinal agents is vital. In manufacturing laboratories, pharmacists often perform physical and chemical analyses either in the course of developing dosage forms of new products or in the control of standard products. In small laboratories, the responsibility for performing analyses may be delegated entirely to pharmacy staff members. However, even if pharmacists are not conducting analyses, they should at a minimum understand the basic principles involved in the standardization and control of the medicinal agents dispensed. The use of an analytical method is justified only after it has been proved to be valid, accurate, and selective. **Drug control** is the most important goal for a medication that may be taken by patients. Control is a method used to eliminate or reduce the potential harm of the drug distributed. Drug control is a means for providing knowledge, understanding, judgments, procedures, skills, and ethical standards that assure optimal safety in distribution and use of medication.

Control of the Drug-Use Process

When multiple institutions such as hospitals, clinics, nursing homes, and drug stores (community pharmacies) are involved jointly in manufacturing, repackaging, and relabeling of drugs, they fall under the jurisdiction of the federal Food, Drug, and Cosmetic Act and, thus, government regulation. Control of quality is essential in the formulation, manufacture, and distribution of pharmaceutical products. This control serves to provide and maintain the desired features of purity, potency, and stability. These must fall within established levels so that all merchandise meets professional requirements, legal standards, and also additional standards that the management of a firm may adopt. The control of quality is the principle adopted by the Pharmaceutical Manufacturers Association, which applies equally to any institution whether a drug manufacturer or a pharmacy. Whatever control system is devised, it must be adequate and effective in attaining its purposes.

Pharmaceutical production presents many problems and conditions that make it a complicated operation, especially when the quantity prepared is large. **Quality control** must be built into the manufacturing process itself; it is not something that can be added after the product is made. Quality control is an organized effort of all individuals directly or indirectly involved in the production, packaging, and distribution of quality medications, which are safe, effective, and acceptable. Its ultimate success depends upon the cooperation of all individuals. In hospital or community pharmacies, quality control should encompass not only formulation, compounding, and dispensing, but must also include packaging, purchasing, storage, and distribution of medication to the ultimate user, the patient. The total control of quality for drugs is a pharmacy department responsibility, but the responsibility for auditing the control system and evaluating product quality is that of a **quality control unit,** sometimes referred to as **assay and control.** This unit is independent and reports to the director of pharmacy services. The assay and control, or quality control, unit may consist of a registered pharmacist supervisor and technicians, depending upon the scope of service. The supervisor of the quality control unit should have the authority to approve, reject, or order the reprocessing of products or procedures.

Professional Organizations

Professional people in the pharmacy, like those in other businesses, have created organizations or associations to advance the purposes of their professions. The most important organizations in the pharmacy profession are discussed in the following sections.

American Association of Colleges of Pharmacy

The **American Association of Colleges of Pharmacy (AACP),** established in 1900, represents all 88 pharmacy colleges and schools in the United States and is the national organization representing the interests of pharmaceutical education and educators. The AACP publishes the *American Journal of Pharmaceutical Education* and a monthly newsletter, as well as other publications.

American Association of Pharmaceutical Scientists

The **American Association of Pharmaceutical Scientists (AAPS),** formerly an academy of the American Pharmacists Association, represents pharmaceutical scientists employed in academia, industry, government, and other research institutions. The AAPS publishes the journals *Pharmaceutical Research, Pharmaceutical Development and Technology,* and *Journal of Pharmaceutical Marketing and Management,* as well as a newsletter.

American Association of Pharmacy Technicians

The **American Association of Pharmacy Technicians (AAPT),** formerly called the APT, was founded in 1979. It

is a national organization and has chapters in many states. It represents pharmacy technicians and promotes certification of technicians. The association has established a Code of Ethics for Pharmacy Technicians.

American College of Clinical Pharmacy

The **American College of Clinical Pharmacy (ACCP)** is a professional and scientific society that provides leadership, education, advocacy, and resources for clinical pharmacists.

American Council on Pharmaceutical Education

Founded in 1932, the **American Council on Pharmaceutical Education (ACPE)** is the national accrediting agency for pharmacy education programs recognized by the Secretary of Education.

American Pharmacists Association

The largest of the national pharmacy organizations, the **American Pharmacists Association (APhA)** consists of three academies: the Academy of Pharmacy Practice and Management (APhA-APPM), the Academy of Pharmaceutical Research and Science (APhA-APRS), and the Academy of Students of Pharmacy (APhA-APS). The APhA publishes the bimonthly *Journal of the American Pharmacists Association,* the monthly *Pharmacy Today Newsletter,* and the monthly *Journal of Pharmaceutical Sciences.* The APhA also operates a political action committee, or PAC. According to the APhA, its mission is "to advocate the interests of pharmacists; influence the profession, government, and others in addressing essential pharmaceutical care issues; promote the highest professional and ethical standards; and foster science and research in support of the practice of pharmacy."

American Society of Health-System Pharmacists

The **American Society of Health-System Pharmacists (ASHP)** is a large organization that represents pharmacists who practice in hospitals, health maintenance organizations (HMOs), long-term care facilities, home care agencies, and other institutions. The ASHP is a national accrediting organization for pharmacy residency and pharmacy technician training programs. The ASHP publishes the *American Journal of Health-System Pharmacy.*

Pharmacy Technician Certification Board

The Pharmacy Technician Certification Board (PTCB) publishes the Pharmacy Technician Certification Examination (PTCE). The PTCE is taken voluntarily by any pharmacy technician who wishes to be certified in the United States. This organization also oversees a recertification program for technicians.

Pharmacy Technician Educators Council

The **Pharmacy Technician Educators Council (PTEC)** is an association of educators who prepare people for careers as pharmacy technicians. Its official publication is the *Journal of Pharmacy Technology*.

United States Pharmacopeia

The **United States Pharmacopeia (USP)** is a nonprofit organization that sets standards for the identity, strength, quality, purity, packaging, and labeling of drug products. The USP provides drug information online.

Code of Ethics

A code of ethics serves to encourage respect and fair treatment for all patients. The following are basic principles that make up a code of ethics:

- Hold the health and safety of each patient to be of primary consideration.
- Form a professional relationship with each patient.
- Honor the autonomy, values, and dignity of each patient.
- Respect and protect the patient's right of confidentiality.
- Respect the rights of patients to receive pharmacy products and services, and ensure that these rights are met.
- Observe the law, preserve high professional standards, and uphold the dignity and honor of the profession.
- Continuously improve levels of professional knowledge and skills.
- Cooperate with colleagues and other health care professionals so that maximum benefits to patients can be realized.
- Contribute to the health care system and to the health needs of society.
- Never condone dispensing, promoting, or distributing of drugs or medical devices that do not meet the standards of law or that lack therapeutic value for the patient.
- Be fair and reasonable when it comes to the amount charged for medications and services.

JOB OPPORTUNITIES

Good job opportunities are expected for full-time and part-time work in the future, especially for pharmacy technicians with formal training or previous experience. Job openings for pharmacy technicians will result from the expansion of retail pharmacies and other employment settings and from the need to replace workers who leave the field. Employment of pharmacy technicians is expected to grow much faster than the average for all occupations through 2010 as a result of the increased pharmaceutical needs of a larger and older population. The increased numbers of middle-aged and elderly people, who, on average, use more prescription drugs than do younger people, will spur demand for pharmacy technicians in all practice settings. With advances in science, newer medications are becoming available to treat more conditions. Cost-conscious insurers, pharmacies, and health systems will continue to emphasize the role of pharmacy technicians. As a result, pharmacy technicians will assume responsibility for more routine tasks previously performed by pharmacists. Pharmacy technicians also will need to learn and master new pharmacy technology as it surfaces. For example, robotic machines are used to dispense medicine into containers, and pharmacy technicians must oversee the machines, stock the bins, and label the containers. Thus, although automation is increasingly being incorporated into the job, it will not necessarily reduce the need for pharmacy technicians.

SUMMARY

The foundation of pharmaceutical care has come a long way in a little more than a century. All of the following have been seen: the continued specialization of pharmacists in specific disease conditions, the growing trend for certification of pharmacy technicians, the rapid dissemination of technology to facilitate the provision of care and a shift in the composition of its workforce. It remains clear, however, that pharmacy will remain an integral part of our health care delivery system and an exciting career choice for its practitioners.

CRITICAL THINKING

1. Describe the factors that make an occupation a profession.
2. Discuss the value of professional organizations and the role they play within a profession.
3. Explain the importance of a code of ethics. How does this relate to the profession of pharmacy practice?

REVIEW QUESTIONS

1. The national testing of a pharmacy technician is adminis-
   tered by the
   A. Illinois Council of Health-System Pharmacists.
   B. American Society of Health-System Pharmacists.
   C. Pharmacy Technician Certification Board.
   D. National American Pharmacy Technicians.

2. A pharmacy technician is recertified by
   A. completing 10 hours of credit every 2 years in
      pharmacy-related study.
   B. completing 10 contact hours of credit that must be in
      pharmacy law.
   C. completing 20 hours of credit every 2 years in pharmacy-
      related study.
   D. completing 40 hours of credit; it is not required for
      recertification.

3. Pharmacists are those who are educated and licensed to
   A. dispense drugs and provide drug information.
   B. dispense information but not drugs.
   C. dispense alternate remedies rather than the drugs
      prescribed.
   D. test pharmacy technicians and provide their certification.

4. The most important goal for patients' medication is
   A. that it is inexpensive.
   B. drug control.
   C. that it is easy to open.
   D. drug therapy.

5. Pharmacy technicians perform some routine tasks, such as
   A. prescribing medications.
   B. counting tablets and labeling bottles.
   C. referring questions to medical assistants.
   D. counting patients and giving out free samples.

6. Of the questions on the Pharmacy Technician Certification
   Exam, 64% concern
   A. medication distribution and inventory control.
   B. the Pharmacy Technician Certification Board.
   C. pharmacy operations.
   D. assisting the pharmacist in serving patients.

7. AAPT stands for
   A. American Association of Pharmaceutical Terminology.
   B. Automatic Accreditation of Pharmacy Technicians.
   C. American Association of Pharmacy Technicians.
   D. American Association of Pharmaceutical Torts.

8. Which of the following organizations gives national accred-
   itation for pharmacy technicians training programs?
   A. PTCB
   B. ASHP
   C. PTEC
   D. APhA

9. To pass the Pharmacy Technician Certification Exam, one
   must have a score of at least
   A. 350.
   B. 450.
   C. 650.
   D. 900.

10. All of the following are the basic principles of a code of
    ethics for pharmacy technicians, except
    A. honor the autonomy, values, and dignity of each patient.
    B. contribute to the health care system and social health
       needs.
    C. condone the dispensing, promoting, or distributing of
       drugs that lack therapeutic value.
    D. respect the rights of patients to receive pharmacy prod-
       ucts and services.

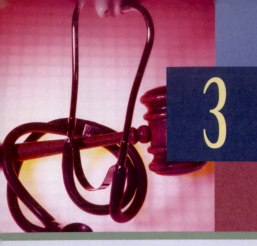

Pharmacy Law and Ethics for Technicians

OBJECTIVES

Upon completion of this chapter, the reader should be able to

1. Explain the various types of law.
2. Discuss violations of the law related to the field of pharmacy.
3. Differentiate among state and federal pharmacy laws.
4. Explain the Controlled Substances Act and Schedule drugs.
5. Discuss the Drug Listing Act of 1972.

6. Discuss the Orphan Drug Act of 1983.
7. Explain the Occupational Safety and Health Administration (OSHA).
8. State the regulations of the new Health Insurance Portability and Accountability Act (HIPAA).

GLOSSARY

accessory Any individual who helps a person to violate the law either directly or indirectly.

administrative law Regulations set forth by governmental agencies, such as the Internal Revenue Service (IRS) and the Social Security Administration (SSA).

bioethics A discipline dealing with the ethical and moral implications of biological research and applications.

case law Law established by judicial decision in legal cases and used as legal precedent.

civil law Rules and regulations that govern the relationship between individuals within society.

common law Derives authority from ancient usages and customs affirmed by court judgments and decrees.

GLOSSARY continued

constitutional law Deals with interpretation and implementation of the United States Constitution.

crime A violation of the law.

criminal An individual who violates the law.

criminal law Rules and regulations that govern the relationship of the individual to society as a whole.

ethics The branch of philosophy that deals with the distinction between right and wrong and with the moral consequences of human actions.

felony A serious crime, such as murder, kidnapping, assault, or rape, that is punishable by imprisonment for more than 1 year.

international law Law based on treaties and other agreements between two or more countries.

judicial law Rules and regulations resulting from court decisions.

law A principle or rule that is advisable or obligatory to observe.

misdemeanor A less serious crime, punishable by a fine or imprisonment for less than 1 year.

National Drug Code (NDC) A unique and permanent product code assigned to each new drug as it becomes available in the marketplace; it identifies the manufacturer or distributor, the drug formulation, and the size and type of its packaging.

National Formulary (NF) A database of officially recognized drug names.

orphan drug A drug that is developed for small populations of people in need of the drug.

regulatory law Regulations set forth by governmental agencies. It is also called administrative law.

standard code sets Under HIPAA, "codes used to encode data elements, tables of terms, medical concepts, diagnostic codes, or medical procedure." A code set includes the codes and descriptors of the codes.

standards Established by authority, custom, or general consent as a model or example; something set up and established by authority as a rule for the measure of quantity, weight, extent, value, or quality.

statutes Rules and regulations resulting from decisions by legislatures.

statutory law The body of laws enacted by a legislative body with the power to make law.

tort A civil wrong committed against person or property.

United States Pharmacopeia (USP) A nonprofit organization that sets standards for the identity, quality, purity, packaging, and labeling of drug products.

OVERVIEW

Pharmacy technicians must be familiar with the legal requirements that relate to their daily professional activities. The laws relevant to the practice of pharmacy may come from different sources, such as the U.S. Food and Drug Administration (FDA), the State Board of Pharmacy, and the Drug Enforcement Administration (DEA). Moreover, laws may appear in different forms, such as statutes, regulations, or court decisions. There are several types of law. **Civil law** governs the relationship between individuals within society. For example, a person or a patient can sue the pharmacy or the pharmacist. **Criminal law** governs the relationship of the individual to society as a whole. For example, if a pharmacist is practicing pharmacy without a license, then he or she is criminally liable and may be prosecuted by the government. In addition, **judicial law** results from court decisions, whereas a **statute** results from action by the legislature. Each type of law is applicable to pharmacists and pharmacy practice. Federal rules primarily relate to the drug products, whereas state rules primarily relate to the people who practice pharmacy and the sites where they perform their professional duties. Criminal law governs intent to defraud pharmacy customers by cheating the customer with regard to drug quality or pricing or misleading a customer as to the facts about their prescriptions. In this chapter, laws, ethics, and different terms that are essential knowledge for pharmacy technicians are discussed. Civil law governs pharmacists who do not act in a professional manner with their customers, including areas such as libel, slander, violation of privacy, or unintentional (personal) bodily injury. Pharmacy technicians should be familiar with the legal system and understand some of its terminology as related to their profession (Table 3-1).

LAW AND ETHICS IN PHARMACY

Laws, standards, and ethics can exercise controls on pharmacy and drugs. A **law** is a rule or regulation established by a governing body. Laws are enacted both to protect society and to maintain order and standards of living. Violation of a law can result in criminal penalties. **Ethics** is the study of values or principles governing personal relationships. These values and principles are used to determine whether actions are right or wrong. Ethics are based on morals, particular behaviors or rules of conduct that are formed through the influences of family, culture, and society. **Standards** are guidelines for practice established by professional organizations. Professionals in a particular area of practice share a common philosophy (a basic viewpoint or shared beliefs, concepts, attitudes, and values). This common philosophy dictates the etiquette, or standards of behavior, considered appropriate for that profession. The philosophy and etiquette established within a profession drive the standards that are established for the profession. Pharmacists and pharmacy technicians are responsible for upholding legal and ethical standards in their profession.

TABLE 3-1.   Legal Terms to Know

Assumption of risk	This refers to a patient who does not follow medical advice, and, therefore, becomes responsible for any problems that occur as a result of his or her decision.
Defendant	The person or group against whom charges are brought in a court action.
Deposition	An oral testimony taken by a court reporter at a location outside the courtroom, subject to the same requirements for truth as court testimony.
Interrogatory	A written set of questions that must be answered under oath as if in a court, within a specific period.
Jurisdiction	The power, right, and authority given to a court to hear a case and to make a judgment.
Litigant	A party to a lawsuit.
Litigation	A lawsuit or a contest in court.
Plaintiff	The person who files a lawsuit initiating a civil legal action. In criminal actions, the prosecution (government) is the plaintiff, acting on behalf of the people.
Statute of limitations	The law that limits the period during which a person can sue. The period varies from 1 to 3 years.
Subpoena	A court order that requires an individual to appear as a witness in court or to make himself or herself available to be deposed.

GOVERNING BODIES

Laws are created and upheld by federal, state, and local government. In the United States the federal government is divided into three branches:

1. The legislative branch consists of the Congress (i.e., the House of Representatives and the Senate). This branch is responsible for creating laws.
2. The executive branch consists of the president and vice president, cabinets, and various smaller organizations. This branch of government enforces law.
3. The judicial branch consists of the Supreme Court and lower federal courts. This branch interprets laws.

The federal government creates, issues, and interprets laws for the general population. State and local governments are responsible for determining the specifics of certain laws within their jurisdictions.

Regulatory agencies are government-based departments that create specific rules about what is and is not legal within a specific field or area of expertise. The regulatory agency for the field of pharmacy is the U.S. Food and Drug Administration (FDA), which is a branch of the U.S. Department of Health and Human Services. Among other things, the FDA regulates all drugs with the exception of illegal drugs. All legislation pertaining to drug administration is initiated, implemented, and enforced by the FDA. The FDA is responsible for the approval of drugs, over-the-counter (OTC) and prescription drug labeling, and standards for drug manufacturing.

TYPES OF LAW

As society grows and changes, laws change to conform to current realities and to try to govern future realties. The main types of law are constitutional, statutory, administrative, common, and international.

Constitutional Law

In the broadest sense, **constitutional law** deals with the interpretation and implementation of the U.S. Constitution. This type of law deals with the fundamental relationships within our society such as relationships among states, relationships among states and the federal government, and the rights of the individual with state and federal governments.

Statutory Law

Statutory law is the body of laws enacted by a legislative body with the power to make law. In the federal government this legislative body is Congress.

Administrative Law

Administrative law is the rules and regulations established by agencies of the federal government. This law is also called **regulatory law**. Administrative law agencies are given authority by Congress to write these rules.

Common Law

Common law, also known as **case law**, is law created by judges based upon previous court decisions. Areas of common law include contracts, property law, domestic law, and torts. A **tort** is a civil wrong committed against a person or property (a law related to personal injury). A tort is the most common civil claim in medical law.

International Law

International law is based on treaties and other agreements between two or more countries. International law defines the

TABLE 3-2.	Violations of Pharmacy Laws	
VIOLATION	**DEFINITION**	**EXAMPLE**
Fraud	Dishonest and deceitful practices undertaken to induce someone to part with something of value or legal right.	A pharmacist or a technician promises patients "miracle cures" or accepts fees from patients for spiritual powers to heal.
Libel	Defamatory writing, such as published material or pictures that injures the reputation of another.	A pharmacy advertises that a competing pharmacy does not stock medications of the same quality.
Slander	Defamatory spoken words that jeopardizes someone's reputation or means of livelihood.	A pharmacy worker tells a customer that another pharmacy's staff are not qualified.
Negligence	Failure to use a reasonable amount of care to prevent injury or damage to another.	A pharmacist or technician fails to exercise ordinary care, and a patient is harmed.
Abuse	The improper use of equipment, a substance (such as a drug), or a service (such as a program).	A patient is harmed because a pharmacy worker gives them the wrong substance, strength, amount, or type of medication.

rules and principles governing the relations between nations, specifically the rights between several countries or countries and the citizens of other countries.

VIOLATIONS OF THE LAW

A violation of the law is a **crime**. A crime can be classified as either a **misdemeanor** (a less serious crime, punishable by a fine or imprisonment for less than 1 year) or a **felony** (a serious crime, such as murder, kidnapping, assault, or rape that is punishable by imprisonment for more than 1 year). An example of a misdemeanor in a pharmacy setting would be theft, such as by shoplifting. An example of a felony in the pharmacy setting would be illegal selling of drugs, burglary of the pharmacy, or arson.

The individual in violation of the law is called a **criminal**. An individual who helps someone commit a crime is called an **accessory**. An accessory can aid the perpetrator of a crime either directly or indirectly.

Violations of pharmacy laws are punishable by fines or by the revocation or suspension of a license to practice. Some state laws specify that violations of the pharmacy act are punishable as misdemeanors. Boards of pharmacy are authorized to make rules and regulations for the enforcement and administration of the pharmacy law. The board is an administrative agency, not a legislative one. It is important to understand various violations of the law, which are defined in Table 3-2.

PHARMACY LAW AND REGULATION AT THE STATE LEVEL

Regulation of pharmacy practice is primarily a function of the state and not of the federal government. Its basis is in the power of the state for protecting the health, safety, and welfare of its citizens. Pharmacy laws of different states are different, but they are based on the same principles, objectives, and goals of pharmaceutical practice. State pharmacy law requires minimal qualifications for a class of individuals who are involved with pharmacy practice. No one may practice pharmacy without a license, except those exempted by the state legislation that creates the license requirement. Any individuals who are qualified to be licensed must successfully complete the requirements of the board of pharmacy. The pharmacy board is a subagency of the licensing division of the health department. Once licensure is gained, it is not revoked easily. The state can suspend, revoke, or terminate an individual's license but only after due process and for just cause as set out in the appropriate legislation. Licensed pharmacists have gained a profession, the practice of which is safeguarded by the federal and state constitutions as a property right. In most states, certificates of registration are granted for 1 or 2 years. Under special circumstances, certificates of registration or pharmacy licenses may be canceled or revoked. The National Association of Boards of Pharmacy (NABP) has developed a Model State Pharmacy Practice Act (MSPPA). This act provides a greater degree of uniformity between states but still offers flexibility to the states that adopt it. The MSPPA is organized by articles that deal with various aspects of regulating pharmacy practice.

PHARMACY LAW AND REGULATION AT THE FEDERAL LEVEL

Pharmacy practice is regulated by a series of rules, regulations, and laws that are enforced by local, state, and federal governments. In 1906, the U.S. Congress passed the first important law to regulate the development, compounding, distribution, storage, and dispensing of drugs.

The Pure Food and Drug Act of 1906

The Pure Food and Drug Act of 1906 prohibited interstate distribution or sale of adulterated and misbranded food and drugs. The 1906 act was believed to be inadequate for the following reasons:

1. It did not include cosmetics.
2. It did not provide authority to ban unsafe drugs.
3. A manufacturer could make false statements about a drug.
4. Labels were not required to identify contents of medications.

In 1912, Congress addressed the false statement problem and included within the definition of misbranding false or fraudulent claims for the curative powers of drugs. Labeling was first regulated by the Sherley Amendment to the act, which Congress enacted during 1912. A deficiency in this revision was that the enforcement agency was required to show deliberate fraud to establish a violation.

The Food, Drug, and Cosmetic Act of 1938

In 1938, further amendments were made to the Pure Food and Drug Act. The Food, Drug, and Cosmetic Act of 1938 created the FDA and required pharmaceutical manufacturers to file New Drug Applications with the FDA. Under this act, manufacturers must be concerned with the purity, strength, effectiveness, safety, and packaging of drugs. Foods and cosmetics are also regulated. By this act, the FDA has the power to approve or deny new drug applications and even to conduct inspections to ensure compliance. The FDA approves the investigational use of drugs on humans and ensures that all approved drugs are safe and effective.

The Durham-Humphrey Amendment of 1951

During the 1940s, the FDA began to use internal regulations to create classifications of prescription (legend drugs) and nonprescription (OTC) drugs. This process did not work very well. Therefore, in 1951, Senator Hubert Humphrey, a pharmacist from Minnesota, and Congressman Carl Durham, a pharmacist from North Carolina, supported legislation to establish clear criteria for such decisions. The Durham-Humphrey Amendment of 1951 prohibits dispensing of legend drugs without a prescription. Nonlegend, OTC drugs were not restricted for sale and use under medical supervision.

The Kefauver-Harris Amendment of 1962

The federal Food, Drug, and Cosmetic Act was amended again with the Kefauver-Harris Amendment of 1962 to require that drug products, both prescription and nonprescription, must be effective and safe. Prescription drug advertising was placed under supervision of the FDA and qualifications of drug investigators were subjected to review.

These amendments provided for registration of manufacturers and inspection of manufacturing sites, and they required an unprecedented program of accountability from manufacturers.

The Medical Device Amendments of 1976

In 1976 the Medical Device Amendments were enacted. These amendments required manufacturers to register and list their products, to follow good manufacturing practices during the making of these products, and to report device failures. Before new devices were marketed, they had to be reviewed by a panel of scientists to ensure their accuracy and preciseness to deliver the intended results.

The Dietary Supplement Health and Education Act of 1994

In 1994, Congress passed the Dietary Supplement Health and Education Act to clarify the regulatory framework applicable to nutritional supplements and to create specific labeling requirements. The products covered by this act are vitamins, minerals, herbs, botanicals, amino acids, other dietary supplements intended to increase total dietary intake, concentrates, metabolites, constituents, extracts, or any combination of the above. These supplements come in different types, including capsules, powders, softgels, gelcaps, tablets, and liquids. This act placed the burden of proof squarely on the FDA, meaning that supplements whose safeness was questioned had to be proved harmful by the FDA.

The Comprehensive Drug Abuse Prevention and Control Act of 1970

This act, also called the Controlled Substances Act (CSA), directs the manufacture, distribution, and dispensing of controlled substances that have the potential for addiction and abuse. This law replaced most previous narcotic and drug abuse control laws. It is enforced by the DEA, which is part of the U.S. Department of Justice. Under the jurisdiction of the CSA, drugs with potential for abuse are classified into five Schedules: I, II, III, IV, and V. Drugs in Schedule I have the highest potential for abuse and addiction, and those in Schedule V have the least potential.

Schedule I

Schedule I agents have a high potential for abuse, and they are not accepted for medical use in the United States. Properly registered people may use Schedule I substances for research purposes.

Schedule II

Schedule II agents also have a high potential for abuse, but they are currently accepted for medical use in the United

TABLE 3-3. Drug Schedules

SCHEDULE	ABUSE POTENTIAL	PRESCRIPTION REQUIREMENT	EXAMPLES
I	High abuse potential; no accepted medical use	No prescription permitted	Heroin, LSD, marijuana, mescaline, and peyote
II	High abuse potential; accepted medical use	Prescription required; no refills permitted without a new written prescription	Cocaine, codeine, methamphetamine (Desoxyn®), methadone hydrochloride (Methadose®), morphine (Astramorph®), opium (deodorized), methylphenidate (Ritalin®), and secobarbital (Seconal®)
III	Moderate abuse potential; accepted medical use	Prescription required; 5 refills permitted in 6 months	Certain drugs compounded with small quantities of narcotics; also other drugs with high potential for abuse (Tylenol® with Codeine tablets), and certain barbiturates
IV	Low abuse potential; accepted medical use	Prescription required; 5 refills permitted in 6 months	Barbital, chloral hydrate (Noctec®), diazepam, (Valium®), chlordiazepoxide (Librium®), and pentazocine hydrochloride (Talwin®)
V	Low abuse potential; accepted medical use	No prescription required for individuals 18 or older	Cough syrups with codeine, diphenoxylate hydrochloride with atropine sulfate (Lomotil®), and kaolin/pectin/opium (Parepectolin®)

States. The abuse of these drugs may result in severe psychological or physical dependence. The broad categories of Schedule II drugs include opiates and opium derivatives, derivatives of cocoa leaves, and certain central nervous system stimulants and depressants. The quantity of the substance in a drug product often determines the schedule that will control it. For example, amphetamines and codeine usually are classified in Schedule II; however, specific products containing smaller quantities of Schedule II substances, most often in combination with a noncontrolled substance, are controlled by Schedules III and IV.

Schedule III

Schedule III agents have accepted medical uses in the United States. They have a lower potential for abuse than Schedule I and II drugs. Schedule III drugs contain limited quantities of certain narcotic and non-narcotic drugs.

Schedule IV

Schedule IV agents have a low potential for abuse relative to those in Schedule III. Schedule IV drugs are generally long-acting barbiturates, certain hypnotics, and minor tranquilizers.

Schedule V

Schedule V agents have the lowest abuse potential of the controlled substances and consist of preparations containing limited quantities of certain narcotic drugs, generally used for antitussive and antidiarrheal purposes. Schedule V drugs are OTC preparations that may be sold without a prescription. Diphenoxylate hydrochloride with atropine sulfate (Lomotil®), which is listed as a Schedule V drug, is an exception—it

requires a prescription. Paregoric now is restricted to prescription sales only and is included in Schedule III. Table 3-3 shows drug schedules and some examples.

Registration

Individuals who manufacture, dispense, or distribute any controlled substance are obligated to register with the DEA unless they are exempted. Registrations vary in length from 1 to 3 years. Most pharmacy registrations will be issued for 3 years. A DEA number must be assigned to those who are registered under the law as manufacturers, distributors, wholesalers, and practitioners such as physicians, dentists, veterinarians, scientists, pharmacies, and hospitals. Pharmacies must register with the DEA to dispense controlled substances, but pharmacists do not have to register. The one exception is that a pharmacist who owns a pharmacy as a sole proprietor must be registered. Applications for re-registration are mailed by the DEA to each registered person approximately 60 days before the expiration date of the registration. The DEA can suspend or revoke a registration if the registrant has falsified his or her application or has been convicted of a felony under the federal or a state controlled substances act.

Record-Keeping

Any pharmacy that handles controlled substances must keep complete and accurate records of all drugs received and dispensed. The records must be kept for 2 years. Some states require that the records must be kept for at least 5 years. Schedule II drug records must be kept separately from all other records. Any record that includes controlled substances must be made available for inspection by DEA officials.

Inventory

The CSA requires each registrant to make a complete and accurate record of all stocks of controlled substances on hand every 2 years. When the inventory of Schedule II controlled substances is done, an exact count or measure must be made.

Prescriptions

A prescription for a controlled substance must be issued by a practitioner for a valid medical purpose. If a practitioner attempts to resupply office stock by writing prescriptions for such a purpose but rather is using the substance to maintain drug-dependent individuals who do not have legitimate prescriptions, then this is a violation of the law. No prescription for a Schedule II controlled substance may be refilled. Prescriptions for Schedule III or IV controlled substances may be refilled if authorization is given by a practitioner. These prescriptions may not be filled or refilled more than 6 months after the date issued, nor can they be refilled more than five times after the date issued. After 6 months or after five refills, the practitioner may renew the prescription. Pharmacies must keep Schedules II, III, IV, and V controlled substances in a locked cabinet. A pharmacy that wants to dispose of any excess or undesired stock of a controlled substance must contact the nearest DEA office and request the necessary form (DEA Form 41). A cover letter from the pharmacy must be attached to the report explaining that the controlled substances are not requested and the pharmacy wishes to dispose of them. If a controlled substance is lost at any pharmacy, the nearest DEA office must be notified of the theft or significant loss upon discovery by submission of a DEA Form 106.

The Poison Prevention Packaging Act of 1970

The Poison Prevention Packaging Act authorized the Consumer Product Safety Commission to create standards for child-resistant packaging. This act requires that most OTC and legend drugs be packaged in child-resistant containers. These containers cannot be opened by 80% of children younger than age 5 but can be opened by 90% of adults (see Figure 3-1). Drugs dispensed for use by patients in a hospital or a nursing home may not be required to be in child-resistant containers because the patients usually do not have access to them.

The Drug Listing Act of 1972

Under this act, each new drug is assigned a unique and permanent product code, known as a **National Drug Code (NDC)**, that identifies the manufacturer or distributor, the drug formulation, and the size and type of its packaging. Using this code, the FDA is able to maintain a database of drugs by use, manufacturer, and active ingredients and of newly marketed, discontinued, and remarketed drugs. The NDC for one product may not be used for another if any

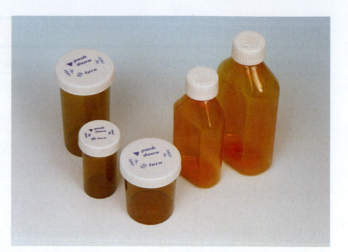

Figure 3-1. Drugs must be packaged in child-resistant containers.

changes occur in product characteristics. A new NDC number must be assigned to the new product version.

The Orphan Drug Act of 1983

The Orphan Drug Act of 1983 offers federal financial incentives to commercial and nonprofit organizations to develop and market drugs previously unavailable in the United States. Before a new drug can be marketed, substantial evidence of both safety and effectiveness is required. The procedure is difficult, lengthy, and extremely expensive. Thus, valuable new drugs with efficacy for a disease that affected only a small number of persons were not being developed because drug companies did not want to invest the millions of dollars and years of research necessary to secure approval for these drugs. A drug that falls into this category is called an **orphan drug**. Orphan drugs are used to treat diseases that affect fewer than 200,000 people in the country. The Orphan Drug Act offers tax breaks and a 7-year monopoly on drug sales to induce companies to undertake the development and manufacturing of such drugs. Since the act went into effect in 1983, more than 100 orphan drugs have been approved, including those for the treatment of conditions such as acquired immunodeficiency syndrome (AIDS), cystic fibrosis, blepharospasm (uncontrolled rapid blinking), and snake bites.

The Drug Price Competition and Patent-Term Restoration Act of 1984

The Drug Price Competition and Patent-Term Restoration Act of 1984 was largely consumer-oriented and designed to lower drug prices by providing a mechanism to increase competition in the drug industry. This law provides abbreviated New Drug Applications and an accelerated procedure for approval of generic versions (pertaining to a substance, product, or drug that is not protected by trademark) of approved drugs whose safeguard protection is about to expire.

The Prescription Drug Marketing Act of 1987

The Prescription Drug Marketing Act of 1987 deals with safety and competition issues raised by secondary markets for drugs, and it prohibits the reimportation of a drug into the United States by anyone but the manufacturer. This act also prohibits the sale or trading of drug samples, the distribution of samples to persons other than those licensed to prescribe them, and the distribution of samples except by mail or by common carrier.

The Anabolic Steroids Control Act of 1990

The Anabolic Steroids Control Act of 1990 became effective in February 1991 and placed anabolic steroids under the regulatory provisions of the CSA. Anabolic steroids are hormonal substances that are related to testosterone, estrogen, progestins, and corticosteroids, which promote muscle growth. These agents are used occasionally by athletes to increase physical performance. This act is significant because some observers believe that it reflects an essential change of direction for drug abuse control.

The Omnibus Budget Reconciliation Act of 1990

The Omnibus Budget Reconciliation Act of 1990 (OBRA '90) requires pharmacists to offer to discuss information about new and refill prescriptions with Medicare and Medicaid recipients (patients). OBRA '90 is decreased in terms of state entitlements to reimbursement from the federal government. This law requires states that seek such reimbursement to adopt programs that directly affect the pharmacy profession. With few exceptions, only costs for drugs that are approved as "safe and effective" will be reimbursed. States must require pharmacists who provide services under the program to give consulting services. Matters that may be discussed in counseling should include the following information:

- Name and description of medication
- Dosage form, dosage, route of administration, and duration of drug therapy
- Common severe side effects or adverse effects
- Interactions (with other drugs or food) and therapeutic contraindications
- Self-monitoring of the medication therapy
- Proper storage
- Action in the event of a missed dose
- Special directions for and precautions to be taken by the patient

The Occupational Safety and Health Act of 1970

The Occupational Safety and Health Act was signed by President Nixon in 1970. The act is administered by the Occupational Safety and Health Administration (OSHA), which is a part of the U.S. Department of Labor. OSHA's mission is to ensure workplace safety and a healthy environment within the workplace. The medical industry became involved in OSHA-related publicity in the late 1980s, when the threat of human immunodeficiency virus (HIV) infection extended to health care workers. Viral hepatitis and other pathogens already were concerns of health care workers, but when HIV, the virus that causes AIDS, was identified, action was needed to better protect individuals who cared for patients with these infectious diseases. OSHA's Final Ruling on Bloodborne Pathogens became fully effective in July 1992. The act requires medical facilities to comply with the Bloodborne Pathogens Standard and to be able to prove that compliance to OSHA inspectors if necessary. Common OSHA violations include the following: no eyewash facilities available, no labeling or improper labeling of hazardous chemicals, no documentation of initial employee training, no documentation of annual employee training, no annual hazard assessment performed, no proof of destruction of hazardous waste, no Emergency Action Plan in the facility, no Written Exposure Control Plan, OSHA Form 300A not posted during required period, and no records of hepatitis B vaccinations on declaration forms. Nuclear pharmacy is probably the first specialty area in the pharmacy profession for which a special regulation at the state level has been established. Most regulations make it unlawful for any person to provide nuclear pharmaceutical services unless under the supervision of a qualified nuclear pharmacist. In nuclear medicine, exposure to chemotherapy requires special precautions and safety procedures.

The Health Insurance Portability and Accountability Act of 1996

The Health Insurance Portability and Accountability Act (HIPAA) was signed into law in August 1996. It amends the Internal Revenue Service Code of 1986, also known as the Kassebaum-Kennedy Act. HIPAA was one of the last acts of the Clinton Administration. Its Administrative Simplification provision is composed of four parts, each of which has generated various rules and standards. Even more confusing, the rules have different compliance deadlines. The Transactions Rule was published on August 12, 2000; however, compliance dates for this section have been set for 2005. The Privacy Rule was finalized on August 14, 2002, and denoted a compliance deadline of April 14, 2003. The Security Rule was finalized and published on February 13, 2003, with implementation dates for 2004. The four parts of Administrative Simplification are the following:

1. Electronic Health Transaction Standards: Health organizations must adopt **standard code sets** to be used in all health transactions. For example, coding systems that describe diseases, injuries, and other health problems, as well as their causes, symptoms, and actions taken, must become uniform. All parties to any transaction must use and accept the same coding. This standardization is

intended to reduce mistakes, duplication of effort, and costs. Fortunately, the code sets proposed as HIPAA standards are already used by many health plans, clearinghouses, and providers, which should ease the transition.

2. Unique Identifiers: Current systems in place allow the use of multiple identification numbers when organizations deal with each other, which is seen as being confusing, conducive to error, and costly. The expectation is that with HIPAA standard identifiers, these problems will be reduced.

3. Security and Electronic Signature Standards: The Security Standard mandates safeguards for physical storage and maintenance, transmission, and access to individual health information. It applies not only to the transactions adopted under HIPAA but also to all individual health information that is maintained or transmitted; however, the Electronic Signature standard applies only to the transactions adopted under HIPAA.

4. Privacy and Confidentiality Standards: The Privacy Standards limit the nonconsensual use and release of private health information, now termed *protected health information;* give patients new rights to access their medical records and to know who else has accessed them; restrict most disclosure of health information to the minimum needed for the intended purpose; establish new criminal and civil sanctions for improper use or disclosure of health information; and establish new requirements for access to records by researchers and others.

FEDERAL REGULATORY AGENCIES

The FDA oversees all domestic and imported food, bottled water, and wine beverages with less than 7% alcohol. It is also responsible for cosmetics, medicines, medical devices, radiation-emitting products, and even the feed and drugs used for farm animals. The Centers for Disease Control and Prevention (CDC) oversees all foods and food-borne diseases. The Drug Enforcement Administration (DEA) oversees controlled substances, including the investigation and prosecution of individuals who grow or manufacture substances for illegal distribution. Each one of these agencies is further discussed in the following paragraphs.

Food and Drug Administration

The FDA controls all drugs for legal use. It is a branch of the U.S. Department of Health and Human Services. All laws pertaining to drug administration are initiated, implemented, and enforced by the FDA.

Centers for Disease Control and Prevention

The CDC is a federal agency that provides facilities and services for the investigation, identification, prevention, and control of disease. It provides statistics and information to health professions about the treatment of common and rare diseases worldwide. Its primary function is to issue regulations for infection control. It was established in 1946 as the Communicable Disease Center and became the Centers for Disease Control in 1970; the words "and Prevention" were added in 1992, but Congress requested that "CDC" remain the agency's initials. This agency also has been deeply involved in the war against HIV infection and AIDS.

Drug Enforcement Administration

The mission of the DEA is to enforce controlled substances laws and regulations and to prosecute both individuals and organizations who grow, manufacture, or distribute illegal substances. The DEA also targets people who use violence to coerce others to help them in their illegal activities and disseminates information about illegal substances to educate and inform the populace, who can then, in turn, help the DEA in its efforts. The DEA also interfaces with other governments to assist in the global enforcement of laws that regulate those who traffic drug and drug-related items.

DRUG RECALLS

The medical staff of the FDA determines the health hazard potential of a product and assigns a drug recall classification. Drug recalls are divided into three classes:

Class I: The use or exposure to the product will cause severe adverse reactions or death.

Class II: The use or exposure to the product may cause temporary or medically reversible adverse health hazards.

Class III: The use or exposure to the product is not likely to cause adverse health hazards.

DRUG STANDARDS

Drug standards are the set of requirements for the formulation of drug substances, ingredients, and dosage forms. Drugs stocked in the pharmacy must be compendia drugs, and a drug formulary or list of drugs stocked by the pharmacy must be maintained. Pharmaceutical services must be under the general supervision of a licensed pharmacist. The pharmacist must schedule regular visits to the facility to supervise the drug handling and administration procedures. At least monthly, he or she must review the drug regimen of each patient and report any discrepancies or irregularities to the administrator and the medical director. This is a significant requirement in terms of patient safety and professional integrity. These drug standards are contained in the

United States Pharmacopeia (USP) and the **National Formulary (NF)**, published by the U.S. Pharmacopeial Convention, Inc.

THE ETHICAL FOUNDATION OF PHARMACY

Ethics concerns the thoughts, judgments, and actions about issues that have the greater implications of moral right and wrong. A pharmacy technician is an integral member of the health care team in general and the pharmacy team specifically. Providing information about the risks and side effects of drug regimens is an ethical responsibility of physicians, pharmacists, and nurses. It is grounded in the principle of respect for the distinctive capacity of humans to make their own choices about their own lives. Patients must be aware of the benefits and risks of drugs that they may be taking.

Bioethics is a discipline dealing with the ethical and moral implications of biological research and applications, especially as they relate to life and death. These include pharmacology, anatomy, physiology, pathology, and biochemistry. This is a new area of ethics resulting from genetic research in the current era.

SUMMARY

The control of drugs in the practice of pharmacy is governed by laws, regulations, standards, and ethics. There are several types of law: civil, criminal, and judicial. Pharmacy technicians should understand the different terminology used in law and which punishments may be given for certain violations. The regulation of pharmacy practice is primarily a function of the state and not of the federal government. There may be some differences in pharmacy law among the different states. The U.S. Congress passed the first important federal law governing pharmacy, the Pure Food and Drug Act, in 1906. The Controlled Substances Act (CSA) governs the manufacture, distribution, and dispensing of substances that have the potential for addiction and abuse. Under this act, drugs are classified into five Schedules. Since 1970, Congress has passed several important laws: the Poison Prevention Packaging Act to prevent and protect children from accidental poisoning (child-resistant packaging), the Orphan Drug Act to provide research for new drugs needed by fewer people, the Occupational Safety and Health Act, and the Health Insurance Portability and Accountability Act (HIPAA).

CRITICAL THINKING

1. Explain why it is necessary to uphold laws and ethical standards in the field of pharmacy. What do these laws prevent? What could be the result if these laws did not exist?

2. Research a legal case in your area involving violation of the laws regulating pharmacy. What was the violation? What were the arguments in the case? What was the outcome of the case?

3. Why is privacy such an important issue in health care and the field of pharmacy? Explain how the latest HIPAA regulations help protect a patient's privacy.

REVIEW QUESTIONS

1. Standards of behavior considered appropriate within a profession are called
   A. etiquette.
   B. ethics.
   C. philosophy.
   D. morals.

2. The drugs with the highest potential for abuse and addiction are classified as which of the following Schedule?
   A. I
   B. II
   C. IV
   D. V

3. Which of the following agencies oversees controlled substances and prosecutes individuals who illegally distribute them?
   A. FDA
   B. CDC
   C. HIPAA
   D. DEA

4. Which of the following laws offers federal financial incentives to commercial and nonprofit organizations to develop and market drugs that were previously unavailable in the United States?
   A. Drug Listing Act
   B. Orphan Drug Act
   C. Poison Prevention Packaging Act
   D. Controlled Substances Act

5. The FDA is a branch of which department that controls all drugs for legal use?
   A. U.S. Department of Health
   B. U.S. Department of Health and Human Services
   C. U.S. Department of Agriculture
   D. U.S. Department of Labor

6. A less serious crime, punishable by a fine or imprisonment for less than 1 year, is called a/an
   A. felony.
   B. assault.
   C. misdemeanor.
   D. slander.

7. The pharmacy practice regulation is primarily a function of the
   A. state.
   B. federal government.
   C. Board of Pharmacy.
   D. U.S. Department of Health and Human Services.

8. A list of officially recognized drug names is known as the
   A. National Pharmacopeia.
   B. U.S. Drug Code.
   C. National Formulary.
   D. International Pharmacopeia.

9. An example of a criminal law being broken would be which of the following?
   A. A pharmacy technician packaging drug products
   B. A patient suing the pharmacist
   C. A pharmacist giving out free information
   D. A pharmacist practicing without a license

10. The three branches of the federal government include all of the following, except
    A. regulatory.
    B. judicial.
    C. executive.
    D. legislative.

11. Assumption of risk refers to a patient who
    A. continues to drink alcohol when it interacts with their prescription medication.
    B. smokes cigarettes while pregnant against physician advice.
    C. is a diabetic and does not watch his or her diet carefully.
    D. does all of the above.

12. An example of a crime occurring in the pharmacy setting, which would be considered a misdemeanor, is
    A. shoplifting.
    B. arson.
    C. burglary.
    D. selling legend drugs without a prescription.

13. Failure to use a reasonable amount of care to prevent injury or damage to a pharmacy's customers would result in a charge of
    A. libel.
    B. slander.
    C. negligence.
    D. abuse.

14. In most states, pharmacists are usually given certificates of registration, which are granted for a period of
    A. 10 to 12 years.
    B. 10 to 12 months.
    C. 1 to 2 years.
    D. 3 to 5 years.

15. Which type of scheduled drugs has a high potential for abuse but is currently accepted for medical treatment in the United States?
    A. Schedule I
    B. Schedule II
    C. Schedule III
    D. Schedule IV

4

Pharmaceutical Terminology and Abbreviations

OBJECTIVES

Upon completion of this chapter, the reader should be able to

1. Describe the origin of medical language.
2. Explain the components of a medical term and use basic prefixes, suffixes, and combining forms to build medical terms.
3. Define basic terms and abbreviations used in pharmacy.
4. Explain the rules for forming and spelling medical terms.
5. Describe common symbols used in medicine.
6. Identify common abbreviations used in prescriptions.
7. Explain why pharmacy technicians must know medical terminology.
8. Describe general abbreviations used in measurement.
9. Give five examples of roots.
10. Define general numerical prefixes.

GLOSSARY

abbreviations Shortened forms of words.

brand name A word, symbol, or device assigned to a product by its manufacturer, registered or not registered, as a trademark of its identity.

chemical name Drug name derived from the chemical composition of the drug.

combining form A root with an added vowel (known as a *combining vowel*) that connects the root with the suffix or the root to another root.

generic name The name that the manufacturer uses for a drug.

prefix A part of a word structure that occurs before or in front of the word and modifies the meaning of the root.

root The main part of a word that gives the word its central meaning.

suffix A word ending that modifies the meaning of the root.

trade name A drug name, followed by the symbol (®), that indicates that the name is registered to a specific manufacturer or owner and that no one else can use it.

OVERVIEW

Medical terminology is the language of medicine that is used in all areas of the health care industry. Medical terminology is derived primarily from Greek and Latin prefixes, roots, and suffixes. (These are called *word parts*.) Many new terms are derived from the universal language, which is English. Most terms related to diagnosis and surgery have Greek origins, and most anatomic terms come from Latin. Memorizing these word parts and rules for creating words will aid the student to understand medical terminology. By learning how word parts are combined, it is possible to determine the meaning of medical words. The ability to understand and define the parts of the medical term will make understanding the whole word easier, therefore, enhancing the ability to communicate precisely with other health care professionals.

WORD PARTS

Most terms have three components: root, suffix, and prefix. The ability to use these common roots, suffixes, and prefixes, called *word building,* is an essential skill needed by a pharmacy technician. Pharmacy technicians must be familiar with word building, common medical terms, and abbreviations and must understand general pharmacology terms and concepts.

Root

The main part of a word that gives the word its central meaning is its **root**. Word parts can be added to the root to offer more specific meanings to words. For example *brady* is a prefix meaning "slow" and *cardi* is a root meaning "heart." If the two word parts are placed together to form the word *bradycardia*, then the meaning is "slowness of the heart." All

---

TABLE 4-1. Commonly Used General Roots

ROOT	MEANING	EXAMPLE	ROOT	MEANING	EXAMPLE
Acu	Abrupt, sudden	Acute	Lingua	Tongue	Sublingual
Adeno	Gland	Adenoid	Mal	Bad	Malpractice
Adipo	Fat	Adipose	Mast, mamm	Breast	Mastectomy
Aero	Air	Aerosol	Melano	Black	Melanoma
Alb	White	Albumin	Meter	Measure	Thermometer
Ambulo	Walk	Ambulatory	My	Muscle	Myalgia
Andro	Male	Androgen	Nas	Nose	Nasal
Angio	Vessel	Angiogram	Necro	Dead	Necrosis
Arthr	Joint	Arthritis	Nephr	Kidney	Nephrosis
Brady	Slow	Bradycardia	Ocul	Eye	Ocular
Bucc	Inside of cheek	Buccal	Odont	Shaped like a tooth	Orthodontist
Canc	Crab	Cancer	Onc	Tumor	Oncology
Carcin	Crab, cancer	Carcinogen	Ophthalm	Eye	Ophthalmoscope
Cardi	Heart	Cardiology	Optic	Eye	Optician
Cereb	Brain	Cerebrum	Oste	Bone	Osteoarthritis
Chemo	Chemistry	Chemotherapy	Ot	Ear	Otalgia
Chol	Bile	Cholangiogram	Patho	Disease	Pathology
Cyst	Urinary bladder	Cystoscopy	Phleb, ven	Vein	Phlebotomy, venipuncture
Cyt	Cell	Cytology	Procto	Rectum	Proctologist
Dactyl	Finger	Syndactylism	Psych	Mind	Psychology
Dermat	Skin	Dermatology	Ren	Kidney	Renal
Encephal	Brain	Electroencephalogram	Rhino	Nose	Rhinovirus
Erythro	Red	Erythrocyte	Spir	Breathing	Spirometer
Gastr	Stomach	Gastric acid	Thrombo	Blood clot	Thrombolysis
Gluco	Sugar	Glucose	Tom, tome	Cut	Phlebotomy
Hemo	Blood	Hematoma	Tox, toxo	Poisonous	Toxic, toxicology
Hepat	Liver	Hepatoma	Uro	Urine	Urology
Hydro	Water	Hydrocephalus	Uter/o, hyster	Uterus	Intrauterine, hysterectomy
Lachry	Tear	Lachrymal fluid			
Lacto	Milk	Lactose	Vaso	Blood vessel	Vasoconstriction
Lapar	Abdomen	Laparoscope	Xantho	Yellow	Xanthin
Laryng	Larynx (voice box)	Laryngitis	Xero	Dry	Xeroderma
Leuko	White	Leukemia	Zyme	Ferment	Enzyme

medical terms have at least one root. The root typically identifies the body part, disease, disorder, or color. The following are examples of roots:

- *hepat* = liver
- *cardi* = heart

Other examples of roots are shown in Table 4-1.

Suffix

A word ending that modifies the meaning of the root is called a **suffix**. The root to which a suffix is attached may need a combining vowel. Not all words have a suffix. An example of a word with a suffix is *pharmacology*. *Pharmaco-* is the root and *-logy* is the suffix. Most medical terms have a suffix. Examples of suffixes are the following:

- *-itis* = inflammation; for example, arthritis = inflammation of the joint
- *-logy* = study of; for example, pathology = study of diseases

- *-plasty* = surgical repair; for example, rhinoplasty = surgical repair of the nose

Other examples of general suffixes are shown in Table 4-2.

Prefix

A structure at the beginning of a word that modifies the meaning of the root is a **prefix**. Not all medical words have a prefix, but every medical word has a root and ending, which is either a suffix or another root, that is itself a word. *Hyperglycemia* is an example of a word containing a prefix. *Hyper-* is the prefix, *glyc-* is the root, and *-emia* is the suffix. Some examples of prefixes follow:

- *poly-* = many; for example, polycystic = many cysts
- *sub-* = below, under; for example, sublingual = below the tongue
- *peri-* = around; for example, perianal = around the anus

Table 4-3 shows general prefixes and Table 4-4 shows general numerical prefixes.

TABLE 4-2. Commonly Used General Suffixes

SUFFIX	MEANING	EXAMPLE	SUFFIX	MEANING	EXAMPLE
-ac	Pertaining to	Cardiac	-oid	Resembling, like	Mucoid
-al	Pertaining to	Esophageal	-oma	Tumor	Melanoma
-algia	Pain	Neuralgia	-opia	Vision	Diplopia
-ary	Pertaining to	Pulmonary	-osis	Condition, abnormal condition	Cyanosis
-cele	Hernia	Hydrocele			
-centesis	Surgical puncture to remove fluid	Amniocentesis	-partum	Birth, labor	Postpartum
			-pathy	Disease	Osteopathy
-cyte	Cell	Erythrocyte	-penia	Deficiency, decreased number	Leukocytopenia
-dipsia	Thirst	Polydipsia			
-ectomy	Excision, surgical removal	Hysterectomy	-pepsia	Digestion	Dyspepsia
			-pexy	Surgical fixation	Mastopexy
-emesis	Vomiting	Hyperemesis	-philia	Attraction to	Chromophilia
-emia	Blood condition	Leukemia	-phobia	Fear	Aerophobia
-genic	Producing, forming	Carcinogenic	-phonia	Sound, voice	Aphonia
-gram	Record, picture	Electrocardiogram	-plasty	Surgical repair	Rhinoplasty
-graph	Instrument for recording	Electrocardiograph	-ptosis	Drooping, sagging	Blepharoptosis
			-rrhage	Bursting forth of blood	Hemorrhage
-graphy	Process of recording	Sonography	-rrhea	Flow, discharge	Diarrhea
-iasis	Pathological condition	Cholelithiasis	-sclerosis	Hardening	Arteriosclerosis
-iatry	Treatment	Psychiatry	-scope	Instrument to view	Laryngoscope
-ic	Pertaining to	Cephalic	-scopy	Process of viewing	Endoscopy
-itis	Inflammation	Arthritis	-stasis	Control, stopping, stop	Hemostasis
-lepsy	Seizure	Epilepsy	-stenosis	Narrowing	Tracheostenosis
-logist	Specialist	Neurologist	-stomy	Creation of an artificial opening	Colostomy
-logy	Study of	Biology			
-lysis	Destruction, breaking down	Neurolysis	-therapy	Treatment	Hydrotherapy
			-tomy	Incision	Craniotomy
-lytic	Reduce, destroy	Hemolytic	-tripsy	Crushing, rubbing	Lithotripsy
-malacia	Softening	Osteomalacia	-trophy	Nourishment, development	Atrophy
-megaly	Enlargement, enlarged	Acromegaly			
-meter	Instrument to measure	Cytometer	-tropia	Turning	Exotropia
-metry	Process of measuring	Pelvimetry	-uria	Urine, urination	Nocturia

TABLE 4-3.   Commonly Used General Prefixes

PREFIX	MEANING	EXAMPLE	PREFIX	MEANING	EXAMPLE
A-	Without, not, no	Aphasia	Macro-	Large	Macrocyte
Ab-	Away from	Abduct	Mal-	Bad, poor	Malaise
Ad-	Toward	Adduct	Meso-	Middle	Mesoderm
Ante-	Before, forward	Anteflexion	Meta-	Change, beyond, after	Metastasis
Auto-	Self	Autoimmune	Micro-	Small	Microscope
Bio-	Life	Biology	Multi-	Many	Multilingual
Brady-	Slow	Bradycardia	Neo-	New	Neonatal
Circum-	Around	Circumcision	Nulli-	None	Nullipara
Con-	Together	Congenital	Para-	Near, beside, abnormal, alongside	Parathyroid
Contra-	Against	Contraindication			
Dia-	Complete, through	Diarrhea	Per-	Through	Perforated
Dys-	Bad, abnormal, painful	Dysuria	Peri-	Around, surrounding	Pericardium
Ecto-	Out, outside	Ectopic	Poly-	Many, excessive	Polycystic
En-	In, within, inward	Encapsulated	Post-	Behind, after	Postpartum
Endo-	Into, within	Endoscopic	Pre-	Before, in front of	Premature
Epi-	Upon, above	Epidermic	Pro-	Before	Prognosis
Eu-	Good, normal, well	Euphoria	Re-	Again, back	Reactive
Ex-, exo-	Out, away from	Excision	Retro-	Behind, backward	Retrograde
Extra-	Outside	Extracellular	Sub-	Below, under, beneath	Sublingual
Hyper-	Excessive, above	Hyperglycemia	Super-	Above, over	Superficial
Hypo-	Below, deficient, under	Hypotension	Supra-	Above, on top of, upper	Suprarenal
In-	Not, into, in	Infusion	Syn-	Together, with, union	Syndactylism
Infra-	Below, inferior	Infracostal	Tachy-	Fast	Tachypnea
Inter-	Between	Interfemoral	Trans-	Across	Transhepatic
Intra-	Within, into, inside	Intradermal	Ultra-	Beyond, excessive	Ultrasound
Iso-	Same, equal	Isograft			

TABLE 4-4.   General Numerical Prefixes

PREFIX	MEANING	EXAMPLE
Semi-	Half	Semicircular
Hemi-	Half	Hemiplegia
Mono-	One, single	Mononucleus
Uni-	One	Unipolar
Bi-	Two, double, both	Bilateral
Di(plo)-	Two, double	Diplococci
Tri-	Three	Tricuspid
Tetra-	Four	Tetratomic
Quadr-	Four	Quadriplegia
Penta-	Five	Pentadactyl
Quint-	Five	Quintipara
Hexa-	Six	Hexastrol
Sexta-	Six	Sextan
Hepta-	Seven	Heptachromic
Septa-	Seven	Septuplets
Octa-	Eight	Octarius
Enne-	Nine	Ennead
Non(i)-	Nine	Nonipara
Deca-	Ten	Decameter
Deci-	One-tenth	Deciliter
Hecto-	One hundred	Hectogram
Centi-	One-one hundredth	Centimeter
Kilo-	One thousand	Kilogram
Milli-	One-one thousandth	Milliliter

Combining Form

A **combining form** is a root with an added vowel (known as a *combining vowel*) that connects the root with the suffix or with another root. The most common combining vowel is *o*, followed by *i*, and then *e*. A combining vowel has no meaning of its own; it only joins one word part to another and is used to ease pronunciation. The following are examples of combining forms:

- *hepat/o* = liver; for example, hepat*o*megaly = enlargement of the liver
- *cardi/o* = heart; for example, cardi*o*pathy = disease of the heart
- *gastr/o* = stomach; for example, gastr*o*tomy = incision into the stomach

Tables 4-5 and 4-6 show general combining forms and general combining forms for colors, respectively.

Often a medical term is formed from two or more roots; this is called a *compound word*. The following are examples of compound words:

- *gastroenterologist* = a physician who is a specialist for conditions of the stomach and intestinal tract
- *electrocardiogram* = written record of the electrical impulses of the heart

TABLE 4-5. General Combining Forms

COMBINING FORM	MEANING	EXAMPLE	COMBINING FORM	MEANING	EXAMPLE
Abdomin/o	Abdomen	Abdominocentesis	Mamm/mast/o	Breast	Mastectomy
Aden/o	Gland	Adenectomy	Men/o	Menses, menstruation	Menarche
Angi/o	Vessel	Angiogram	My/o	Muscle	Myalgia
Arteri/o	Artery	Arteriograph	Myel/o	Spinal cord, bone marrow	Myelitis
Arthr/o	Joint	Arthroscopy			
Ather/o	Fatty, porridge-like	Atherosclerosis	Nas/o	Nose	Nasal
Balan/o	Glans penis	Balanoplasty	Nat/o	Birth	Prenatal
Bronch/o	Bronchus	Bronchoscope	Necr/o	Death	Necrosis
Bucc/o	Cheek	Buccal	Nephr/o	Kidney	Nephrotomy
Burs/o	Bursa, sac	Bursitis	Neur/o	Nerve	Neuropathy
Carcin/o	Cancer, cancerous	Carcinogenic	Noct/o	Night	Nocturia
Cardi/o	Heart	Cardiologist	Ocul/o	Eye	Interocular
Carp/o	Wrist	Carpal	Olig/o	Scanty, few	Oligouria
Cephal/o	Head	Cephalodynia	Oophor/o	Ovaries	Oophorectomy
Cerebr/o	Cerebrum, brain	Cerebral	Orch/orchid/o	Testes	Orchidoplasty
Chol/e	Gall, bile	Cholelithiasis	Oste/o	Bone	Osteoarthritis
Cost/o	Rib	Intercostal	Ot/o	Ear	Otalgia
Crani/o	Cranium (skull)	Craniotomy	Phleb/o	Vein	Phlebotomy
Cyst/o	Urinary bladder	Cystoscopy	Phren/o	Diaphragm	Phrenoplegia
Cyt/o	Cell	Cytology	Proct/o	Rectum	Proctologist
Derm/ dermat/o	Skin	Dermatologist	Psych/o	Mind	Psychiatrist
			Pulmon/o	Lungs	Pulmonary
Encephal/o	Brain	Hydrencephalitis	Py/o	Pus	Pyorrhea
Electr/o	Electricity, electrical activity	Electroencephalogram	Ren/o	Kidney	Renal
			Rhin/o	Nose	Rhinoplasty
Enter/o	Intestines	Enteritis	Salping/o	Fallopian tubes	Salpingotomy
Esophag/o	Esophagus	Esophageal	Sperm/ spermat/o	Sperm, spermatic cord	Spermatolysis
Gastr/o	Stomach	Gastrectomy			
Gingiv/o	Gums	Gingivitis	Spir/o	Breathe, breath	Spirometer
Gynec/o	Woman	Gynecomastia	Spleen/o	Spleen	Splenectomy
Hem/hemat/o	Blood	Hematolysis	Stern/o	Sternum	Sternal
Hepat/o	Liver	Hepatoma	Stomat/o	Mouth	Stomatitis
Hist/o	Tissue	Histology	Ten/tendin/o	Tendon	Tenalgia
Hydr/o	Water	Hydrocele	Thorac/o	Thorax (chest)	Thoracocentesis
Hyster/o	Uterus	Hysterectomy	Thromb/o	Clot	Thrombocyte
Kerat/o	Cornea	Keratotomy	Tox/o	Poison, toxic	Toxicology
Lacrim/o	Tear duct, tears	Lacrimal	Tympan/o	Eardrum	Tympanometer
Lact/o	Milk	Lactose	Ur/o	Urine	Urology
Lapar/o	Abdomen	Laparoscopy	Vas/o	Vessel	Vasectomy
Laryng/o	Larynx (voice box)	Laryngitis	Vertebr/o	Vertebrae	Vertebral
Lingu/o	Tongue	Sublingual	Xer/o	Dry	Xerosis
Lip/o	Fat	Lipoma			

TABLE 4-6. General Combining Forms for Colors

COMBINING FORM	MEANING	EXAMPLE	COMBINING FORM	MEANING	EXAMPLE
Chlor/o	Green	Chloremia	Melan/o	Black	Melanoma
Cyan/oB	Blue	Cyanotic	Poli/o	Gray	Poliomyelitis
Erythr/o	Red	Erythroderma	Rhod/o	Red	Rhodotoxin
Leuk/leuc/o	White	Leukocyte	Xanth/o	Yellow	Xanthine

To define a medical term a meaning needs to be applied to each word part in the term. Typically, when translating a medical term, one should begin with the suffix, then go back to the beginning of the term. This rule does not always apply to all medical terms.

RULES FOR FORMING AND SPELLING MEDICAL TERMS

A combining vowel usually is used to join a root to another root, even when the second root begins with a vowel:

- *oste + arthr + itis = oste/o/arthr/itis*
- root + root + suffix
- bone + joint + inflammation = inflammation of the bone and joint

A combining vowel also is used to connect a root with a suffix that begins with a consonant:

- *cardi + megaly = cardi/o/megaly*
- root + suffix
- heart + enlargement = enlargement of the heart

A combining vowel is not used before a suffix that begins with a vowel:

- *hyster + ectomy = hyster/ectomy*
- root + suffix
- uterus + excision = excision of the uterus

If a root ends in a vowel and the suffix begins with the same vowel, the final vowel is dropped from the root and a combining vowel is not used:

- *cardi + itis = card/itis*
- root + suffix
- heart + inflammation = inflammation of the heart

Occasionally, when a prefix ends in a vowel and the root begins with a vowel, the final vowel is dropped from the prefix:

- *para + enter + al = par/enter/al*
- prefix + root + suffix
- alongside + intestine + pertaining to = pertaining to alongside the intestine

ABBREVIATIONS

Abbreviations are shortened forms of words representing commonly used medical terms. Many such abbreviations are used in all areas of health care practice. It is important for the pharmacy technician to be familiar with the most common abbreviations used for writing prescriptions (see Table 4-7), the abbreviations associated with various measurements (see Table 4-8), and general medical abbreviations (see Table 4-9). Tables 4-10 through 4-20 list common abbreviations related to each body system.

TABLE 4-7. Abbreviations Commonly Used in Prescriptions

ABBREVIATION	MEANING	ABBREVIATION	MEANING
a̅ a̅, aa	Of each	IM	Intramuscular
a.c.	Before meals	inj.	Inject
ad	To, up to	IV	Intravenous
AD	Right ear (auris dextra)	liq.	Liquid
ad lib	As desired	mixt	Mixture
AM, a.m.	Morning	mist.	A mixture
amt	Amount	noc., noct.	Night
aq.	Water	non rep	Do not repeat, no refills
AS	Left ear (auris sinestra)	NPO	Nothing by mouth (nulla
AU	Both ears (auris uterque)		per os)
b.i.d., BID	Twice a day	O.D.	Right eye
b.i.n.	Twice a night	oint	Ointment
c̅	With	O.S.	Left eye
cap, caps	Capsule	OU	Both eyes, each eye
comp	Compound	p.c.	After meals
d	Day	per	Through or by
dil.	Dilute	p.m.	Afternoon
disp	Dispense	p.o.	By mouth
elix.	Elixir	p.r.	Through the rectum
hr	Hour	p.r.n., PRN	As needed
h.s.	Hour of sleep (bedtime)	p.v.	Through the vagina

Continues

TABLE 4-7. Abbreviations Commonly Used in Prescriptions, cont'd

ABBREVIATION	MEANING	ABBREVIATION	MEANING
pulv.	Powder	sp.	Spirits
q	Every	s.o.s.	If necessary
q.d.	Every day	Stat	Immediately
q.h.	Every hour	Supp.	Suppository
q2h	Every 2 hours	Syr.	Syrup
q.i.d., QID	Four times a day	Top.	Topically
Qn	Every night	Tab.	Tablet
q.o.d.	Every other day	t.i.d., TID	Three times a day
q.s., q.v.	As much as you wish	tr., tinct.	Tincture
$\overline{S}$	Without	u.d.	As directed
Sig.	Write on label	vo	Verbal order
Sol.	Solution	x	Times

TABLE 4-8. Abbreviations Commonly Used for Measurements

ABBREVIATION	MEANING	ABBREVIATION	MEANING
°C	Celsius	mEq	Milliequivalent
cc	Cubic centimeter (1 cc = 1 mL)	mg	Milligram
cm	Centimeter (2.5 cm = 1 inch)	mL	Milliliter
°F	Fahrenheit	No.	Number
fl	Fluid	oz	Ounce
g, gm	Gram	Ss	One-half
gtt	Drops	T	Temperature
lb	Pound	tbs, tbsp	Tablespoon
kg	Kilogram (1 kg = 2.2 lb)	tsp	Teaspoon
L	Liter	w/v	Weight in volume
mcg	Microgram		

TABLE 4-9. General Medical Abbreviations

ABBREVIATION	MEANING	ABBREVIATION	MEANING
AP	Anterior-posterior	D&C	Dilatation and curettage
BE	Barium enema	DOB	Date of birth
BP	Blood pressure	DPT	Diphtheria-pertussis-tetanus
Bx	Biopsy	Dx	Diagnosis
C	Carbon	EEG	Electroencephalogram
Ca	Calcium, cancer	EENT	Eyes, ears, nose, throat
CAD	Coronary artery disease	EKG	Electrocardiogram
C&S	Culture and sensitivity	FBS	Fasting blood sugar
cath.	Catheter	Fe	Iron
CBC	Complete blood count	FUO	Fever of unknown origin
CC	Chief complaint	GI	Gastrointestinal
CHF	Congestive heart failure	GU	Genitourinary
c/o	Complains of	Gyn	Gynecology
CO	Carbon dioxide	H	Hydrogen
COPD	Chronic obstructive pulmonary disease	H&P	History and physical
CVA	Cerebral vascular accident	Hgb	Hemoglobin
CXR	Chest x-ray	HBV	Hepatitis B virus

Continues

TABLE 4-9. General Medical Abbreviations, cont'd

ABBREVIATION	MEANING	ABBREVIATION	MEANING
HCT	Hematocrit	Pt	Patient
Hg	Mercury	R	Respirations, right
Hib	*Haemophilus influenzae* type B	r	Take
Hx, hx	History	RBC	Red blood cell
I	Iodine	rbc	Red blood count
IM	Intramuscular	R/O	Rule out
IUD	Intrauterine device	ROM	Range of motion
IV	Intravenous	SOB	Shortness of breath
K	Potassium	T	Temperature
LMP	Last menstrual period	TIA	Transient ischemic attack
MI	Myocardial infarction	Tx	Treatment
MMR	Measles-mumps-rubella	UA	Urinalysis
N	Nitrogen	UTI	Urinary tract infection
Na	Sodium	VS, v.s.	Vital signs
NPO	Nothing by mouth	WBC	White blood cell
OB	Obstetrics	wbc	White blood count
P	Pulse	WNL	Within normal limits
PERRLA	Pupils equal, round, reactive to light and accommodation	wt	Weight
		y/o, yo	Years old
PO	Orally		

TABLE 4-10. Abbreviations Related to the Integumentary System

ABBREVIATION	MEANING
Bx	Biopsy
Derm	Dermatology
SC, sub-Q, SQ, sub CU, Subq.	Subcutaneous

TABLE 4-11. Abbreviations Related to the Musculoskeletal System

ABBREVIATION	MEANING
C1, C2, ... C7	Individual cervical vertebrae
Ca	Calcium
CTS	Carpal tunnel syndrome
EMG	Electromyography
Fx	Fracture
Ortho	Orthopedics
ROM	Range of motion
SLE	Systemic lupus erythematosus

TABLE 4-12. Abbreviations Related to the Eye

ABBREVIATION	MEANING
Ast	Astigmatism
IOP	Intraocular pressure
OD	Right eye
OS	Left eye
OU	Both eyes
REM	Rapid eye movement
VA	Visual acuity
VF	Visual field

TABLE 4-13. Abbreviations Related to the Nervous System

ABBREVIATION	MEANING
AD	Alzheimer's disease
ALS	Amyotrophic lateral sclerosis
CAT	Computed axial tomography
CNS	Central nervous system
CP	Cerebral palsy
CSF	Cerebrospinal fluid
CT	Computed tomography
CVA	Cerebrovascular accident
EEG	Electroencephalogram
LP	Lumbar puncture
MRI	Magnetic resonance imaging
MS	Multiple sclerosis
TIA	Transient ischemic attack

TABLE 4-14. Abbreviations Related to the Ear

ABBREVIATION	MEANING
AD	Right ear
AS	Left ear
AU	Each ear
EENT	Eyes, ears, nose, and throat
Oto	Otology

TABLE 4-15. Abbreviations Related to the Endocrine System

ABBREVIATION	MEANING
ACTH	Adrenocorticotropic hormone
BMR	Basal metabolic rate
DI	Diabetes insipidus
DM	Diabetes mellitus
FBS	Fasting blood sugar
FSH	Follicle-stimulating hormone
GH	Growth hormone
GTT	Glucose tolerance test
IDDM	Insulin-dependent diabetes mellitus
K	Potassium
Na	Sodium
PRL	Prolactin
TFT	Thyroid function test

TABLE 4-16. Abbreviations Related to the Cardiovascular System

ABBREVIATION	MEANING
AF	Atrial fibrillation
AS	Aortic stenosis
ASD	Atrial septal defect
BP	Blood pressure
CAD	Coronary artery disease
CHD	Coronary heart disease
CHF	Congestive heart failure
ECG, EKG	Electrocardiogram
ECHO	Echocardiography
MI	Myocardial infarction
MVP	Mitral valve prolapse
PDA	Patent ductus arteriosus
PVC	Premature ventricular contraction
VT	Ventricular tachycardia

TABLE 4-17. Abbreviations Related to the Digestive System

ABBREVIATION	MEANING
BE	Barium enema
EUS	Endoscopic ultrasound
GERD	Gastroesophageal reflex disease
GI	Gastrointestinal
IBS	Irritable bowel syndrome

TABLE 4-18. Abbreviations Related to the Urinary System

ABBREVIATION	MEANING
ADH	Antidiuretic hormone; vasopressin
ARF	Acute renal failure
BUN	Blood urea nitrogen
Cath	Catheter
CFR	Chronic renal failure
HD	Hemodialysis
IVP	Intravenous pyelogram
KUB	Kidney, ureter, and bladder
PKU	Phenylketonuria
UA	Urinalysis
UTI	Urinary tract infection

TABLE 4-19. Abbreviations Related to the Reproductive System

ABBREVIATION	MEANING
AB	Abortion
AIDS	Acquired immunodeficiency syndrome
BPH	Benign prostatic hyperplasia
CS, C-section	Cesarean section
CX	Cervix
D&C	Dilation and curettage
ECC	Endocervical curettage
EMB	Endometrial biopsy
FHT	Fetal heart tones
FSH	Follicle-stimulating hormone
GYN	Gynecology
HCG	Human chorionic gonadotropin
HIV	Human immunodeficiency virus
HSV	Herpes simplex virus
LH	Luteinizing hormone
Multip	Multipara
Pap smear	Papanicolaou smear (test for cervical of vaginal cancer)
PMS	Premenstrual syndrome
PSA	Prostate-specific antigen
STD	Sexually transmitted disease

TABLE 4-20. Poisons and Their Antidotes

POISON	ANTIDOTES
Acetaminophen	N-Acetylcysteine
Benzodiazepines	Flumazenil
Carbon monoxide	Oxygen
Cyanide	Amyl nitrate
Iron	Deferoxamine
Methanol	Ethanol
Opiates	Naloxone
Organophosphates	Atropine or pralidoxime

DRUG NAMES

Throughout the process of development, drugs may have several names assigned to them: a chemical name, a generic (nonproprietary) name, an official name, and a trade or **brand name**. This naming convention is confusing unless the pharmacy technician has a clear understanding of the different names used. The most commonly used name is the **generic name**. This is the name the manufacturer uses for a drug, and it is the same in all countries. The **trade name** is followed by the symbol (r), which indicates that the name is registered to a specific manufacturer or owner and that no one else can use it. The **chemical name** is derived from the chemical composition of the drug. This name may be hyphenated and is usually long. Table 4-21 shows the most commonly used trade names of medications and their corresponding generic names.

TABLE 4-21.   Trade Names and Generic Names of Commonly Used Drugs

TRADE NAME	GENERIC NAME	TRADE NAME	GENERIC NAME
Abelcet®	Amphotericin B, liposomal	Corlopam®	Fenoldopam
Achromycin®	Tetracycline	Coumadin®	Warfarin
Acti-12®	Hydroxocobalamin (Vitamin B_{12})	Crystodigin®	Digitoxin
Activase®	Alteplase, recombinant	Cytotec®	Misoprostol
Adalat®	Nifedipine	Decadron®	Dexamethasone
Advil®	Ibuprofen	Deltasone®	Prednisone
Aerolate SR®	Theophylline	Demerol®	Meperidine
Airet®	Albuterol sulfate	Depakene®	Valproic acid
Alazine®	Hydralazine HCl	Dia Beta®	Glyburide
Aldomet®	Methyldopa	Diabinese®	Chlorpropamide
Alka-Seltzer®	Aspirin	Diamox®	Acetazolamide
Allegra®	Fexofenadine HCl	Didrex®	Benzphetamine HCl
Zyloprim	Allopurinol	Dilantin®	Phenytoin
Altracin®	Bacitracin	Diprolene®	Betamethasone
Amerge®	Naratriptan	Dramamine®	Dimenhydrinate
Amoxil®	Amoxicillin	Dulcolax®	Bisacodyl
Amphojel®	Aluminum hydroxide	Duricef®	Cefadroxil
Ancef®	Cefazolin	Dyazide®	Hydrochlorothiazide
Anzemet®	Dolasetron	Effexor®	Venlafaxine
Apresoline®	Hydralazine	Elavil®	Amitriptyline
Atarax®	Hydroxyzine	Eramycin®	Erythromycin stearate
Ativan®	Lorazepam	Ery-Tab®	Erythromycin base
Axid®	Nizatidine	Exna®	Benzthiazide
Bactrim®	Sulfamethoxazole	Flagyl®	Metronidazole
Benadryl®	Diphenhydramine	Floxin®	Ofloxacin
Bentyl®	Dicyclomine	Fluothane®	Halothane
Beta Cort®	Betamethasone valerate	Folvite®	Folic acid
Biaxin®	Clarithromycin	Fortaz®	Ceftazidime
Biomox®	Amoxicillin trihydrate	Fosamax®	Alendronate sodium
Brethine®	Terbutaline	Fungizone®	Amphotericin B
Bufferin®	Aspirin	Gantrisin®	Sulfisoxazole
BuSpar®	Buspirone	Garamycin®	Gentamicin
Calderol®	Calcifediol	Gee-Gee®	Guaifenesin
Capoten®	Captopril	Genevax-HIV®	Human immunodeficiency virus vaccine
Carafate®	Sucralfate	Gen-K®	Potassium chloride
Cardizem®	Diltiazem	Genprin®	Aspirin
Catapres®	Clonidine	Glucotrol®	Glipizide
Ceclor®	Cefaclor	Haldol®	Haloperidol
Cefzil®	Cefprozil	Hexadrol®	Dexamethasone
Celexa®	Citalopram	Hismanal®	Astemizole
Cipro®	Ciprofloxacin	Humatin®	Paromomycin sulfate
Claritin®	Loratadine	Humulin®	Insulin
Cleocin®	Clindamycin	Hycort®	Hydrocortisone, topical
Compazine®	Prochlorperazine	Hytrin®	Terazosin
Corgard®	Nadolol	Ilosone®	Erythromycin estolate

Continues

TABLE 4-21. Trade Names and Generic Names of Commonly Used Drugs, cont'd

TRADE NAME	GENERIC NAME	TRADE NAME	GENERIC NAME
Ilotycin®	Erythromycin base	Tega-Cort®	Hydrocortisone, topical
Impril®	Imipramine HCl	Tegopen®	Cloxacillin sodium
Inderal®	Propranolol	Tegretol®	Carbamazepine
Indocin®	Indomethacin	Terramycin®	Oxytetracycline HCl
Integrilin®	Eptifibatide	Tobrex®	Tobramycin
Isoptin®	Verapamil	Tofranil®	Imipramine
Kantrex®	Kanamycin sulfate	Totacillin®	Ampicillin, oral
Keflex®	Cephalexin	Trilafon®	Perphenazine
Kefzol®	Cefazolin	Tums®	Calcium carbonate
Kenalog®	Triamcinolone	Tylenol®	Acetaminophen
Klonopin®	Clonazepam	Tyzine®	Tetrahydrozoline HCl, nasal
Lanoxin®	Digoxin	Ultiva®	Remifentanil HCl
Lasix®	Furosemide	Ultram®	Tramadol
Levate®	Amitriptyline HCl	Uritrol®	Furosemide
Lipitor®	Atorvastatin	Urobak®	Sulfamethoxazole
Lopid®	Gemfibrozil	Valisone®	Betamethasone valerate
Lopressor®	Metoprolol	Valium®	Diazepam
Maxalt®	Rizatriptan	Vancocin®	Vancomycin
Mefoxin®	Cefoxitin	Vasomax®	Phentolamine
Mellaril®	Thioridazine	Vasotec®	Enalapril
Micronase®	Glyburide	V-cillin K®	Penicillin V potassium
Minipress®	Prazosin	Velosef®	Cephradine
Motrin®	Ibuprofen	Velosulin®	Insulin injection
Mycostatin®	Nystatin	Ventolin®	Albuterol
Mylicon®	Simethicone	Vermox®	Mebendazole
Naprosyn®	Naproxen sodium	Vibramycin®	Doxycycline
Nebcin®	Tobramycin	Virilon®	Methyltestosterone
Nizoral®	Ketoconazole	Vivarin®	Caffeine
Omnicef®	Cefdinir	Vivol®	Diazepam
Oretic®	Hydrochorothiazide	Volmax®	Albuterol sulfate
Pepcid®	Famotidine	Vontrol®	Diphenidol
Phenergan®	Promethazine	Wellferon®	Interferon alfa-N1
Prilosec®	Omeprazole	Westcort®	Hydrocortisone valerate
Prinivil®	Lisinopril	Wycillin®	Penicillin G procaine
Procardia®	Nifedipine	Xalatan®	Latanoprost
Pronestyl®	Procainamide	Xanax®	Alprazolam
Prozac®	Fluoxetine	Xylocaine®	Lidocaine HCl, local
Proventil®	Albuterol	YF-Vax®	Yellow fever vaccine
Regitine®	Phentolamine	Yocon®	Yohimbine HCl
Resectisol®	Mannitol	Yohimex®	Yohimbine HCl
Retrovir®	Zidovudine	Zantac®	Ranitidine
Rhinocort®	Budesonide, nasal	Zarontin®	Ethosuximide
Robitussin®	Guaifenesin	Zestril®	Lisinopril
Rocephin®	Ceftriaxone	Zetar®	Coal tar
Rufen®	Ibuprofen	Zetran®	Diazepam
Septra®	Trimethoprim	Zincate®	Zinc sulfate
Silapap® children's	Acetaminophen	Zithromax®	Azithromycin
Stadol®	Butorphanol	Zocor®	Simvastatin
Synthroid®	Levothyroxine	Zoloft®	Sertraline HCl
Tagamet HB®	Cimetidine	Zomig®	Zolmitriptan
Talwin®	Pentazocine	Zonalon®	Doxepin, topical
Tamoxifen®	Tamoxifen citrate	Zorprin®	Aspirin
Tapazole®	Methimazole	Zovirax®	Acyclovir
Tavist®	Clemastine fumarate	Zyloprim®	Allopurinol
Teargen®	Artificial tears solution	Zyban®	Bupropion HCl
Tebamide®	Trimethobenzamide HCl	Zyrtec®	Cetirizine HCl
Tebrazid®	Pyrazinamide		

APOTHECARY SYMBOLS

The definitions of apothecary symbols are not absolute; many of them have more than one meaning when used in different contexts. The symbols used most commonly in medicine are shown in Table 4-22.

SUMMARY

The pharmacy technician must be able to communicate precisely with other professionals and specialists in different fields of health care. Therefore, he or she should be familiar with medical terminology, abbreviations, and symbols. In medical terminology commonly encountered in the practice of pharmacy extensive use is made of Greek and Latin roots, prefixes, and suffixes. Pharmacy, of course, is the practice of dispensing drugs and information about drugs. A clear understanding of what a drug is involves an understanding of its uses and of terms related to drug uses, including diagnosis, disease, trauma, prevention, treatment, generic name, and trade name. The technician must be familiar with many abbreviations used on prescriptions and medication orders, including ones used to specify amounts, bodily functions and conditions, dosage forms and delivery systems, drugs, drug references, time, administration time, administration sites, and parts of the body. A technician must also be familiar with common symbols for weights and measures of drugs to avoid serious medication errors.

TABLE 4-22.   Symbols Commonly Used in Medicine

SYMBOL	MEANING	SYMBOL	MEANING
□	Left	°	Hours
®	Right	1°	Primary
>	Greater than	2°	Secondary
<	Less than	℥	Teaspoonful, 5ml (dram)
=	Equal to		
↑	Increase	℔	Minim
↓	Decrease	#	Pound
∅	None	×	Times (as in two times a week)
Δ	Change		
'	Minutes	♀	Female
"	Seconds	♂	Male

REVIEW QUESTIONS

1. The abbreviation *AU* means
   A. both eyes.
   B. left eye.
   C. right ear.
   D. both ears.

2. The suffix *-dipsia* means
   A. pain.
   B. thirst.
   C. vomiting.
   D. seizure.

3. Which of the following suffixes means "pain"?
   A. -cele
   B. -lepsy
   C. -lysis
   D. -algia

4. When the combining form *xer/o* is used, it means that
   A. the object is blue.
   B. the object is oily.
   C. the object is dry.
   D. something is poisonous.

5. The most common combining vowel is
   A. i.
   B. a.
   C. o.
   D. e.

6. Which of the following abbreviations means "every day"?
   A. q.d.
   B. q.i.d.
   C. q.e.d.
   D. b.i.d.

7. The underlined portion of the word <u>hypo</u>lipemia represents which of the following word parts?
   A. Suffix
   B. Prefix
   C. Root
   D. Combining form

8. The prefix *milli-* means
   A. one-thousandth.
   B. many.
   C. one-hundredth.
   D. one-tenth.

9. The abbreviation *mist* means
   A. liquid.
   B. ointment.
   C. a mixture.
   D. solution.

10. The abbreviation *s.o.s.* means
    A. immediately.
    B. suppository.
    C. solution.
    D. if necessary.

11. Which of the following prefixes means "bad, difficult, painful"?
    A. Ex-
    B. Dis-
    C. Dys-
    D. Meta-

12. The abbreviation *q.o.d.* means
    A. every other day.
    B. twice a day.
    C. four times a day.
    D. every hour.

13. The brand name of nizatidine is
    A. Nizoral®.
    B. Ativan®.
    C. Axid®.
    D. Atarax®.

14. The generic name of Ventolin® is
    A. phentolamine.
    B. cephradine.
    C. lisinopril.
    D. albuterol.

15. The generic name of Zorprin® is
    A. methimazole.
    B. alprazolam.
    C. aspirin.
    D. allopurinol.

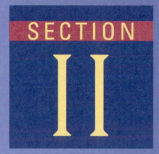

The Science of Pharmacology

Dosage Forms and Administration of Medications

OBJECTIVES

Upon completion of this chapter, the reader should be able to

1. Differentiate chemical names, generic names, and trade names of drugs.
2. Describe dosage forms of drugs.
3. Explain the significance of medication errors.
4. Summarize methods of administering medications.
5. Describe the basic equipment for parenteral administration.
6. Explain transdermal drug delivery.
7. Define oxygen therapy.
8. Describe rectal administration.
9. List the sites suitable for subcutaneous and intramuscular injections.

GLOSSARY

ampule A sealed glass container that usually contains a single dose of medicine. The top of the ampule must be broken off to open the container.

aromatic water A mixture of distilled water with an aromatic volatile water.

buccal Pertaining to the inside of the cheek.

buffered tablet A tablet that prevents ulceration or irritation of the stomach wall.

caplet A tablet shaped like a capsule.

capsule A solid dosage form in which the drug is enclosed in either a hard or soft shell of soluble material.

cream A semisolid emulsion of either the oil-in-water or the water-in-oil type, ordinarily intended for topical use.

elixir A clear, sweetened, hydroalcoholic liquid intended for oral use.

emulsion A system containing two liquids that cannot be mixed together in which one is dispersed, in the form of very small globules, throughout the other.

enteric-coated tablet A tablet covered in a special coating to protect it from stomach acid, allowing the drug to dissolve in the intestines.

fluidextract A pharmacopeial liquid preparation of vegetable drugs, made by filtration, containing alcohol as a solvent or as a preservative or both.

gavage Feeding with a stomach tube.

gel A jelly or the solid or semisolid phase of a colloidal solution.

gelcap An oil-based medication that is enclosed in a soft gelatin capsule.

granule A very small pill, usually gelatin- or sugar-coated, containing a drug to be given in a small dose.

induration An excessive hardening or firmness of any body site. It is one of the signs of inflammation.

GLOSSARY continued

intradermal injection Between the layers of the skin. A dose of an agent administered between the layers of the skin.

intramuscular injection Inside a muscle. Normally used in the context of an injection given into a muscle.

intravenous injection Into a vein. Most commonly used in the context of an injection given directly into a vein.

liniment A liquid preparation for external use, usually applied by friction to the skin.

lozenge A small, disk-shaped tablet composed of solidifying paste containing an astringent, an antiseptic, or an oil-based drug used for local treatment of the mouth or throat. It is held in the mouth until dissolved. Also known as a troche.

mixture A mutual incorporation of two or more substances, without chemical union, in which the physical characteristics of each of the components are retained.

ointment A semisolid preparation that usually contains medicinal substances and is intended for external application.

oral Pertaining to the mouth. Medication given by mouth.

parenteral Administration by some means other than through the gastrointestinal tract; referring particularly to introduction of substances into an organism by intravenous, subcutaneous, intramuscular, or intramedullary injection.

pill A small, globular mass of soluble material containing a medicinal substance to be swallowed.

plaster A solid preparation that can be spread when heated and that becomes adhesive at the temperature of the body.

powder A dry mass of minute separate particles of any substance.

solution A liquid dosage form in which active ingredients are dissolved in a liquid vehicle.

spirits An alcoholic or hydroalcoholic solution of volatile substances.

subcutaneous injection The administration of medication by means of a needle and syringe into the layer of fat and blood vessels beneath the skin.

sublingual Pertaining to the area under the tongue.

suppository A small, solid body shaped for ready introduction into one of the orifices of the body other than the oral cavity (e.g., rectum, urethra, or vagina), made of a substance, usually medicated, that is solid at ordinary temperature but melts at body temperature.

suspension A liquid dosage form that contains solid drug particles floating in a liquid medium.

sustained release (SR) A capsule with a controlled release of the dosage over a special period of time.

syrup A liquid preparation in a concentrated aqueous solution of a sugar used for medicinal purposes or to add flavor to a substance.

tablet A solid dosage form containing medicinal substances with or without suitable diluents.

tincture An alcoholic solution prepared from vegetable materials or from chemical substances.

topical Pertaining to a drug that is applied to the surface of the body.

troche A small, disk-shaped tablet composed of solidifying paste containing an astringent, antiseptic, or oil-based drug used for local treatment of the mouth or throat. It is held in the mouth until dissolved. Also known as a lozenge.

vial A small glass or plastic bottle intended to hold medicine.

wheal An intensely itchy skin eruption larger than a hive.

Z-track method A method of intramuscular injection of medication in which the skin must be pulled to one side before the tissue is grasped for the injection of such medication. It is used when a drug is highly irritating to subcutaneous tissues or has the ability to permanently stain the skin.

OVERVIEW

Any medication has the potential to cause serious harm to the patient. Therefore, the process of dispensing and administering medication orders must always be performed with great care. Each member of the health care team involved in medication administration must be constantly vigilant to prevent errors and deliver quality patient care. The pharmacy technician must be familiar with many different forms of medication as well as with their routes of administration, doses, and strengths. A medication should never be given until its purpose, possible side effects, precautions, and recommended dosages are known. Safeguarding the patient during this process involves using the Seven Rights of Medication Administration.

DRUG NAMES

It is not unusual for each drug entity to be known by several designations. Usually, a single drug may have up to three names: chemical, generic, and trade. The first type of name, usually applied to compounds of known composition, is the chemical name. For substances of plant or animal origin that cannot be classified as pure chemical compounds, scientific identification is given in terms of precise biochemical or zoological names. These names are generally not useful to the physician, the pharmacist, or other users of the drug. When a new drug has been proved to be useful through successive research stages to the point at which it appears that it may become a marketable product, a trade name is developed by the manufacturer. Properly registered trade names become the legal property of their owners, are protected by copyright laws, and cannot be used freely in the public domain. These two types of names do not fulfill the need for a single, simple, informative designation available for unrestricted public use. The nonproprietary name is the only name intended to function in this capacity. The nonproprietary name often is referred to as the generic name. A generic name is the official name of the drug. This name is much simpler than the chemical name, and it is not protected by copyright. The use of generic names is encouraged over use of trade names to avoid confusion.

DRUG SOURCES

There are basically five sources of drugs: plant, animal (including humans), mineral or mineral products, synthetic (chemical substances), and engineered (investigational drugs). Today, chemicals and even human tissues such as those used in stem-cell therapy can be manipulated to create new drug sources.

Plant Sources

Plant sources are grouped by their physical and chemical properties. Alkaloids are organic compounds combined with acids to make a salt. Nicotine, morphine sulfate, and atropine sulfate are examples of these chemical compounds. An important cardiac glycoside is digoxin. Digoxin is made from digitalis, a derivative of the foxglove plant.

Animal Sources

Animal sources, such as the body fluids and glands of animals, can act as drugs. The drugs obtained from animal sources include enzymes such as pancreatin and pepsin. Hormones such as thyroid and insulin are also from animal sources.

Mineral Sources

Minerals from the earth and soil are used to provide inorganic materials unavailable from plants and animals. They are used as they occur in nature. Examples include iron, potassium, silver, and gold, which are used to prepare medications. Sodium chloride (table salt) is one of the best-known examples in this category. Gold is used to prevent severe rheumatoid arthritis, and coal tar is used to treat seborrheic dermatitis and psoriasis.

Synthetic Sources

New drugs may come from living organisms (organic substances) or nonliving materials (inorganic substances). These drugs are called synthetic or manufactured drugs. They have evolved from the application of chemistry, biology, and computer technology to the creation of new drugs. Because they are not found in nature, these medications come from artificial substances. Common examples of synthetic drugs include meperidine (Demerol®), sulfonamides, and oral contraceptives. Certain organic drugs such as penicillin are semisynthetic and are made by altering their natural compounds or elements. Some drugs are both organic and inorganic, such as propylthiouracil, which is an antithyroid hormone.

Engineered Sources

The newest area of drug origin is gene splicing or genetic engineering. The newer forms of insulin for use in humans have been produced with this technique.

MEDICATION ERRORS

Any incorrect or wrongful administration of a medication may result in serious untoward effects for the patient. Mistakes may be made in prescribing, administering, or dispensing a medication. These errors include the following:

- The wrong patient
- The incorrect route
- The incorrect drug
- The incorrect dose
- The incorrect time
- The incorrect technique
- The incorrect information on the patient's chart

Causes of medication errors may include difficulty in reading handwritten orders, confusion about different drugs with similar names, differences between pharmaceutical and generic names, or lack of information about a patient's drug allergies or sensitivities.

A medication error must be reported as soon as it is noticed, and the patient must be monitored to see if any adverse reaction to the medication develops. Medication errors must be documented in the medical record with the signature of the person who made the error. If the pharmacy technician or nurse follows the Seven Rights of Medication Administration and dispensing guidelines, medication errors should not occur (see Figure 5-1).

- *Right Patient:* Always verify that you have the right patient. Ask the patient to tell you his or her name, and check the patient's identification band if available, especially if the patient's mental status is decreased.
- *Right Drug:* Be sure that the correct drug has been selected before you administer the drug. The label should be checked three times: when the medication is taken from the drawer or cabinet, when the medication is removed from the bottle, and when the medication is returned to storage. Make sure generic names and pharmaceutical names are for same medication.
- *Right Dose:* Be sure that the patient receives the right dose. Giving less medication may be ineffective; giving too much may result in harm to the patient.
- *Right Time:* Give medications to the patient at the proper time. Ensure that directions, such as before or after meals, with milk, etc., are adhered to.
- *Right Route:* Follow the manufacturer's instructions when administering the medication to ensure that it will have the desired effect. The effectiveness of the drugs depends on the correct route of administration.
- *Right Technique:* Always use the proper administration technique.
- *Right Documentation:* After a medication is given, document it immediately in the patient's medical record. The following information must be included: date, time given, name of the medication, administration route, dosage of medication, and patient reaction.

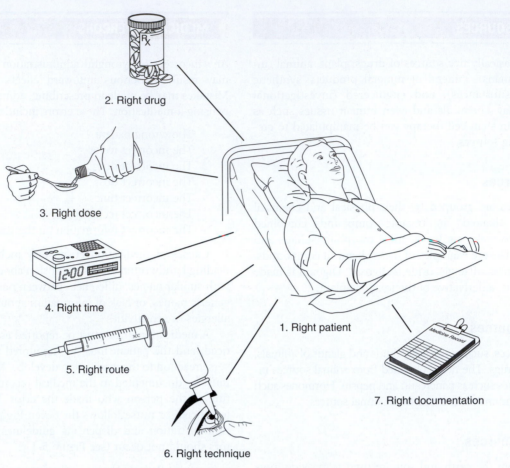

2. Right drug

3. Right dose

4. Right time

1. Right patient

5. Right route

7. Right documentation

6. Right technique

Figure 5-1. The Seven Rights of Medication Administration.

The signature of the person who gave the medication must accompany the documentation.

Unfortunately, mistakes and errors may occasionally be made. When the pharmacy technician or the nurse has doubts, administration of a drug should be delayed until specifically authorized by the prescriber.

DOSAGE FORMS OF DRUGS

Pharmaceutical principles are the underlying physiochemical principles that allow a drug to be incorporated in a pharmaceutical dosage form such as tablets and solutions. These principles apply whether the drug is extemporaneously compounded by the pharmacist or manufactured for commercial distribution as a drug product. Drug dosage forms are classified according to their physical state and chemical composition. They may include gases, liquids, solids, and semisolids. Some substances can undergo a change of state or phase, from solid to liquid states (melting) or from liquid to gaseous states (vaporization). Certain drugs are soluble in water, some are soluble in alcohol, and others are soluble in a mixture of liquids.

Solid Drugs

The route for administering a medication depends on its form, its properties, and the effects desired. Intermolecular forces of attraction are stronger in solids than in liquids or in gases. Solid drugs include tablets, pills, plasters, capsules, caplets, gelcaps, powder, granules, troches, or lozenges (see Figure 5-2).

Tablet

A **tablet** is a pharmaceutical preparation made by compressing the powered form of a drug and bulk filling material under high pressure (see Figure 5-2). Special forms of tablets include sublingual tablets and enteric-coated tablets. Most tablets are intended to be swallowed whole for dissolution and absorption from the gastrointestinal tract. Some are intended to be dissolved in the mouth, dissolved in water, or inserted as suppositories. Many times tablets are mistakenly called pills. Tablets come in various sizes, shapes, colors, and composition. The various forms of tablets include chewable, sublingual, buccal, enteric-coated, and buffered tablets. Chewable tablets must be chewed. They contain a flavored or sugar base. Chewable tablets are commonly used for antacids and antiflatulents and for children who cannot swallow med-

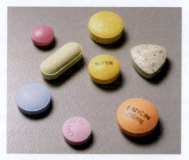

A. Tablets

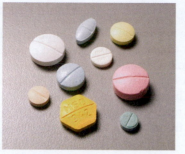

B. Scored tablets

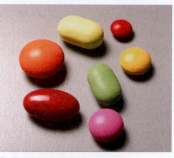

C. Enteric-coated tablets

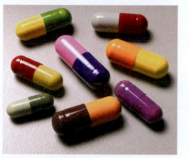

D. Capsules

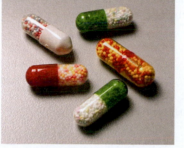

E. Controlled release capsules

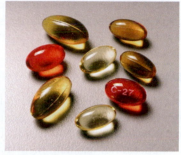

F. Gelatin capsules

Figure 5-2. Solid dosage forms.

ication. Sublingual tablets must be dissolved under the tongue for rapid absorption. An example is nitroglycerin for angina pectoris. Buccal tablets are placed between the cheek and the gum until they are dissolved and absorbed. A **enteric-coated tablet** has a special coating to protect against stomach acid, allowing the drug to dissolve in the alkaline environment of the intestines. A **buffered tablet** can prevent ulceration or severe irritation of the stomach wall. Antacids have been added to reduce irritation to the stomach by the active ingredients. Some tablets are coated with a volatile liquid that is meant to dissolve in the mouth, such as antacid tablets.

Pill

A single-dose unit of medicine made by mixing the powdered drug with a liquid such as syrup and rolling it into a round or oval shape is called a **pill**.

Plaster

Any composition of a liquid and a powder that hardens when it dries is called a **plaster**. Plasters may be solid or semisolid. An example is the salicylic acid plaster used to remove corns.

Capsule

A **capsule** is a medication dosage form in which the drug is contained in an external shell (see Figure 5-2). Capsule shells are usually made of hard cylindrical gelatin and enclose or encapsulate powder, granules, liquids, or some combinations of these. Liquids may be placed in soft gelatin capsules, such as vitamin E capsules and cod liver oil capsules. They are

used when medications have an unpleasant odor or taste. Capsules can be pulled apart, and the entire contents can be added as powder to food for individuals who have difficulty swallowing. Some forms of capsules come with a controlled-release dosage and are used over a defined period of time. These are called **sustained-release (SR)** or timed-release capsules. These drugs should never be crushed or dissolved, because this would negate their timed-release action.

Caplet

A **caplet** is shaped like a capsule but has the form of a tablet. The shape and film-coated covering make swallowing easier.

Gelcap

A **gelcap** is an oil-based medication that is enclosed in a soft gelatin capsule (see Figure 5-2).

Powder

A drug that is dried and ground into fine particles is called a **powder**. An example is potassium chloride powder (Kato powder).

Granule

A small pill, usually accompanied by many others encased within a gelatin capsule is called a **granule**. In most cases, granules within capsules are specially coated to gradually release medication over a period of up to 12 hours (see Figure 5-2).

Troche or Lozenge

A hard or semisolid dosage form containing a medication intended for local application in the mouth or throat is called a **troche** or **lozenge**. These are flattened disks. Typically, a troche is placed on the tongue or between the cheek and gum and left in place until it dissolves. The medications most commonly administered by means of troches include cough suppressants and treatments for sore throat.

Semisolid Drugs

Semisolid drugs are often used as topical applications. These drugs are soft and pliable. Semisolid drugs include suppositories, ointments, and gels.

Suppository

A bullet-shaped dosage form intended to be inserted into a body orifice is called a **suppository**. Suppositories contain medication usually intended for a local effect at the site of insertion. Suppositories maintain their shape at room temperature but melt or dissolve when inserted. The most common sites of administration for suppositories are the rectum, vagina, and urethra.

Ointment

An **ointment** is a semisolid, greasy medication intended for external application, usually by rubbing (see Figure 5-3). Medications that may be administered in ointment form include anti-inflammatory drugs, topical anesthetics, and antibiotics. Examples are zinc oxide ointment and Ben-Gay® ointment.

Cream

A **cream** is a semisolid preparation that is usually white and nongreasy and has a water base. It is applied externally to the skin or administered via an applicator intravaginally.

Gel

A **gel** is a jelly-like substance that may be used for topical medication. Some gels have a high alcohol content and can cause stinging if applied to broken skin.

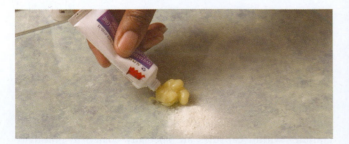

Figure 5-3. Semisolid dosage forms.

Liquid Drugs

Liquid preparations include drugs that have been dissolved or suspended. Examples of liquid drugs are syrups, spirits, elixirs, tinctures, fluidextracts, liniments, emulsions, solutions, mixtures, suspensions, aromatic waters, sprays, and aerosols. They are also classified by site or route of administration such as local (topical) on or through the skin, through the mouth, through the eye (ophthalmic), through the ear (otic), or through the rectum, urethra, or vagina. Liquid drugs may also be administered systemically by mouth or by injection throughout the body (see Figure 5-4).

Syrup

A drug dosage form that consists of a high concentration of a sugar in water is called a **syrup**. It may or may not have medicinal substances added (e.g., simple syrup and ipecac syrup).

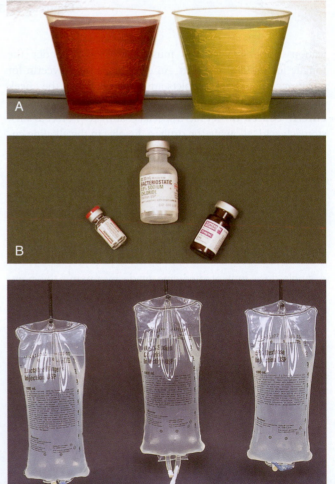

Figure 5-4. Liquid dosage forms.

Solution

A **solution** is a drug or drugs dissolved in an appropriate solvent. An example of a solution is normal saline.

Spirit

An alcohol-containing liquid that may be used pharmaceutically as a solvent is called a **spirit**. It is also known as an essence (e.g., essence of peppermint and camphor spirit).

Elixir

A drug vehicle that consists of water, alcohol, and sugar is known as an **elixir**. It may or may not be aromatic and may or may not have active medicinal properties. Their alcohol content makes elixirs convenient liquid dosage forms for many drugs that are only slightly soluble in water. In these cases, the drug is first dissolved in alcohol, and the other elixir components are added. All elixirs contain alcohol (e.g., terpin hydrate elixir and phenobarbital elixir). Elixirs differ from tinctures in that they are sweetened. They should be used with caution in patients with diabetes or a history of alcohol abuse. Some pediatric medications retain the name of elixir, although they no longer contain alcohol.

Tincture

A **tincture** is an alcoholic preparation of a soluble drug, usually from a plant source. In some cases, the solution may also contain water (e.g., iodine, tincture, and digitalis tincture).

Fluidextract

A concentrated solution of a drug removed from a plant source by mixing ground parts of the plant with a suitable solvent, usually alcohol, and then separating the plant residue from the solvent is called a **fluidextract**. Typically, 1 ml (1 cc) contains 1 g of the drug. Fluidextracts are not intended to be administered directly to a patient. Instead, they are used to provide a source of drug in the manufacture of final dosage forms. Only vegetable drugs are used (e.g., glycyrrhiza fluidextract).

Liniment

A **liniment** is a mixture of drugs with oil, soap, water, or alcohol, intended for external application with rubbing. Most liniments are counterirritants intended to treat muscle or joint pain (e.g., camphor liniment and chloroform liniment).

Emulsion

A pharmaceutical preparation in which two agents that cannot ordinarily be combined are mixed is called an **emulsion**. In the typical emulsion oil is dispersed inside water. Most creams and lotions are emulsions (e.g., Petrogalar Plain®).

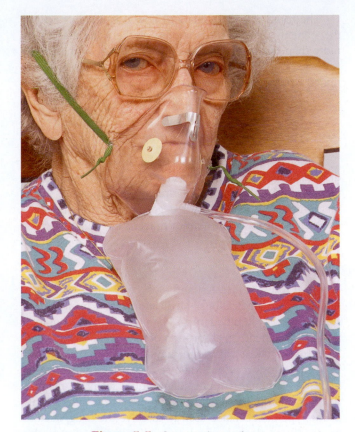

Figure 5-5. Gaseous dosage forms.

Mixture and Suspension

In a **mixture** or a **suspension** an agent is mixed with a liquid but not dissolved. These preparations must be shaken before being taken by the patient. An example is milk of magnesia.

Aromatic Water

In pharmacy, a mixture of distilled water with an aromatic volatile oil is called an **aromatic water**. Aromatic waters may be used for medicinal purposes (e.g., peppermint water and camphor water).

Gaseous Drugs

Pharmaceutical gases include the anesthetic gases such as nitrous oxide and halothane. Compressed gases include oxygen for therapy (see Figure 5-5) or carbon dioxide.

PRINCIPLES OF DRUG ADMINISTRATION

The chosen route of drug administration determines the rate and intensity of the drug's effect. A drug prepared for one route but administered by another route may not have any effect at all and is potentially dangerous. Each route requires different dosage forms.

The route of a drug refers to how it is administered to the patient. Certain medications can be administered by more than one route, whereas others must be administered via a specific route. The route of administration is determined by a number of factors:

- The action of medication on the body
- The physical and emotional state of the patient
- The characteristics of the drug

Other factors, such as age (pediatric and geriatric), the disease being treated, and the absorption, distribution, metabolism, and elimination of drugs, are important. Three methods of administration are generally used: oral, parenteral, and topical (the skin or mucous membranes).

Oral Route

The **oral** route is the safest and most convenient route chosen for most medications. Medication taken by mouth is solid (tablet) or liquid (syrup). The presence or lack of food in the stomach affects absorption of many oral medications. Some drugs taken with food may have a slow absorption rate. Oral drugs may be swallowed or may be taken by the buccal or sublingual route. Many liquid forms of medications can also be taken by the oral route. These differ mainly in the type of substance used to dissolve the drug, such as water, oil, or alcohol, which were discussed earlier in this chapter. Generally, oral medications should be taken with enough water to send the drug to the stomach. Liquid medications are ideal for children. Solid drugs should not be given to children until they are old enough to safely swallow them without the danger of aspiration. Oral syringes are an ideal way to administer liquid medications to children (see Figure 5-6). Liquid medications that may stain the teeth can be taken through a straw. If the patient has been vomiting or is nauseated, an alternative route of administration might be necessary.

Basic Equipment Needed for Oral Administration

Three measuring devices are used in the administration of oral medications:

The medicine or water cup
The medicine dropper/oral syringe
The calibrated spoon

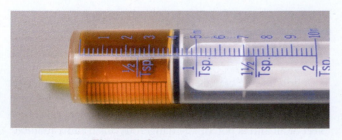

Figure 5-6. Liquid oral syringe.

The medicine cup may be calibrated in fluid ounces, fluidrams, cubic centimeters (cc), milliliters (ml), teaspoons, or tablespoons. The medicine dropper may be calibrated in milliliters, minims, or drops (see Figure 5-7). Calibrated spoons are usually marked up with $\frac{1}{4}$ teaspoon and 1 cc measurements, up to two teaspoons (10 cc). Syringes are usually marked up with $\frac{1}{2}$ cc increments.

Sublingual Route

Drugs given via the **sublingual** route are held under the tongue until completely dissolved (see Figure 5-8). This method is used when rapid action is desired; for example, ergotamine tartrate (Ergostat®) for migraines and nitroglycerin for angina pectoris can be administered by the sublingual route.

Buccal Route

For administration of drugs via the **buccal** route, the medication is placed between the gum and cheek, and left there until it is dissolved (see Figure 5-9). Oxytocin, used for inducing labor, may be administered by the buccal route, but it is not often administered this way.

Parenteral Route

Administration of drugs other than through the digestive system is called **parenteral**; thus, a medication bypasses the gastrointestinal tract, such as with drugs given by injection. Medications are injected into the tissues of the body with a syringe and a needle for rapid effect and absorption. There are four main categories for parenteral administration according to the site of the injection. Drugs may be injected into muscles, veins, skin (intradermal or subcutaneous), and the spinal column.

Basic Equipment Needed for Parenteral Medication Administration

Two types of needles are available (disposable and nondisposable) for giving medications via the parenteral route. The most commonly used are the disposable needles. Gauge (G) of a needle is determined by the diameter of the lumen or opening at its beveled tip. Needle gauges range in size from 16 to 30 G, and needle lengths vary from $\frac{3}{8}$ inch to 2 inches. The larger the gauge is, the smaller is the diameter of its lumen. Various sizes and types of needles are shown in Figure 5-10.

Needles consist of four parts: the needle, the needle cover, the hub, and the syringe (see Figure 5-11).

Syringes

Both disposable and nondisposable syringes are available. Disposable syringes are sterilized, prepackaged, nontoxic,

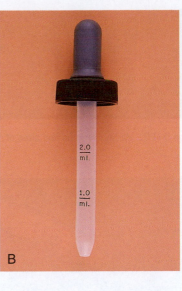

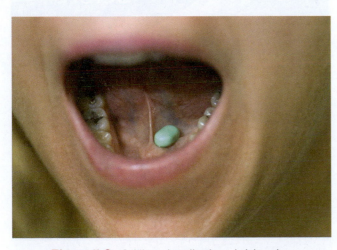

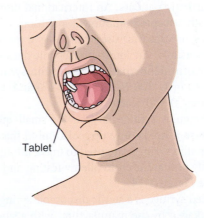

Figure 5-7. Tools to administer liquid dosages.

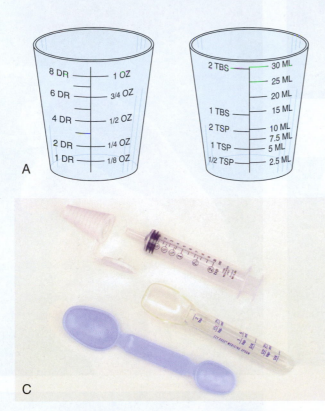

Figure 5-8. Sublingual medication administration.

Figure 5-9. Buccal medication administration.

nonpyrogenic, and ready for use. The size of the syringes varies from ½ to 50 cc. The 1-, 3-, and 5-cc syringes are the ones most commonly used.

A disposable syringe and needle unit consists of a syringe with an attached needle. Syringes are named according to their sizes and uses. In general there are two types of syringes: hypodermic and prefilled.

Hypodermic syringes are available in sizes of 3, 5, 10, 20, and 60 cc. These are typically used for intramuscular or subcutaneous injections. They are also used for venipuncture, medical, surgical treatment, aspiration, irrigations, and **gavage** (tube-to-stomach) feedings. There are several types of hypodermic syringes, which include needleless, insulin, and tuberculin. Another type of syringe, called the injector pen, is used most commonly for insulin administration.

Retractable needle cover syringes are used for prevention of needle sticks, as required by Occupational Health and Safety Administration (OSHA) standards. These syringes

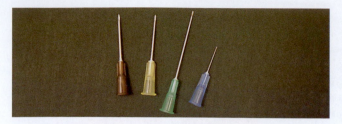

Figure 5-10. Various lengths and sizes of needles.

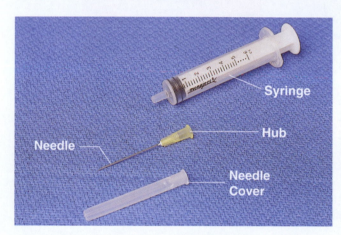

Figure 5-11. Parts of a syringe.

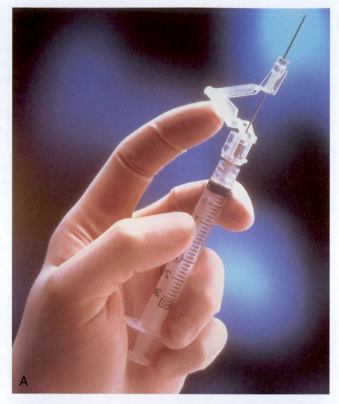

A

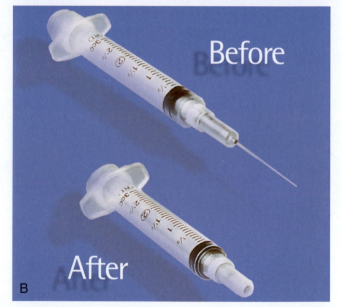

B

Figure 5-12. Safety syringes. (A. Courtesy of Becton Dickinson. B. Courtesy of Retractable Technologies.)

come with retractable needle covers to prevent needle sticks from contaminated syringes (see Figure 5-12).

The insulin syringe is calibrated in units (U) specifically for use of diabetic patients. An international unit (IU) is an internationally accepted amount of a substance (for example, vitamins or vaccines) used simply as a means of standardizing measures. An international unit does not have a specific, uniform definition of size. Insulin syringes are labeled as U-40 or U-100 (see Figure 5-13) and come in the following sizes: 0.3, 0.5, and 1.0 cc.

The tuberculin syringe is used for small quantities of drugs, because it holds only up to 1.0 ml of injectable material. Tuberculin syringes are used to inject minute amounts intradermally and are used in allergy testing and allergy injections (see Figure 5-14).

A prefilled syringe is a sterile disposable syringe and needle unit packaged by the manufacturer with a single dose of medication inside and ready to administer (see Figure 5-15). These syringes are meant for one-time use only and should be properly disposed of after medication administration.

Medication Containers

Medications prescribed for injection are available in different containers such as ampules, vials, and sterile cartridges with premeasured medication.

An **ampule** is a small, hermetically sealed glass container that usually holds a single dose of medication (see Figure

5-16B). Ampules have a neck with a scored weak point that is broken just before use. A **vial** is a small bottle with a rubber stopper, through which a sterile needle is inserted to withdraw a dose of the medication inside. There are two types of vials: single and multiple dose. A multiple-dose vial may contain varying numbered doses of a drug. Vials vary in size from 2 ml to 100 or more doses (see Figure 5-16A).

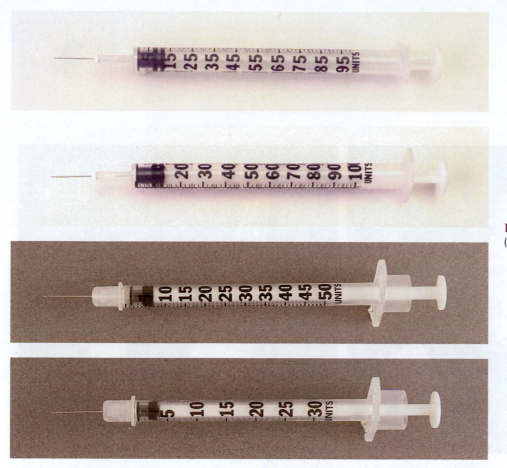

Figure 5-13. Insulin syringes. (Courtesy of Becton Dickinson.)

Because multidose vials are used more than once, extreme caution must be taken every time a needle is inserted into the medication to protect it from contamination, which could cause serious infections in future patients. If at any time the technician thinks that an error has been made or suspects possible contamination, the vial should be discarded. Unused medication should never be returned to the vial.

Parenteral Medication Forms

Parenteral forms of medication can be selected when a rapid response time to medication is desired or if the patient is not able to take the medication orally. Injectable drug forms may be available as a solution or a powder. A solution is a mixture of one or more substances dissolved in another substance. A solution is usually a fluid to form a homogeneous mixture.

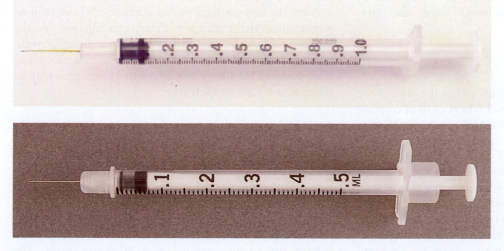

Figure 5-14. Tuberculin syringe. (Courtesy of Becton Dickinson.)

Figure 5-15. Prefilled, single-dose syringe. (Courtesy of Roche Laboratories, Inc.)

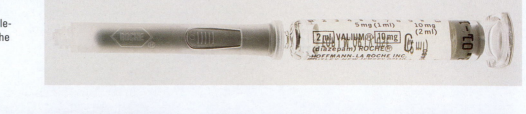

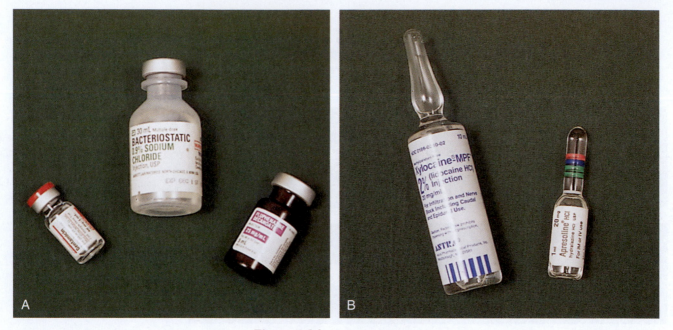

A

B

Figure 5-16. Vials and ampules.

A powder consists of dry particles of medications. The powder itself cannot be injected. It must be reconstituted to a liquid for injection. A diluent such as sterile water is added to the powder and mixed well.

Parenteral Administration Routes

Parenteral medication can be administered via different routes such as intravenous, intramuscular, subcutaneous, intradermal, epidural or subarachnoid space, and intra-articular.

Intradermal Injection

An **intradermal injection** is given within the skin. If the injection is given correctly, a small **wheal** (a skin eruption that may follow injection of an antigen) occurs on the skin. A ³/₈-inch, 27- or 28-G needle is used for intradermal injections. The angle of insertion is 15 degrees, almost parallel to the skin surface (Figure 5-17). The common site of injection is the center of the forearm. The other sites that may be used are the upper chest and back areas. Skin tests for allergies and tuberculin tests are the most common uses for intradermal injections. One method of tuberculin screening is the tine test, which is administered with individually packaged disposable sterile stamps with four or six prongs on the end that have been treated with tuberculin solution. The tine test is not as accurate as the Mantoux (purified protein derivative [PPD]) intradermal screening test. With the Mantoux test, a 0.1-ml solution of PPD is injected into the intradermal layers. The site is then monitored after 48 to 72 hours. The result is considered positive if the **induration** is more than 10 mm in diameter. Allergy skin testing involves intradermally injecting a small amount of antigen and later examining the test site for a visible reaction. This test is more accurate than the scratch test. Extracts are injected into the intradermal layer of the skin, with the usual sterile technique, in a dose of 0.1 to 0.2 ml. When intradermal injections are used for allergy testing, 10 to 15 allergens may be tested at one time on each arm.

Subcutaneous Injections

A **subcutaneous injection** is given just below the skin and the layer of fatty tissue called adipose tissue. The most common sites for subcutaneous injections are the deltoid area, anterior thigh, abdomen, and upper back. The angle of insertion is 45 degrees for local anesthetics, allergy treatments, and epinephrine (see Figure 5-18); however, insulin and heparin are usually injected at a 90-degree angle. The

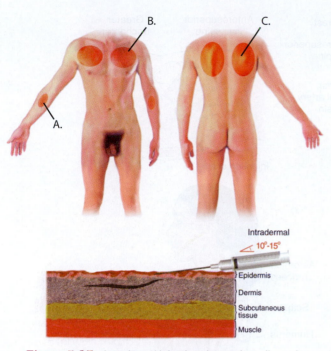

Figure 5-17. Intradermal injection sites and needle angle.

amount of drug administered through the subcutaneous route should not be more than 2 ml.

Intramuscular Injection

A drug is injected into a muscle (**intramuscular injection**) for the following reasons: the drug will irritate the skin tissues, a more rapid absorption is desired, and the volume of the medication to be injected is large. The preferred sites are the gluteus, deltoid, and vastus lateralis muscles of the adult. The vastus lateralis is part of the quadriceps muscle in the thigh and is also considered the safest site of administration for infants (see Figure 5-19). The angle of insertion is 90 degrees. The deltoid site is acceptable for adults and older children. Muscles can absorb a greater amount of fluid than is usually given by subcutaneous administration. Dosage may vary from 0.5 to 5 ml. In adults, up to 2 ml of medication can be injected into the deltoid muscle, whereas up to 5 ml can be injected into the vastus lateralis and gluteal sites. Infants and children should be given no more than 2 ml in the vastus lateralis or ventrogluteal sites. The needle should be 1 to 3 inches in length or sometimes can be longer, especially for obese patients. The recommended gauge of the needle ranges from 20 to 23.

Some drugs injected intramuscularly are irritating to skin tissue. Therefore, the injection must be given in a way to prevent any leakage back from the deep muscle into the upper subcutaneous layers. For these, the **Z-track method**, which displaces the upper tissue laterally before the needle is inserted, is used (see Figure 5-20). The sites of injections for many medications that require administration with the Z-track method should not be massaged after injection, because massaging will encourage the spread of the medication.

Intravenous Injection

Intravenous injection is used during emergency situations, when immediate effects are required, or when drugs or fluids are being administered by infusion. Sometimes large doses of medication must be given, either every few hours or over a long period of time. The rate of absorption and the onset of action by medication administered intravenously are faster. Needles for intravenous injections are generally inserted into the smallest veins and as close to the hands as possible (see Figure 5-21). The metacarpal, dorsal, basilic, and cephalic veins are commonly used in adults. Veins commonly used in infants and children include the scalp vein in the temporal area and veins in the dorsum of the foot and the back of the hand. Peripheral veins used in adults include the back of the hand, arm and forearm, and dorsal plexus of the foot. If an intravenous infusion is required for more than 2 to 3 days, a cardiovascular catheter is required.

Pump Systems

Medication can be administered via a pump to provide a continuous flow into the patient's system. Pumps are electronic

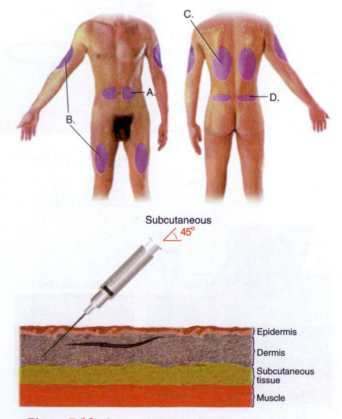

Figure 5-18. Subcutaneous injection sites and needle angle.

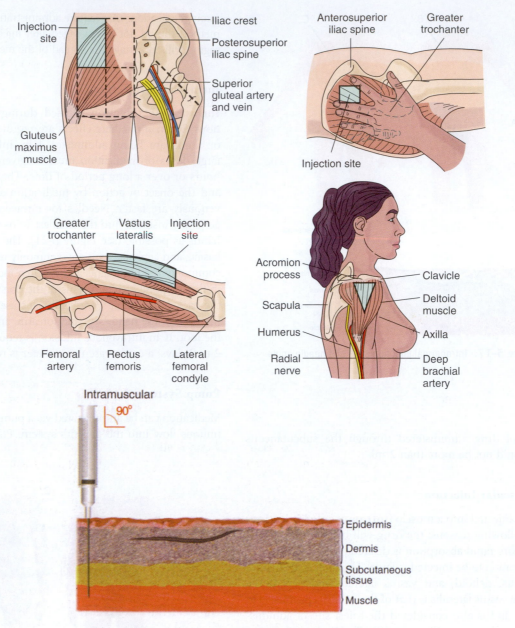

Intramuscular

Figure 5-19. Intramuscular injection sites and needle angle.

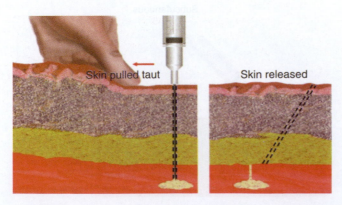

Figure 5-20. Z-track method of intramuscular injection.

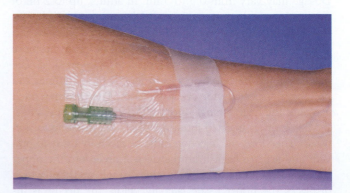

Figure 5-21. Intravenous injection.

devices that force a precisely measured amount of intravenous fluid into a patient's vein over a predetermined amount of time. The pump is a very popular way of administering a constant dose of insulin to a diabetic patient. Infusion pumps are used for administration of most intravenous medications in institutional and home settings. These devices create a positive pressure of 10 to 25 pounds per square inch. They offer more accurately controlled rates of infusion than other devices. The infusion pumps flow at 999 ml/hr, providing a higher rate of infusion and higher pressure.

Urethral Route

A solution is instilled into the urinary bladder using a catheter.

Topical Route

Topical medications are applied to the surface of the body. The effects of topically administered drugs are usually local. The vast majority of drugs applied to the skin are not designed to produce systemic effects. For instance, topical anesthesia is the application to the skin of a drug that temporarily deadens nerve sensations. Skin medication forms include lotions, liniments, ointments, and transdermal patches. Lotions are often used to control itching. Calamine lotion is an example. Some lotions are used to relieve congestion and pain in muscles and joints. After applying the lotion, the area may be covered with a thick cloth to retain heat. Liniments (emulsions) have a higher portion of oil than do lotions. They are often used to protect dried, cracked, or fissured skin. Ointments are applied to dry, scaly areas with little or no hair and can exert a prolonged effect.

Transdermal Patches

Certain medications can be absorbed slowly through the skin to create a constant, time-released systemic effect. For example, transdermal patches are dosage forms that release minute amounts of drug at a consistent rate (see Figure 5-22). As the drug is released from the patch, it is absorbed into the skin and carried off by the capillary blood supply. Examples of drugs administered transdermally include nitroglycerin, estrogen, testosterone, nicotine, and scopolamine.

Mucous Membrane Routes

Some mucous membranes are selected for their ability to absorb medication for a local or systemic effect. The most commonly used methods are buccal, sublingual, rectal, and respiratory for a systemic effect. Other routes, such as ophthalmic, otic, nasal, vaginal, or urethral, are used for their local effects. The systemic effects of the sublingual and buccal routes are discussed earlier in this chapter.

Inhalation Administration

The act of drawing breath, vapor, or gas into the lungs is called inhalation. Inhalation therapy may involve the administration of medicines, water vapor, and gases such as oxygen, carbon dioxide, and helium. The medication is inhaled to achieve local effects within the respiratory tract through aerosols (see Figure 5-23), nebulizers, Spinhalers, or metered-dose inhalers. Medications that are administered through inhalers include bronchodilators, mucolytic agents, and steroids.

Oxygen is another medication that is administered by the inhalation route. When oxygen is to be administered, the dosage is based on individual needs. Oxygen is a drug; it needs to be prescribed according to the flow rate, concentration, method of delivery, and length of time for administration. Oxygen is ordered as liters per minute (LPM) and as percentage of oxygen concentration (%). Oxygen toxicity may develop when 100% oxygen is breathed for a prolonged period. A high concentration of inhaled oxygen causes alveolar collapse, intra-alveolar hemorrhage, hyaline membrane formation, and disturbance of the central nervous system and retrolental fibroplasias in newborns. There are several ways to use oxygen. The most commonly prescribed methods are the use of nasal cannulas and masks.

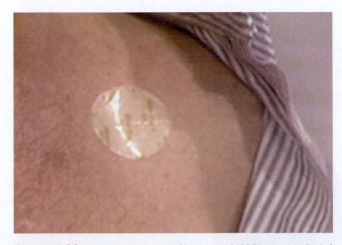

Figure 5-22. Transdermal patch. (Courtesy of 3M Pharmaceuticals.)

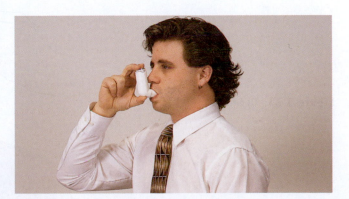

Figure 5-23. Inhaler.

Spray and Aerosol

A liquid or fine powder that is sprayed in a fine mist is called an aerosol. The most commonly used aerosols are respiratory treatments for asthma and the skin sprays. Although most aerosolized medicines are liquids, some are powders whose particles are small enough to pass through the spray apparatus.

Ophthalmic Administration

Drops and ointments instilled into the eye are generally absorbed slowly and affect only the area in contact. The medications are placed between the eyeball and the lower lid (see Figure 5-24). Ophthalmic preparations must be sterile to prevent eye infections and should be isotonic to minimize burning. Medications in ophthalmic preparations include antibiotics, antivirals, decongestants, artificial tears, and topical anesthetics.

Otic Route

Localized infection or inflammation of the ear is treated by dropping a small amount of a sterile medicated solution into the ear. Very low dosages of medication are required, and the manufacturer must indicate that the medication is meant for otic usage. In children younger than 3 years of age, gently pull the earlobe down and back; in adults, gently pull the earlobe up and out (see Figure 5-25). The patient must remain on that side for 5 minutes to allow the medication to coat the surface of the inner ear canal. The use of ear drops is usually contraindicated if the patient has a perforated eardrum.

Nasal Route

Nasal solutions act locally to treat minor congestion or infection. The medication should be drawn up in the dropper and held just over one nostril, and then the required number of nose drops should be administered (see Figure 5-26). If a nasal spray is used, the patient sits upright, one nostril is blocked, and the tip of the nasal spray is inserted into the nostril. As the patient takes a deep breath, a puff of spray is squeezed into the opposite nostril.

Nasal decongestant sprays are often misused by patients. Nasal medications are commonly used for blocked nasal passages (decongestants) and nosebleeds (hemostatics).

Vaginal Route

Vaginal suppositories, tablets, creams, and fluid solutions are used to treat local infections. Medications are deposited into the vagina. Douches may be used as anti-infectives. Local contraceptives are available as creams and foams. Vaginal instillation is most effective if the patient is lying down. Creams are instilled with applicators.

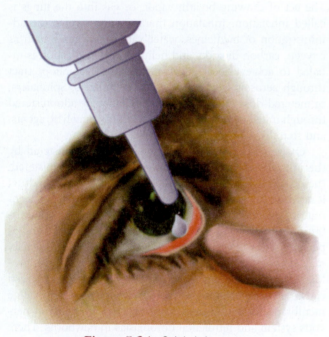

Figure 5-24. Ophthalmic route.

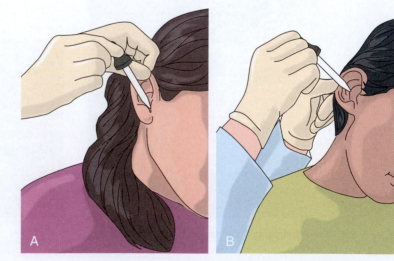

Figure 5-25. Otic route.

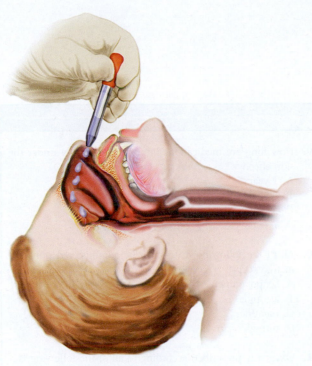

Figure 5-26. Nasal route.

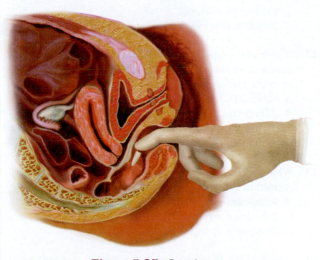

Figure 5-27. Rectal route.

Rectal Route

Rectal medications are useful if the patient is nauseated, vomiting, or unconscious. Manufacturers supply rectal medications in the form of gelatin or cocoa butter-based suppositories, which melt in the warmth of the rectum and release the medication, or in the form of enemas as a solution (see Figure 5-27). Suppositories may be used to soften the stool or stimulate evacuation of the bowel. The best time to administer a rectal drug intended for a systemic effect is after a bowel movement or enema. An enema is the means of delivering a solution or medication into the rectum and colon. An enema is used to cleanse the lower bowel in preparation for radiography, proctoscopy, sigmoidoscopy,

and surgery. A Fleet Ready-To-Use Enema promotes bowel evacuation by softening the feces and stimulating peristalsis. The Fleet Ready-To-Use Enema does not cause burning, irritation, or dehydration and does not interfere with the absorption of vitamins or the actions of drugs.

Implants

Insertion of medication by surgery under the skin is accomplished via implants. Female contraception involves surgically inserting hormone-containing rods (e.g., Norplant) beneath the skin of the forearm. Once implanted the medication slowly and consistently releases enough hormones to prevent conception. The rods may be removed if the woman wants to reestablish fertility. If left in place, implants may be effective for up to 5 years.

SUMMARY

Administering a dose of a drug is one of the most important tasks in medicine. The safe administration of drugs requires knowledge of the drug being given and the proper route of administration, following the Seven Rights of Medication Administration. When medication errors occur, the person administering the medication must report and document the error. Drugs may be administered by oral, parenteral, topical, and other routes. Oral administration of drugs is the easiest, safest, and most commonly used route. The medication is placed in the mouth and swallowed into the stomach for absorption in the gastrointestinal tract. Medication may be administered rectally by either suppository or enema. Parenteral administration of medications requires special processes that must be carried out while sterile technique is maintained. Injections may be given into the dermis of the skin, into the subcutaneous tissue, into the muscles, or into the veins. Administering an intravenous injection is an advanced skill, and each route of administration requires special expertise to be sure that the medication reaches the desired location. Syringes come in nondisposable and disposable types of various sizes. Parenteral medications come in vials, ampules, and prefilled syringes. Topical medication administration results in absorption of the drug through the skin or mucous membranes. Topical medications are used for local effects. Some drugs are absorbed through mucous membranes via the eyes, ears, nose, vagina, and respiratory tract.

CRITICAL THINKING

1. Why is it important to administer a medication via the proper route? Please explain your answer. Choose one route of administration and research a drug that needs to be administered using this route.
2. What is the most common reason for medication administration errors? Explain how this error can be prevented.

Explain what procedures need to be followed if an error in medication administration occurs.

3. How does the form of the drug affect the method through which it is administered? Choose a dosage form and explain why it is administered in a particular way.

REVIEW QUESTIONS

1. Needle gauges are determined by which of the following?
   A. The size of the shaft
   B. The diameter of the lumen
   C. The length of the hilt
   D. The size of the syringe

2. The angle of insertion for intradermal injections is which of the following degrees?
   A. 90
   B. 45
   C. 30
   D. 15

3. Which of the following is an important cardiac glycoside?
   A. Nicotine
   B. Digoxin
   C. Morphine sulfate
   D. Atropine sulfate

4. Tablets are mistakenly called
   A. pills.
   B. powders.
   C. buffered.
   D. gelcaps.

5. Which of the following is an example of semisolid drugs?
   A. Caplets
   B. Gelcaps
   C. Gels
   D. Granules

6. The best time to administer a rectal drug intended for a systemic effect is
   A. early morning.
   B. after dinner.
   C. after a bowel movement.
   D. bedtime.

7. Which of the following needles are used for prevention of needle sticks and are required by OSHA standards?
   A. Hypodermic
   B. Retractable needle cover
   C. Insulin
   D. Prefilled

8. A wheal occurs on the skin from which of the following injections?
   A. Intradermal
   B. Intramuscular
   C. Subcutaneous
   D. Z-track

9. How long are medications implanted surgically under the skin effective?
   A. 1 year
   B. 3 years
   C. 5 years
   D. 7 years

10. All of the following drugs may be administered transdermally, except
    A. scopolamine.
    B. atropine.
    C. nicotine.
    D. nitroglycerin.

11. Oxygen is prescribed according to all of the following factors except
    A. flow rate.
    B. age of patient.
    C. method of delivery.
    D. length of time of administration.

12. Which of the following would require an injection of medication at an angle of insertion of 15 degrees, almost parallel to the skin surface?
    A. Tuberculin test
    B. Allergy treatments
    C. Allergy tests
    D. A and C

13. Which of the following syringes are calibrated in units?
    A. Insulin syringes
    B. Needleless syringes
    C. Tuberculin syringes
    D. Disposable syringes

14. Which of the following types of injections is inserted just below the surface of the skin and forms a wheal?
    A. Subcutaneous
    B. Intradermal
    C. Intramuscular
    D. Z-track

15. Which of the following is the route of administration of a drug that is placed between the gums and the cheek?
    A. Transdermal
    B. Sublingual
    C. Buccal
    D. Topical

6

Drug Interaction

OBJECTIVES

Upon completion of this chapter, the reader should be able to

1. Explain drug interaction.
2. List factors that may cause drug interaction.
3. Describe synergism, potentiation, and antagonism.
4. Describe the relationship between drug abuse and drug interaction.
5. Explain cytochrome P-450.
6. Describe the role of alcohol consumption in drug interaction.
7. List factors that may reduce the risk of drug interaction.
8. Explain the importance of patient education.
9. Describe how drug interaction may be prevented.

GLOSSARY

antagonism When two drugs act to decrease the effects of each other.

cytochrome P-450 A system of enzymes that contributes to drug interactions.

drug interaction An interference of a drug with the effect of another drug, nutrient, or laboratory test.

potentiation One drug prolongs the effects of another drug.

synergism The cooperative effect of two or more drugs given together to produce a stronger effect than that of either drug given alone.

OVERVIEW

Many patients are treated with two or more drugs that may interact to alter the effects of each. Some drug-related problems develop unexpectedly and cannot be predicted. On the other hand, many drugs have known pharmacological effects, and specific actions may reasonably be anticipated. Therefore, drug therapy becomes more complicated when more than one drug is being administered. It is essential that complete and current medication records be maintained for patients. It is also important that drug therapy be closely monitored and supervised so that problems can be prevented or detected at an early stage in their development. The pharmacist is in a unique position to meet these needs. Many drug-related problems are caused by drug interaction. Pharmacy technicians must be familiar with this important matter and understand factors that may have an effect on different agents.

MECHANISM OF DRUG INTERACTION

A **drug interaction** is an interference of a drug with the effect of another drug, nutrient, or laboratory test. In addition, a drug interaction is possible if a food interferes with the action of a drug. Drug interaction is usually the result of a patient's receiving more than one drug concurrently. Surgical patients commonly receive more than 10 drugs, and these patients often experience the effects of several drugs at once. Multiple-drug administration is also common for patients hospitalized for infections and other disorders. Furthermore, patients may have more than one unrelated disorder, which means that they need simultaneous treatment with two or more drugs. Drug interactions may occur at any step in the passage of a drug through the body—during its liberation, absorption, distribution, biotransformation, or excretion. Metabolism of medications will be discussed in Chapter 19. To understand the mechanism of drug interaction, discussion of synergism, potentiation, and antagonism is essential.

Synergism

Synergism refers to the cooperative effect of two or more drugs given together to produce a stronger effect than that of either drug given alone. When two drugs with similar actions are taken, the effect of the drugs will be double. Synergism is the working together of two drugs to produce a stronger effect than that expected for each drug when taken alone. Sometimes synergism is desirable, for example, the mixture of meperidine (Demerol®) for pain and promethazine (Phenergan®), which is used as an antiemetic and sedative. Synergism is dangerous when the drug combination produces undesirable effects that can be dangerous to the body. An example is the combination of warfarin sodium (Coumadin®) and aspirin, which causes an excessive risk of hemorrhage because the two together can potentiate blood loss.

Potentiation

Potentiation occurs as one drug prolongs the effects of another drug. An example is the combination of acetaminophen (Tylenol®) and codeine for pain relief or fever reduction. Desirable potentiation is a wanted effect used to build up a drug level in the body or to prolong its effect; for instance, the combination of penicillin and probenecid is given to prolong the excretion time of penicillin in the body. When toxic effects occur from drug potentiation, the potentiation is undesirable. An example is the use of cimetidine (Tagamet®) for a stomach disorder and theophylline to assist in relieving asthma. Cimetidine increases serum levels of theophylline.

Antagonism

Antagonism occurs when two drugs decrease the effects of each other. An example is ibuprofen and aspirin, which, when taken together, stop each other's action. Antagonism may be desirable to stop the effects of a medication. Another example is the use of activated charcoal to stop the effect of syrup of ipecac for a drug overdose or poisoning. Undesirable antagonism is the unwanted cancellation of action of drugs. An example is in the use of tetracycline and antacids together, tetracycline is partially absorbed from the stomach and upper gastrointestinal tract. Therefore antacids can inhibit the gastric absorption of tetracycline.

CAUSES OF DRUG INTERACTION

A number of factors may be associated with drug interaction. These include multiple pharmacological effects, multiple prescribers, nonprescription drug use, patient noncompliance, and drug abuse.

Multiple Pharmacological Effects

Many drugs used currently have the capacity to influence many physiological systems. For example, combined therapy with a phenothiazine antipsychotic (such as chlorpromazine), a tricyclic antidepressant (amitriptyline), and an antiparkinson agent (trihexyphenidyl) is used in some patients. Each of these agents has a different primary effect; however, all three possess anticholinergic activity. Even though the anticholinergic effect of any one of the drugs may be slight, the additive effects of the three agents may be significant.

Multiple Prescribers

Sometimes an individual may see more than one physician or two or more specialists in addition to a family physician. Thus, it is difficult for any one of these physicians to be aware of all the drugs that have been prescribed by the others for this patient. For example, one prescriber may give an antihistamine to a patient and another physician may prescribe an antianxiety agent, with the possible consequence of an excessive depressant effect.

Nonprescription Drug Use

Sometimes patients neglect to mention the nonprescription medications that they have purchased when their physician questions them about medications they are taking. When patients are taking some over-the-counter drugs such as antacids, analgesics, and laxatives for long periods in a routine manner, they do not consider them to be drugs. Therefore, interactions may occur. Many individuals have their prescriptions filled at their local pharmacy but purchase nonprescription drugs elsewhere, thus making identification of potential problems extremely difficult for the pharmacist as well as for the physician. For these reasons, patients should be encouraged to obtain both their prescription and nonprescription medications at a pharmacy.

Patient Noncompliance

For a variety of reasons, many patients do not take medication in the manner intended by the prescriber. Sometimes, those who are taking several medications may be confused because of inadequate instruction. Older patients who may be taking five or six medications can forget to take them. Upon realizing they have forgotten to take a dose of medication, some patients double the next dose to make up for missing one.

Drug Abuse

The tendencies of some individuals to abuse or deliberately misuse drugs also may lead to increased incidence of drug interactions. Opioids, barbiturates, analgesics, and amphetamines are among the agents most often abused, and the inappropriate use of these drugs can result in a number of problems, including an increased potential for drug interaction.

PATIENT VARIABLES THAT AFFECT DRUG INTERACTION

Many factors can influence the response to a drug in humans. These factors may predispose a patient to the development of adverse effects to a drug, and it can be anticipated that many of these considerations also apply to the development of drug interactions. Examples of these factors follow.

Age

Age is always an important factor in the risk of drug interaction. Studies indicate that there is an increased incidence of adverse drug reactions in both young and elderly patients, and, thus, the occurrence of drug interactions also is highest in these patient groups.

Drug-related problems in young patients are encountered most commonly in newborn infants. Newborn infants do not have fully developed enzyme systems. A system of enzymes called **cytochrome P-450** has been identified as the factor that contributes to many drug interactions. Cytochrome P-450 plays a key role in the oxidative biotransformation of drugs. The enzymes are involved in the metabolism of certain drugs. Newborn infants also have immature renal function, which plays a part in drug-related problems.

Most elderly patients have at least one chronic illness, for example, diabetes or hypertension. Renal disorders may also contribute to an altered drug response, and increased sensitivity to the action of certain drugs occurs with advancing age. The factor of age also has a role in the absorption, distribution, metabolism, and excretion of certain drugs, which increases the possibility of adverse drug reactions and drug interactions.

Genetic Factors

Genetic factors may be responsible for the development of an unexpected drug response in some patients. For example, isoniazid is metabolized by an acetylation process, the rate of which appears to be under genetic control. Some patients metabolize isoniazid rapidly, whereas others metabolize it slowly. Isoniazid may cause peripheral neuritis in a number of patients, and this effect has been noted most commonly in slow acetylators (persons whose metabolism of substances derived from the radicals of acetic acid is slow). Isoniazid may inhibit the metabolism of phenytoin, which can result in nystagmus, ataxia, and lethargy.

Diseases and Conditions of Patients

Some diseases may influence patient responses to a particular drug. Impaired renal function and hepatic function are the most important conditions that may alter drug activity and cause drug interactions.

Diet

Food often may affect the rate and extent of absorption of drugs from the gastrointestinal (GI) tract. For example, many antibiotics should be given at least 1 hour before or 2 hours after meals to achieve optimal absorption. The type of food may be important for the absorption of concurrently administered drugs. For example, dietary items such as milk and other dairy products that contain calcium may decrease the absorption of tetracycline and fluoroquinolone derivatives by forming a complex with them in the GI tract that is absorbed poorly. Grapefruit juice has been found to affect many different drugs—specifically those drugs that are metabolized by cytochrome P-450 in the liver and wall of the

GI tract. Based on current data, the following drugs should not be given concurrently with grapefruit juice:

- estrogens
- cyclosporine
- midazolam
- triazolam
- all calcium channel blockers
- simvastatin (Zocor®)

The toxicity of some drugs increases when the drugs interact with foods such as wine, cheese, or yogurt. Any patient taking a monoamine oxidase (MAO) inhibitor (an antidepressant) should avoid these foods because of potential toxic effects. Medications that stimulate the central nervous system may cause a toxic stimulation if caffeine or caffeine-containing foods are also consumed. The combination of potassium-sparing diuretics and salt substitutes can result in dangerously high blood potassium levels. Aluminum-based antacids taken with citrus juices (such as orange juice) result in excess absorption of the aluminum. Vegetables such as broccoli, cabbage, or Brussels sprouts may inactivate anticoagulants such as warfarin sodium, because they contain vitamin K. Table 6-1 shows some examples of the most common food and drug interactions that are considered to be of greatest clinical significance. For more information about common drug and food interactions, refer to the *Physician's Desk Reference* and other reference books.

TABLE 6-1. Clinically Significant Drug and/or Food Interactions

DRUGS	INTERACTING DRUGS AND FOOD	NATURE OF INTERACTION
Acetaminophen	Carbamazepine	Increases acetaminophen breakdown; increases risk of hepatotoxicity
	Oral contraceptives	Decreases acetaminophen effects
Aminoglycosides	Penicillins	Decreases aminoglycoside effects
Anticholinergics (cholinergic-blocking agents)	Antacids	Decreases absorption of anticholinergics
	Antihistamines	Increases anticholinergic side effects
	Corticosteroids	Increases intraocular pressure
Anticoagulants (oral)	Aspirin	Increases effects of anticoagulants by decreasing plasma protein binding
	Oral contraceptives	Decreases anticoagulant effects
	Thyroid preparations	Increases anticoagulant effects
Antidepressants	Oral contraceptives	Decreases antidepressant effects
Antidiabetic drugs	Alcohol	Possible disulfiram-like syndrome
	Anticoagulants	Increases hypoglycemic action
	Estrogens	Decreases hypoglycemic effects
Antihypertensives	Garlic	Increases antihypertensive effects
Antipsychotic agents (phenothiazines)	Alcohol	Potentiates action of phenothiazines
	Lithium	Increases extrapyramidal effects
	MAO inhibitors	Increases phenothiazine effects
Aspirin	Alcohol, ethyl	Increases risk of GI bleeding associated with use of aspirin
	Antacids	Decreases salicylate levels due to increased rate of renal excretion
	Ascorbic acid (vitamin C)	Increases effects of aspirin
Atenolol	Anticholinergics	Increases effects of atenolol
Benzodiazepines	Antacids	Decreases absorption of benzodiazepines
	Opiates	Additive central nervous system effects
	Oral contraceptives	Increases benzodiazepine effects
β-Adrenergic blocking agents	Anesthetic agents	Increases depression of myocardium
	Aspirin	Decreases action of β-adrenergic blocking agents by inhibiting prostaglandin
	Epinephrine	Increases blood pressure
Calcium channel blockers (CCBs)	Cimetidine	Increases effects of CCBs
	Fentanyl	Severe hypotensive crisis
	Ranitidine	Increases effects of CCBs

Continues

TABLE 6-1.   Clinically Significant Drug and/or Food Interactions, cont'd

DRUGS	INTERACTING DRUGS AND FOOD	NATURE OF INTERACTION
Cephalosporins	Alcohol	Disulfiram-type responses
	Aminoglycosides	Increases risk of nephrotoxicity
	Antacids	Decreases effects of cefaclor, cefdinir, and cefpodoxime
Ciprofloxacin	Aluminum and magnesium hydroxides	Reduces ciprofloxacin absorption
	Iron supplements	Reduces ciprofloxacin absorption
Clonidine	Propranolol	Rapid discontinuation can cause hypertensive crisis
Digoxin	Antacids	Decreases digoxin levels; administer at least 1.5 hours before antacids
	Ibuprofen	Increases risk of digoxin toxicity
	Insulin	Use with caution because of effects on potassium levels
Diuretics	Anticholinergics	Increases thiazide effects
	Corticosteroids	Enhances potassium loss
Potassium-sparing	Indomethacin	Decreases diuretic effects
	Potassium supplements	Hyperkalemia
Doxycycline	Carbamazepine	Decreases doxycycline effect
	Phenobarbital	Decreases doxycycline effect
	Phenytoin	Decreases doxycycline effect
Estrogen	Barbiturates	Decreases estrogen effects
	Rifampin	Decreases estrogen effects
Heparin	Aspirin	Because of increased platelet aggregation by aspirin, concomitant use may increase risk of bleeding
	Garlic	Increases antiplatelet effects
	Nonsteroidal anti-inflammatory drugs	Increases risk of bleeding
Hypoglycemics (oral)	Aspirin	Increases hypoglycemic action
Insulin	Alcohol	Increases hypoglycemic effect and risk of insulin shock
	Propranolol	Inhibits rebound of serum glucose after insulin-induced hypoglycemia
	Tetracyclines	Increases hypoglycemic effects
Isoniazid	Corticosteroids	Decreases isoniazid effects
Nifedipine	Cimetidine	May cause up to an 80% increase in nifedipine blood levels, which can result in hypotensive crisis
Nitroglycerin	Aspirin	May cause hypotension
Nonsteroidal anti-inflammatory drugs (NSAIDs)	Aspirin	May decrease serum levels of NSAIDs
	Loop diuretics	Decreases NSAID effects
	Phenobarbital	Decreases NSAID effects
Oral contraceptives	Penicillins	Decreases contraceptive effects
	Phenobarbital	Decreases contraceptive effects
	Tetracyclines	Decreases contraceptive effects
Penicillins	Antacids	Decreases penicillin effects
	Aspirin	Increases penicillin effects
	Tetracyclines	Decreases penicillin effects
Propranolol	Indomethacin	Decreases propranolol effects
	Nicotine	Decreases propranolol serum levels
Spironolactone	Aspirin	Decreases diuretic effect
Sulfonamides	Anticoagulants	Increases sulfonamide effects
	Aspirin	Increases sulfonamide effects
	Diuretics, thiazide	Increases risk of thrombocytopenia
Tetracyclines	Antacids	Decreases tetracycline effects
	Iron preparations	Decreases tetracycline effects
	Lithium	May increase or decrease tetracycline effects
Theophylline	Barbiturates	Decreases theophylline levels
	Caffeine	Increases theophylline levels
	Nicotine	Decreases theophylline levels

Continues

TABLE 6-1.   Clinically Significant Drug and/or Food Interactions, cont'd

DRUGS	INTERACTING DRUGS AND FOOD	NATURE OF INTERACTION
Thyroid hormones	Estrogens	Decreases thyroid effects
	Salicylates	Decreases thyroid effects by competing with thyroid-binding sites on proteins
	Soy	Decreases absorption of thyroid hormones so space at least 2 hours apart
Warfarin	Amiodarone	Increases warfarin effect
	Carbamazepine	Decreases warfarin effect
	Erythromycin	Increases warfarin effect
	Phenobarbital	Increases warfarin effect

Alcohol Consumption

Chronic use of alcoholic beverages may increase the rate of metabolism of drugs such as warfarin, phenytoin, and tolbutamide, probably by increasing the activity of liver enzymes. However, in contrast, acute use of alcohol by individuals who are not alcoholics may cause inhibition of hepatic enzymes.

Concurrent use of alcoholic beverages with sedatives and other depressant drugs could result in an excessive depressant response. The use of such combinations on a regular basis cannot be a reason for failing to exercise the caution that must be observed if problems are to be averted.

Smoking

A number of investigations have suggested that smoking increases the activity of drug-metabolizing enzymes in the liver, with the result that certain therapeutic agents such as diazepam, theophylline, chlorpromazine, and amitriptyline are metabolized more rapidly, and their effect is decreased. This response may be more pronounced in young and middle-aged individuals than in older patients.

REDUCING THE RISK OF DRUG INTERACTION

Reduction of the risk of drug interactions is a challenge that includes a number of considerations. Although they could be applied to drug therapy in general, the following guidelines to reduce and manage drug interactions are offered to assist health professionals who have the responsibility of selecting and monitoring therapeutic regimens.

Identify Patient Risk Factors

Factors such as age, the nature of the patient's medical problems (e.g., impaired renal function), dietary habits, smoking, and problems such as alcoholism will influence the effects of certain drugs. These factors should be considered during the initial patient interview.

Obtain a Drug History

An accurate and complete record of the prescription and nonprescription medications a patient is taking as well as herbal products and dietary supplements must be obtained. Numerous interactions have resulted from a lack of awareness of prescription medications prescribed by another physician or nonprescription medications the patient did not consider important enough to mention.

Be Knowledgeable About the Actions of Drugs

Knowledge of the properties, including the primary and secondary pharmacological actions of each of the agents used or being considered for use, is essential if the interaction potential is to be assessed accurately.

Consider Therapeutic Alternatives

In the majority of cases, two drugs that are known to interact can be administered concurrently as long as adequate precautions are taken, for example, closer monitoring of therapy or dosage adjustments to compensate for the altered response. However, if another agent with similar therapeutic properties and a lesser risk of interacting is available, it should be used.

Refrain from Administering Complex Therapeutic Regimens

The number of medications used should be kept to a minimum. In addition, the use of medications or dosage regimens that require less frequent administration may help avoid interactions that result from an alteration of absorption, for example, when a drug is administered close to mealtime.

Educate the Patient

Most patients know little about their illnesses and the benefits or problems that could result from drug therapy. Individuals who are aware of and understand this information can be expected to comply better with the instructions for administering medications and be more attentive to the development of symptoms that could be early indicators of drug-related problems. Patients should be encouraged to ask questions about their therapy and to report any excessive or unexpected responses. There should be no uncertainty on the part of patients about how to use their medications in the most effective and safest way.

SUMMARY

Some drug-related problems develop unexpectedly and cannot be predicted; many others are related to known pharmaceutical actions of the drugs and can be reasonably anticipated. However, as drug therapy becomes more complex and because many patients are being treated with two or more drugs, the ability to predict the magnitude of a specific action of any given drug diminishes. Maintaining complete and current medication records for patients is essential. The pharmacist is in a unique position to meet these needs to supervise drug therapy and prevent problems. Many drug-related problems are caused by drug interactions. A number of factors may be associated with drug interactions. Multiple prescribers, consumption of nonprescription drugs, patient noncompliance, drug abuse, and patient variables (such as age, genetic factors, diseases, diet, alcohol consumption, and smoking) are factors that are known to cause drug interactions.

Pharmacists, physicians, and other health care workers can prevent some of these problems by being knowledgeable about the actions of drugs, considering therapeutic alternatives, refraining from administering complex therapeutic regimens, and educating the patient. The pharmacist has a valuable opportunity to make a significant contribution to further enhance the efficacy and safety of drug therapy.

CRITICAL THINKING

1. Choose one of the causes of drug interaction and develop a plan to prevent the interaction from occurring.
2. Elderly patients often take many different medications. What are some strategies for working with this patient population to prevent adverse drug interactions?

REVIEW QUESTIONS

1. The cooperative effect of two or more drugs given together to produce a stronger effect than that of the drugs given alone is known as
   A. potentiation.
   B. synergism.
   C. antagonism.
   D. noncompliance.

2. Drug-related problems in young patients are encountered most commonly in which of the following age group?
   A. Newborns
   B. School age
   C. Toddlers
   D. Teenagers

3. Many antibiotics should be given at least how long before or after meals?
   A. 30 minutes before or 30 minutes after
   B. 60 minutes before and 60 minutes after
   C. 60 minutes before and 90 minutes after
   D. 60 minutes before and 120 minutes after

4. Surgical patients commonly receive more than how many medications?
   A. 2
   B. 5
   C. 7
   D. 10

5. Which of the following is not an example of drug antagonism?
   A. Diazepam and acetaminophen
   B. Ibuprofen and aspirin
   C. Tetracycline and antacids
   D. Charcoal and ipecac

6. Chronic use of alcoholic beverages may increase the rate of metabolism of which of the following drugs?
   A. Penicillin
   B. Erythromycin
   C. Warfarin
   D. Vitamin C

7. Any patient taking a monoamine oxidase (MAO) inhibitor should avoid which of the following foods?
   A. Seafood
   B. Yogurt
   C. Tea
   D. Broccoli

8. Genetic factors may be responsible for developing which of the following?
   A. Sexually transmitted diseases
   B. Unexpected drug response in a particular patient
   C. Eating disorders
   D. Phobias

Continues

9. Which of the following enzymes has been identified as the factor that may contribute to many drug interactions?
   A. Lipase
   B. Pepsin
   C. Enterokinase
   D. Cytochrome P-450

10. Which of the following drugs should be avoided concurrently with grapefruit juice?
    A. Triazolam
    B. Aspirin
    C. Alcohol
    D. Tetracycline

11. _____ occurs as one drug prolongs the effects of another drug.
    A. Potentiation
    B. Prolongation
    C. Extension
    D. Impotentiation

12. Newborn infants are most at risk for drug interaction because of their
    A. large skulls.
    B. large hearts.
    C. immature bone marrow function.
    D. immature renal function.

13. Many patients do not consider _____ to be drugs.
    A. antibiotics
    B. over-the-counter medications
    C. probiotics
    D. amphetamines

14. Smoking _____ the activity of drug-metabolizing enzymes in the liver, resulting in a decreased effect of drugs such as diazepam and theophylline.
    A. decreases
    B. potentiates
    C. increases
    D. inhibits

Hospital and Retail Pharmacy

Hospital Pharmacy

7

OBJECTIVES

Upon completion of this chapter, the reader should be able to

1. Describe the organizational structure of the hospital and the pharmacy department.
2. Explain medication orders.
3. Define floor stock.
4. Discuss the patient prescription system.
5. Explain unit dose.
6. Describe sterile products.
7. Define automation.
8. Name five roles and duties of pharmacy technicians in the hospital pharmacy.
9. Describe the policy and procedure manual.
10. Explain the benefits of the policy and procedure manual.
11. Name four regulatory agencies that oversee hospital pharmacy practice.

GLOSSARY

Centers for Medicare & Medicaid (CMS) An organization that inspects and approves institutions to provide Medicaid and Medicare services.

computerized physician order entry system (CPOE) A computerized system in which the physician inputs the medication order directly for electronic receipt in the pharmacy.

GLOSSARY continued

controlled substance medication order An order for medication (generally narcotics) that requires monitored documentation of procurement, dispensing, and administration.

demand/stat medication order An order for medication to be given in rapid response to a specific medical condition.

Department of Health (DPH) An organization that oversees hospitals, including the pharmacy department.

emergency medication order An order for a medication to be given in response to a medical emergency.

floor stock system A system of drug distribution in which drugs are issued in bulk form and stored in medication rooms on patient care units.

group purchasing Many hospitals working together to negotiate with pharmaceutical manufacturers to get better prices and benefits based upon the ability to promise high committed volumes.

hospital pharmacy The provision of pharmaceutical care within an institutional or hospital setting.

independent purchasing The director of the pharmacy or buyer directly contacts and negotiates pricing with pharmaceutical manufacturers.

inventory turnover rate A mathematical calculation used to determine the number of times the average inventory is replaced over a period of time, usually annually.

investigational medication order An order for a medication given under direction of research protocols that also require strict documentation of procurement, dispensing, and administration.

Joint Commission on Accreditation of Healthcare Organizations (JCAHO) An organization that surveys and accredits health care organizations.

just in time (JIT) system An inventory control system in which stock arrives just before it is needed.

medication order The written order for particular medications and services to be provided to a patient within an institutional setting; medication orders are written by physicians, nurse practitioners, or physician's assistants.

patient prescription system A system of drug distribution in which a nurse supplies the pharmacy with a transcribed medication order for a particular patient and the pharmacy prepares a 3-day supply of the medication.

policy Statement of the definite course or method of action selected to support goals of the overall organization.

policy and procedure manual A formal document specifying guidelines for operations of an institution.

PRN (as needed) medication order An order for medication to be given in response to a specific defined parameter or condition.

procedure Statement of a series of steps to implement the policies of the department or organization.

scheduled intravenous (IV)/total parenteral nutrition (TPN) solution order An order for medication given via an injection; these medications are to be prepared in a controlled (sterile) environment.

scheduled medication order An order for medication that is to be given on a continuous schedule.

State Board of Pharmacy (BOP) An agency that registers pharmacists and pharmacy technicians.

sterile product A substance that contains no living microorganisms.

unit-dose drug distribution system A system for distributing medication in which the pharmacy prepares single doses of medications for a patient for a 24-hour period.

OVERVIEW

In the hospital setting, the practice of pharmacy combines support, product, clinical, and educational services to provide all-encompassing medical care. Dispensing processes have become much more sophisticated than in the past in response to the need to handle a variety of different types of medication orders. The unit-dose system of drug distribution has become the preeminent method used by hospital pharmacies, reducing errors, cost, unused medication, and drug inventories. Hospital pharmacies control the cost of their inventories either by purchasing directly from pharmaceutical manufacturers or by using group purchasing, which involves many hospitals negotiating volume purchases together. The advent of pharmacy automation has increased the volume of medication transactions while maintaining accuracy. Robots are being used for many of the dispensing activities formerly done only by pharmacists or pharmacy technicians. Many of the duties once exclusively performed by pharmacists, including compounding, administering medication, and inspecting the drug stocks of the nursing units, can now be performed by the pharmacy technician. Because of these changes in responsibilities, the need for a policy and procedure manual to improve hospital pharmacy management has increased greatly. Because it is monitored by several governmental agencies, the hospital pharmacy staff must adhere to the policies and procedures contained in its manual, while being able to accommodate the regularly changing needs of the patient. Because of the increased elderly population and the number of new medications being introduced, the future of the hospital pharmacy looks very bright.

WHAT IS HOSPITAL PHARMACY?

In the simplest terms **hospital pharmacy**, in today's practice setting, can be defined as the provision of pharmaceutical care within an institutional or hospital setting. The practice of pharmacy within an institution comprises several types of services:

- Support services—ordering and properly storing medications and maintaining an inventory of pharmaceuticals and associated medical supplies, billing for services, and installing and maintaining computer systems
- Product services—dispensing, preparing, and processing medication orders for inpatients and maintaining required patient records and drug control records
- Clinical services—managing the formulary system, evaluating drug use, and reviewing drug orders for appropriateness
- Educational services—providing education about medications to pharmacy staff, other health care professionals, the public, and patients and their caregivers

Hospital pharmacy practice now encompasses all aspects of drug therapy through the total continuum of medical care.

ORGANIZATION OF THE HOSPITAL

The structure of a hospital or a health care system varies greatly from organization to organization. The basic structure includes a board of directors, who are responsible for the overall governance of the organization. Answering to the board are several layers of management. The primary leadership position is chief executive officer (CEO). This position may also be called hospital director or hospital president. Depending upon the size of the hospital, a senior vice president or chief operating officer (COO) who answers to the CEO may be present. The CEO usually works with the medical staff leadership and the COO with the operating staff leadership, which both consist of vice presidents, functional department heads, assistant department heads, and supervisors. At the vice president level, there may be positions such as chief financial officer (CFO), director of nursing (many times this position is called vice president of patient care services), and vice president of professional or clinical services, and chief information officer (CIO). The functional directors are the directors of departments with a specific function or specialty. These are usually departments such as radiology, respiratory care, dietary services, pharmacy, environmental services, plant operations, medical records, finance and accounting, and many more.

In the preceding description, there is no mention of the medical staff, who are ultimately responsible for the diagnosis and treatment of the patients within the hospital. The medical staff members have a unique relationship with the hospital in that they are not employees of the hospital. They function as independent medical practitioners in private practice. Often they perform procedures in the hospital, but their income is derived through their office practices. The medical staff has a unique structure that links it to the hospital's organization. There is a chief of staff or a medical director who is elected by the medical staff of the hospital. This person acts as the liaison with the hospital director or CEO. A medical staff executive committee is elected to govern the medical staff. This committee is composed of functional medical department (e.g., medicine, surgery, cardiology, and pediatrics) chairpersons or chiefs of services and the medical director or chief of staff. This committee is responsible for overseeing the activities of the medical staff. It recommends the granting of clinical privileges to medical staff members and conducts quality assurance processes to ensure that the medical staff is providing appropriate medical care. The committee functions are performed through the formation of specific committees to oversee credentialing, pharmacy and therapeutics, and quality assurance. There is also a joint conference committee that is established and composed of representatives from the board of directors, the hospital executive staff, and the medical staff. Meetings of this committee are generally convened when there are issues to be addressed between the medical staff and the hospital administration and the board of directors. A sample organizational chart for an institutional setting is shown in Figure 7-1.

ORGANIZATION OF THE HOSPITAL PHARMACY

The pharmacy department within an institution is responsible for all aspects of drug use. These include product-related services, clinical services, support services, and educational services. The personnel in a hospital pharmacy are classified into three categories:

- Professional—all pharmacists and management
- Technical—pharmacy technicians involved in the drug-related processes
- Support—nonlicensed personnel involved in providing services that support the drug-related processes and/or management functions

All hospital pharmacies have a leadership position in the department, usually titled director of pharmacy. This individual is responsible for all the pharmacy services provided in or by the organization. The rest of the department's structure depends on the size of the organization. Smaller hospitals may have a small staff, consisting of a pharmacy director and a staff pharmacist. As the size of the institution grows, additional pharmacists may be added along with pharmacy technicians. Larger hospital systems will have many different positions categorized by functions:

1. Management—almost always pharmacists
   a. Director
   b. Manager
   c. Supervisor—may have a technician supervisor supervising technicians

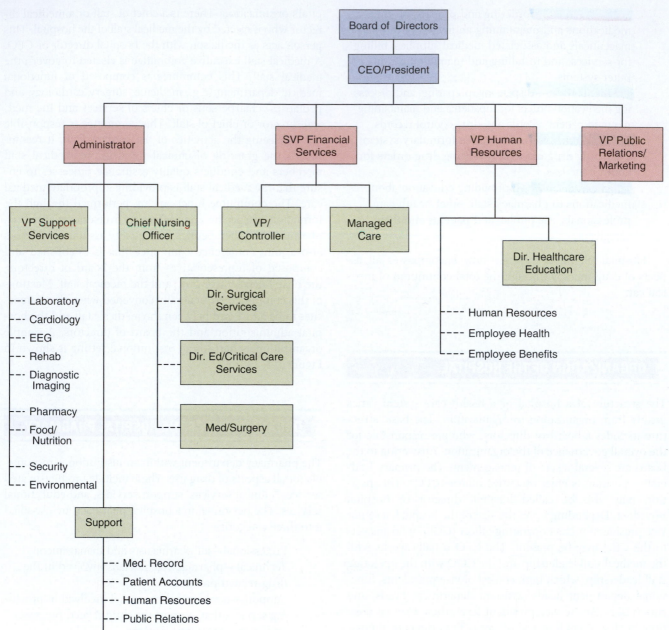

Figure 7-1. Sample organizational chart for a hospital.

2. Dispensing and preparation
   a. Pharmacist—unit dose, satellite
   b. Technician—unit dose, cart fill, medication and supply delivery
   c. Central intravenous (IV) admixture and sterile processing
   d. Controlled drug storage and distribution
3. Support—generally nonpharmacists
   a. Department secretary
   b. Buyer
   c. Biller
   d. Systems analyst

4. Clinical
   a. Clinical coordinator
   b. Clinical pharmacist
   c. Clinical specialist
5. Education and research
   a. Drug information specialist
   b. Research coordinator

As the pharmacy department becomes more involved in the provision of direct patient care, many departments are beginning to redesign their organizational structure to support the practices of the future.

MEDICATION ORDERS

The practice of hospital pharmacy begins with the **medication order** generated by the physician. In the hospital pharmacy the medication order is the equivalent to the prescription in the retail pharmacy. All medications, including prescription and over-the-counter (OTC), ordered in a hospital require a medication order. The medication fulfillment process begins in the pharmacy department when a copy of the original medication order is received in the department. The original physician's order can be a carbon copy or an electronically scanned copy.

The medication order must contain the following information (see Figure 7-2):

- Patient's name, height, weight, medical condition, and known allergies
- Dosage schedule
- Instructions for preparing the drugs
- The exact dosage form of the drug
- The dosage strength
- Directions for use
- Route of administration

Pharmacists and technicians must be able to distinguish between various types of orders that are written on the

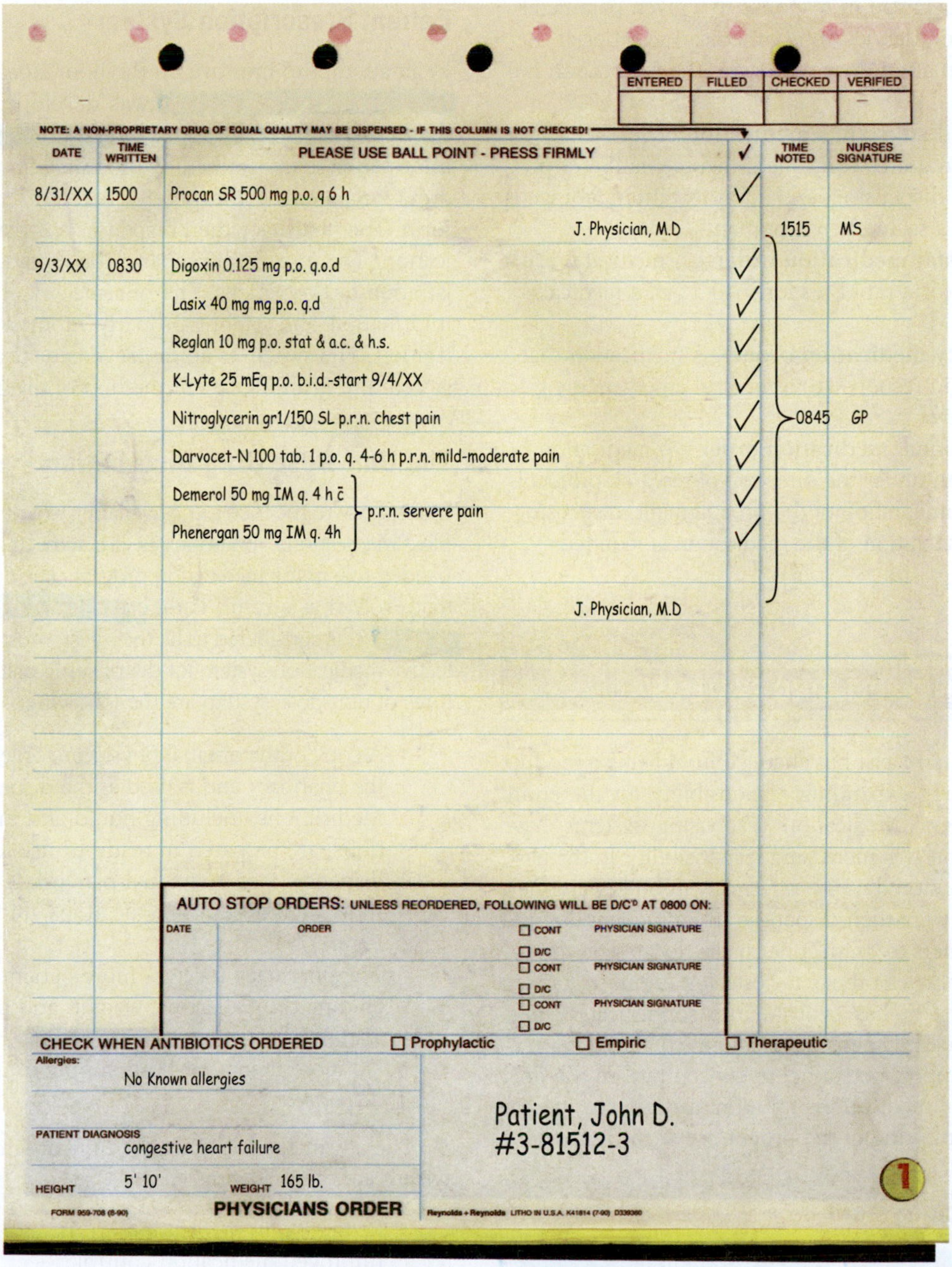

		ENTERED	FILLED	CHECKED	VERIFIED
					—

NOTE: A NON-PROPRIETARY DRUG OF EQUAL QUALITY MAY BE DISPENSED - IF THIS COLUMN IS NOT CHECKED!

DATE	TIME WRITTEN	PLEASE USE BALL POINT - PRESS FIRMLY	✓	TIME NOTED	NURSES SIGNATURE
8/31/XX	1500	Procan SR 500 mg p.o. q 6 h	✓		
		J. Physician, M.D		1515	MS
9/3/XX	0830	Digoxin 0.125 mg p.o. q.o.d	✓		
		Lasix 40 mg mg p.o. q.d	✓		
		Reglan 10 mg p.o. stat & a.c. & h.s.	✓		
		K-Lyte 25 mEq p.o. b.i.d.-start 9/4/XX	✓		
		Nitroglycerin gr1/150 SL p.r.n. chest pain	✓	0845	GP
		Darvocet-N 100 tab. 1 p.o. q. 4-6 h p.r.n. mild-moderate pain	✓		
		Demerol 50 mg IM q. 4 h c̄ } p.r.n. servere pain	✓		
		Phenergan 50 mg IM q. 4h	✓		
		J. Physician, M.D			

AUTO STOP ORDERS: UNLESS REORDERED, FOLLOWING WILL BE D/C'D AT 0800 ON:

DATE	ORDER		
		☐ CONT ☐ D/C	PHYSICIAN SIGNATURE
		☐ CONT ☐ D/C	PHYSICIAN SIGNATURE
		☐ CONT ☐ D/C	PHYSICIAN SIGNATURE

CHECK WHEN ANTIBIOTICS ORDERED   ☐ Prophylactic   ☐ Empiric   ☐ Therapeutic

Allergies: No Known allergies

PATIENT DIAGNOSIS   congestive heart failure

HEIGHT   5' 10'   WEIGHT   165 lb.

Patient, John D.
#3-81512-3

FORM 959-708 (6-90)   **PHYSICIANS ORDER**   Reynolds + Reynolds LITHO IN U.S.A. K41814 (7-90) D336060

Figure 7-2. Sample physician's order.

medication order because there may be many orders on this document that do not pertain to the pharmacy. Diet, laboratory, radiology, and physical activity orders are a few examples of nonmedication orders. A variety of types of medication orders may also be encountered. The types of orders are the following:

- **Scheduled medication order**—A medication that is given on a continuous schedule according to the medication order
- **Scheduled intravenous (IV)/total parenteral nutrition (TPN) solution order**—A medication that is given by the injectable route and must be prepared in a controlled environment
- **PRN (as needed) medication order**—A medication that may be given in response to a given parameter or condition defined in the medication order. If the defined situation does not occur, the medication is not given.
- **Controlled substance medication order**—A narcotic that requires controlled documentation of procurement, dispensing, and administration. Storage is usually in a secured environment.
- **Demand/stat medication order**—A medication that is needed for a rapid response to a given medical condition
- **Emergency medication order**—A medication that is needed in response to a medical emergency, e.g., cardiac arrest
- **Investigational medication order**—A medication that is given under the direction of research protocols. Strict documentation of the procurement, dispensing, and administration of the medication is required.

MEDICATION DISPENSING SYSTEMS

The role of the pharmacist has changed from being a product dispenser to having expanding responsibility for the entire medication process. Medication dispensing systems have changed to support this increasing responsibility. In the past, medications were stored in the pharmacy in bulk quantities. The medications were then dispensed in bulk quantities and multidose containers to "mini" pharmacies located on the patient care units. Nurses prepared doses for administration to patients. This system has evolved into sophisticated unit-dose and automated dispensing processes to allow pharmacists and their support personnel to concentrate on the final preparation of the medications for administration to the patient and the monitoring of the proper use of medications.

The Floor Stock System

In the **floor stock system**, the role of the pharmacy in the medication process is product related only. Drugs are purchased in bulk and multidose dosage forms. The drugs are

issued to patient care units via a bulk drug order form and are stored in medication rooms. Once placed in the medication room, drugs for administration to patients are prepared by a nurse. A medication could be used for more than one patient. In this system the nurse is responsible for most of the steps in the medication process.

The disadvantages of this system are the following:

- Potential for medication errors
- Potential for drug diversion and misappropriation resulting in economic loss
- Increased inventory needs
- Inadequate space for medication storage on the patient care unit

Patient Prescription System

In an attempt to improve on the floor stock system, the **patient prescription system** was developed. In this system the nurse orders medications on a specific patient form. The information is transcribed by the nurse from the medication order prepared by the physician to this medication order form. The pharmacy then dispenses a 3-day supply of medication. The nurse still prepares the medications for administration to the patient. The pharmacy still has little patient information and cannot properly monitor medication utilization. The system is an improvement over the floor stock system but is an inefficient method of drug distribution.

The Unit-Dose Drug Distribution System

In response to the increasing availability of new and more complex medications, pharmacists are expected to play an expanded role in the medication process. The distribution system that evolved as a result is the **unit-dose drug distribution system**. It is considered to be the safest, most efficient, most effective medication system for distributing medications. The features of unit-dose system are the following:

- A copy of the original physician's order is received by the pharmacy and is used as the dispensing document.
- Medications, including liquid and injectable medications, are prepared in ready-to-use forms and are dispensed per individual patient.
- Individual doses of medications are labeled (see Figure 7-3).
- The pharmacy receives more patient information, including drug allergies, weight, and possibly a medication history.
- No more than a 24-hour supply of medication is dispensed.

The advantages of using the unit-dose drug distribution system are the following:

- Reduction in medication errors
- Improved medication control
- Decreased overall cost of medication distribution
- More precise medication billing

- Reduction in medication credits (medications returned unused)
- Reduced drug inventories

STERILE PRODUCTS

The term **sterile product** is usually associated with drugs that are administered by injection. A sterile product contains no living microorganisms. The need for sterility is based on the fact that through injection the major body defense mechanisms are bypassed. The greatest protection against infection is the intact skin. Even products that are administered to porous, membranous tissues must be sterile. An example of this is ophthalmic preparations, ointments, solutions, and suspensions. In the hospital, a majority of patients will receive a medication that is administered by injection. Because of improvements in manufacturing processes and technology, most products requiring sterility are prepared commercially. When a product of this nature that is not available commercially is required, the responsibility for preparing the med-

ication resides in the pharmacy department. The pharmacy department will do the following:

- Ensure that the person preparing these products is properly and carefully trained in the use of aseptic technique.
- Prepare the product in an environment (clean room and laminar flow hood) that will prevent contamination (see Figure 7-4).
- Prepare the product using aseptic technique to prevent contamination.
- Ensure that all contents of the preparation are chemically, physically, and therapeutically compatible.
- Ensure that the product is stable over the time it is to be used.
- Ensure that the prepared product is stored under proper conditions.
- Ensure that the product is labeled properly.
- Keep records of preparation.
- Use proper quality control processes to ensure that a proper preparation has been produced.

Handwashing is a very important procedure for preventing contamination. In preparing sterile products, the primary concern must be safety and accuracy.

INVENTORY CONTROL

The director of pharmacy is responsible for maintaining an adequate medication inventory and establishing specifications for the procurement of all drugs, chemicals, and biologic agents related to the practice of pharmacy. This duty is usually delegated to a pharmacy buyer or pharmacy technician. Customers of pharmacy services expect to have drugs quickly, cheaply, of high quality, and that have been stored properly. In the hospital pharmacy the pharmacy and therapeutics committee determines which medications will be purchased and maintained in stock.

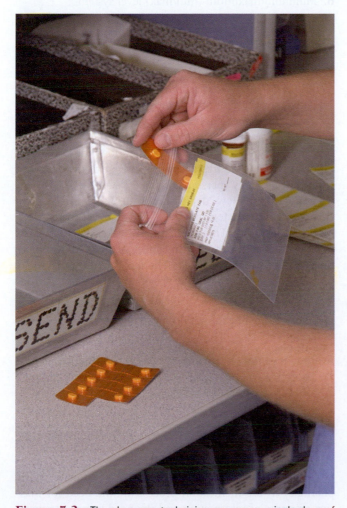

Figure 7-3. The pharmacy technician prepares a single dose of medication for the hospital patient in the unit-dose system.

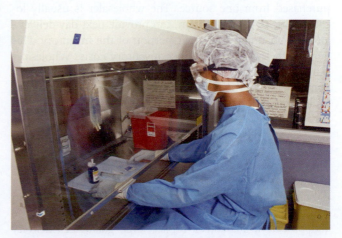

Figure 7-4. Sterile products must be prepared in an aseptic environment.

Purchasing Systems

The hospital must then decide on the system of purchasing the medications. The two types of systems are the following:

1. **Independent purchasing:** The director of pharmacy or pharmacy buyer will contract directly with pharmaceutical manufacturers to negotiate prices and other conditions affecting purchases from that manufacturer. Larger institutions are more likely to use the independent purchasing system because they can offer larger committed volumes independent of other institutions. Smaller hospitals will form coalitions to achieve the larger committed volumes needed to obtain competitive prices.
2. **Group purchasing** (group purchasing organization [GPO]): This type of purchasing involves the collaboration of many hospitals in negotiations with pharmaceutical manufacturers to achieve advantageous pricing and other benefits. The main advantage of this process is that the manufacturer offers more competitive pricing because of the promise of high committed volumes.

Modes of Purchasing

The next consideration is to determine the method of acquisition of the pharmaceuticals. There are three modes of purchasing:

1. Direct purchasing from the pharmaceutical manufacturer
2. Purchase from a wholesaler
3. Purchase from a prime vendor

Direct Purchasing

Direct purchasing eliminates the middle man and handling fees but requires a significant commitment of time, larger inventories, and more storage space. Purchases must be made from many vendors.

Wholesaler Purchasing

Purchasing from a wholesaler means that many items are purchased from one source. The wholesaler is usually located close to the institution, can provide next day delivery, and will maintain the larger portion of the inventory. This enables the hospital to reduce inventory costs. Wholesaler purchasing also reduces the need for a large commitment of personnel to support the purchasing process. The primary disadvantage is higher costs of pharmaceuticals.

Prime Vendor Purchasing

The prime vendor system of purchasing is a relationship established between the hospital and a single wholesaler. A contract is established, stipulating a committed volume of purchases. In return the vendor will charge a highly competitive service fee and provide a guaranteed service level, guaranteed delivery schedule, and a guarantee that individual or group contract prices will be the base price. A contract with a prime vendor may be an independent agreement with the hospital or an agreement made through the GPO. Generally the GPO is better able to negotiate a competitive contract. The prime vendor system has the advantages of both the direct and wholesaler purchasing processes without the disadvantages. To reduce inventory costs most pharmacy departments will attempt to have a **just-in-time (JIT) inventory** system. In this system sufficient inventory is maintained for the pharmacy to function until the next reorder period. With the prime vendor system this reorder period could be as little as 24 hours.

Inventory Management

The pharmacy department must select a method of inventory management. The types of inventory management are the following:

1. Order book system
2. Inventory record card system
3. ABC inventory system
4. Economic order quantity (EOQ)/economic order value (EOV) system
5. Computerized inventory system
6. Minimum/maximum (min/max) level system

In general, most of these systems require a large commitment of personnel. The EOQ/EOV systems are mathematical equations with parameters that are not easily obtained, rendering them unusable in the normal hospital. The inventory record card system, minimum/maximum level system, and ABC inventory system are laborious manual record-keeping processes. Most hospital pharmacies use the order book system or the computerized inventory system. The computerized inventory system can also be laborious; however, this problem is being addressed by the use of bar coding and wireless technology (personal digital assistants [PDAs]).

Many pharmacy departments use the **inventory turnover rate** to determine the effectiveness of their inventory control system. This is a mathematical calculation of the number of times the average inventory is replaced over a period of time, usually annually. The target figure is 10 to 12 times per year. This generally means that the entire inventory value is turned over once a month:

Inventory turnover rate = Purchases for period/
Average inventory for period

Average Inventory = Beginning inventory for period +
Ending inventory for period/2

AUTOMATION

Some disadvantages of the increased involvement of the pharmacy in the medication process are the need for massive amounts of information and the need to process many transactions quickly. The advent of automation (pharmacy information systems) has greatly enhanced the ability of pharmacies to achieve these requirements (see Figure 7-5). Automation provides the ability to rapidly process large volumes of medication orders accurately and quickly. From the automated processing of medication orders, patient profiles are generated, medication labels are produced, medication fill lists are produced, medication administration records are produced, and medication charges are processed.

Clinical screening can occur to check for drug interactions, drug allergies, and dosage ranges. Reports can also be generated to produce data to monitor appropriate drug utilization. Utilization and usage data from the pharmacy information system can be used to order and maintain a medication inventory. One of the problems identified with this process is the medication order. It is a document handwritten by the physician, nurse practitioner, or physician's assistant that is prone to error because the handwriting may be illegible. Currently, in many facilities, the physician rather than the pharmacy staff is responsible for entering medication orders into the hospital information system. This type of system is generically called a **computerized physician order entry system (CPOE)**.

Many unit-dose systems use the 24-hour medication cart exchange process. These carts contain a 24-hour supply of medication for each patient on a patient care unit. The carts are usually filled by a pharmacy technician and checked by a pharmacist. A robotic device interfaced with the pharmacy information system will fill each patient medication tray in the cart. This robotic device is also capable of returning credited medication to proper stock locations. Automation is also used to create point-of-service storage cabinets that are interfaced with the pharmacy information system. Use of these cabinets eliminates the medication cart-filling process. An example of this type of automation is the automated dispensing cabinet. Many fear that the use of automation will decrease the need for pharmacy personnel. However, these devices require human intervention for appropriate use. The

pharmacy technician of the future will be controlling these machines and providing proper maintenance, repair, and quality assurance processes. If mechanical failure occurs, manual backup processes must be in place, and human intervention will be needed to repair failed mechanical systems. Human intervention can never be replaced.

THE ROLES AND DUTIES OF PHARMACY TECHNICIANS IN HOSPITALS

The increasing complexity of health care in the modern hospital is creating ever-greater demands for the hospital pharmacy to broaden its scope of services. New health care legislation and rapid changes in health care technology are imposing new demands on hospital pharmacies, which result in a need for increased manpower. The scope of pharmaceutical services being provided in most hospitals is limited largely by personnel shortages. The time of the hospital pharmacist can be freed to a great extent by delegation of routine tasks to the pharmacy technician, under the supervision of the pharmacist. Supportive hospital pharmacy personnel are used in most hospitals today. Therefore, it is essential to understand the roles and duties of the technician in the hospital setting, as listed in the following:

- Maintenance of medication records
- Preparing unit doses
- Compounding medications
- Packaging
- Administration of medication
- Preparing and delivering prescriptions to patients who are out of the hospital, such as those in nursing homes, hospice, and rehabilitation facilities
- Computer data input
- Inspecting nursing unit drug stocks
- Inventory maintenance
- Preparation of labels
- Maintaining privacy
- Communication skills
- Working safely

Maintenance of Medication Records

An important part of the job of the pharmacy technician is to accurately maintain the patient records on the pharmacy information system. Records should include the patient's weight, height, diagnosis, treatment, therapy, diet plans, blood and laboratory test results, and the name of the primary physician. Maintaining up-to-date records allows the pharmacist to provide better care and counseling of the patient.

Preparing Unit Doses

The pharmacy technician is responsible for preparing the unit doses for individual patients each day. The technician will

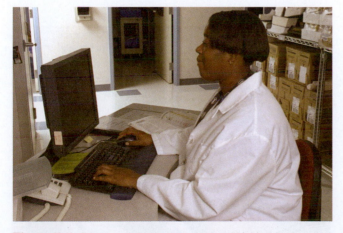

Figure 7-5. Pharmacy information systems within the hospital allow processing of massive amounts of information, resulting in quicker and more efficient service.

prepare each day's doses of medication for all patients and place them in a unit-dose cart to be delivered to the patient care areas of the hospital. The cart must be checked by the pharmacist before being delivered to the patient care floors.

Compounding Medications

In some circumstances a drug may need to be created from a prepared recipe (see Figure 7-6). If a written procedure exists for preparation of a drug, then the pharmacy technician can prepare it. This process is called compounding. To create a compound drug, the technician must be able to clearly understand the formula and be able to adjust it to increase or decrease amounts as necessary. A sound understanding of mathematical principles is required.

Packaging

Many drugs have to be placed in proper containers to remain active and potent. The pharmacy technician must be aware of these characteristics of drugs to properly choose the appropriate containers for dispensing and storing them.

Administration of Medication

The administration of medication is the method in which pharmacy technicians prepare, provide, and deliver prescriptions. Prescriptions are delivered to the hospital floor and nursing stations as well as outside the hospital to nursing homes and rehabilitation centers. Steps for the administration of medication to patients in the hospital setting are discussed below.

Preparing and Delivering Outpatient Prescriptions

Some hospitals are affiliated with facilities outside of the hospital itself such as nursing homes and rehabilitation centers. The pharmacy technician is responsible for preparing the medications these facilities need and for delivering them to the facilities in a timely manner.

Computer Data Input

Data entry is an important part of the pharmacy technician's job. Accurate entry of new data into the computer system and maintenance of records within the system are important. The pharmacy then can be run efficiently because patient records are accurate, inventory is maintained at appropriate levels, and billing can be done in an accurate and timely manner.

Inspecting Nursing Unit Drug Stocks

Nursing unit drug stocks must be maintained by the pharmacy. The technician is responsible for inspection of unit drug stocks for proper storage conditions, appropriate inventory, and replacement of expired or damaged stock.

Inventory Maintenance

Ordering and maintenance of stock levels is often the responsibility of the pharmacy technician. As discussed earlier many inventory systems are available for use within the pharmacy. Regardless of the system used the technician must ensure that stock levels are appropriate to allow the pharmacy to operate efficiently without having to borrow stock or order stock at higher prices. When stock is delivered, it must be checked and verified against the order. Receipt of the order must be clearly marked on the invoice. All orders must be appropriately stored within the pharmacy (see Figure 7-7). Any damaged goods or expired drugs must be returned or properly disposed of.

Preparation of Labels

Each filled medication order must be appropriately labeled (see Figure 7-8). The label should contain the name of the patient the drug is prescribed for, the patient's medical record number, the patient's room number, the name of the prescriber, the date of dispensing, the name of the drug, the strength of the drug, the quantity of the drug dispensed,

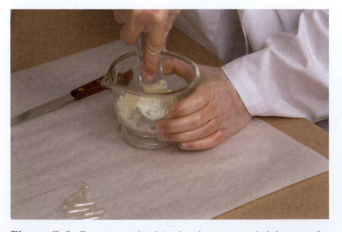

Figure 7-6. To compound a drug the pharmacy technician must be able to accurately follow written procedures and formulas.

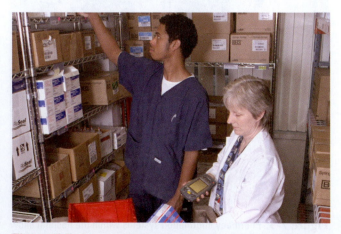

Figure 7-7. Proper maintenance of inventory levels is necessary to allow the pharmacy to run efficiently.

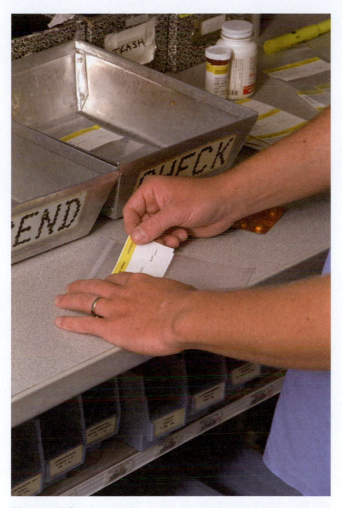

Figure 7-8. Each filled medication order must be appropriately labeled.

dosage directions, and expiration date. The label should also contain the initials of the person dispensing the drug. Proper labeling on medications is critically important. A great deal of care should be taken in this task. The label should be checked and rechecked against the medication order. All labels must be checked and initialed by the pharmacist before the medication leaves the pharmacy.

Maintaining Privacy

The pharmacy technician is legally bound to uphold the privacy of all patients. New standards for maintaining a patient's privacy have been implemented with regulations in Health Insurance Portability and Accountability Act (HIPAA). Please review Chapter 3 for more information.

Communication Skills

Communication skills are very important in the field of pharmacy. The pharmacy technician will need to accurately communicate with patients as well as other health care workers. Communication skills will be discussed in more detail in Chapter 16.

Working Safely

For the health and safety of pharmacy personnel a safe working environment must be maintained. Work areas should be clean, and accidental exposures to harmful substances should be avoided. Emergency and exposure treatment plans should be in place. The pharmacy technician should be aware of and quickly be able to respond to any unsafe condition. Workplace safety is discussed in more detail in Chapter 14.

THE POLICY AND PROCEDURE MANUAL

Hospitals today are very complex organizations. In addition, the hospital may be a member of an integrated health care delivery system. This complexity dictates that the hospital and all its departments must have a set of standard operating statements to operate effectively and efficiently. The regulatory and quasi-legal organizations that oversee hospitals require a manual to fulfill this need. In support of the hospital and health care delivery system, the pharmacy department must develop guideline for operations. This document is formally called the **policy and procedure manual**, and contains the following:

- **Policy:** A statement of the definite course or method of action selected to support the goals of the overall organization. It is a general plan that provides a framework for action.
- **Procedure:** A statement of a series of steps to implement the policies of the department or organization.

The policy and procedure statements of the manual should answer the following questions:

- What action must be undertaken?
- What is its purpose (why must it be done)?
- When must it be done?
- Where must it be done?
- Who should do it?
- How must it be done?

The policy and procedure manual document provides a standard direction for operating and functioning within an organization and its specific departments.

The Need for Policies and Procedures

The primary reason for developing policies and procedures is that regulatory agencies such as the Food and Drug Administration (FDA) and state boards of pharmacy, governing the delivery of pharmaceutical services, require that certain policies and procedures be developed, and many times prescribe the content of the document. The Joint Commission on

Accreditation of Healthcare Organizations (JCAHO) and the American Society of Health-System Pharmacists (ASHP) are quasi-legal organizations that have defined a standard of practice for pharmacy departments which includes certain policies and procedures with a defined content. The pharmacy director is responsible for initiating and developing the policies and procedures for the pharmacy department. This is done in cooperation with and with the approval of the hospital director, CEO, or president, and the pharmacy and therapeutics committee. It should be continually revised to reflect changes in procedures and organization. All pharmacy personnel should be familiar with the contents of the manual. The minimum standard for pharmacies in the hospital includes the following:

1. Preparation of a comprehensive operations manual
2. Clearly defined lines of authority and areas of responsibility
3. Written job descriptions that are developed and revised as needed
4. Manual revisions that include continuing changes
5. Familiarization of all personnel with the contents of the manual
6. Obtaining of input from other disciplines

Policies and procedures should relate to the selection, distribution, and safe and effective use of drugs in the facility. They should be established by the combined effort of the director of pharmaceutical services, the medical staff, the nursing service, and the administration. Examples of organizations requiring polices and procedures are the following:

- Food and Drug Administration: Investigation of drug policies and procedures in hospital pharmacies and drug recall policies and procedures.
- Drug Enforcement Administration: Policies and procedures to show proper handling of controlled substances.
- Occupational Safety and Health Administration: Policies and procedures that ensure the health and safety of people in the workplace.
- Joint Commission on Accreditation of Healthcare Organizations: Policies and procedures that guide the pharmacy department in providing safe, effective, and cost-effective drug therapy.
- American Society of Health-System Pharmacists: Policies and procedures showing implementation of its guidelines and standards of practice.

Benefits of a Policy and Procedure Manual

The primary benefit of having a policy and procedure manual is to document compliance with accrediting, certifying, and regulatory bodies. The second most beneficial effect of having a policy and procedure manual is to create a more effective departmental management program. Other benefits include the following:

- Establishing standards of practice for delivering pharmaceutical services
- Coordinating use of resources
- Improving intradepartmental relationships
- Providing consistency in orientation and training of personnel
- Providing a reference guide to all personnel in the performance of daily activities
- Creating a positive work environment including increased job satisfaction and productivity

A department with a functioning policy and procedure manual will function more efficiently and effectively.

Contents of a Policy and Procedure Manual

The purpose of a policy and procedure manual is to provide an authoritative source for organizational and departmental policies and procedures. In it standards of operation are identified, and it is a guide and reference for personnel in the performance of their daily duties. The pharmacy director is responsible for creating the manual. Each employee is responsible for becoming familiar with its content. It is beyond the scope of this chapter to give examples of specific policies and procedures. Policies and procedures will be either administrative or professional. Administrative policies and procedures are related to the control of resources (human resources, financial resources, supplies and equipment, job descriptions, and the physical plant) and relationships with other departments and administration. Professional policies and procedures pertain either directly or indirectly to patient care services. This section should represent the major portion of the manual. It should include all dispensing and clinical functions. A list of the topics contained in a policy and procedure manual is found in Table 7-1.

Writing Policies and Procedures

Writing of polices and procedures is imperative for a hospital. Either the hospital administration or the pharmacy and therapeutics committee should approve all pharmacy policies and procedures. The information should be clear, direct, and simple. Creative writing techniques should not be used in writing policies and procedures. The policies and procedures should be developed with the input of all affected parties and the staff of other departments. The content, format, and design of the policy and procedure manual will vary with each organization. There is general information that should be included in each policy and procedure manual. A system of indexing of each policy and procedure must be created. It is also imperative that a method of tracking origination date, reviews, and revisions of policies and procedures be established. Because the practices of medicine and pharmacy are ever-changing, the policy and procedure manual should always be in a state of development. Thus, it would be beneficial to have a dedicated staff member who is skilled in the process of creating and managing a policy and procedure manual. The person(s) writing policies and procedures should be able to think analytically. The policy and proce-

TABLE 7-1. Hospital Pharmacy USA—Policy and Procedure Manual

SECTION 1: INTRODUCTION	SECTION 2: ORGANIZATIONAL STRUCTURE	SECTION 3: ADMINISTRATION	SECTION 4: CLINICAL PHARMACY	SECTION 5: DISPENSING	SECTION 6: DRUG DISTRIBUTION SYSTEMS	SECTION 7: SAFE USE OF MEDICATIONS	SECTION 8: PHARMACY COMMUNICATIONS	SECTION 9
Purpose Hospital	Hospital Pharmacy	Develops budget Purchasing and inventory control	Patient care Research	Inpatients Outpatients	Floor stock Unit doses			Index
Mission/vision statement		Medical service representative and pharmacy relations	Teaching	Ancillary supplies	Automation			
Pharmacy		Drug charges	Pharmacy and therapeutic committee	Controlled substances	Mixed systems			
Mission/vision statement		Pharmacy policy and procedure manual	Formulary	After hours				
Scope of practice		Accreditation— JCAHO Physical plant and facilities	Drug research studies Drug utilization and evaluation	Intravenous admixtures Pharmacist and radioisotopes				
		Professional practices and relations	Pharmacy library— drug information center	Prepackaging				
		Preparation of annual report		Manufacturing —bulk and sterile				
		Human resources Job descriptions Performance evaluations Quality improvement						

dure manual should inform and guide but not suppress professional judgment, personal initiative, or creativity.

A copy of the policy and procedure manual needs to be located in each area of the pharmacy department so that it will be available to any department employee. The document should start with a policy title followed by a policy statement. The next section of the document should contain the step-by-step procedure for placing the policy into operation. A section should be devoted to references to source material used in the creation of the policy and procedure. Signatures indicating proper approvals should be obtained after the policies and procedures have been defined.

Review and Revision of a Manual

The information in the policy and procedure manual must be current and reliable. It must be flexible and change accordingly; thus, the manual must be readily revisable. The entire contents should be reviewed or revised at least annually. Reasons for this are to ensure currency and conformity with new laws, rules, and regulations of government agencies and to ensure that the standards of the Joint Commission on Accreditation of Healthcare Organizations are met. Policies and procedures that clearly identify the method for handling revisions in the manual should be established. These should address who can initiate change, how change is accomplished, who reviews and comments on change, and how to process revision of material no longer in effect.

REGULATORY AGENCIES THAT OVERSEE HOSPITAL PHARMACY

The agencies that oversee all aspects of hospital operations, including the pharmacy department, are as follows:

- **Joint Commission on Accreditation of Healthcare Organizations (JCAHO):** This organization surveys and accredits health care services. All health care organizations must undergo this accreditation process every 3 years. JCAHO identifies specific guidelines for every department within the hospital.
- **State Board of Pharmacy (BOP):** This agency registers pharmacists and pharmacy technicians. Currently only 20 states require that pharmacy technicians be certified and registered with the BOP.
- **Centers for Medicare & Medicaid (CMS):** The CMS inspects and approves hospitals to provide care for Medicaid patients. Approval by this organization is required to receive reimbursement for any patients covered by Medicaid.
- **Department of Health (DPH):** This organization oversees hospitals including the pharmacy department. Hospitals undergo inspections by the DPH to assure compliance with laws concerning hospital practice.

FUTURE OF HOSPITAL PHARMACY

With the aging of the population and the increasing number of medications being produced by research, an increasing need for pharmacy services in all settings will be seen. Trends for the future include the following:

1. Continuing expansion of the responsibilities of pharmacy technicians to allow pharmacists to concentrate on direct patient care activities.
2. An increasing need for education of both pharmacists and pharmacy technicians.
3. An increasing need for pharmacists and pharmacy technicians to obtain the skills necessary to work directly with patients.
4. An increasing multiprofessional approach to providing patient care, thus requiring better communication skills.
5. Increasing use of automation to perform routine tasks and to handle the massive amounts of information and documentation that must occur as a result of providing patient care. Automation will also be used to make patient information available in the multiple settings in which patient care will be delivered.

The future of pharmacy is bright for those who choose pharmacy as a profession. It is the responsibility of those in the field now to prepare for the requirements of the future directions of pharmacy.

SUMMARY

Pharmacy practice in the institutional setting includes support, product, clinical, and educational services. The basic structure of the hospital organization includes a board of directors, who are responsible for the overall governance of the organization. The personnel in a hospital pharmacy are classified into three categories: professional, technical, and support staff. The pharmacy director is responsible for all pharmacy services. The practice of hospital pharmacy begins with the medication order generated by the physician. Medication dispensing may be done by automated machines, and technical personnel such as pharmacy technicians must finalize the preparation of the medications. The term sterile product is usually associated with drugs that are administered by injection. The pharmacy director is responsible for maintaining an adequate medication inventory. This duty is usually delegated to a pharmacy buyer or pharmacy technician. In support of the hospital and health care delivery system, the pharmacy department must develop a guideline for operations, which is called the policy and procedure manual. The primary reason for this manual is that regulatory agencies require certain policies and procedures.

CRITICAL THINKING

1. Compare and contrast methods of inventory management. What method do you feel has the most advantages? Why?
2. Research the use of automation within the pharmacy. What impact do you think automation will have on the future of pharmacy?

REVIEW QUESTIONS

1. Creating a medication from a formula is called
   A. compounding medications.
   B. administration of medications.
   C. responsibility for all pharmacy services.
   D. inventory maintenance.

2. The pharmacy practice in the hospital comprises all of the following, except
   A. educational services.
   B. product services.
   C. engineering services.
   D. clinical services.

3. In the hospital pharmacy, the medications that are purchased and stocked are determined by
   A. the pharmacy buyer and the pharmacy technician.
   B. the pharmacy supervisors.
   C. the pharmacists on staff.
   D. the pharmacy and therapeutics committee.

4. In preparing sterile products, the primary concern must be
   A. safety and accuracy.
   B. saving time and speeding.
   C. availability and productivity.
   D. cost.

5. The disadvantages of the floor stock system include all of the following, except
   A. the potential for drug diversion and misappropriation resulting in economic loss.
   B. decreased inventory needs.
   C. inadequate space for medication storage on the patient care unit.
   D. the potential for scheduling errors.

6. Which of the following personnel will be running the automation machines?
   A. The pharmacy technician
   B. The secretarial department
   C. The pharmacist
   D. The supervisor

7. CPOE means
   A. certified physician-ordered examination.
   B. computerized physician order entry.
   C. computerized patient order entry.
   D. certified physician order entry.

8. Providing a policy and procedure manual is a responsibility of the
   A. pharmacy technician.
   B. pharmacy director.
   C. director of the hospital.
   D. director of human resources.

9. The Centers for Medicare & Medicaid (CMS) inspects and approves hospitals to provide care for
   A. elderly patients.
   B. Medicaid patients.
   C. only inpatients.
   D. only pregnant patients.

10. Setting up unit doses is a responsibility of the
    A. pharmacy technician.
    B. nurse.
    C. pharmacy director.
    D. support staff.

11. The basis for the practice of hospital pharmacy begins with the
    A. providing pharmacy technician.
    B. medication order.
    C. emergency department.
    D. administration of medication.

12. The unit dose is considered to have all of the following characteristics, except
    A. it is safest.
    B. it is the most efficient.
    C. it is the cheapest.
    D. it is the most effective.

Continues

13. All of the following are among the three modes of purchasing, except
A. purchase from wholesaler.
B. purchase from a second vendor.
C. purchase from a prime vendor.
D. purchase from the pharmaceutical manufacturer.

14. The inventory turn over rate equals
A. purchases for period plus average inventory for period.
B. purchases for previous year divided by average inventory of this year.
C. purchases for period divided by average inventory for period.
D. beginning inventory for period plus ending inventory for period.

15. The provision of pharmaceutical care in the institutional setting is known as
A. nuclear pharmacy.
B. hospital pharmacy.
C. retail pharmacy.
D. mail-order pharmacy.

Retail (Community) Pharmacy

OUTLINE

Overview
The Prescription
    Processing Prescriptions—Dispensing
Organization of the Retail Pharmacy
    Prescription Counter and Consulting Area
    Transaction Windows
    Storage
    Refrigeration
    Computer Systems
    Equipment
    Customer Pick-Up
    Cash Register
    Controlled Substances
    Purchasing and Inventory Control

The Professional Characteristics of Pharmacy Technicians
    Accountability
    Ethical Standards and Professional Behavior
    Communication Skills
    Teamwork
    Ability to Handle a Fast Pace and Stress
Summary

OBJECTIVES

Upon completion of this chapter, the reader should be able to

1. Explain prescriptions, their uses, requirements, and components.
2. Discuss how prescriptions are processed, received, and checked.
3. Describe the ways prescriptions are numbered, dated, and labeled.
4. Demonstrate the ways prescriptions are compounded and dispensed.
5. List various points involved in packaging and delivering prescriptions.
6. Identify methods for recording and filing prescriptions.
7. Explain requirements for refilling prescriptions.
8. Identify the various areas and equipment used in the pharmacy.
9. Describe controlled substances and methods for their handling.

GLOSSARY

drive through An external site at a pharmacy that can be accessed by driving up in the car.
inscription Medication prescribed.
legend drug A medication that may be dispensed only with a prescription; also know as prescription drug.
over-the-counter (OTC) A medication that may be purchased without a prescription directly from the pharmacy.

pharmacy compounding The preparation, mixing, assembling, packaging, or labeling of a drug or device.
professionalism The following of a profession as an occupation. A person who conforms to the rules and standard of their chosen profession.
signa Directions for patient.
subscription Dispensing directions to pharmacist.
superscription Rx symbol.

OVERVIEW

There are more than 60,000 community pharmacies across the United States. They are the primary providers of pharmaceuticals and pharmaceutical care services to patients. Community pharmacies are found in a variety of locations such as shopping centers, grocery stores, department stores, and medical office buildings. These are classified into two main categories: independent pharmacies or chain pharmacies. Independent pharmacies are owned by local individuals. On the contrary, chain pharmacies are usually regionally or nationally based, such as Walgreens and Eckerd. Giant regional or national mass merchandisers such as Wal-Mart or Kmart also have pharmacies inside most of their stores. Pharmacists in the community pharmacy provide several important functions:

1. They provide distribution of prescribed drug products.
2. They are caretakers of the nation's drug supply.
3. They compound prescriptions to meet the specific needs of individual patients.
4. They educate the public to maximize the intended benefits of drug therapy while minimizing unintended side effects and adverse reactions.

Recent studies indicate the pharmacy technician of today is involved in more areas of pharmacy practice than ever before. In addition to assisting with outpatient prescription dispensing, many community pharmacy technicians participate in purchasing, inventory control, billing, and repackaging products.

THE PRESCRIPTION

An order for medication issued by a physician, dentist, or other licensed medical practitioner is called a prescription. In certain states, nurse practitioners and even pharmacists can issue prescriptions with certain restrictions. The prescription order is a part of the professional relationship among the prescriber, the pharmacist, and the patient. It is the pharmacist's responsibility in this relationship to provide quality pharmaceutical care that meets the medication needs of the patient. The pharmacist or pharmacy technicians not only must be precise in the manual aspects of filling the prescription order but also must provide the patient with the necessary information and guidance to assure the patient's compliance in taking the medication properly. There are two broad legal classifications of medications: those that can be obtained only by prescription and those that may be purchased without a prescription. The latter are termed *nonprescription drugs* or **over-the-counter (OTC)** drugs. Medications that may be dispensed legally only by prescription are referred to as prescription drugs or **legend drugs**. Prescriptions may be written by the prescriber and given to the patient for presentation at the pharmacy, telephoned or sent directly to the pharma-

cist by means of a fax machine, or sent electronically from a physician's computer to a pharmacist's computer. The component parts of a prescription include the following:

- Address of the prescriber's office
- Name and address of the patient
- Date
- Medication prescribed (**inscription**)
- Rx symbol (**superscription**)
- Dispensing directions to pharmacist (**subscription**)
- Directions for patient (**signa**)
- Refill and special labeling
- Prescriber's signature and license or Drug Enforcement Agency (DEA) number

An example of a physician's prescription is shown in Figure 8-1.

Processing Prescriptions—Dispensing

Proper procedures and correct steps for processing prescriptions and dispensing include receiving, reading and checking, numbering and dating, labeling, preparing, packaging, rechecking, delivering and patient counseling, recording and filing, pricing, and refilling.

Receiving the Prescription

The pharmacy technician receives the prescription order directly from the patient. This is a good opportunity to enhance

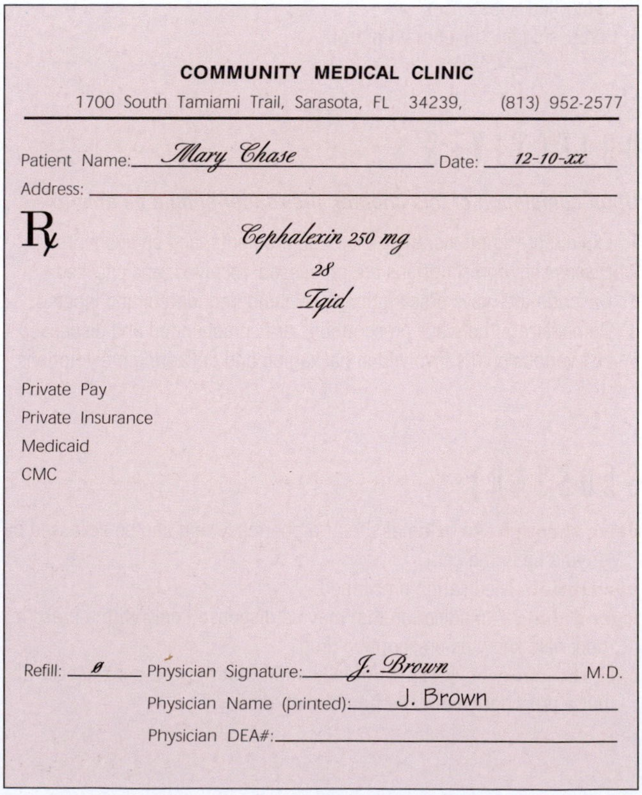

COMMUNITY MEDICAL CLINIC
1700 South Tamiami Trail, Sarasota, FL 34239,   (813) 952-2577

Patient Name: _Mary Chase_   Date: _12-10-xx_
Address: _____

℞   *Cephalexin 250 mg*
                              28
                           Tgid

Private Pay
Private Insurance
Medicaid
CMC

Refill: _0_   Physician Signature: _J. Brown_   M.D.
              Physician Name (printed): _J. Brown_
              Physician DEA#: _____

Figure 8-1. Prescription.

the pharmacist- or the technician-patient relationship and facilitates the gathering of essential information from the patient, such as a history of diseases and other drugs being taken. This information is critical for the provision of quality pharmaceutical care. The technician can also obtain the patient's correct name, address, and other necessary information and determine whether the patient's medications are provided through insurance coverage. Pharmacy technicians should ask the patient whether he or she wishes to wait, call back, or have the medication delivered. Many pharmacists try to price prescriptions before dispensing, especially for unusually expensive medication, to avoid subsequent questions concerning the charge.

Reading and Checking

Pharmacy technicians should read the prescription completely and carefully to be sure the ingredients or quantities prescribed are clear. The pharmacy technician should take the time to update the patient's profile. From the computer, the technician should determine the compatibility of the newly prescribed medication with other drugs being taken by the patient. The technician should determine whether drug-food or drug-disease interactions are possible. If some part of the information is illegible or if it appears that an error has been made, the technician should notify the pharmacist. Then the pharmacist should consult another pharmacist or the prescriber. Unfamiliar or unclear abbreviations represent a source of errors in interpreting and filling prescriptions. The pharmacist must take great care and use his or her broad knowledge of drug products to prevent dispensing errors. The amount and frequency of a dose must be noted carefully and checked. In determining the safety of the dose of a medicinal agent, the age, weight, and condition of the patient, dosage form prescribed, possible influence of other drugs being taken, and the frequency of administration all must be considered.

Numbering and Dating

It is a legal requirement that the prescription order be numbered and that the same number be placed on the label. This numbering helps to identify the bottle or package. Consecutive numbers are assigned by prescription computers or manually by use of numbering machines. Including the date the prescription is filled on the label is also a legal requirement. This information is important in determining the appropriate refill frequency and patient compliance and can be used as an alternate means of locating the prescription order if the prescription number is lost by the patient.

Labeling

The prescription label may be typewritten or prepared by computer, using the information entered by the pharmacist or pharmacy technician. Figure 8-2 shows a computer-prepared prescription, including the label.

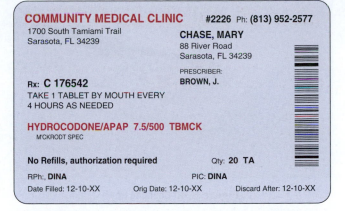

Figure 8-2. Computer-prepared prescription and label.

A prescription should have a professional-appearing label. The size of the label used should be appropriate to the size of the prescription container. The name, address, and telephone number of the pharmacy are all legally required to appear on the label. The prescription number, prescriber's name, patient's name, directions for use, and date of dispensing also are legally required. The patient's name and address and strength of the medication are also commonly included. Some state laws require that the name or initials of the pharmacist dispensing the medication appear on the label. Auxiliary labels (also known as strip labels) are used to emphasize important aspects of the dispensed medication, including its proper use, handling, storage, refill status, and necessary warnings or precautions. Certain medications must be taken with food, may make the patient sensitive to sunlight, or may change the color of urine. Auxiliary labels are available in various colors to give them special prominence. Figure 8-3 shows some examples of pharmacy auxiliary labels.

Preparing

Most prescriptions call for dispensing of medications already prefabricated into dosage forms by pharmaceutical

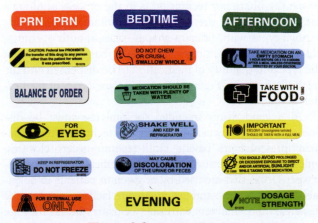

Figure 8-3. Auxiliary labels.

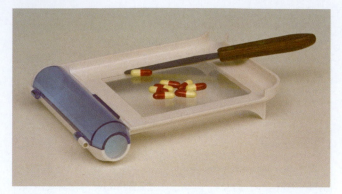

Figure 8-4. Counting tray.

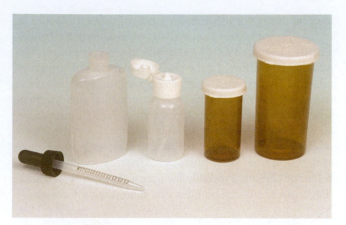

Figure 8-5. Various types of medication containers.

manufacturers. In filling prescriptions with prefabricated products, the pharmacist should compare the manufacturer's label with the prescription to be certain it is the correct medication. Medications that show signs of poor manufacture or deterioration or for which the stated expiration date on the label has passed should never be dispensed.

Tablets, capsules, and some other solid, prefabricated dosage forms usually are counted in the pharmacy using a device that is called the counting tray, which is shown in Figure 8-4. This device facilitates the rapid and sanitary counting and transferring of medication from the stock packages to the prescription container. To prevent contamination of capsules and tablets, the counting tray should be wiped clean after each use, because powder, especially from uncoated tablets, tends to remain on the tray.

Some prescriptions may require compounding, but these represent only a small percentage of the total. The pharmacist must have the knowledge and skills needed to prepare them accurately. **Pharmacy compounding** is defined as the preparation, mixing, assembling, packaging, or labeling of a drug or device. Extemporaneous compounding is essential in the course of professional practice to prepare drug formulations in dosage forms or strengths that are not otherwise commercially available.

Packaging

When the pharmacy technician is in the process of filling a prescription, he or she may select a container from among various types with different shapes, sizes, mouth openings, colors, and compositions. Selection is based primarily on the type and quantity of medication to be dispensed and the method of its use. Figure 8-5 shows some types of medication containers.

All legend drugs intended for oral use must be dispensed by the pharmacist or pharmacy technician to the patient in containers having child-resistant safety closures, unless the prescriber or the patient specifically requests otherwise. Drugs that are used by or given to patients in hospitals, nursing homes, and extended-care facilities need not be dispensed in containers with safety closures unless they are intended for patients who are leaving the confines of the in-

stitution. Examples of child-resistant containers are shown in Figure 8-6.

Rechecking

The pharmacist must recheck every prescription that has been dispensed for verification. All details of the label should be rechecked against the prescription order to verify directions, patient's name, prescription number, date, and prescriber's name. Rechecking is especially important for those drug products available in multiple strengths.

Delivering and Patient Counseling

The pharmacist should personally present the prescription medication to the patient or his or her family member unless it is to be delivered to the patient's home or workplace. There has been an increased awareness that labeling instructions are often inadequate to ensure the patient's understanding of his or her medication. The prescriber and the

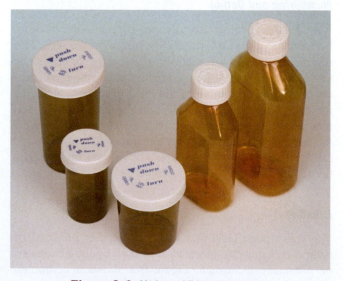

Figure 8-6. Various child-resistant caps.

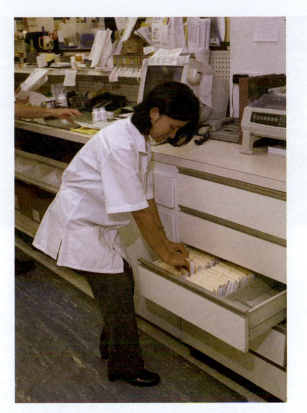

Figure 8-7. Prescription filing system.

pharmacist share the responsibility for ensuring that the patient receives specific instructions, precautions, and warnings for safe and effective use of the prescribed drugs.

Recording and Filing

A record of the prescriptions dispensed is maintained in the pharmacy through the use of computers and hard copy prescription files. Many chain drug stores have central computer systems today, which allows pharmacists from any place in the system to access a patient's record and refill a prescription previously dispensed at another store. There are various types of units available to keep original prescription orders. Metal or cardboard units, which conveniently store approximately 1000 prescriptions, are commonly used (see Figure 8-7). Partitioned drawers often are used for filing. The least common method of filing is microfilming of prescriptions.

Pricing

The pharmacy is a business practice. The pharmacy technician must assist in the financial aspects of this practice so that the business is maintained and makes a fair profit. A method of pricing prescriptions should be established to ensure the profitable operation of the prescription section. The charge applied to a prescription should cover the costs of the ingredients, which include the container and label, the time of the pharmacist or pharmacy technician and auxiliary

personnel involved, the cost of inventory maintenance, and operational costs of the pharmacy. It is obvious that pricing the prescription must provide a reasonable margin of profit on investment.

Refilling

The prescriber must provide instruction for refilling a prescription by indicating on the original prescription the number of appropriate refills. The number of refills of prescriptions for noncontrolled medications is not limited by federal law. State laws may impose such limits. On the other hand, the refilling of prescriptions for controlled agents is strictly regulated. No prescription should be renewed indefinitely without the patient being reevaluated by the prescriber to assure that the medication as originally prescribed remains the drug of choice. The maintenance of accurate records of refilling is important not only for complying with federal and state laws, but also for providing information on the patient's medication history.

ORGANIZATION OF THE RETAIL PHARMACY

Most retail pharmacies have a consistent layout and floor plan. Specific areas are designated for a particular task to be performed. There are also areas for interaction between the patient and the pharmacist or pharmacy technician. All areas of the pharmacy are designed to achieve a particular goal in providing services.

Prescription Counter and Consulting Area

Almost all community pharmacies have similar floor plans and are generally organized into two areas: the front area and the prescription processing area. OTC drugs, cosmetics, and other merchandise items are located in the front area. Only authorized individuals are able to enter the prescription processing areas. The prescription counter is an area that a pharmacist or a technician can use to prepare prescriptions. The consultation area is strictly for the pharmacist's use to counsel patients privately. The technician must always remember that he or she is not legally permitted to counsel patients about medications. This is the role and responsibility of the pharmacist. By state regulations, a description of the space and equipment is required. Figures 8-8 and 8-9 show the front and prescription dispensing areas of community pharmacies.

Transaction Windows

The customer drops off the prescription, new hard copy (or Rx) or refill, or verbally asks for a refill. The technician will obtain all personal information that is required for a hard copy prescription. The technician must put the information in the computer before starting the order. When the information for

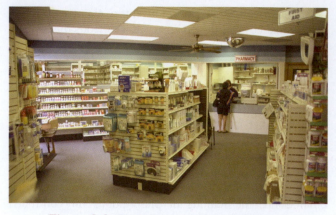

Figure 8-8. The front area of the retail pharmacy.

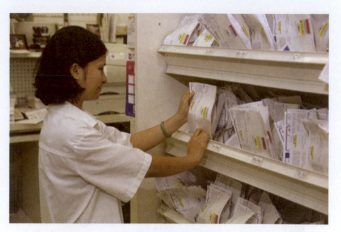

Figure 8-10. Prescription storage area.

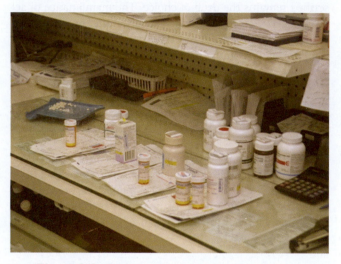

Figure 8-9. The dispensing area of the retail pharmacy.

the prescription has been entered, the order goes to be filed. The community pharmacy is different from the hospital pharmacy. Technicians in the community pharmacy interact with patients as customers. Therefore, customer service is one of the most important aspects in the community pharmacy, and technicians must have strong interpersonal skills. Customers can also pick up their prescription in this area.

Storage

When prescriptions are completed and customers do not pick them up right away, they should be placed in a specific area or on shelves. For storage, prescriptions should be alphabetized by the name of the patient (see Figure 8-10).

Refrigeration

Each pharmacy must have a refrigerator to store drugs that are required to be kept at temperatures between 2 and 8°C. It must be used exclusively for medications. No food or beverages are permitted to be stored in any refrigerator in which medication is stored.

Computer Systems

The use of computers is now standard in pharmacy practice because of the expanded informational needs of the pharmacist. Another factor is the increased amount of paperwork required in practice. Computer systems are essential for promoting efficiency by offering improving technology and expanding databases that provide needed support. Most chain pharmacies are linked together by dedicated telephone lines or satellites, thus facilitating the sharing of information between pharmacies.

There are three areas in the pharmacy in which computerized systems can be used:

- Prescription dispensing and associated record maintenance
- Clinical support and accounting
- Business management

Many insurance and prescription plans now require on-line verification and authorization before the dispensing of any medication. Pharmacists and pharmacy technicians can now use the Internet to obtain and download information about disease states and drug therapy for their patients.

Equipment

Pharmacy technicians need to be familiar with computer hardware and software that applies to the pharmacy environment. Many popular software programs exist, and these are discussed elsewhere in this book. As for hardware, pharmacy computer systems include a monitor, CPU, keyboard, mouse, scanner, modem, printer, and even robotic machinery that handles prescription counting, filling, labeling, and packaging. Pharmacy technicians will need to become proficient in use of all of these types of equipment.

Customer Pick-Up

Some community pharmacies have **drive-through** windows that allow customers or patients to drop-off prescriptions or purchase their medications (see Figure 8-11). Pharmacy

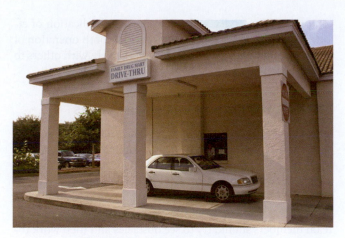

Figure 8-11. Drive-through window.

technicians need to make sure that the correct person is receiving his or her order and not another person's order. The technician must ask if the patient has any questions about the prescription for the pharmacist. The pharmacist should be available for consultation.

Cash Register

The technician may ring up prescriptions and other items such as OTC products into the cash register and accept payment for their purchase. Cash register machines are connected into the pharmacy's computer and can provide prices automatically by using bar code scanners. The pharmacy technician must handle payments properly (see Figure 8-12). For cash payments, he or she must count the payment in the presence of the customer, confirming the amount verbally.

Controlled Substances

The more dangerous substances on drug schedules are called *controlled substances* and are kept in a locked storage cabinet under the pharmacist's supervision. The pharmacy technician must take direction from the pharmacist about

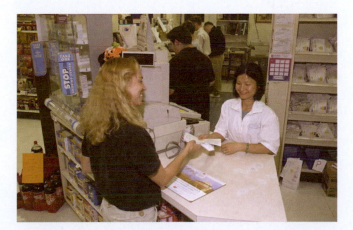

Figure 8-12. Pharmacy technicians must also be able to operate the cash register to take customers' payments.

which controlled substances he or she may handle in preparation of distribution to customers. All controlled substances require prescriptions, and repeated checking of the products, labeling, packaging, and the customer who receives them must be performed for error-free handling.

Purchasing and Inventory Control

The pharmacy technician often orders products for use or sale. He or she may work alone with a purchasing agent or deal directly with pharmaceutical or medical supply companies on matters such as price. The technician must complete a purchase order that includes the product name, amount, and price. The order is then transmitted directly to manufacturers. Although selection of drugs must always remain the responsibility of the pharmacist, purchase orders may be prepared by a pharmacy technician. When pharmaceutical products are received, the technician must carefully check the product against the purchase order. Damaged products must be reported without delay and returned to the manufacturer. The pharmacy technician must check all products for expiration dates.

■ **THE PROFESSIONAL CHARACTERISTICS OF PHARMACY TECHNICIANS**

The pharmacy technician must maintain a professional manner in all aspects of the job. A professional is held accountable for his or her actions while on the job, must maintain an ethical standard of behavior, must clearly and concisely communicate with customers and other health care providers, and must be able to work as a team member and in a fast paced environment.

Accountability

Pharmacy technicians must understand the boundaries of what they can and cannot do legally. They must be accountable for their performance and also their mistakes. An error, even a small one, can have disastrous consequences for a patient, a customer, or the pharmacy itself. The pharmacy technician must develop work habits to ensure accuracy and expect to be held responsible for what he or she does on the job. The technician must always double-check everything to avoid mistakes.

Ethical Standards and Professional Behavior

Ethics is the study of moral values or principles, and a professional is an individual qualified to perform the activities of a specific occupation. **Professionalism** goes beyond the knowledge, skills, and abilities required to perform those activities. The pharmacy technician, as a professional, represents the profession of pharmacy. He or she must always be courteous and listen with focus. The technician must respect the privacy of patients and keep all information confidential. The most important character traits of a good pharmacy technician are honesty, organization, reliability, and dependability. The pharmacist must be able to count on the technician to maintain confidentiality and privacy of patients and behave ethically, even when not under direct supervision, because of the higher level of trust needed to provide excellent patient care. The HIPAA privacy rule became effective on April 14, 2001, and all health care facilities needed to become compliant by April 14, 2003. This rule sets national standards for the protection of health information of patients. To become compliant, the covered entities are required to implement standards to protect individually identifiable health information and guard against the misuse of that information. The Health Insurance Portability and Accountability Act (HIPAA) was drafted to help ensure the confidentiality of medical records, which was discussed in Chapter 2. The privacy rule does not replace federal, state, or other laws that grant individuals even greater privacy protection. Therefore, pharmacy technicians must always keep in mind that they must maintain confidentiality and privacy of patients.

Communication Skills

One of the fundamental skills that the pharmacy technician must acquire to function successfully in the pharmacy is effective verbal communication. Verbal communication is either oral (spoken) or written. Written communication has traditionally been thought of as being more formal than oral conversation. Today, however, with the increasing use of e-mail, written communication is often as informal as oral communication.

Nonverbal communication is easy to understand, and one needs only to pay attention to the other party to interpret what is being conveyed. Facial expression, eye contact, and body position are all methods of communicating without using words. Listening to the words and the tone of voice is important. The pharmacy technician must always use a nonjudgmental expression and tone of voice. Communication skills are covered in more depth in Chapter 16.

Teamwork

A pharmacy technician needs to be genuinely interested in helping people and be warm and caring. He or she should be able to put the needs of others first. An effective health care team working together does not just happen. To be effective, team members work together to provide appropriate care for each patient. Each member of the team must be committed to problem solving, focusing on the patient, and communicating. A team approach to patient care ensures comprehensive service without expensive duplication of effort. Teamwork is also necessary for the smooth operation of the entire pharmacy. Technicians work closely with others to perform their duties.

Ability to Handle a Fast Pace and Stress

A pharmacy technician's ability to learn new ideas, modify his or her thinking, adapt to new situations, and handle stress in the pharmacy is an increasingly important skill in today's evolving and complex health care delivery system. Most difficult problems can be solved if one steps back and looks at the situation from the other person's point of view. Team members should try to see obstacles and then work together to move past the problem. A team member in the pharmacy should expect to work in a high stress environment. The pharmacy technician must handle any workload and other specific situations in a professional manner.

SUMMARY

As the practice of pharmacy has developed, so have the roles of the pharmacy technician. Technicians will regularly receive and review new and refill prescriptions and handle dispensing, labeling, record keeping, pricing, patient profiles, purchasing, billing, phone calls, cash registers, receiving, and inventory. The computer will be a major part of their daily routines. Technicians will be accountable for all of these tasks, trying to perform them with as few errors as possible, in addition to maintaining high ethical and professional standards, having strong communication skills, and being good team players who can handle the high pace and high stress of their jobs. The number of prescriptions dispensed in the United States has rapidly increased, as have the different settings in which the pharmacists practice. To keep up with the rising demand for pharmaceutical products and services, technicians will play a much greater role to support pharmaceutical care.

CRITICAL THINKING

1. Why are privacy and confidentiality so important in the field of health care and pharmacy?
2. Why are controlled substances more heavily regulated than other types of medications?
3. Describe the characteristics that a pharmacy technician should possess. Why are these important?

REVIEW QUESTIONS

1. Prescribed medication is also called
   A. superscription.
   B. subscription.
   C. inscription.
   D. legend drug.

2. Auxiliary labels are used to emphasize
   A. important aspects of aseptic technique.
   B. important characteristics of the dispensed medication.
   C. that technicians complete the dispensed medication.
   D. that technicians satisfy the customers.

3. Child-resistant containers are used in which of the following conditions?
   A. Dispensed medications for patients in the hospital
   B. Dispensed medications for patients in nursing homes
   C. The dispensing of all legend drugs
   D. Dispensed drugs for extended-care facilities

4. Which of the following areas in the community pharmacy is the most important?
   A. Customer service area
   B. Consultation area
   C. Drive-through area
   D. All of the above

5. The pharmacy technician may do which of the following?
   A. Count or pour medications
   B. Empty returned medications to stock containers
   C. Take prescriptions over the phone
   D. Counsel a patient

6. Refills for a prescription may be completed when the
   A. prescription is lost.
   B. refill blank is filled in.
   C. refill blank is left blank.
   D. pharmacist tells the technician to refill the prescription.

7. Which of the following is correct in regard to a prescription?
   A. It must include the full first and last name of the patient.
   B. It must include the patient's social security number.
   C. It must include the pharmacy technician's signature.
   D. It must include the pharmacist's signature.

8. Pharmacists in the community pharmacy provide several important functions, including all of the following, except
   A. provide distribution of prescribed drug products.
   B. compound prescriptions to meet the specific needs of individual patients.
   C. dispense Schedule I drugs in certain situations without a prescription.
   D. educate the public to maximize the intended benefits of drug therapy.

9. In certain states, nurse practitioners and _____ can issue prescriptions with certain restrictions.
   A. medical assistants
   B. pharmacy technicians
   C. pharmacists
   D. respiratory technologists

10. The component parts of a prescription include all of the following, except
    A. date.
    B. medication prescribed (inscription).
    C. dispensing directions to the pharmacist (subscription).
    D. prescriber's signature and tax identification number.

11. With use of the computer, who should determine the compatibility of a newly prescribed medication with other drugs being taken by the patient?
    A. Pharmacy technician
    B. Cardiovascular technician
    C. Medical assistant
    D. Nurse

12. Tablets, capsules, and some other prefabricated dosage forms usually are counted in the pharmacy using a device called the _____.
    A. scanner
    B. tray
    C. counter
    D. dispensary

13. Unless the prescriber or patient requests otherwise, all legend drugs intended for oral use must be dispensed by the pharmacy technician to the patient in containers having
    A. tinted plastic to avoid sunlight damage.
    B. a chemical packet to keep contents dry.
    C. a device inside to remove the medication for use.
    D. a safety closure.

14. The pharmacy technician is legally permitted to counsel patients about medications in which situation?
    A. If it is a medical emergency.
    B. If the patient is younger than 18.
    C. If the pharmacist feels he or she is knowledgeable enough.
    D. Never.

15. One concern about the use of drive-through windows is
    A. that the correct person receives his or her order and not someone else's order.
    B. that patients may not be able to hear what the pharmacy technician tells them.
    C. that they close too early on a regular basis.
    D. that medication could be easily stolen through the window.

Continues

16. The more dangerous drug schedule substances are called _____.
    A. legend drugs
    B. narcotics
    C. hallucinogenics
    D. controlled substances

17. Products that are damaged must be
    A. destroyed immediately.
    B. reported without delay and returned to the manufacturer.
    C. repackaged after removing the damaged portion.
    D. tested to see if they are still able to be sold.

18. OTC drugs require
    A. no prescription.
    B. just a permission slip from the physician.
    C. tinted containers to protect from light.
    D. a legal prescription.

19. Auxiliary labels are also known as
    A. prescriber labels.
    B. strip labels.
    C. record labels.
    D. direction labels.

20. Pharmacy compounding is defined as
    A. the prevention of contamination of capsules and tablets.
    B. the transfer of medication from stock packages to the prescription container.
    C. the preparation, mixing, assembling, packaging, or labeling of a drug or device.
    D. the formulation of dosage forms that are requested by the patient.

Advanced Pharmacy

9

OBJECTIVES

Upon completion of this chapter, the reader should be able to

1. Define long-term care.
2. Explain long-term pharmacy organization.
3. Describe the "nursing home" and the responsibility of the pharmacy.
4. List the most common high-technology therapies.
5. Explain total parenteral nutrition.

6. Describe hospice.
7. Identify the role of clinical pharmacies in ambulatory care.
8. Name the advantages of mail-order pharmacy.
9. Explain the importance of health and safety in nuclear pharmacy.

GLOSSARY

enteral nutrition Feedings given into the gastrointestinal system. Although normal eating qualifies as enteral nutrition, the term is usually applied to specially prepared liquid feedings.

hospice Originally a facility, usually within a hospital, intended to care for the terminally ill, in particular, by providing physical comfort to the patient and emotional support and counseling to the patient and the family.

long-term care A range of health and health-related support services.

long-term care pharmacy organization An organization involving a licensed professional pharmacy or practice that provides medications and clinical services to long-term care facilities and their residents.

mail-order pharmacy A licensed pharmacy that uses the mail or other carriers (e.g., overnight carriers or parcel services) to deliver prescriptions to patients.

nuclear pharmacy A pharmacy that is specially licensed to work with radioactive materials. Previously called radiopharmacy.

parenteral nutrition A combination of amino acids, dextrose, fats, vitamins, minerals, electrolytes, and water administered intravenously. Parenteral nutrition is capable of providing all the nutrients needed to sustain life.

radiopharmaceutical A drug that is or has been made to be radioactive. Although a few radiopharmaceuticals are used to treat diseases (e.g., radioactive iodine), most are used as diagnostic agents.

reagent kit Vials containing particular compounds, usually in freeze-dried form used in nuclear pharmacy.

starter kit A group of medications provided to a hospice patient by the hospice pharmacy to provide a "start" in treatment for most urgent problems that can develop during the last days or weeks of life.

total parenteral nutrition (TPN) An intravenous feeding that supplies all the nutrients necessary for life.

OVERVIEW

Today the role of the pharmacist is expanding. The rapid development of new drugs and drug delivery systems, changes in the health care delivery system, an increase in the acuity of illness of institutionalized patients, and increased emphasis on patient outcomes and quality of health care have contributed to the evolution of pharmacy practice. The primary goal is to reduce health care costs and increase the overall quality of life for the patient. Pharmacy technicians must be trained, skillful, and knowledgeable in these areas, because many of the drug preparation and distribution tasks of pharmacists have been delegated to trained pharmacy technicians. Pharmacy technicians work under the direct supervision of a pharmacist. Pharmacy technicians are trained to work in various care delivery areas, including inpatient care, home care, ambulatory care, and more advanced areas, such as nuclear medicine and chemotherapy.

LONG-TERM CARE PHARMACY SERVICES

Long-term care is defined as a range of health and health-related support services, and it has become an important issue in the total health care system. There are now more long-term facility beds than acute care beds. Future emphasis will be to increase the number of facilities and beds in long-term care, whereas those of acute care will be reduced. With advances in medical sciences and technologies, people are living longer. Prolongation of life expectancy has created a totally new set of problems for the health care system. There has been a rapid rise in the number of people with chronic disease conditions, with associated social and emotional problems, that require a different management approach. The recipients may be people of any age, such as children with congenital anomalies, young adults with lengthy recovery periods from trauma, and frail elderly persons with chronic diseases and multifaceted changes associated with aging (e.g., mental or physical impairment). The goal of long-term care is to enable a person to maintain the maximal possible level of functional independence. The same forces affecting acute care also have had an impact on the growth of long-term care.

The numbers and size of long-term care facilities have increased. There are various types of long-term care facilities, with nursing homes, including skilled-nursing facilities and intermediate-care facilities, being among the most common, and an increasing number of alternative-care sites such as those that offer board and care. Many patients in these facilities are treated with long-term and multiple drug therapy. There are an increasing number of patients being admitted to long-term care facilities who require high-technology pharmacy services. Because of limited resources, most long-term care facilities will contract out dispensing and clinical pharmacy services, meaning that they will pay another company to take care of most patient medications. The licensed professional pharmacy or practice that provides medications and clinical services to long-term care facilities and their residents is called a **long-term care pharmacy organization**. A pharmacist or pharmacy technician does not have to physically be present at the facility during all hours; however, pharmacy services must be made available 24 hours a day.

Pharmacists perform two types of functions for long-term care: distributive and consultant. The distributive pharmacist is responsible for ensuring that patients receive the correct medicines that were ordered. This job is mainly done outside the long-term care facility. The impact and savings of the use of consultant pharmacist services in long-term care have been documented. The role of the pharmacist has been shown to decrease overall medication costs, adverse drug reactions and interactions, medication errors, the length of hospitalization, and mortality rates of long-term care patients. The consultant pharmacist in long-term care is, in many ways, like a hospital pharmacy director, because he or she must supervise all aspects of the comprehensive pharmaceutical services delivered to patients. The consultant pharmacist interacts with doctors, nurses, and other health professionals. The consultant pharmacist is responsible for several different nursing homes or other facilities and may only visit each at certain weekly or monthly intervals. Newer standards, such as the Omnibus Budget Reconciliation Act of 1990 (OBRA '90), and impending national health care reform initiatives require the pharmacist to assume greater responsibility and participation in long-term facility care. In addition to maintaining a safe drug distribution and control system, pharmacists are asked to apply this knowledge by reviewing drug regimens, providing cost containment, participating in patient care and related committees, and developing pharmacy policies and procedures.

HOME HEALTH CARE PHARMACY

Home health care services is one of the fastest growing parts of the health care market. Today, most serious medical conditions and problems are treated outside the hospital setting, many times at home. Home health care is an important part of the continuum of care. The growth of this system is related to several factors, such as the increase in the number of elderly persons, patient preference, lower costs, improvement of technology, managed care, and physician acceptance. The services rendered are performed under the supervision of individuals licensed to provide such services or care in accordance with the laws of the state in which the care is given. A state-licensed administrator assumes responsibility for facility operations, including the quality of health care rendered to the clients. The

TABLE 9-1. Sources of Payment for Home Care	
PAYMENT SOURCE	**PERCENT**
Medicare	39.0
Medicaid	27.2
Private insurance	12.0
Out-of-pocket	20.5
Other and unknown	1.3
Total	100.0

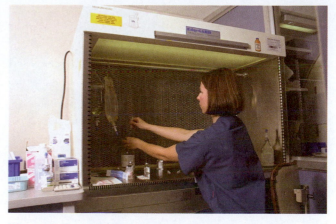

Figure 9-1. Home infusion therapy is one of many expanding areas for pharmacy practice the pharmacy technician can work in.

major services provided in nursing homes include nursing care, personal care, and residual care. Nursing procedures require the professional skills of a registered nurse or a licensed practical nurse. These skills include administering medication, giving injections, placing catheters, and performing other procedures ordered by the physician. Posthospital care after strokes, heart disease, or orthopedic procedures is available.

Several types of home health care services may be available. These include the following:

- Pharmaceutical services
- Nursing services
- Personal care services
- Rehabilitation services
- Home medical supply services

The use of home care is a viable alternative that is safe and cost effective. It is also mutually satisfying to the patient and caregiver. The major sources of payment for home care are Medicare and Medicaid (see Table 9-1).

There are many home health care products and services provided by pharmacies today. These services include provision of durable medical supplies, orthopedic supplies, oxygen therapy, wound care, artificial limbs, medical devices, prescription medications, and infusion therapy (intravenous [IV] and nutritional therapy). For patients with multiple conditions that require monitoring of treatment beyond high-technology therapy, the home care providers and the patient's regular physician will continue to be involved. The technician can assist the pharmacist in these services. The most common high-technology therapies include the following:

- IV antibiotic therapy
- Chemotherapy
- Pain medication
- Total parenteral nutrition
- Enteral nutrition
- Renal dialysis
- Respiratory and ventilation therapy

High-technology home care requires close collaboration of the physician, the pharmacist, the registered nurse, and, depending on the type of therapy, the medical supply company.

HOME INFUSION PHARMACY

Home infusion pharmacy is a unique practice for pharmacists and pharmacy technicians. In this type of practice, infusion therapies are prepared and dispensed to patients in the home. In the acute care and home IV therapy environment, substantial pharmacy effort is devoted to the preparation of sterile products for IV and other parenteral administration (see Figure 9-1). Home infusion pharmacy service includes preparation of IV solutions, other injectable drugs, and enteral nutrition therapy. This type of service involves the safe compounding of an IV solution and its delivery to the patient. Equipment and supplies needed to infuse the solution are also provided. Home infusion pharmacies may be used in different areas, such as community pharmacies, long-term care pharmacies, and hospital pharmacies.

Several types of infusion therapies are prescribed for home infusion, depending on the conditions of patients. These therapies include antibiotic therapy, pain management therapy, hydration therapy, total parenteral nutrition therapy, and cytotoxic cancer chemotherapy agents. Drugs added to IV solutions can be degraded by the diluting solution and by the effects of light, heat, and the storage environment. Drugs mixed in an IV solution also can interact with each other, leading to decreased effectiveness or to toxicity. The IV admixture itself may be contaminated through manipulation, leading to bacterial growth and transmission of bacteria to the patient. Some new biotechnology-derived drugs have very short periods of stability and may require special techniques for dilution and dispersion. Accuracy of preparation supports delivery of the labeled amount and ensures consistency from dose to dose and from patient to patient. In the past, IV solutions were prepared by nurses on the patient care units, but this practice is no longer recommended.

There is a variety of equipment found in home infusion pharmacy such as automated compounding and dispensing devices, horizontal and vertical laminar flow hoods, a

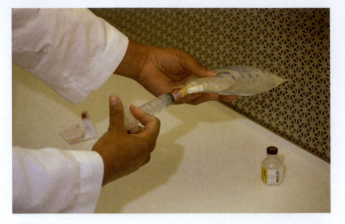

Figure 9-2. Preparation of intravenous medications within a sterile environment is one of the primary responsibilities of the pharmacy technician working in home infusion pharmacy.

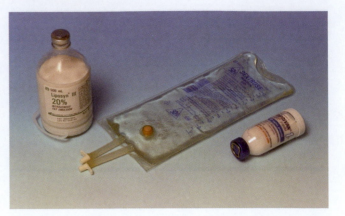

Figure 9-3. Total parenteral nutrition (TPN) consists of amino acid (protein), dextrose (carbohydrate), fats, electrolytes, vitamins, trace elements, and medication (e.g., insulin and heparin).

refrigerator with a locked compartment for storage of drugs, computer hardware, and printers. Supplies found in home infusion pharmacy include syringes, needles, dispensing pins, IV solution containers, filters, transfer sets, IV tubing, alcohol preparation pads, gloves, masks, gowns, beard and shoe covers, and others.

One of the main duties of the pharmacy technician in home infusion pharmacy is the processing of equipment and supply orders. The pharmacy technician must be familiar with vascular access and vascular access devices, infusion devices, and other IV delivery systems. The pharmacy technician performs the compounding of sterile products and handling of home infusion equipment and supplies (see Figure 9-2).

He or she must have knowledge and skills specific to home infusion therapies and nutritional products, sterile compounding, aseptic technique, pharmaceutical calculations, and computer skills and understanding of the laws and regulations pertaining to home infusion pharmacy. The pharmacy technician may be responsible for compounding, equipment and supplies, and computer functions in home infusion pharmacy. Pharmacy technicians must be familiar with nutrition therapy. There are two types of nutritional therapy provided by home infusion pharmacy: parenteral and enteral.

In **parenteral nutrition** therapy, nutrients are delivered directly into the bloodstream. **Total parenteral nutrition (TPN)** consists of amino acid (protein), dextrose (carbohydrate), fats, electrolytes, vitamins, trace elements, and medication (e.g., insulin and heparin) (see Figure 9-3). TPN formulations are highly complex, and proper mixing is important. A safe and effective order of mixing ingredients should be followed. TPN formulations for home infusion are usually prepared several days before they are administered.

In **enteral nutrition** therapy, foods and nutrients are delivered into the gastrointestinal (GI) tract through a tube. This process is called tube feeding and is the most common

home infusion nutritional therapy. Enteral nutrition can be used to supplement oral or parenteral nutrition, or it can be used to meet the patient's entire nutritional needs. Patients with swallowing problems resulting from conditions such as stroke, dementia, trauma, cancer, or acquired immunodeficiency syndrome (AIDS) are candidates for home enteral nutrition. Feeding tubes placed into the stomach through the nose are used for short-term therapy of up to 3 to 4 weeks. Feeding tubes placed into the stomach or small intestine through the skin are used for long-term enteral therapy. Various enteral feeding routes are shown in Figure 9-4.

HOSPICE PHARMACY

Hospice is an organized program of services to meet the medical, physical, emotional, spiritual, and social needs of a patient who is terminally ill, in both the hospital and home setting. Hospice care focuses on the patient's comfort rather than on a cure for the disease. Hospice care allows the patient to live the remainder of his or her life as free from pain and other symptoms as possible. Hospice serves all types and ages of patients. Hospice services are provided in various settings. The preferred setting is in the patient's home. An inpatient hospice facility may provide a safe and comfortable alternative. Funding for hospice programs comes from Medicare, Medicaid, and private insurance. For a patient to be eligible for hospice care under Medicare, a physician must certify that death is expected within 6 months. The average length of stay in hospice is 51 days. Hospices are licensed by the state department of health. Hospice recognizes dying as part of the normal process of living and focuses on maintaining the quality of life. Hospice affirms life and neither hastens nor postpones death. The philosophy of hospice is that through appropriate care and the promotion of a caring community sensitive to their needs, patients and

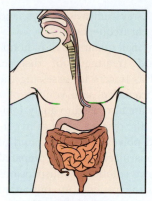

Nasogastric Route

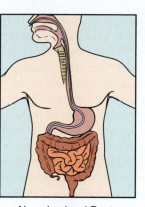

Nasoduodenal Route

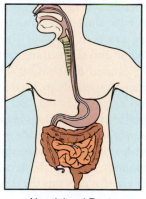

Nasojejunal Route

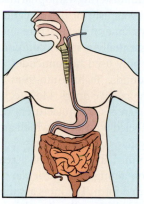

Esophagostomy Route

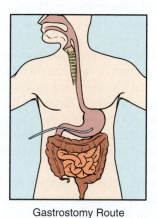

Gastrostomy Route

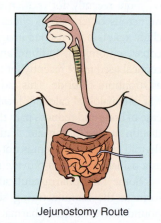

Jejunostomy Route

Figure 9-4. Enteral feeding routes.

their families may be free to attain a degree of mental and spiritual preparation for death that is satisfactory to them. Hospice offers palliative care to terminally ill people and support to their families without regard to age, sex, nationality, race, creed, sexual orientation, disability, diagnosis, availability of primary caregiver, or ability to pay.

Pharmacists have become involved in hospice by providing needed medications and pharmaceutical care services to patients who are terminally ill or nearing the end of life. A pharmacy must prepare and dispense medications, medication-related equipment and supplies, and pharmaceutical care

services to hospice patients at home or in an inpatient facility. A hospice pharmacy can be part of a traditional community pharmacy, in which hospice is a part of its business, or it can be a pharmacy that services only hospice patients. Hospice pharmacy services can be divided into two areas: clinical services and dispensing services. Clinical services include pain management, symptom management, medication monitoring, drug regimen review, drug information services, and formulary development and management. Dispensing services include medications and related equipment and supplies, sterile IV infusion compounding (pain, hydration, and chemotherapy), starter kits, and 24-hour on-call coverage. A **starter kit** is a group of medications that is given to a hospice patient by the hospice pharmacy to provide a "start" in treatment for most urgent problems that can develop during the last days or weeks of life. Patients may suffer from pain, fever, nausea, vomiting, anxiety, agitation, increased secretions, and constipation.

AMBULATORY CARE PHARMACY

The provision of ambulatory care services increased dramatically during the 1980s and mid- to late 1990s. Traditionally, most outpatient care has been provided in hospital-based facilities and, in most cases, on the campuses of such hospitals. During the 1980s and 1990s, the health care industry experienced explosive growth in the type of ownership of facilities in which ambulatory care was offered. Various designations are used to categorize patients: institutionalized, noninstitutionalized, inpatient, outpatient, bedridden, and ambulatory. One of the most significant trends in health care has been the emphasis on shorter hospital stays and on outpatient care. Ambulatory patients are those who are able to walk and who are responsible for obtaining their medication, storing it, and taking it. Ambulatory care has become the standard for health care delivery. The term *ambulatory care* includes a range of services such as outpatient pharmacies, emergency departments, primary care clinics, specialty clinics, ambulatory care centers, and family practice groups. At present, ambulatory care services provide radiation therapy, dialysis centers, diagnostic imaging, mobile imaging, rehabilitation, free-standing ambulatory surgery, urgent care, wound care, sleep study laboratories, infusion/chemotherapy, ambulatory clinical pharmacy, and endoscopy centers.

The increase in ambulatory care services has greatly expanded the opportunities for ambulatory care pharmacy practitioners. Clinical pharmacists practice in various primary care clinics. The clinical pharmacist improves drug therapy documentation, improves patient compliance, decreases duplicate prescriptions, and prevents the risk of overdosage. The pharmacy clinic provides refills to drop-in patients. Patients are referred by physicians to clinical pharmacists, who provide physical assessment, order laboratory tests, alter dosages, and change medications. One of the most successful pharmacist-managed ambulatory clinics has been the anticoagulation clinic. The value of clinical pharmacists in the chronic management of patients with hypertension, diabetes, and allergies of patients receiving anticoagulation therapy is obvious. One of the most important aspects of ambulatory care practice is the involvement of the clinical pharmacist in drug therapy decisions. This requires that the pharmacist be available and accessible when the patient is being seen. It is clear that successful ambulatory care pharmacy services must be comprehensive and continual. Clinical pharmacy services must be provided 80% to 90% percent of the time.

MAIL-ORDER PHARMACY

Mail-order pharmacy is defined as a pharmacy that dispenses maintenance medications to patients through mail delivery. It is one of the fastest growing areas in pharmacy practice. It is offered by most health plans today as an option to the traditional retail pharmacy for obtaining prescriptions. Medications are sent to patients through mail or delivery services. Mail-order pharmacy is a unique setting for pharmacists and pharmacy technicians. Staff members consist of licensed pharmacists, registered nurses, and technicians. Mail-order pharmacies provide services to all 50 states. Therefore, they operate at a high volume, which results in discounts and is more economical for patients. Mail-order pharmacies can serve more patients, particularly those who have chronic illnesses such as diabetes, high blood pressure, depression, heart disease, arthritis, or gastrointestinal disorders. The need for medication can be predicted, and the supply can be easily maintained by mail delivery. Medication, that is required regularly for the treatment of a chronic condition is called a maintenance medication. In most cases, mail-order pharmacies contract with health insurers and fill prescriptions at discounted rates for members of those plans.

NUCLEAR PHARMACY

Nuclear pharmacy is a branch of pharmacy that deals with the provisions of services related to radiopharmaceuticals. A **radiopharmaceutical** is a radioactive drug that is used in the diagnosis and treatment of disease. A radiopharmaceutical consists of both a drug component and a radioactive component. The drug component is responsible for localization in specific organs or tissues. The radioactive component contains radioactive elements. The three types of radiation that can be released by a radionuclide are alpha, beta, and gamma. Gamma radiation is the most penetrating type of radiation. It differs from alpha and beta radiation, because it is electromagnetic, whereas they are particulate.

Gamma radiation differs from X-rays, ultraviolet rays, and visible light only in wavelength (or frequency).

Nuclear medicine uses very small quantities of radionuclides for the diagnosis and treatment of disease. Radiopharmaceuticals are used as tracers for assessing the structure, function, secretion, excretion, and volume of a particular organ or tissue. They are also used to analyze biological specimens; to treat specific diseases such as hyperthyroidism, thyroid cancer, and polycythemia vera; and to alleviate bone pain. Most radiopharmaceuticals are prepared as sterile, pyrogen-free intravenous solutions or suspensions to be administered directly to the patient. An important component of nuclear medicine is imaging, which involves administering radiopharmaceuticals to a patient orally, intravenously, or by inhalation to localize a specific organ or system and its structure and function. Nuclear pharmacy is essentially a sterile compounding practice. The most commonly used radionuclides are iodine and technetium compounds. Technetium-99m (^{99m}Tc) is used in about 80% of radioactive drugs. Most technetium compounds are used for diagnosis. Manufacturers develop compounds that can be labeled with ^{99m}Tc, which are used for imaging various organ systems or tissues. These compounds are often available in a form that is known as a **reagent kit**. Reagent kits are vials containing the particular compounds, usually in freeze-dried form. The kit is a multidose vial that contains the compound (ligand) as it is labeled.

Iodine-131 (^{131}I) is used for treatment of hyperthyroidism or, more recently, for ovarian and prostate cancer. There are numerous other radionuclides used in medicine. These include xenon (a gas used to image the lungs), thallium, gallium, cobalt, chromium, indium, and strontium. A radiopharmaceutical used more recently for treatment is strontium-89 (^{89}Sr) as strontium chloride. This radionuclide emits beta radiation. ^{89}Sr, an analog of calcium, localizes in areas of metastatic disease of bone and reduces pain through the effect of the beta radiation at the tumor site. Unlike the use of ^{131}I to destroy thyroid cancer, this agent is not used to cure cancer, but rather as a palliative agent to provide relief from pain.

Some radiopharmaceuticals are prepared in their final form at the manufacturing site, whereas others are compounded in a nuclear pharmacy or nuclear medicine department. There are several levels of sophistication to compound these agents, such as simple addition of radioactive pertechnetate to the reagent kit vial, radiolabeling of autologous blood cells, custom radiolabeling of peptides and antibodies, and rapid hot laboratory chemical compounding of short-lived positron-emitting radiopharmaceuticals. Because the radionuclides commonly used in radiopharmaceuticals have short half-lives, most radiopharmaceuticals must be prepared on the day of use. Nuclear pharmacy involves the procuring, storage, compounding, dispensing, and provision of information about radiopharmaceuticals and is one possible area of specialization for both pharmacists and pharmacy technicians (see Figure 9-5). To practice nuclear pharmacy, pharmacists must have specialized training in several areas, such

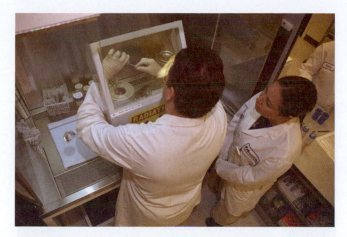

Figure 9-5. Nuclear pharmacy is another area of specialization for pharmacy technicians to work in.

as nuclear physics, radiation detection instrumentation, radiochemistry, and radiation protection.

Experience in a practice site is essential as well. The level of knowledge and experience necessary, as well as services provided, vary with the practice site. Most nuclear pharmacists practice in a centralized commercial nuclear pharmacy. Most practitioners in this setting have a professional degree, whereas nuclear pharmacists in an institutional site commonly have received an advanced degree (MS). The basic functions are similar; however, the pharmacist in the larger hospital may be more involved with clinical service, investigational products, and teaching. The pharmacist in a centralized nuclear pharmacy inherently spends considerable time preparing and dispensing radiopharmaceuticals, because one pharmacy generally services 10 to 15 hospitals and clinics.

Guidelines for Practice of Nuclear Pharmacy

The practice of nuclear pharmacy is a specialized field of pharmacy that requires specific guidelines and regulations. The nine general areas involved in nuclear pharmacy practice are the following:

1. Procurement
2. Compounding
3. Quality assurance
4. Dispensing
5. Distribution
6. Health and safety
7. Provision of information and consultation
8. Monitoring patient outcome
9. Regulations

Procurement

Procurement of radiopharmaceuticals and other drugs, supplies, and materials necessary for nuclear pharmacy practice involves determining product specifications, initiating

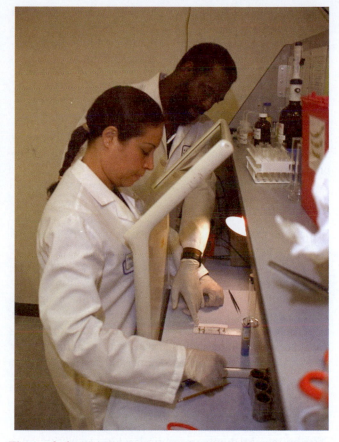

Figure 9-6. One of the primary duties within nuclear pharmacy is that of compounding radiopharmaceuticals.

purchase orders, receiving shipments, maintaining inventory, and storing materials under proper conditions. Although these tasks appear similar to those involved in community and hospital pharmacy practice, the special characteristics of and requirements associated with radiopharmaceuticals present some unique demands. For example, radiopharmaceuticals or radioactive components, because of their short half-lives, are not available through conventional wholesalers; rather, they typically are ordered directly from the manufacturers. Receipt of radioactive materials involves following regulatory procedures for opening packages, including performing surveys for radioactive contamination. Inventory control of radioactive materials is complicated by their distinctive, continuous radioactive decay. Fortunately, repetitive manual calculations have been replaced by computer programs developed for this purpose.

Compounding

Compounding of radiopharmaceuticals involves various activities ranging from relatively simple tasks such as reconstituting reagent kits with ^{99m}Tc sodium pertechnetate to complex tasks (see Figure 9-6). Compounding of radiopharmaceuticals requires receipt of a valid prescription or drug order; appropriate components, supplies, and equipment; a suitable environment, especially for sterile dosage forms; appropriate record keeping; and verification of the compounding procedure, storage conditions, and expiration.

Quality Assurance

Quality assurance of radiopharmaceuticals involves performing the appropriate chemical, physical, and biological tests on radiopharmaceuticals to ensure the suitability of the products for use in humans.

Dispensing

Dispensing radiopharmaceuticals occurs upon the receipt of a valid prescription or drug order. In contrast to traditional pharmacy practice, radiopharmaceuticals are rarely dispensed directly to patients; rather, they are dispensed to hospitals or clinics for administration to patients by trained health professionals. Radiopharmaceuticals generally are dispensed in unit doses ready for administration to the patient. In addition to radiopharmaceuticals, certain other drugs, such as those used in pharmacological intervention studies, often are dispensed by nuclear pharmacists.

Distribution

Distribution of radiopharmaceuticals within an institution is subject to institutional policies and procedures, generally involving lead-lined boxes or other shielded containers labeled with identifying information (see Figure 9-7).

Distribution of radiopharmaceuticals from a centralized nuclear pharmacy to other institutions is subject to local, state, and federal regulations, including those promulgated by state boards of pharmacy, the U.S. Department of Transportation, and the U.S. Nuclear Regulatory Commission (NRC). These requirements generally relate to packaging, labeling, shipping papers, other record keeping, and personnel training.

Health and Safety

Health and safety are crucial elements of nuclear pharmacy practice. Radiation safety standards, including limits for radiation doses, levels of radiation in an area, concentrations of radioactivity in air and waste water, waste disposal, and precautionary procedures have been established and are enforced by the NRC. Although radiation protection may be the most visible and most regulated, other aspects of health and safety are also important. Hazardous chemicals, such as chromatography solvents, must be stored, handled, and disposed of using proper techniques, personal protective devices, containers, and environment. Biological specimens, such as blood samples obtained for preparation of labeled red and white blood cells, must be handled as potentially infectious, using standard precautions. Last, physical exertion, such as lifting heavy lead shields, must be done with appropriate care.

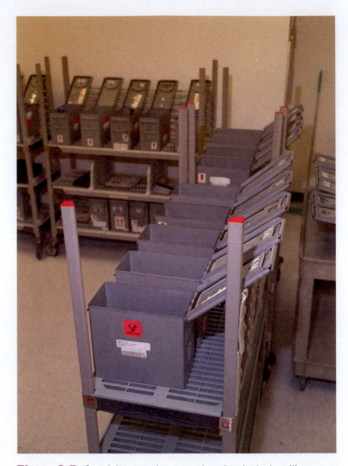

Figure 9-7. Special precautions must be taken in the handling, care, storage, and distribution of radioactive materials.

Provision of Information and Consultation

Provision of information and consultation is a highly important function of nuclear pharmacists. Using both oral and written communication skills, nuclear pharmacists convey their expert knowledge to physicians, technologists, pharmacy technicians, patients, and others. The nuclear pharmacist should provide appropriate types of information, including the biological effects of radiation, radiation physics and radiation protection, radiopharmaceutical chemistry, radiopharmaceutical compounding, and quality assurance.

Monitoring Patient Outcome

Monitoring patient outcome is an important component in pharmaceutical care. A nuclear pharmacist can assist to ensure that patients are referred for appropriate nuclear medicine procedures. Evaluating the safety and efficacy of radiopharmaceutical and ancillary medications is important, as is ensuring that patients receive proper preparation before receiving radiopharmaceuticals. A nuclear pharmacist must be sure that clinical problems associated with the use of the radiopharmaceuticals are prevented or

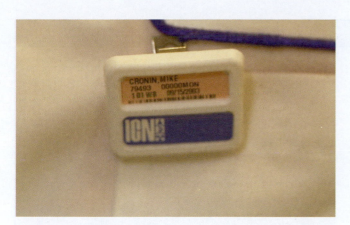

Figure 9-8. Staff within the nuclear pharmacy must wear devices to monitor the amount of radiation exposure they experience while on the job.

recognized, investigated, and rectified. He or she must be administering therapeutic or diagnostic radiopharmaceuticals and ancillary medications and performing nuclear medicine procedures.

Regulations

Regulation of nuclear pharmacy practice is the responsibility of the NRC. This commission issues licenses and has regulatory authority for functions relating to by-products of radioactive materials; however, individual states are responsible for regulating accelerator-produced materials in a manner similar to their regulation of X-ray–producing machines. The primary responsibility of the NRC is to provide for the safety of workers and the general public exposed to radiation and to protect their health and minimize danger to life and property. Badges must be worn by all health care professionals who work with radiation, and the badges are monitored monthly (see Figure 9-8). The responsibility of employing organization is to ensure that no worker is exposed to higher levels of radiation than those approved by the NRC, to maintain a radiation safety committee, to monitor and control patient exposure, and to provide lead shielding to protect all vulnerable body parts.

SUMMARY

Because of advances in medical science and technology, people are living longer, resulting in the need for more long-term care than ever before. Long-term pharmacy organizations have been created to provide medications and clinical services to these long-term care facilities. In addition, home health care services have expanded to include pharmaceutical, nursing, personal care, rehabilitation, and home medical supply services. High-technology home care includes administration of IV antibiotics, chemotherapy, pain medications, TPN, and enteral nutrition; renal dialysis; respiratory and ventilation therapy; and even hospice services for the terminally ill. Clinical pharmacists are routinely involved in drug therapy decisions for ambulatory care practices. Mail-order pharmacies, which dispense medications through mail delivery, have become one of the fastest growing areas in pharmacy. One possible area of specialization is nuclear pharmacy, which involves the procuring, storage, compounding, dispensing, and provision of information about radiopharmaceuticals. With so much growth in advanced pharmacy, it is essential that pharmacy technicians be trained in all areas that reflect the growing needs of the public.

CRITICAL THINKING

1. Research one of the areas of advanced practice discussed in the chapter. What are the educational requirements for working in this field? What are the primary duties of the pharmacy technician in this field? Of the pharmacist in this field?
2. Of the areas of advanced pharmacy practice discussed in this chapter, what field do you think will experience the most growth in the future? Why?

REVIEW QUESTIONS

1. NRC is the abbreviation for
   A. The Nuclear Regulatory Commission.
   B. The Nuclear Registry Center.
   C. Nuclear Remission Cancer.
   D. Nuclear Register Consulting.

2. The major services provided in nursing homes include
   A. assuring the patient's comfort rather than caring for their disease.
   B. satisfying Medicare requirements for palliative care to the terminally ill.
   C. meeting the physical, emotional, and spiritual needs of a patient.
   D. nursing care.

3. Compounding of radiopharmaceuticals requires
   A. payment in advance.
   B. a patient's insurance card.
   C. receipt of a valid prescription.
   D. technicians who are nationally certified.

4. One of the fastest growing areas in pharmacy is
   A. health care administration.
   B. mail-order.
   C. traditional.
   D. all of the above.

5. Home health care services include
   A. nursing.
   B. pharmaceutical.
   C. rehabilitation.
   D. all of the above.

6. Home infusion pharmacy includes
   A. radiography.
   B. enteral nutrition therapy.
   C. physical therapy.
   D. hydrotherapy.

7. At present, ambulatory care services provide
   A. surgery.
   B. sleep study laboratory.
   C. pharmacy.
   D. all of the above.

8. Which of the following patients are the best candidates for home enteral nutrition therapy?
   A. Those who have cancer
   B. Those who suffered from a stroke
   C. Those who are nauseated
   D. Those who have bone fractures

9. Which of the following emissions from the decay of radionuclides is most commonly used in nuclear medicine imaging?
   A. Beta
   B. Gamma
   C. Alpha
   D. X-ray

10. Which of the following radionuclides is most commonly used in nuclear pharmacy practice?
    A. ^{99m}Tc
    B. ^{133}Xe
    C. ^{123}I
    D. ^{67}Ga

11. Radiopharmaceutical agents can be administered
    A. intravenously.
    B. orally.
    C. by inhalation.
    D. all of the above.

12. The major source of payment for home care is
    A. Medicaid.
    B. private insurance.
    C. Medicare.
    D. A and C.

13. All of the following equipment can be found in home infusion pharmacy, except
    A. horizontal laminar flow hoods.
    B. refrigerators with locked compartments.
    C. automated compounding.
    D. rehabilitation equipment.

14. Total parenteral nutrition (TPN) formulations for home infusion are usually prepared how long before they are administered?
    A. Less than 1 hour
    B. Several hours
    C. Several days
    D. Several years

15. Which of the following is one of the fastest growing parts of the health care market?
    A. Home nuclear pharmacy
    B. Home health care services
    C. Home mental care services
    D. All of the above

Extemporaneous Prescription Compounding

OBJECTIVES

Upon completion of this chapter, the reader should be able to

1. Demonstrate the use of a class A prescription balance, a counter balance, and a solution balance.
2. Describe extemporaneous compounding.
3. Describe the difference between a solution, a suspension, an ointment, and a cream.
4. Use the proper technique for measuring liquid volumes.
5. Explain the proper technique for weighing pharmaceutical ingredients.
6. State the ingredients found in an enteral solution.
7. Name the most common and important equipment for extemporaneous compounding.
8. Explain different meanings of compounding terms used by different pharmacists.
9. Identify the different types of graduates and which one is more accurate.

GLOSSARY

class A prescription balance A two-pan device that may be used for weighing small amounts of drugs (not more than 120 g).

compounding slab A plate made of ground glass with a hard, flat, and nonabsorbent surface for mixing compounds.

conical graduates Devices used for measuring liquids that have wide tops and wide bases and taper from the top to the bottom.

counter balance A device capable of weighing much larger quantities, up to about 5 kg. It is a double-pan balance.

cylindrical graduates Devices used for measuring liquids that have narrow diameters that are the same from top to base.

electronic balance A two-pan device that may be used for weighing small amounts of drugs (not more than 120 g).

extemporaneous compounding The preparation, mixing, assembling, packaging, and labeling of a drug product based on a prescription order from a licensed practitioner for the individual patient.

geometric dilution When mixing agents, the medicament is first mixed with an equal weight of diluent. A further quantity of diluent equal in weight to the mixture is then incorporated. This process is repeated until all the diluent has been mixed in.

levigate To grind into a smooth substance with moisture.

meniscus Meaning "moon-shaped body"; indicates that the level of the liquid will be slightly higher at the edges.

mortar A cup-shaped vessel in which materials are ground or crushed.

pestle A solid device that is used to crush or grind materials in a mortar.

pipette A long, thin, calibrated hollow tube, which is made of glass used for measuring liquids.

solution A liquid dosage form in which active ingredients are dissolved in a liquid vehicle.

solvent The liquid substance in which another substance is being dissolved.

GLOSSARY continued

suspension A liquid dosage form that contains solid drug particles floating in a liquid medium.

tablet triturate Solid, small, and usually cylindrically molded or compressed tablets.

tare The weight of an empty capsule used to compare with the full capsule.

triturate To reduce a fine powder by friction.

OVERVIEW

Compounding has always been a basic part of pharmacy practice. The equipment or techniques, drugs, and dosage forms used are the variables. Manufacturing is the mass production of compounded prescription products for resale to pharmacies and is regulated by the Food and Drug Administration (FDA). Today, on many occasions, the pharmacist or technician may practice this ancient art. Good manufacturing practices are the standards of practice used in the pharmaceutical industry and are regulated by the FDA. Community pharmacists must comply with state board of pharmacy regulations and guidelines to ensure a quality product, which includes using proper materials, weighing equipment, documented technique, and dispensing and storage instructions. The liability of compounding is no greater than the risk of filling a prescription for a manufactured product, because the pharmacist must ensure that the correct drug, dose, and directions are provided.

EXTEMPORANEOUS COMPOUNDING

Extemporaneous compounding is the preparation, mixing, assembling, packaging, and labeling of a drug product based on a prescription order from a licensed practitioner for the individual patient. The pharmacist is responsible for preparing a quality pharmaceutical product, providing proper instructions about its storage, and advising the patient of any adverse effects. Compounding may have different meanings for different pharmacists, including the following:

- The preparation of oral liquids, topical preparations, and suppositories
- The conversion of one dose or dosage form into another
- The preparation of select dosage forms from bulk chemicals
- The preparation of intravenous admixtures, parenteral nutrition solutions, and pediatric dosage forms from adult dosage forms
- The preparation of radioactive isotopes
- The preparation of cassettes, syringes, and other devices with drugs for administration in the home setting

Equipment

The correct equipment is important when compounding. Therefore, pharmacy technicians should be familiar with those pieces of equipment that are necessary for compounding drugs. Many state boards of pharmacy have a required minimum list of equipment for compounding prescriptions. These pieces of equipment vary according to the amount of material needed and the type of compounded prescription. There are several conventional pieces of equipment and instruments that a pharmacist or pharmacy technician may use for the operation of compounding. These include balances, forceps, spatulas, a compounding slab, mortar and pestle, graduates, and pipettes.

Class A Prescription Balance

Each pharmacy is required to have a **class A prescription balance** and/or an **electronic balance** (see Figure 10-1). Class A balances have a sensitivity requirement of 6 mg. This piece of equipment is a two-pan balance that may be used for weighing small amounts of drugs (not more than 120 g).

Counter Balance

A **counter balance** is capable of weighing larger quantities, up to about 5 kg. It is a double-pan balance. A counter balance is not indicated for prescription compounding. It is used for measuring bulk products.

Weights

Good-quality weights are essential, and they should be stored appropriately. Weights made from corrosion-resistant metals, such as brass, are preferred (see Figure 10-2). Metric weights are in the front row and apothecary weights are in the back row. When transferring weights, you should always be careful not to drop them, and you should always use forceps.

Spatulas

Spatulas are available in stainless steel, plastic, or hard rubber (see Figure 10-3). Spatulas are used to transfer solid ingredients, such as ointments and creams, to weighing pans. Spatulas are also used to mix compounds on an ointment slab. They must be clean and have indented edges.

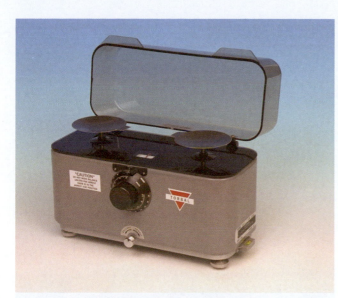

Figure 10-1. Class A prescription balance.

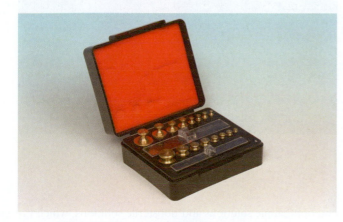

Figure 10-2. Weights used in pharmacy practice.

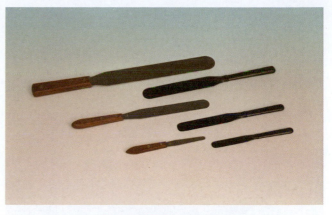

Figure 10-3. Spatulas.

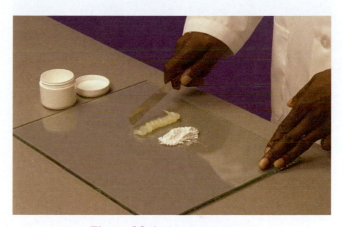

Figure 10-4. Compounding slab.

Compounding Slab

The **compounding slab** is a plate made of ground glass with a hard, flat, and nonabsorbent surface for mixing compounds (see Figure 10-4). Compounding slabs are also called ointment slabs.

Mortar and Pestle

A **mortar** is a cup-shaped vessel in which materials are ground or crushed by a **pestle** in the preparation of drugs. Mortars and pestles are available in three types: glass (see Figure 10-5B), Wedgwood, and porcelain (see Figure 10-5A), which is quite similar to Wedgwood in use and appearance. Glass mortars are preferred for mixing liquids and semisoft dosage forms. Advantages of glass mortars and pestles are that they are nonporous and nonstaining.

Graduates and Pipettes

To measure liquids you need equipment, which consists of conical graduates, cylindrical graduates, pipettes, or syringes. **Conical graduates** have wide tops and wide bases and taper from the top to the bottom (see Figure 10-6). They are easier to clean than cylindrical graduates. **Cylindrical graduates** are designed with a narrow diameter that is the same from top to base. Cylindrical graduates are more accurate than conical graduates (see Figure 10-7). These types of graduates are generally calibrated in metric units (cubic centimeters), and conical graduates are mostly calibrated in both metric and apothecary units. Both types of graduates are used in different sizes, ranging from 5 mL to >1,000 mL (1 liter). The smallest graduate available should always be used to measure a particular volume of liquid. Measuring of volumes that are less than 20% of the capacity of the graduate should be avoided, because the accuracy is unacceptable. A **pipette** can be used for measurement of volumes of liquids <1.5 mL. This device is a long, thin, calibrated, hollow tube that is made of glass. There are two types of pipettes: mouth or auto-pipettes.

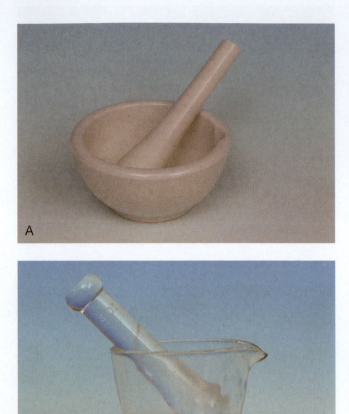

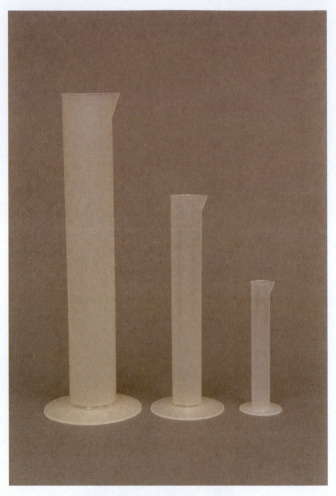

Figure 10-7. Cylindrical graduates.

Figure 10-5. (A) Porcelain mortar and pestle. (B) Glass mortar and pestle.

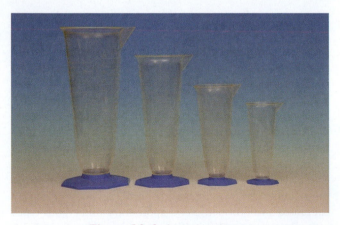

Figure 10-6. Conical graduates.

COMPOUNDING SOLUTIONS

A **solution** is a liquid dosage form in which active ingredients are dissolved in a liquid vehicle. This vehicle is known as a **solvent**. There are two types of solutions: sterile parenteral

and ophthalmic solutions and nonsterile solutions, which include oral, topical, or otic solutions. Liquids are the most common form of compounded medications. Solutions are the easiest of the dosage forms to compound extemporaneously, as long as a few general rules are followed:

1. Each drug is dissolved in the solvent in which it is most soluble. Therefore, the solubility characteristics of each drug or chemical must be known.
2. If an alcoholic solution of a poor water-soluble drug is used, an aqueous solution is added to the alcoholic solution to maintain as high an alcohol concentration as possible.
3. The salt form of the drug and not the free-acid or base form, which both have poor solubility, is used.
4. When a salt is added to a syrup, the salt should be dissolved in a few milliliters of water first and then the syrup added to volume.
5. The proper vehicle, such as syrup, elixir, aromatic water, or purified water, must be selected.
6. Flavoring or sweetening agents are prepared ahead of time.

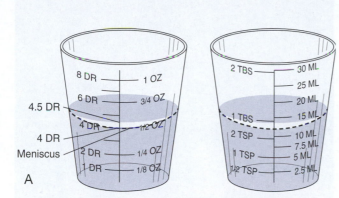

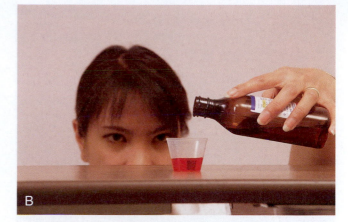

Figure 10-8. (A) Meniscus. (B) Liquids should be poured and measured at eye level.

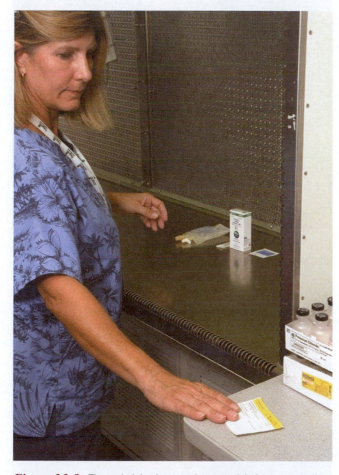

Figure 10-9. The technician is preparing materials for compounding.

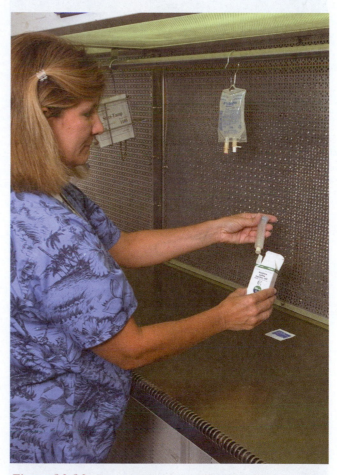

Figure 10-10. The technician is removing the medication sample.

Compounding of solutions generally takes time. The pharmacy technician must not rush. All equipment should be gathered before compounding begins. Liquid volumes are easier to measure than solid volumes, which must be weighed. It is good practice to select a container that will be at least half full when measuring. The upper surface of the liquid in the container will be a **meniscus**, or moon-shaped body. This means that the level of the liquid will be slightly higher at the edges (see Figure 10-8A). Therefore, the level should not be measured by looking down on the graduate. The eyes must be level with the liquid, and the level of the liquid should be read at the bottom of the meniscus (see Figure 10-8B). Figures 10-9 through 10-14 show the steps involved to compound a solution.

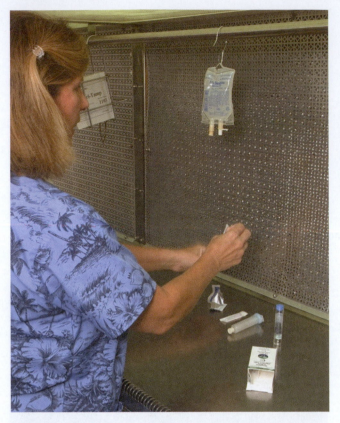

Figure 10-11. The technician is cleaning the vial with alcohol.

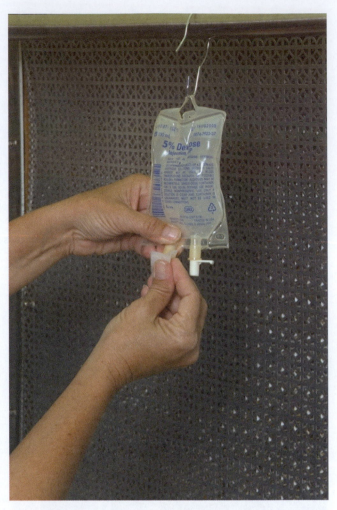

Figure 10-12. The technician is cleaning the bag of solution with alcohol.

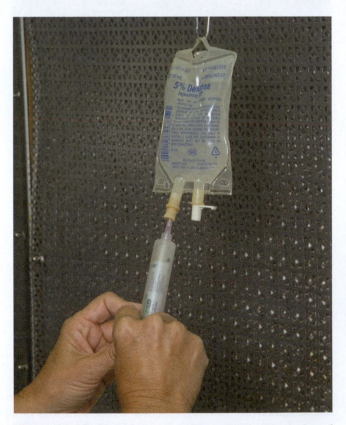

Figure 10-13. The technician is adding medication into the bag of solution for compounding.

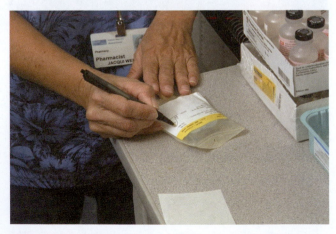

Figure 10-14. The technician is labeling the compounded solution.

COMPOUNDING SUSPENSIONS

A **suspension** is a liquid dosage form that contains solid drug particles floating in a liquid medium. Suspensions are easy to compound; however, physical stability of the final product after compounding is problematic. The insoluble powders are **triturated** (reduced to a fine powder by friction). A small portion of liquid is used to **levigate** the powder (grind into a smooth surface with moisture), and the powders are triturated until a smooth paste is formed. The levigating agent is added slowly and mixed deliberately. The vehicle containing the suspending agent is added in divided portions. A high-speed mixer greatly increases the dispersion and the final mixture is transferred to a "light" bottle for dispensing to the patient. All suspensions should be dispensed with an auxiliary label reading "Shake Well." Suspensions are not filtered. The water-soluble ingredients, including flavoring agents, are mixed in the vehicle before mixing with the insoluble ingredients. The steps performed to compound a suspension are illustrated in Figures 10-15 through 10-21.

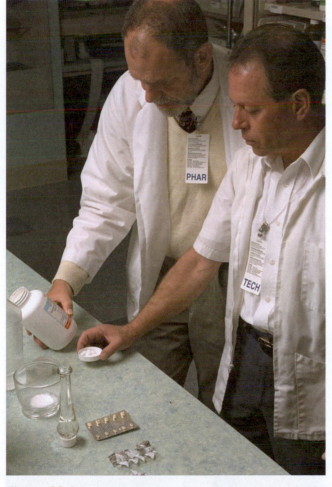

Figure 10-15. The technician and pharmacist are checking the dosage of tablets for compounding.

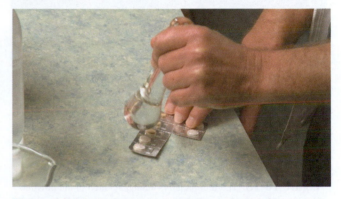

Figure 10-16. The technician is grinding the tablets into a powder.

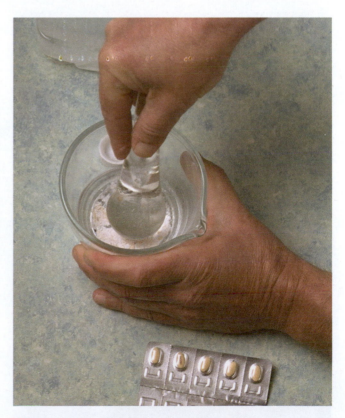

Figure 10-17. The technician is further grinding the powdered tablets.

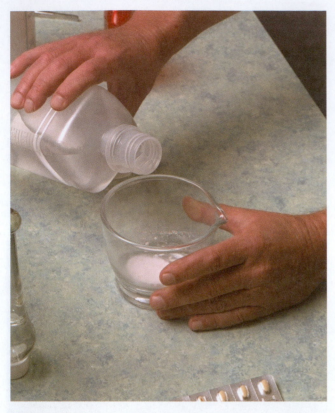

Figure 10-18. The technician is adding solution to the powder.

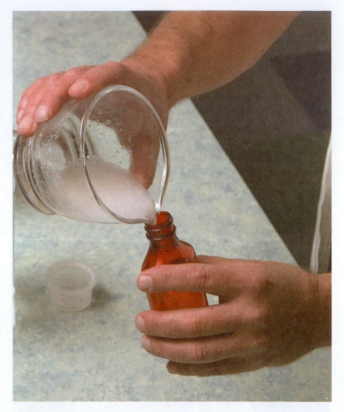

Figure 10-19. The compounded suspension is being poured into the patient's bottle.

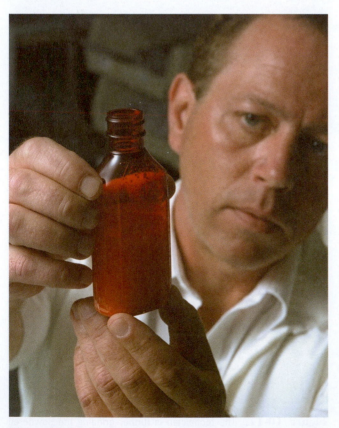

Figure 10-20. The technician is verifying the amount of the solution at eye level.

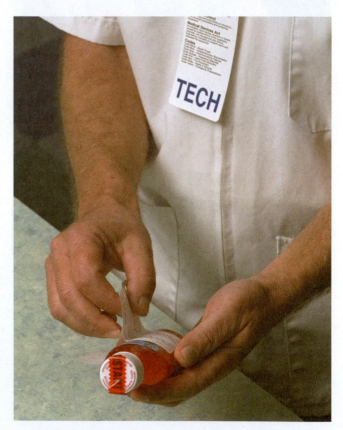

Figure 10-21. The technician is labeling the bottle.

COMPOUNDING OINTMENTS, CREAMS, PASTES, AND GELS

Ointments, creams, pastes, and gels are semisolid dosage forms intended for topical application to the skin or mucous membranes. Ointments are characterized as being oily. Creams are generally oil-in-water or water-in-oil emulsions, and pastes are characterized by their high content of solids. Gels consist of suspensions made up of either small inorganic particles or large organic molecules interpenetrated by a liquid. These dosage forms are generally applied externally. They may act solely on the surface of the skin to produce a local effect (e.g., an antifungal agent), or they can release the medication that penetrates into the skin (e.g.,

cortisol cream). These semisolid dosage forms may release medication for systemic absorption through the skin (e.g., nitroglycerin).

Ointments are oil-based, whereas creams are water-based. Drugs that are in powder or crystal forms, such as hydrocortisone, salicylic acid, or precipitated sulfur, are often ordered to be mixed into ointment or cream bases. Mixing can be done in a mortar or on an ointment slab. Liquids are incorporated by gradually adding them to an absorption-type base and mixing. Insoluble powders are reduced to a fine powder and then are added to the base, using geometric dilution. Water-soluble substances are dissolved with water and then are incorporated into the base. The final product should be smooth and free of any abrasive particles. The steps followed to compound an ointment are shown in Figures 10-22 through 10-27.

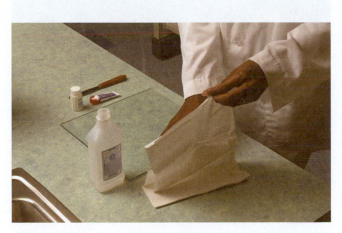

Figure 10-22. The technician is cleaning the glass slab for compounding an ointment.

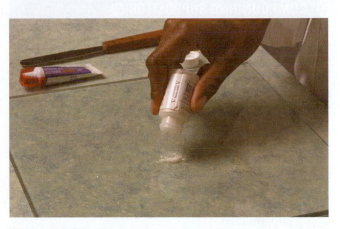

Figure 10-23. The technician is pouring the desired amount of powder to compound into ointment.

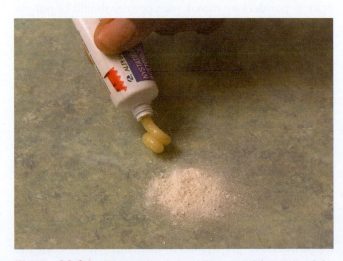

Figure 10-24. The technician is adding a partial amount of the cream needed to make the ointment.

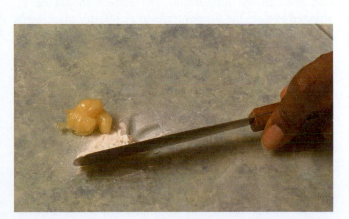

Figure 10-25. The technician is mixing the powder into the cream.

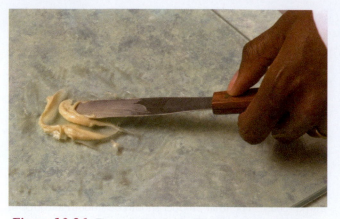

Figure 10-26. The technician is blending the powder and cream.

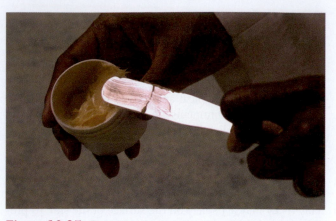

Figure 10-27. The technician is putting the blended ointment into the patient's ointment container.

COMPOUNDING SUPPOSITORIES

Suppositories are solid bodies of various weights, sizes, and shapes. They are adapted for introduction into the rectal, vaginal, or urethral orifices of the human body. Suppositories are used to deliver drugs for local or systemic effects. There are three common suppository bases:

1. Cocoa butter (theobroma oil), which melts at body temperature. It is a fat-soluble mixture of triglycerides that is most often used for rectal suppositories.
2. Polyethylene glycol (Carbowax) derivatives are water-soluble bases suitable for vaginal and rectal suppositories.
3. Glycerinated gelatin is a water-miscible base often used in vaginal and rectal suppositories.

The first step to prepare suppositories is the choice of a proper mold. Suppository molds can be made of rubber, plastic, brass, stainless steel, or other suitable material (see Figure 10-28). If appropriate, a "Refrigerate" label should appear on the container. Regardless of the base or medication used in the formulation, the patient should be instructed to store the suppositories in a cool, dry place. Steps for compounding suppositories are highlighted in Figures 10-29 through 10-34.

COMPOUNDING POWDERS

Powder dosage forms are used when drug stability or solubility is a concern. These dosage forms may also be used when the powders are too bulky to make into capsules and when the patient has difficulty swallowing a capsule. Powder dosage forms may be unpleasant-tasting medications. Blending of powders may be accomplished by using

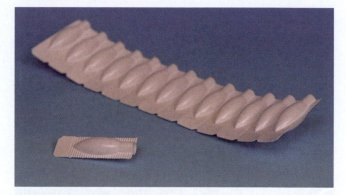

Figure 10-28. Suppository mold.

trituration in a mortar, stirring with a spatula, and sifting. **Geometric dilution** should be used if needed. When heavy powders are mixed with lighter powders, the heavier powder should be placed on top and then blended. When two or more powders are mixed, each powder should be pulverized separately to about the same particle size before they are blended together.

PREPARATION AND FILLING OF CAPSULES

Capsules are solid forms in which the drug is enclosed within either a hard or soft soluble container or shell. The shells are usually made from a suitable gelatin. Hard gelatin capsules may be manually filled for extemporaneous compounding. Capsule sizes for oral administration in humans range from number 5, which is the smallest, to number 000, the largest. Number 0 is usually the largest oral size suitable for patients. For preparation of hard and soft capsules, the correct size must be determined by trying different sizes,

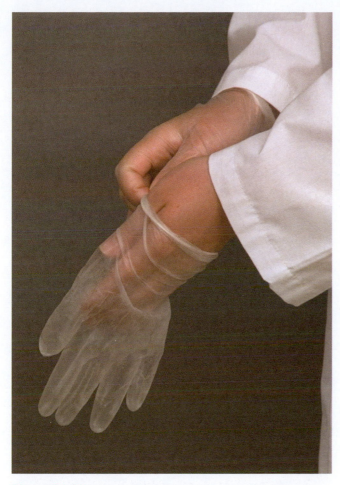

Figure 10-29. The technician is putting on gloves for the procedure of compounding suppositories.

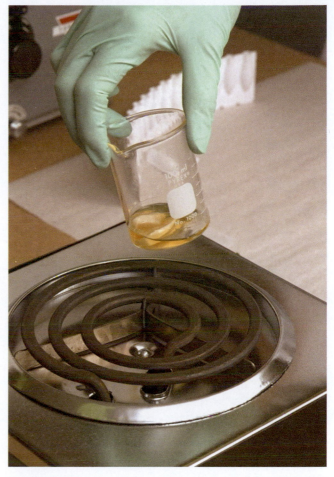

Figure 10-31. The technician is melting the base material that will be combined with the powder.

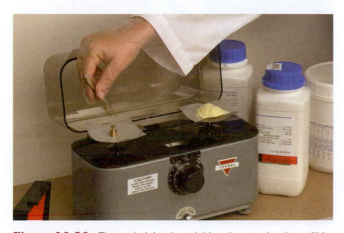

Figure 10-30. The technician is weighing the powder that will be compounded into suppositories.

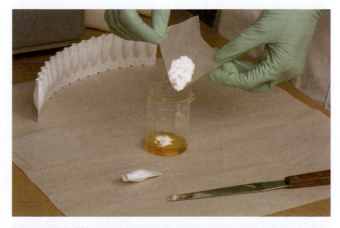

Figure 10-32. The technician is adding the powder to the melted base material.

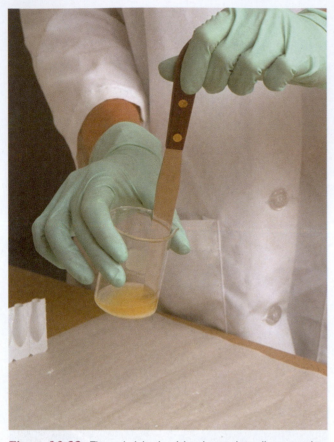

Figure 10-33. The technician is mixing the two ingredients together.

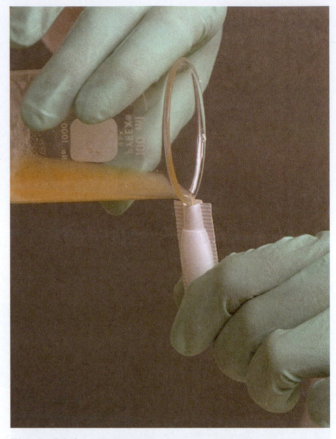

Figure 10-34. The technician is pouring the mixture into the suppository mold.

weighing, and choosing the appropriate size. Before capsules are filled with the medication, the body and cap of the capsule are separated. Filling is accomplished by using the "punch" method. The powder formulation is compressed with a spatula on a pill tile. The empty capsule body is repeatedly pressed into the powder until full. The capsule is then weighed to ensure an accurate dose. An empty **tare** capsule (the weight of an empty capsule used to compare to the full capsule) of the same size is placed on the pan containing the weights. For a large number of capsules, capsule-filling machines can be used for small-scale use to save time. The capsule is wiped clean of any powder or oil and dispensed in a suitable prescription vial. Figures 10-35 through 10-43 illustrate the steps involved to compound a capsule.

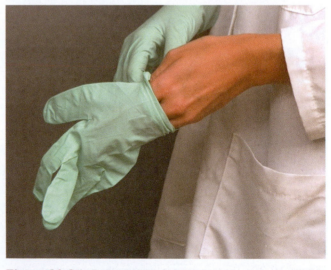

Figure 10-35. The technician is putting on gloves for the capsule compounding procedure.

COMPOUNDING TABLET TRITURATES

Tablet triturates are solid and small and are usually cylindrically molded or compressed tablets. Tablets are made of powders created by moistening the powder mixture with alcohol and water. They are used for compounding potent drugs in small doses. Tablet triturates are made in special molds consisting of a pegboard and a corresponding perforated plate. In addition to the mold, a diluent, usually a mixture of lactose, sucrose, and a moistening agent, is used. Moistening agents are usually a mixture of ethyl alcohol and

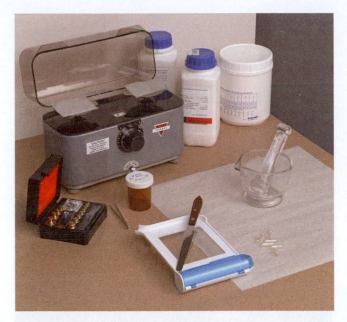

Figure 10-36. The technician has prepared all the materials needed to compound capsules.

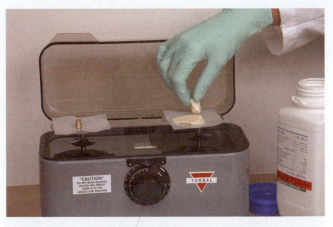

Figure 10-37. The technician is weighing the base material to be ground into powder for compounding capsules.

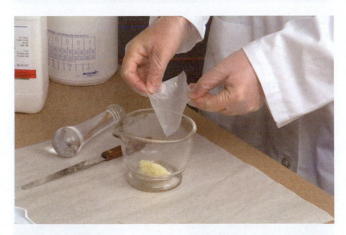

Figure 10-38. The technician is putting the weighed base material into a mortar for grinding.

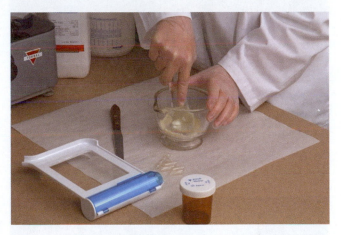

Figure 10-39. The technician is grinding the base material into a powder inside the mortar with the pestle.

water. The diluent is triturated with the active ingredients, and then a paste is made by using the alcohol and water mixture. This paste is spread into the mold, and the tablets are punched out and remain on the pegs until dry.

COMPOUNDING PARENTERAL PRODUCTS

The extemporaneous compounding of sterile products is no longer confined only to the hospital environment. The term *sterile* indicates there are no living microorganisms present. There are two types of product, either sterile or nonsterile. Sterility can be achieved through heat, gas, or filtration methods. Extemporaneous compounding of sterile products is now done by community pharmacists engaged in home care practice. The pharmacy technician is an integral part of the production of parenteral products, both in hospitals and in the home care industry. Preparation of sterile products requires special skills and training. Provision of this service without proper training should not be attempted. Sterile products must be prepared in a clean room, using aseptic technique (discussed in Chapter 13). Dry powders of parenteral drugs for reconstitution are used for drug products that are unstable as solutions. It is important to know the correct diluents that can be used to yield a solution. Drug solutions for parenteral administration may also be further diluted before administration.

Intravenous Admixtures

Hospital pharmacists are actively involved in compounding admixtures for daily intravenous (IV) therapy. They calculate

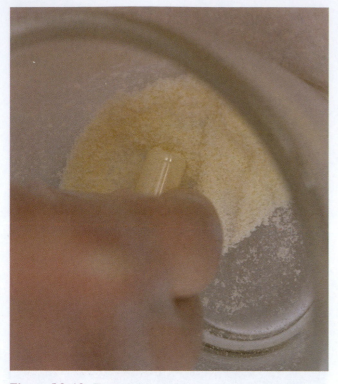

Figure 10-40. The technician is "punching" the powdered mixture into the empty capsule shell.

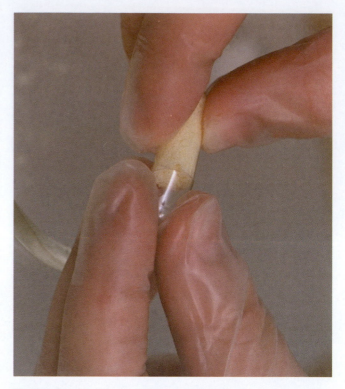

Figure 10-41. The technician is putting the two capsule halves together.

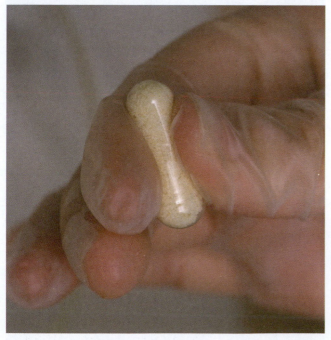

Figure 10-42. The technician is checking to see that the capsule is full of powdered mixture.

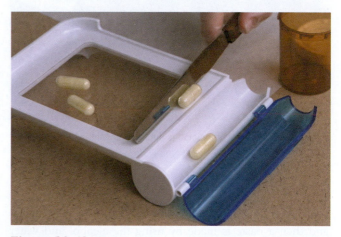

Figure 10-43. The technician is counting the compounded capsules for dispensing.

amounts for antibiotic piggybacks, total parenteral nutrition solutions, IV additives, and many others and compound and dispense the medications, which are generally administered by the nursing staff. The IV admixture products are sterile drugs. Minimal requirements include proper equipment and supplies, laminar airflow hoods, and a clean room, proper documentation of all products made, quality control, proper storage (both at the facility and in transport to the patient's home), and proper labeling of the prescription product. Preparation of sterile products and the laminar airflow clean bench will be discussed in Chapter 13. Figures 10-44 through 10-49 show the steps involved to prepare an intravenous admixture.

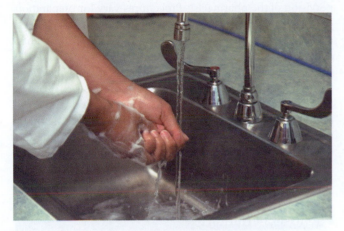

Figure 10-44. The technician is washing his hands before the intravenous admixture compounding procedure.

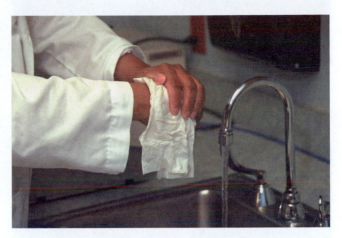

Figure 10-45. The technician is drying his hands.

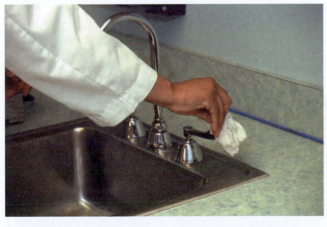

Figure 10-46. The technician is using the hand-drying towel to shut off the water faucet, avoiding any contamination to his hands.

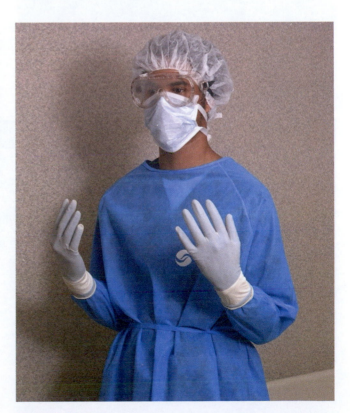

Figure 10-47. The technician is fully prepared for the sterile procedure.

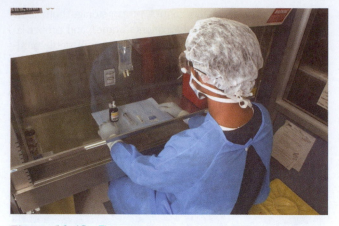

Figure 10-48. The technician is ready to perform sterile compounding of the intravenous admixture under the laminar airflow hood.

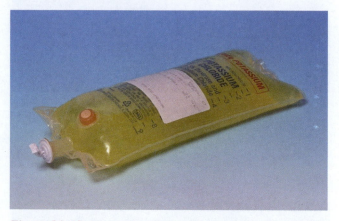

Figure 10-49. The compounded intravenous admixture is complete.

SUMMARY

Extemporaneous compounding is providing pharmacists with a unique opportunity to practice their time-honored profession. It will become an even more important part of pharmacy practice in the future, including those involved in community, hospital, nursing home, home health care, and specialty practices. The pharmacy technician must be trained and skilled to compound medication under the supervision of the pharmacist. Procedures vary for preparation of different extemporaneous compounds, such as powders, capsules, solutions, suspensions, suppositories, ointments, and creams. The extemporaneous compounding of sterile products is no longer confined only to the hospital environment. It is now done by community pharmacists engaged in home care practice. Quality control and proper documentation of all products are essential. Preparation of sterile products requires special skills and training. A clean room and the use of aseptic technique are very important to minimize contamination.

CRITICAL THINKING

1. Explain why it is important to follow the order precisely when compounding medications. What are the dangers of carelessness in compounding?
2. Why must some medications be prepared in a sterile environment? What are the dangers of preparing this medication without using proper sterile technique?

REVIEW QUESTIONS

1. When measuring the amount of liquid in a graduate, at what level of the meniscus do you read?
   A. Bottom
   B. Front
   C. Back
   D. Top

2. An ingredient dissolved in a solution is known as a
   A. solute.
   B. solvent.
   C. suspension.
   D. precipitate.

3. Which of the following equipment can be used for weighing larger quantities?
   A. Counter balance
   B. Class A prescription balance
   C. Slab
   D. Graduate

4. Avoid measurement of volumes that are less than 20% of the capacity of the graduate, because
   A. contamination is more possible.
   B. calibration is incorrect.
   C. measurement requires more timing.
   D. accuracy is unacceptable.

Continues

5. A semisolid, external dosage form with an oily base is called
   A. a suppository.
   B. a cream.
   C. a lotion.
   D. an ointment.

6. Capsule sizes for oral administration in humans range from number 0 to 5. Which of the following capsule sizes is the smallest?
   A. 000
   B. 00
   C. 0
   D. 5

7. The powders in tablets are moistened by mixing with
   A. water.
   B. oil.
   C. water and alcohol.
   D. water, oil, and alcohol.

8. Spatulas are used to
   A. measure bulk products.
   B. transfer solid ingredients for weighing.
   C. grind materials in the preparation of drugs.
   D. measure volumes of liquid.

9. A pipette is used for volumes less than
   A. 15 mL.
   B. 10 mL.
   C. 5 mL.
   D. 1.5 mL.

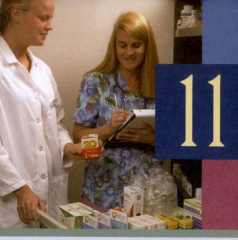

11

Management of Pharmacy Operations

OBJECTIVES

Upon completion of this chapter, the reader should be able to

1. Explain cost analysis and cost control.
2. Discuss the differences between independent, group, and time purchasing.
3. Describe the different types of paperwork used, such as purchase orders and invoices.
4. Detail the types of information specified when medications are ordered from a pharmacy's want book.

5. Explain the steps taken when ordered products are received.
6. Identify the three key components of a modern record-keeping system.
7. List at least five different types of expense accounts.
8. Define inventory and discuss its three major issues.
9. Compare and contrast unit-of-use packaging and batch repackaging.

GLOSSARY

bar coding Placing a code on packaging to help standardize and regulate inventory control.

batch repackaging The reassembling of a specific dosage and dosage form of medication at a given time.

cost analysis All information regarding the disbursements of an activity, department, program, or agency.

cost-benefit analysis The procedure of evaluating costs and benefits of only those programs whose benefits are found to supersede the costs.

cost control The implementation of managerial efforts to achieve cost objectives.

GLOSSARY continued

group purchasing Many hospitals working together to negotiate with pharmaceutical manufacturers to get better prices and benefits based upon the ability to promise high committed volumes.

independent purchasing The director of pharmacy or buyer directly contacts and negotiates pricing with pharmaceutical manufacturers.

inventory The stock of medications a pharmacy keeps immediately on hand.

inventory control Controlling the amount of product on hand to maximize the return on investment.

invoice A form describing a purchase and the amount due.

just-in-time (JIT) system An inventory control system in which stock arrives just before it is needed.

perpetual inventory system An inventory control system that allows review of drug use monthly.

point of sale (POS) master An inventory control system that allows inventory to be tracked as it is used.

prime supplier Establishment of a relationship with a single supplier to obtain lower prices.

time purchase The time that the purchase order was made.

unit-of-use packaging The packaging from bulk containers into patient-specific containers.

want book A list of drugs and devices that routinely need to be reordered.

OVERVIEW

Pharmacy practice has changed dramatically over the last several years. Pharmacists are more likely to be employees rather than owners and to work for large organizations, such as hospitals, chain pharmacies, and managed care pharmacies, rather than in small, independently owned pharmacies. They now have clinically oriented patient care responsibilities, rather than purely distributive duties. Although these changes have been associated with a dramatic decline in the number of pharmacists who own their businesses, they have not affected the number who are managers. In fact, the need for pharmacy managers has increased. This need has occurred because large organizations, such as major hospital pharmacies, managed care pharmacies, and chain pharmacies, need pharmacist managers for coordination and direction.

The need for pharmacist managers has also increased as more dispensing functions are handled by technicians and are being automated. Pharmacist managers are needed to supervise technicians and to manage the increased use of dispensing technology. Pharmacists have also found ownership and management opportunities in a variety of new settings, such as home health care and home intravenous (IV) infusion businesses, long-term care consulting organizations, disease management companies, and pharmaceutical care training companies. Managers are responsible for planning, organizing, and controlling resources so that the organizations in which they are employed meet their goals.

COST ANALYSIS

The most important concerns of pharmaceutical organizations are productivity, quality, service, and price. The pharmacist manager is responsible and accountable for the finances of the pharmacy. In general, the process of control involves the gathering of information and data, the establishment of standards based on this information, and the adjustment of operations to conform to the standards developed. **Cost analysis** involves all information about the financial disbursements of an activity, agency department, or program. **Cost control** is considered to be the implementation of managerial efforts to achieve cost objectives. The extent of the measures used can vary from simple decrees of a new policy or procedure to an entire reorganization of the drug distribution system. For example, a simple decree might be that all photocopying must be submitted to a departmental secretary rather than individuals being allowed to have uncontrolled use of the machine. The cost analysis that precedes a cost control decision also varies greatly in degree of sophistication and can range from an observation, hypothesis, or supposition to complex statistical and probabilistic theories and analyses.

An integral part of the cost control process is the establishment of priorities for the implementation of cost control programs. These priorities should be reevaluated after the information is gathered and the analysis is completed. Naturally, programs for which anticipated cost reductions are high and analysis and implementation costs are low are the most amenable to plans for cost control. An example of such a program is an ongoing drug utilization surveillance program that addresses issues such as the cost of irrational prescribing of antibiotics among hospitalized inpatients. Several factors should be considered when a cost analysis study is performed. These include cost finding, cost factors, and cost-benefit analysis. Generally, cost analysis studies are performed for one of two purposes:

1. To estimate the total cost of an operational or proposed system
2. To compare two or more methods or systems to determine which is more advantageous (profitable)

An example of the first is to determine the total cost of the hospital's drug distribution system, and an example of the second is to determine the cost per dose of the hospital's traditional multidose drug distribution system and then compare it with the results of cost studies of a pilot unit-dose drug distribution system.

Cost Finding

Decisions of cost control should be based on the total cost of a system such as supplies, personnel, overhead, and others. It is especially important to consider and measure all components of total cost. Commonly, indirect costs such as overhead, central pharmacy administration, and fringe benefits are overlooked.

Studies of the second type should be based on evaluation of the effect of differences in systems, equipment, or personnel on costs. This study should be carefully controlled to eliminate sources of bias.

In both types of studies, unit cost should be expressed as a function of a nonmonetary unit of measurement. Familiar units in pharmacy are cost per patient day, cost per item, cost per dose, and cost per unit time.

Cost Factors

The effects of costs in the hospital industry or community pharmacy depend on the following factors:

1. Output or volume
2. Quality of services
3. Scope of services
4. Factor prices
5. Relative efficiency

A change in one of these factors will usually result in a subsequent change in total cost. Generally, the relationship between volume, quality, prices, and cost is direct. An increase in one of these factors will result in an increase in cost.

It is important to understand that if total cost has changed unexpectedly, it is a result of a change in one or more of these factors. In this situation, it is necessary to isolate the factor(s) causing the change, identify the relative effect of each factor, and then correct the problems.

Cost-Benefit Analysis

Cost-benefit analysis is the procedure of evaluating costs and benefits of only those programs whose benefits are found to supersede costs and serves as a tool for cost control. An example is the long-term savings associated with automated billing (decreased personnel costs and increased revenue) that offsets the initial costs of implementation. Another example is a continuing search to attach monetary values to decreased medication errors resulting from unit-dose services. The pharmacist should be able to conduct and evaluate cost-benefit analysis studies and use them as tools for cost control.

PURCHASING PROCEDURES

The complexity of services offered by the pharmacy department will dictate the frequency of involvement that the pharmacy has with the purchasing department. In various types of pharmacies, this complexity will be different, because it depends on the size and type of the pharmacy. In pharmacies with IV programs, central supply services, or other services such as orthopedic assistance, there will be continual involvement with purchasing for buying of equipment and supplies. Pharmacies with limited services may have little involvement, particularly if purchasing of medications is the pharmacy's responsibility. When the pharmacy must order and buy products for use or sale; the procedure is usually carried out in one of the following ways: independent purchasing, group purchasing, or purchasing from prime suppliers.

Independent Purchasing

Independent purchasing means the individual pharmacist or technician works alone and deals directly with representatives of pharmaceutical companies to negotiate price, quantity, and delivery.

Group Purchasing

Because larger purchases generally result in lower prices, groups of buyers who pool their buying power can usually gain lower prices than any of the individual buyers acting alone; this is **group purchasing**. There are costs involved in belonging to a purchasing group, however. These include the direct cost of membership, commonly called an annual fee and a certain loss of control in product selection. The members of the group must meet periodically to evaluate supplier proposals, products, and performance.

Prime Suppliers

Another approach to obtaining lower prices and better service is to establish a relationship with a single supplier for a major portion of the system's purchases; this is the **prime supplier**. In addition to allowing the pharmacy to maintain lower in-house inventory levels, the supplier is expected to provide the following:

- Lower prices
- Extended price protection
- Minimal occurrence of back orders
- Simplified paperwork in purchasing, receiving, and paying for items
- Other special services

Potential disadvantages of using a prime supplier include the following:

- Economic competition may be reduced over a period of time.

- Quality may be inconsistent across the supplier's complete line of products.
- The pharmacy may become overly dependent on the supplier, so that a change in supplier would be disruptive to pharmacy routines.
- Prices may creep upward if inadequate controls are placed on the relationship.

Ordering

Regular drugs, devices, and supplies may be ordered electronically by fax or telephone or online by computer. The order is normally made on a form known as a purchase order. The decision to order a drug or item depends on how well it sells in the pharmacy.

One of the simplest and most widely used methods of inventory control is a **want book**. A want book is simply a list of items that the pharmacy or technician needs to order. Before the operations of most pharmacies and wholesalers were computerized, a want book typically consisted of a notebook kept in a convenient place. Pharmacists or technicians recorded product names or item numbers and quantities to be ordered in the want book as the items were sold or dispensed. The pharmacist or technician in charge of inventory then made orders to the wholesaler or manufacturer directly from the information recorded in the want book. Now, the want book is more likely to be a hand-held electronic device into which item numbers and quantities are entered (see Figure 11-1). The pharmacist or technician records the needed items in this device just as in the notebook, and the order can now be placed electronically.

Information to be specified when ordering includes the following:

- The item name and manufacturer. For a drug product, the generic or brand name must be specified.
- The strength and dosage form of the drug (or size, if ordering a device)
- The quantity of drug dosage forms per package (e.g., bottle of or boxes of 100, package of two or more)
- The type of packaging
- The number of bottles, packages, or devices being ordered

Colored or dated price stickers are another simple and effective manual technique used for ordering. Colored price stickers can be used to indicate the time period during which a product was received. For example, a pharmacy might use blue stickers for products received during the first 6 months of a year, red stickers for products received during the next 6 months, yellow stickers for the first 6 months of the next year, and so on. Because the colors change every 6 months, the manager can readily estimate how long an item has been in inventory by simply glancing at the sticker. The length of time an item has been in inventory gives a rough indication of the quantity of the item needed and whether the item should be discontinued.

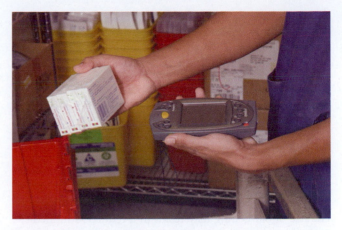

Figure 11-1. Hand-held devices contain the pharmacy want book and make ordering inventory faster and more efficient.

A system of colored or dated price stickers and a want book are sufficient for control of specific types of items. In practice, this control amounts to having minimal amounts of each specific item on hand and eliminating items that do not sell within some predetermined length of time, for example, within 6 to 12 months.

Invoice

An **invoice** is a paper describing a purchase and the amount due. When a **time purchase** is made, that is, when the item is not paid for at the time of purchase, the vendor usually includes a packing slip with delivery of the merchandise. A packing slip describes the item enclosed. The vendor may also enclose an invoice. Invoices should be placed in a special folder until paid. The pharmacy may be making more than one purchase from the same vendor during the month. Some vendors request that payment be made from the invoice; others send a statement later. A statement is a request for payment.

RECEIVING

Receiving is one of the most important parts of the pharmacy operation. When products that have been ordered arrive at the pharmacy, it is essential that a system for checking purchasing and receiving is in place. Generally, the individual who ordered the products should not do the receiving also. All items must be carefully checked against the purchase order. The following procedure should be followed when pharmaceuticals or medical supplies are received:

- They should be verified and compared against the purchase order for name of product, quantity of boxes, and package size and examined for any gross damage of boxes.

■ For drug products the name, brand, dosage form, size of the package, strength, quantity, and expiration date must be checked.

After products are received and checked, they must be placed in an appropriate storage location. Products requiring refrigeration or freezing should be processed first.

Bar Coding

Bar coding is becoming increasingly popular in the pharmacy setting, although its use has been delayed because of the lack of a universal bar code standard for all medications. The use of bar coding may result in a reduction in medication errors, assurance that the identity and dose of the drug are as prescribed for the correct patient, and improved timeliness and accuracy. The advent of the bar coding of pharmaceuticals has required changes in label designs, production processes, and size of packages, but these are all minor setbacks when viewed alongside the overall benefits of the process. By insisting that unit-dose packaging remain the norm for the pharmaceutical industry, the U.S. Food and Drug Administration (FDA) has helped to direct the implementation of bar coding so that patient safety is kept in mind. Not all pharmaceuticals have been brought into the new bar coding system, and there has been a slight decrease in drug availability as a result. However, as conditions improve, bar coding of all pharmaceuticals in a uniform, consistent manner, will help to offer the following:

■ Product-specific manufacturer-generated bar codes
■ Product-specific pharmacy-generated bar codes
■ Pharmacy information system–generated bar codes (that identify a patient and an order number but not a specific medication)

Bar coding saves dollars, time, and, most importantly, lives.

Returning Products

For damaged or incorrect shipments or expired medications, the manufacturer should be notified immediately and a return merchandise authorization should be requested for the return of the rejected shipment.

Drug Recalls

Under the federal Food, Drug, and Cosmetic Act, the FDA can request a recall if a drug manufacturer is not willing to remove dangerous drugs from the market without the FDA's written request. The FDA then monitors company recalls and assesses the adequacy of the firm's action. If the firm does not comply with a recall request, the FDA can seek legal action and force the recall to occur. Products that may be recalled by the FDA without requesting the manufacturer to do so include medical devices, human tissue products, and infant formulas that pose a risk to human health.

After a recall is completed, the FDA makes sure that the product is destroyed or reconditioned and investigates why it was defective in the first place. Many times, however, drugs are recalled by the manufacturers themselves when they find them to be defective. Class I recalls are for dangerous or defective products that could cause serious health problems or death. Class II recalls are for products that may cause temporary health problems or pose a slight threat of a serious nature. Class III recalls are for products unlikely to cause any adverse health reactions, but which violate FDA labeling or manufacturing regulations.

RECORD KEEPING

A modern record keeping system has three key components:

1. A symbol on the outside of the jacket or folder to indicate the active or inactive status of records
2. Safeguards to prevent misfiling
3. A filing technique to allow quick, accurate retrieval and proper refiling

Files may be kept as hard copy (on paper) or on the computer disk. Most medical facilities use a combination of computers and hard copy. The most popular system today is the use of color coding on open shelves. Some records are kept in card or tray files (see Figure 11-2). Regardless of the type or style of filing system equipment, purchasing the best quality is always recommended. Some of the considerations in record keeping are size, type, and volume of records. It is also important to ensure confidentiality requirements and at the same time maximize retrieval speed. At the time of payment, the pharmacy technician should compare the statement with the invoice(s) to verify accuracy and fasten the statement and invoices together. The technician should write the date and check number on the statement and place it in the paid file.

Disbursements are recorded and distributed to specific expense accounts such as the following:

■ Dues and meeting
■ Equipment
■ Insurance
■ Medical supplies
■ Pharmacy expenses
■ Printing, postage, and stationery
■ Rent and maintenance
■ Salaries
■ Taxes and licenses
■ Travel
■ Utilities
■ Miscellaneous

All records for wholesale distributors need to be kept separate and distinct from the records for the rest of the pharmacy operations. Records must be made available for

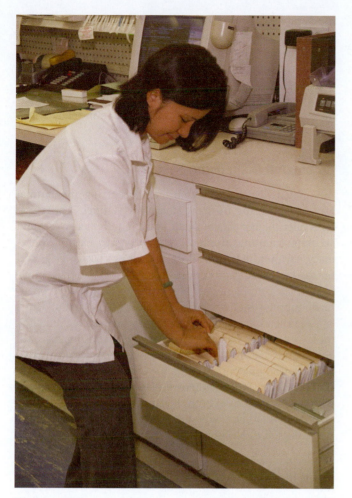

Figure 11-2. An organized filing system is imperative in the pharmacy.

inspection by state and federal agencies, for which they should be centrally maintained. Wholesale records (purchase and sale) must be maintained for a minimum of 2 years from the date of disposition of the prescription drugs. Also, the pharmacy may have to keep required records for more than 2 years after the date of disposition of the prescription drug if notified that an investigation is underway.

■ INVENTORY CONTROL

Inventory control is of vital importance to pharmacies of all types. Inventory is typically a pharmacy's largest asset. Because so much is invested in inventory, proper inventory control has a strong and direct effect on a pharmacy's return on investment.

Inventory control is also important because a pharmacy must have the correct inventory to properly serve its patients. It must have those products that patients need in the quantities in which they need them. This aspect of inventory

control is much harder to quantify and control but equally important. If a community pharmacy does not have the products that its patients need, at the time they need them, it will lose sales. If this happens often, the pharmacy will lose patients. If a hospital pharmacy does not have a needed item, the consequence can range from inconvenience—for items not needed immediately—to physical harm to patients in need of life-saving emergency drugs.

Thus, the two goals of effective inventory control are minimizing total inventory investment and carrying the right mix of products to satisfy patient demand. **Inventory** is a list of articles in stock, with the description and quantity of each. In other words, inventory is the entire stock of products on hand at a given time in the pharmacy. Inventory control is closely associated with the function of purchasing. Inventory control is important to the pharmacist because it is the means by which he or she assures that all medications and products are accounted for and used legitimately, that adequate stocks are available when needed, and that the costs of too large an inventory are avoided. There are several important factors and issues with regard to inventory such as the following:

1. How much inventory should be maintained?
2. When should inventory levels be adjusted?
3. Where should inventory be stored?

In an ideal system, pharmaceutical products would arrive shortly before they are needed (**just-in-time [JIT] system**).

Computerized Inventory System

The traditional purchasing and inventory control system, which is still being used in a majority of pharmacies today, does not involve computers and is considered old-fashioned. It is more expensive and difficult to maintain all information accurately, in addition to being more time consuming. For these reasons, some pharmacists have attempted to implement more sophisticated purchasing and inventory control systems. Computers and computerized inventory systems increase accuracy, generate more data, and require less time compared with traditional systems. Computerized systems have the capability of making it possible for pharmacies to maintain *perpetual* control of inventories. This means that inventories and sales figures for individual products are updated constantly as purchases and sales are made. However, to maintain perpetual control, the pharmacy must update inventory records whenever inventory is purchased and whenever it is sold. Thus, all purchases and sales must be entered into the computer.

Computer systems use sales and inventory information to calculate and record points, to identify low turnover items that should be dropped from inventory, and to generate orders to be sent to wholesalers or manufacturers. The basis of the computerized purchasing and control system is the medication database. The medication master file contains all of the information needed for ordering, inventory, pricing, and distribution of pharmaceuticals. Most computerized systems provide all of the information needed to write a purchase requisition and a few systems actually produce the final purchase order. The real advantage of computerized inventory control systems is the time savings for the pharmacy and the business office.

Perpetual Inventory

Perpetual inventory systems are being used today to show when it is time to reorder materials. These systems allow the pharmacist to review drug use monthly, allowing better monitoring of all information. The computer also enables the monitoring of the budget. Board regulations require that a pharmacist should keep a perpetual inventory of each controlled substance in Schedule II, which has been received, dispensed, or disposed of. This inventory must be reconciled at least every 10 days. The perpetual inventory is a written record of the amount of controlled substances in Schedule II that are physically contained with the pharmacy or pharmacy department. The technician must keep in mind that the computer system is only effective when all input information is accurate.

Expired Stock

Expired, deteriorated, contaminated, or other nonreusable drug products should be removed immediately from usable pharmacy stock and disposed of. Expired drugs should be placed into containers labeled with "Expired Drugs—DO NOT USE" or a similar clearly understood warning. Disposal requirements for most drugs that have an expiration date are listed in the package inserts or on a material safety data sheet (MSDS). Expired drugs and their disposal methods should be documented, regardless of whether they are put into biohazard bags for collection by approved biohazard disposal companies, returned to pharmaceutical representatives, or disposed of in any other way.

Drug Formulary

Drug formularies are lists or catalogs of drugs that are approved for use either within a hospital or for reimbursement by a third-party payer. The purpose of formularies is to eliminate therapeutic duplication and provide patients with the best drug at the lowest cost. In the early days of formularies, they were used by hospitals to control drug inventories and provide prescribers with a list of drugs of choice for various conditions. However, the absence of a drug from the formulary was not usually a great barrier to a prescriber's obtaining it for a patient. A special request could be made by the prescriber to a member of the pharmacy and therapeutic committee of the hospital, and usually the drug would be obtained. When managed-care organizations and pharmacy-benefit management companies began to use formularies, circumventing them became much more difficult. The restrictive use of formularies has led to a number of important ethical questions. For example, does the use of generic over therapeutic substitution violate the autonomy of the patient and/or prescriber? Is the use of such substitution a violation of informed consent? Does the use of formularies violate the ethical principles of beneficence (doing good) and non-malfeasance (avoiding harm)?

Automated Dispensing System

Automated dispensing systems are becoming the normal way of dispensing in many pharmacy settings. These systems offer the benefits of small space requirements, fast and accurate counting, minimal renovations to existing pharmacy surroundings, unit-dose packaging, bar coding, and finished packaging procedures for pills, solids, vials, cups, injectables, ampules, and blister packs. Automated pneumatic tubing systems are also offered by some manufacturers. Alternate care settings and supply logistics are aided by these systems as well, because many of them organize, secure, and track medications for increased customer interaction, medication control, and more efficient use of pharmacy staff members. Most automated dispensing systems comply with the regulations of both the Health Insurance Portability and Accountability Act and the Joint Commission on Accreditation of Healthcare Organizations regulations.

Point of Sale

The **point-of-sale (POS) master** is the most suitable, flexible, and open-ended system on the market. The POS master can increase overall profitability, and it can be installed in all of the computers at the main pharmacy. POS systems can control stock in the pharmacy accurately. The system can handle a significant volume of customers and transactions and all the orders, credits, interstore transfers, and returns. A major benefit of the POS master is that it can cover every area that a user could conceivably be interested in and is driven by practical requests of the users themselves. The POS master can enhance every area of the pharmacy and is really easy to use; it is probably the best system and the best support team for the business.

REPACKAGING

As pharmaceutical manufacturers began to prepare, package, and distribute commonly prescribed medications, the role of pharmacist changed from formulator and packager to repackager of commercially prepared medication. Therefore, the pharmacist and technician repackage bulk containers of medication into patient-specific containers of medication. The amount of medication that is repackaged into the patient container is generally predicated on the course of therapy.

This type of packaging from bulk containers into patient-specific containers is called **unit-of-use packaging**. Unit-of-use packaging, sometimes referred to as "repackaging" is a suitable concept for inpatient or outpatient dispensing. An advantage to this type of dispensing process is that it allows the pharmacist to prepare medications for administration before their use is anticipated. The unit-dose system of dispensing medication in organized health care settings has been the driving force behind repackaging programs as we know them today. Unit-dose distribution is the standard by which all other distribution systems are measured. The single-dose package always contains the dose of the drug for a given patient. A single-dose package may contain two tablets or two capsules in one package or container for a given patient if the dose calls for two tablets or two capsules. Single-unit packages will contain only one tablet or one capsule. One of the major advantages of unit-dose drug distribution systems is that they decrease the total cost of medication-related activities. Repackaging medications in advance of when they are needed allows the pharmacist to take advantage of periods of reduced staff activity to lessen the demands of peak activity.

   Batch repackaging is defined as the repackaging of a specific dosage and dosage form of medication at a given time.

Specific Guidelines for Repackaging

Drug packages must have four basic functions:

1. Protect their contents from deleterious environmental effects.
2. Protect their contents from deterioration resulting from handling.
3. Identify their contents completely and precisely.
4. Permit their contents to be used quickly, easily, and safely.

Manufacturers of repackaging materials and repackaging equipment describe their products based on the type of package that is achievable. There are four classes—A, B, C, or D—with class A being the best and class D the worst. The package types most often found in hospital pharmacy departments include those used for oral solids, oral liquids, injections, respiratory medications, and topical medications.

Compounded and repackaged products typically have short expiration dates ranging from days to months. Expired compounded or repackaged pharmaceuticals cannot be returned and must be disposed of.

Disposal of Drugs

Expired, deteriorated, or contaminated drugs in all pharmacy areas should be considered "nonreusable" and should be removed immediately from usable stock either by direct disposal into the sink, trash, toilet, or biohazard bags or by return to the pharmacy stockroom for credit. Nonreusable drugs may be returned to the stockroom if they are in their original containers and/or the manufacturer can be identified or if they have been repackaged with an automatic tablet counting machine. They should be kept in the stockroom in clearly labeled bins that say "RETURNED FOR CREDIT—DO NOT USE." Drugs that should be disposed of include parenteral medications, oral liquids, ophthalmic solutions/suspensions, nasal solutions, oral solids, ointments, creams, topical solutions, biologicals, suppositories, transdermal patches, insulin, and inhalers.

SUMMARY

Pharmacies survive by providing products and services that their customers need. The managers of any pharmacy should strive to combine their experience, skills, judgment, abilities, and other characteristics to strengthen their organization. Cost control is central to the pharmacy's success, because it serves to achieve the cost objectives that such a complicated endeavor can require. By utilizing the combined strength of other pharmacies and by purchasing products in larger quantities, a pharmacy can greatly control the purchase cost of its medical products. A "want book" is a device that helps to manage routine purchases of products by the pharmacy, based on average sales ratios. With the use of computerized inventory systems, pharmacies will continue to thrive and become even more responsive to the needs of their customers, offering fair prices and availability of the most requested medications.

CRITICAL THINKING

1. What are the advantages of bar coding?
2. Explain cost-benefit analysis.

REVIEW QUESTIONS

1. Pharmacists are now more likely to be
   A. employees rather than owners.
   B. patients rather than experts.
   C. pharmacy technicians rather than medical assistants.
   D. doctors rather than nurses.

2. Cost analysis involves all information of the _____ of an activity, agency department, or program.
   A. control
   B. standards
   C. operations
   D. disbursements

3. Cost factors in hospitals and pharmacies include
   A. quality of the security system.
   B. quality of services.
   C. scope of personnel.
   D. drug displays.

4. Long-term savings is associated with automated billing because of
   A. increased personnel costs and decreased revenue.
   B. interest.
   C. decreased personnel costs and increased revenue.
   D. robotics involved in the process.

5. Independent purchasing means the individual pharmacy may work alone and
   A. deal directly with pharmaceutical representatives.
   B. deal with groups of buyers.
   C. belong to a purchasing group.
   D. have little involvement in pharmacy responsibility.

6. Prime suppliers are expected to provide
   A. higher prices and complex paperwork.
   B. a high quantity of back orders of popular medications.
   C. higher in-house inventory levels.
   D. simplified paperwork in purchasing, receiving, and paying for items.

7. One of the simplest and most widely-used methods of inventory control is a
   A. notebook.
   B. want book.
   C. red book.
   D. inventory book.

8. Under the federal Food, Drug, and Cosmetic Act, the FDA can request a recall if a drug manufacturer is not willing to
   A. give them a small percentage of their sales.
   B. destroy outdated medications.
   C. remove dangerous drugs from the market without the FDA's written request.
   D. monitor competitors' recalls.

9. One of the three key components of a modern record keeping system is
   A. a symbol indicating the status of each record.
   B. safeguards to prevent filing.
   C. a filing technique that allows retrieval only by the physician.
   D. a backup.

10. _____ is of vital importance to pharmacies of all types.
    A. Pharmacy expenses
    B. Stationery
    C. Utilities
    D. Inventory control

11. A JIT or "just-in-time" system means that pharmaceutical products arrive
    A. a few months before they are needed.
    B. the exact day they are needed.
    C. shortly before they are needed.
    D. just before they expire.

12. To maintain perpetual control, the pharmacy must update inventory records
    A. whenever inventory is purchased or sold.
    B. whenever sales figures are updated.
    C. to identify low turnover.
    D. to generate orders.

13. Disposal requirements for most drugs that expire are listed in the package inserts or on _____.
    A. medical safety board servers (MSBS)
    B. material safety data sheets (MSDS)
    C. drug formularies
    D. material stock forms (MSF)

14. Automated dispensing systems utilize _____.
    A. calculators
    B. scanners
    C. hydraulic tubes
    D. robotics

15. The most suitable, flexible, and open-ended dispensing system on the market is the
    A. unit-of-use system.
    B. point-of-sale master.
    C. repackaging system.
    D. batch repackaging system.

12

Financial Management and Health Insurance

OUTLINE

OBJECTIVES

Upon completion of this chapter, the reader should be able to

1. Discuss the financial issues relevant to the practice of pharmacy.
2. Define the key terms of health insurance.
3. Describe four examples of medical insurance coverage and explain their differences.
4. Define third-party billing.
5. Explain legal and ethical issues related to medical insurance and pharmacy.

GLOSSARY

assignment of benefits An authorization to an insurance company to make payment directly to the pharmacy or physician.

beneficiary An individual entitled to receive insurance policy or government program health care benefits.

CHAMPVA Civilian Health and Medical Program of the Veterans Administration; a program to cover medical expenses of the dependent spouse and children of veterans with total, permanent service-connected disabilities.

coinsurance An arrangement in which the insured must pay a percentage of the cost of medical services covered by the insurer.

contract An insurance policy; this is a legally enforceable agreement.

coordination of benefits The prevention of duplicate payment for the same service.

co-payment A patient's payment of a portion of the cost at the time the service is rendered.

deductible A specific amount of money that must be paid each year before the policy benefits begin (e.g., $50, $100, $300, or $500).

dependents The insured's spouse and children under the terms of the policy.

direct costs Costs caused directly by or resulting from providing the service.

eligibility The specific terms of coverage under a policy.

health insurance A contract between a policyholder and an insurance carrier or government program to reimburse the policyholder for all or a portion of the cost of medical care rendered by health care professionals.

GLOSSARY continued

independent practice association (IPA) A type of health maintenance organization (HMO) in which the HMO contracts directly with physicians, who continue in their existing practices.

indirect costs Costs not caused directly by or that do not result from providing the service.

markup method A pricing mechanism in which the price charged to the patient is calculated by adding a percentage markup, in addition to a dispensing fee, to the acquisition cost of the drug.

Medicaid A federal/state medical assistance program to provide health insurance for specific populations.

Medicare A federal health insurance program created as part of the Social Security Act.

overpayment Payment by the insurer or by the patient of more than the amount due.

policy limitation Policies that exclude certain types of coverage.

preauthorization The requirement of notification and permission to receive additional types of services before one obtains those services.

preferred provider organization (PPO) A managed care organization that contracts with a group of providers, who are called *preferred providers*, to offer services to the managed care organization's members.

premium The cost of the coverage that the insurance policy contains; this may vary greatly depending on the age and health of the individual and the type of insurance protection.

professional fee method A set dollar amount added to the ingredient cost to determine prescription price.

sliding scale method Variable markup percentages or professional fees that are used to calculate prescription prices.

subscriber The individual or organization protected in case of loss under the terms of an insurance policy.

third-party payer The fee for services provided is paid by an insurance company and not by the patient.

time limit The amount of time from the date of service to the date (deadline) the claim can be filed with the insurance company.

TRICARE A federally funded comprehensive health benefits program for dependents of personnel serving in the uniformed services.

waiting period The period of time that an individual must wait to become eligible for insurance coverage (e.g., 30 days) before coverage commences or for a specific benefit.

OVERVIEW

The practice of pharmacy is a business as well as a profession, and the details of conducting the business aspects are often the responsibility of the pharmacy technician. Although service to the patient is the primary concern of the medical profession, a pharmacist must charge and collect a fee for such services to continue providing medical care. As a business, a pharmacy must charge competitive and fair prices for services and must receive payment for those services in cash and in a timely fashion. Even a patient or customer with medical insurance should be fully informed about the practice's fees and payment policies. He or she is ultimately responsible for the bill if the insurance company refuses to pay or does not cover the full amount. The purpose of health insurance companies is to help individuals and families offset the costs of medical care. As the cost of medical treatment rapidly increases, insurance companies selling medical insurance policies are considering ways to control the increasing costs for medical insurance and prescription drug insurance. Insurance claims must be submitted for pharmacies to control cash flow, obtain correct reimbursement amounts, honor insurance contracts, and maintain a good relationship with patients. Those that administer the federal government's Medicare program have been asked to electronically transmit insurance claims. Therefore, the pharmacy technician should be familiar with and knowledgeable about all administrative aspects of pharmacies. There are many kinds of insurance coverage available in the United States. Pharmacies that accept patients' insurance and deal with different insurance companies must understand the billing process, and documentation must be accurate.

FINANCIAL ISSUES IN PHARMACY PRACTICE

The cost of pharmaceuticals has increased in the double digits in the past 10 years. This double-digit rate of growth is predicted to continue into the near future. Financial issues in pharmacy practice are always foremost in the minds of people who are responsible for paying and managing these costs.

Decision makers charged with managing pharmacy costs have historically focused on the ingredient cost of the product along with its clinical profile in assessing a product's value. This is often referred to as the "silo" approach to evaluating pharmaceuticals. However, this approach does not consider the impact of the costs of pharmaceuticals on other health care costs such as hospitalizations, physician visits, or other services. All of these are important aspects to consider in capturing the true value of pharmaceuticals. Pharmacoeconomic evaluations have been used as a tool in selecting formulary products, developing treatment guidelines, conducting disease management programs, establishing prior authorization policies, implementing step-therapy programs, and designing prescription drug benefit programs. The economic evaluation of pharmaceuticals and pharmacy services grew out of the need to establish value or to respond to the question of value.

Statements of product or service value center around two attributes: cost and benefit. From the consumer's perspective, the price paid should represent the benefit gained from use of the product or services. Several factors have created the need to monitor the value of pharmaceuticals more closely:

1. Increased cost and, thus, growing concern on the part of payers
2. Increased number of alternatives available to treat illness and disease
3. Growing demand for pharmaceuticals
4. The introduction of high-cost biotechnology products

Higher Expenditures for Drug Therapies

Expenditures for drugs vary widely in organized delivery systems. Most systems still allocate less than 20% of their total expenditures to drug therapies, but some organizations, such as those dealing with patients with acquired immunodeficiency syndrome (AIDS) or oncology patients, may experience higher expenses. All organizations are experiencing growth in expenditures related to new drugs and therapies.

Pharmacies generate revenue that covers only a small portion of drug expenses. Reimbursement for inpatient drug expenses is bundled with overall patient costs and contracts. Organized delivery systems also are often at risk for outpatient drug expenses in newer delivery models. In general, selection of the most effective and least costly alternative is the prudent course of action. Involvement of the pharmacy and therapeutics committee and front-line clinical pharmacists will lead to better patient care and financial outcomes. Balancing effectiveness and cost is perhaps the most challenging part of pharmaceutical care today.

The Cost of Drug Delivery Systems and Personnel

Pharmacy departments are often charged with the responsibility of managing drug and delivery system costs. Systems should be developed to utilize drug and delivery resources in a cost-effective fashion. Daily, weekly, monthly, and quarterly assessments of drug costs and salary costs should be done. Financial management systems in contemporary pharmacies should provide methods of quantifying costs, monitoring financial performance, relating clinical information, and determining data servicing costs.

The pharmacy management team should focus on developing effective strategies to maximize leverage of drug and human resource costs. These include automation of distribution tasks and the use of technicians and other support personnel, when warranted. Attention should also be paid to the level of experience and qualifications of the pharmacist engaged in a particular activity. A mix of specialists, generalists, and support system pharmacists should be hired to meet the organization's needs.

Managing Drug Costs

Two types of strategies can be applied to manage drug costs: administrative control and clinical review. Administrative control is implemented through reductions in drug acquisition costs, inventory management, use of appropriate drug distribution systems, and computerization. Clinical review can be determined by the severity of a disease, duration and continuation of drugs, or the effect of a drug on the patient.

The goal of reducing drug acquisition costs it to provide quality drugs at the lowest possible price. Many chemically identical drug entities, known as generic equivalents, are manufactured and distributed by various drug companies. The U.S. Food and Drug Administration (FDA) requires that drugs and their generic equivalents all act the same in the human body. Therefore, pharmacies can control drug acquisition costs by selecting the least expensive equivalent, whether through internal buying, group purchasing, or negotiation with acceptable vendors.

Cost-benefit analysis, along with other pharmacoeconomic approaches, is a way to analyze the value of the service to the public as a supplement to traditional marketplace value as measured by the prices that the patient or patron is willing to pay. Several factors affect financial issues in pharmacy practice today: The increased cost of prescriptions, the use of new medications, and the aging of the population combine to both enhance the quality of health care and increase inflation.

PRICING

Setting prices is essential to the success of a pharmacy practice. Pricing is the mechanism by which the manager ensures that the pharmacy covers its costs and makes a satisfactory profit. If prices are set too high, consumers may take their business elsewhere. If they are set too low, the pharmacy will not be able to cover its cost of operation. Either way, the pharmacy will not be able to stay in business.

The price of a prescription consists of three components: the cost of the drug dispensed, the cost of dispensing the drug, and net income from dispensing the drug. The cost of the drug is usually referred to as the *ingredient cost* or *product cost*. The cost of dispensing the drug covers expenses such as salaries, rent and utilities, depreciation, and insurance. These expenses may be considered to be service costs because they relate to the service provided rather than to the product. The service cost of dispensing a prescription is called the *cost to dispense*. The *net income* is the amount of profit the pharmacy earns on the prescription.

If the pharmacy is to earn a satisfactory profit, its price must cover its costs plus some surplus for net income. This suggests that pricing should be based primarily on cost factors. However, although costs are important, other factors also play a major role in determining prices.

Service Costs

For setting a correct price of product or service, the pharmacy must have an accurate estimate of the average, or per unit, cost of providing it. Service costs include the expenses directly incurred in providing the product or service and a fair share of expenses incurred indirectly.

To accurately calculate service costs, a pharmacist must understand several different kinds of costs and how they are related. All of a pharmacy's expenses can be classified as either direct or indirect costs.

Direct costs are costs that are caused directly by or result from providing the service. Direct costs of dispensing prescriptions include the costs of prescription labels and containers, patient education materials, pharmacy licenses, and continuing education for pharmacists.

Indirect costs are costs that are not caused directly by or that do not result directly from providing the service. They are costs that the pharmacy would incur even if it did not provide the service in question. Examples include rent, utilities, and a manager's salary. These costs are shared costs or joint costs. They are shared, or joint, in the sense that they are costs necessary to the sale of all of the pharmacy's products and services.

Recommended Strategy for Pricing

A pharmacy needs an overall strategy for setting proper prices. The strategy should ensure that prices are high enough, in aggregate, to cover all costs and include a reasonable profit. At the same time, the strategy must recognize the prices that the pharmacy can change are constrained by demand, competition, pharmacy goals and image, and nonmonetary costs.

To calculate the pharmacy's service cost, the manager must know how much, on average, the pharmacy should make on each prescription or unit of service to break even. The manager must then determine the average amount of net income the pharmacy must make on each prescription or unit of service to meet its overall profit objective. The profit objective is based on the desired return on assets for the pharmacy and is adjusted for competition and the pharmacy's image.

For example, assume that the pharmacy has $200,000 invested in prescription department assets. These would include fixtures, equipment, and prescription inventory. A typical community pharmacy should have a return on assets of at least 12%. To attain this return, a pharmacy with $200,000 in assets would need a $24,000 profit on prescriptions. If the pharmacy expected to dispense 48,000 prescriptions during the year, it would need an average net income of $1.00 per prescription to attain the $24,000 overall profit on prescriptions. If the pharmacy were in an area of high competition, the profit objective may have to be decreased to keep prices competitive. If it had a high-quality, high-service image, the profit objective may be increased and it may charge higher prices.

The manager must periodically evaluate the system to ensure that the pharmacy is making its desired profit. The average dollar margin required should be recalculated at least every 6 months. Changes in competition may also require the manager to reevaluate prices. Changes in prescribing habits and new products require the manager to periodically reevaluate the products in the market-priced and premium categories.

Methods of Calculating Product Prices

Three methods are commonly used to calculate prices for pharmaceutical products: the markup method, the professional fee method, and the sliding scale.

Markup Method

The **markup method** bases price and dollar margin on the ingredient cost of the product dispensed. Consequently, as ingredient cost increases, both price and margin increase proportionately. The markup may be calculated as a percentage of either ingredient cost or price. The following formula is used to calculate price using markup on cost:

$$\text{Price} = \text{Ingredient cost} + (\text{Ingredient cost} \times \text{Markup \%})$$

For example, if the cost of a drug is $35.00 and the markup is 50%, the price would be

$$\text{Price} = \$35.00 + (\$35.00 \times 0.50) = \$52.50$$

A markup system automatically adjusts prices to accommodate changes in ingredient costs. A disadvantage of the markup system is that it subsidizes low-cost products with high-cost ones. For example, if prescription prices are calculated using a markup, low-cost products have margins lower than the pharmacy's price image because consumers are more likely to recognize and react to higher prices on expensive drugs than to lower prices on inexpensive ones.

Professional Fee Method

The **professional fee method** is often used to calculate prescription prices. Almost all third-party prescription programs use this method to reimburse pharmacies for prescriptions. The professional fee is a set dollar amount, which is added to ingredient cost to determine the prescription price. It should be set at a level sufficient to cover the pharmacy's cost to dispense and net income. The fee is the same regardless of the cost of the drug dispensed. For example, if the ingredient cost of a drug is $7.00 and the fee is $8.75, the prescription price would be $15.75. If the ingredient cost is $65.00, the price would be $73.75. Therefore, the professional fee method avoids the markup system's disadvantage of subsidizing low-cost products with high-cost ones.

A disadvantage of the professional fee system is that it produces low gross margin percentages on expensive products. As the cost of prescription products increases, as it has in recent years, the pharmacy's gross margin percentage declines. A related disadvantage is that the professional fee system disregards the costs of carrying inventory. It costs the pharmacy more to invest in and carry expensive drugs. Consequently, the pharmacy requires a higher dollar margin on these items.

Sliding Scale Method

The markup method subsidizes low-cost drugs over expensive ones. The professional fee method disregards the higher inventory carrying costs associated with more expensive products. The **sliding scale method** overcomes both disadvantages by using variable markup percentages or professional fees to calculate prescription prices.

If a markup is used, the size of the percentage markup decreases as drug cost increases. A larger markup is added to the cost of cheaper drugs and a smaller markup is added to the cost of more expensive products. Therefore, the amount by which expensive drugs subsidize cheaper ones is minimized, and the effect of charging higher prices for expensive drugs is moderated.

HEALTH INSURANCE

Health insurance is a contract between a policyholder and an insurance carrier or government program to reimburse the policyholder for all or a portion of the cost of medical care rendered by health care professionals. This care includes care that is medically necessary and preventative treatment. The purpose of health insurance is to help offset some of the high costs accrued from an injury or illness.

Pharmacy technicians should be familiar with some specific terms that are commonly used in health insurance. An overview of terms the pharmacy technician should know and recognize follows:

- **Assignment of benefits**: An authorization to an insurance company to make payments directly to the pharmacy or physician.
- **Overpayment**: Payment by the insurer or by the patient of more than the amount due.
- **Contract**: An insurance policy; this is a legally enforceable agreement.
- **Subscriber**: The individual or organization protected in case of loss under the terms of an insurance policy. The subscriber is known as an insured or a member, policyholder, or recipient. In group insurance, the employer is known as the insured, and the employees are the risks.
- **Dependents**: The spouse and children of the insured who are also covered under the terms of the policy.
- **Policy limitation**: Some patients or individuals have exclusion health insurance policies. Some types of

exclusions are acquired immunodeficiency syndrome (AIDS), attempted suicide, cancer, losses due to injury on the job, and pregnancy.

- **Waiting period**: A waiting period or elimination period is the period of time that an individual must wait to become eligible for insurance coverage (e.g., 30 days) before coverage commences or for a specific benefit (e.g., an employee must wait 9 months before seeking maternity benefits).
- **Time limit**: The time limit is the amount of time from the date of service to the date (deadline) a claim can be filed with the insurance company. Each insurance program has specific time limits that must be adhered to or the insured party will not be able to collect from the insurance company.
- **Eligibility**: The determination of the exact coverage the insured is entitled to. The pharmacy technician may be responsible for checking on a customer's or patient's eligibility of coverage. This can be done over the telephone, via a voice-automated system, by using computer software, over the Internet, or by checking an eligibility list for a managed care plan.
- **Preauthorization**: Many private insurance companies and prepaid health plans have certain requirements that must be met before they will approve diagnostic testing, hospital admissions, inpatient or outpatient surgical procedures, specific procedures, and specific treatment or medications. For example, most outpatient intravenous therapies require a prior approval authorization.
- **Premium**: The premium is the cost of the coverage that the insurance policy contains and may vary greatly depending on the age and health of the individual and the type of insurance protection. The premium may be paid in full or in part by the employer and/or the employee.
- **Beneficiary**: A person designated by an insurance policy to receive benefits or funds.
- **Deductible**: A specific amount of money that must be paid yearly before the policy benefits begin (e.g., $50, $100, $300, or $500). The higher the deductible is, the lower the cost of the policy and the lower the deductible is, the higher the cost of the policy.
- **Coinsurance**: An arrangement in which the insured must pay a percentage of the cost of medical services covered by the insurer.
- **Co-payment**: Most insurance policies have a coinsurance, or cost-sharing, requirement, which is the responsibility of the insured to make a payment of a specified amount, for example, $5 or $10, at the time of treatment or purchase of a prescription. Some policies have both a copayment and coinsurance clause.
- **Coordination of benefits**: This prevents duplicate payment for the same service. For example, if a child

has coverage through both parents' insurance policies, a primary carrier is designated to pay benefits according to the terms of its policy and the secondary plan may cover whatever charges are still left. If the primary carrier pays $145 of a $180 charge, the most the secondary carrier will pay is $35.

Patients may be covered under different types of private, state, or federal programs. Each patient may have a different type of health insurance policy with various benefits. Therefore, the pharmacy technician should be familiar with different types of patient insurance coverage. There are three ways in which a person can acquire health insurance: (1) being included in a group plan (contract or policy), (2) enrolling in a prepaid health plan, and (3) paying the premium on an individual basis.

Group Plan

Any insurance plan by which a group of employees is insured under a single policy issued to their employer with individual certificates given to all insured individuals or their families is classified as a group plan or policy. A group policy usually provides better benefits and offers lower premiums than individual plans.

Prepaid Health Plan

In a prepaid health plan a policyholder or enrolled group of policyholders (subscribers) pay a yearly fee or fixed periodic payments. Providers of services are paid by capitation, which is a system of payments used by managed care plans in which physicians and hospitals are paid a fixed, per capita amount for each patient who registers for a specific period of time, regardless of the type and number of services provided.

Individual Contract

An insurance plan issued to an individual and his or her dependents is considered an individual contract. This kind of policy includes a higher premium, and the benefits are fewer. This type of insurance may also be called *personal insurance*.

TYPES OF HEALTH INSURANCE

Many forms of health insurance coverage are available in the United States. The majority of patients, almost 84%, have coverage from some type of insurance policy or other third-party payer. A **third-party payer** is an individual or corporation that makes a payment on an obligation or debt but is not a party to the contract that created the obligation or debt. To understand third-party payers better, let us first discuss first- and second-party payers. The first party is the person designated in the contract to receive a contracted service, whereas the second party is the person or organization

providing the service. There are three major third-party payers: third-party full-payment groups (private insurance companies), third-party contractual payment groups (Blue Cross®, Medicare, and Medicaid), and the cash payment group. Health insurance may include private insurance, government plans, managed care contracts, and worker's compensation—all referred to as third-party payers.

Private Health Insurance

Numerous private insurance companies across the United States offer health insurance to individuals and groups. They offer a variety of managed care plans. Examples of private insurance include Blue Cross®-Blue Shield®, various health maintenance organizations (HMOs), the Kaiser Foundation, and workers' compensation.

Blue Cross®-Blue Shield® Association

The Blue Cross®-Blue Shield® Association (BCBS) is a nationwide federation of local nonprofit service organizations that offer prepaid health care services to subscribers. Under a prepaid health coverage plan, the carrier will pay for specified medical expenses if premiums are paid in advance. The Blue Cross® part of BCBS covers hospital services, outpatient and home care services, and other institutional care. The Blue Shield® plan covers physician and dental services, vision, and other outpatient benefits. Now, however, both offer full health care coverage for their subscribers. In most states, they have become a single corporation, although in some they remain separate. A variety of plans are offered through BCBS, including individual and family, group, preventative care, and managed care plans. Some local BCBS organizations help the government administer Medicare, Medicaid, and TRICARE programs. There are 86 local BCBS plans in the United States, each with its own claim form. Plans make direct payments to member physicians, but payments may be made to the subscriber (patient) if the physician is a nonmember. Many small groups and individuals who may not be able to get coverage elsewhere can join a BCBS plan. Some plans offer coverage regardless of medical condition during special periods of time. Plans must get permission from the state to raise their rates.

Health Maintenance Organizations

HMOs were the first type of managed care organizations developed to control the expenditure of health care dollars and to manage patient care. The HMO contracts with employers to provide health service for their employees. The member of an HMO selects a primary care physician (PCP) from the medical group. The HMO is responsible for all but limited administrative needs of a PCP, including processing of capitation and fee-for-service checks. The HMO remains a challenging and exciting setting for developing the optimum contribution of drug services to good medical care.

Point-of-Service Point-of-service is an option added to some HMO plans that allows patients to choose a physician outside the HMO network. For this option, patients pay increased deductibles and coinsurance fees.

Kaiser Foundation Health Plan

The Kaiser Foundation Health Plan is a type of prepaid group practice HMO. The Kaiser Foundation was a pioneer of the nonprofit prepaid group practice, beginning in California in 1933. The plan owns its own medical facilities and directly employs physicians and other providers.

Workers' Compensation

All state legislatures have passed workers' compensation laws to protect wage earners against the loss of wages and the cost of medical care resulting from occupational accidents or disease. Compensation benefits include medical care benefits, weekly income replacement benefits for temporary disability, permanent disability settlements, and survivor benefits, when applicable. The providers of service, such as doctors, hospitals, therapists, or pharmacies, accept the workers' compensation payment as payment in full and do not bill the patient. Time limitations are set forth for the prompt reporting of workers' compensation cases. The employee is obligated to promptly notify the employer; the employer, in turn, must notify the insurance company and must refer the employee to a source of medical care. Individuals entitled to workers' compensation insurance are private business employees, state employees, and federal employees such as postal workers, coal miners, and maritime workers. Workers' compensation insurance coverage provides benefits to employees and their dependents if employees suffer work-related injuries, illnesses, or death. When a claim is made, a workers' compensation claim form is completed and sent to the insurance carrier or to the state fund for reimbursement. The injured worker receives no bills and pays no deductible or coinsurance; 100% of medical expenses related specifically to that injury are covered.

Managed Care Programs

During the past six decades, there have been many reforms of the health care system. Medical practices have made transitions from rural to urban, from generalist to specialist, from solo to group practice, and from fee-for-service to capitated reimbursement. The expansion of health care plans to a number of different types of delivery systems that try to manage the cost of health care resulted in managed care. Managed care organizations manage, negotiate, and contract for health care with the goal of keeping costs down. Managed care organizations sign up health care providers who agree to charge a fixed fee for services. These fixed fees are set by the managed care organization or by the governmental agency responsible for managed care.

Independent Practice Association

An **independent practice association (IPA)** is a closed-panel HMO. Instead of maintaining its own staff and clinic buildings, the IPA contracts with independently practicing physicians. The IPA may pay each doctor a set amount per patient in advance (capitation), or the fees charged for services to group members may be billed directly to the IPA rather than to the patient. Fees for services to nonmember patients are handled the same as any other fee for service. The physician may be contracted with several IPAs.

Preferred Provider Organization

In a **preferred provider organization (PPO)**, a type of managed care plan, enrollees receive the highest level of benefits when they obtain services from a physician, hospital, or other health provider designated by their program as a preferred provider. Enrollees receive reduced benefits when they obtain care from a provider who is not designated as a preferred provider by their program. PPO patients may see specialists without prior authorization from their primary care physicians. HMOs offering point-of-service options are more like PPOs.

Government Plans

Government plans sponsor insurance coverage for eligible individuals. The federal government provides coverage under Medicare, Medicaid, TRICARE or CHAMPUS, and CHAMPVA.

Medicare

Medicare is the largest single medical benefits program in the United States. Medicare is a federal program authorized by Congress and administered by the Centers for Medicare & Medicaid Services (CMS). It became a law in 1965 as Title 18 of the Social Security Act. Medicare is a nationwide program that offers the same benefits in all 50 states. It provides health insurance to citizens aged 65 and older and to younger patients who are blind or widowed or who are disabled because of serious long-term illnesses such as kidney failure. There are three distinct parts (A, B, and C) to the Medicare program. Medicare Part A covers hospital, nursing facility, home health, hospice, and inpatient care. Those who are eligible for Social Security benefits are automatically enrolled in Medicare Part A. Medicare Part B covers outpatient health care services, services by physicians, durable medical equipment, and other services and supplies. Medicare Part B does not cover prescriptions. Medicare Part B coverage is optional. Everyone eligible for Part A can choose to enroll in Part B by paying monthly premiums. Deductibles must be met in Parts A and B before payment benefits begin. Medicare pays only a portion of a patient's hospitalization expenses. Some federal employees and former federal employees who are not eligible for Social Security benefits and

Medicare Part A may still enroll in Part B. Many Medicare enrollees also carry private supplemental insurance that pays the deductible and the 20% co-payment. Medicare Part C is Medicare + Choice plans, which were created to offer a number of health care options in addition to those available under Medicare Part A and Part B. These plans receive a fixed amount of money from Medicare to spend on their Medicare members. Some plans may require members to pay a premium similar to the Medicare Part B premium. If the patient chooses coverage under Part C, he or she will not need coverage under Part A and Part B.

Plans available under this program may include the following:

1. Health maintenance organization (HMO)
2. Point-of-service (POS)
3. Private fee-for-service (PFFS)
4. Provider-sponsored organization (PSO)
5. Religious fraternal benefit society (RFBS)
6. Medicare medical savings account (MSA) (pilot program)

If a patient has both Medicare and Medicaid, charges must be filed with Medicare first, and Medicaid is the secondary payer.

Medicaid

In 1965, Congress passed Title 19 of the Social Security Act, setting up a combined federal-state medical insurance program to provide medical care for persons with income below the national poverty level. **Medicaid** is a health benefits program designed for low-income people (those receiving welfare payment or other forms of public assistance), the blind, the disabled, and members of families with dependent children deprived of the support of at least one parent and financially eligible on the basis of income and resources. Each state decides what services are covered and what the reimbursement will be for each service. Two types of co-payment requirements may apply to the Medicaid patient. Some states require a small fixed co-payment paid to the provider at the time of service (e.g., $1.00 or $2.00). This policy was instituted to help pay some of the administrative costs of physicians participating in the Medicaid program. Certain groups of patients may be exempt from this co-payment requirement (e.g., persons under 18 years of age or women receiving prenatal care).

TRICARE

TRICARE is a comprehensive health benefits program offering three (tri) types of plans for dependents of men and women in the uniformed services (military). Under the basic TRICARE program, individuals have the following three options:

- TRICARE standard: fee-for-service (cost-sharing plan)
- TRICARE extra: preferred provider organization plan

- TRICARE prime: health maintenance organization plan with a point-of-service option

TRICARE is a new program that replaced CHAMPUS. CHAMPUS stands for "Civilian Health and Medical Program of the Uniformed Services." CHAMPUS was a health care benefit for families of uniformed personnel and retirees from the uniformed services (the Army, Navy, Air Force, Marines, Coast Guard, Public Health Service, and National Oceanic and Atmospheric Administration).

CHAMPVA

CHAMPVA stands for "Civilian Health and Medical Program of the Veterans Administration." It was created in 1973. CHAMPVA covers the expenses of the families of veterans with total, permanent, service-connected disabilities. It also covers the expenses of surviving spouses and dependent children of veterans who died in the line of duty. Eligibility is determined and identification cards are issued by the nearest Veterans Affairs medical center. The insured persons are then free to choose their own private physicians. Benefits and cost-sharing features are the same as those for CHAMPUS beneficiaries who are military retirees or their dependents and dependents of deceased members of the military.

INSURANCE POLICY

An insurance policy is a legally enforceable agreement. It is also called an insurance contract, regardless of whether the contract is a group, individual, or prepaid contract. There is no standard health insurance contract; however, state laws regulate the way policies are written and minimum requirements of coverage. A policy might also include dependents of the insured, which means the spouse and children of the insured. However, under some contracts, parents and other family members may be covered as dependents. The policy becomes effective only after the company offers the policy and the person accepts it and pays the initial premium.

CLAIM FORM

A claim occurs when patients, having received treatment, wish to receive reimbursement under their insurance policies for charges for treatment. The patient or the billing department sends the claim to the insurance carrier for the amount of the treatment. This is done via a claim form. The most common claim form is the CMS-1500 (12-90), which is illustrated in Figure 12-1. This form was developed by the CMS.

PLEASE
DO NOT
STAPLE
IN THIS
AREA

CARRIER

HEALTH INSURANCE CLAIM FORM

PICA | | | | PICA

1. MEDICARE | MEDICAID | CHAMPUS | CHAMPVA | GROUP HEALTH PLAN | FECA BLK LUNG | OTHER | 1a. INSURED'S I.D. NUMBER (FOR PROGRAM IN ITEM 1)
☐ (Medicare #) | ☐ (Medicaid #) | ☐ (Sponsor's SSN) | ☐ (VA File #) | ☐ (SSN or ID) | ☐ (SSN) | ☐ (ID)

2. PATIENT'S NAME (Last Name, First Name, Middle Initial)

3. PATIENT'S BIRTH DATE MM ‖ DD ‖ YY   SEX   M☐ F☐

4. INSURED'S NAME (Last Name, First Name, Middle Initial)

5. PATIENT'S ADDRESS (No., Street)

6. PATIENT RELATIONSHIP TO INSURED
Self☐ Spouse☐ Child☐ Other☐

7. INSURED'S ADDRESS (No., Street)

CITY | STATE

8. PATIENT STATUS
Single☐ Married☐ Other☐

CITY | STATE

ZIP CODE | TELEPHONE (Include Area Code) ( )

Employed☐ Full-Time Student☐ Part-Time Student☐

ZIP CODE | TELEPHONE (INCLUDE AREA CODE) ( )

9. OTHER INSURED'S NAME (Last Name, First Name, Middle Initial)

10. IS PATIENT'S CONDITION RELATED TO:

11. INSURED'S POLICY GROUP OR FECA NUMBER

a. OTHER INSURED'S POLICY OR GROUP NUMBER

a. EMPLOYMENT? (CURRENT OR PREVIOUS) ☐ YES ☐ NO

a. INSURED'S DATE OF BIRTH MM ‖ DD ‖ YY   SEX   M☐ F☐

b. OTHER INSURED'S DATE OF BIRTH MM ‖ DD ‖ YY   SEX   M☐ F☐

b. AUTO ACCIDENT? PLACE (State) ☐ YES ☐ NO

b. EMPLOYER'S NAME OR SCHOOL NAME

c. EMPLOYER'S NAME OR SCHOOL NAME

c. OTHER ACCIDENT? ☐ YES ☐ NO

c. INSURANCE PLAN NAME OR PROGRAM NAME

d. INSURANCE PLAN NAME OR PROGRAM NAME

10d. RESERVED FOR LOCAL USE

d. IS THERE ANOTHER HEALTH BENEFIT PLAN?
☐ YES ☐ NO *If yes*, return to and complete item 9 a-d.

READ BACK OF FORM BEFORE COMPLETING & SIGNING THIS FORM.

12. PATIENT'S OR AUTHORIZED PERSON'S SIGNATURE I authorize the release of any medical or other information necessary to process this claim. I also request payment of government benefits either to myself or to the party who accepts assignment below.

SIGNED _____ DATE _____

13. INSURED'S OR AUTHORIZED PERSON'S SIGNATURE I authorize payment of medical benefits to the undersigned physician or supplier for services described below.

SIGNED _____

14. DATE OF CURRENT: MM ‖ DD ‖ YY ◀ ILLNESS (First symptom) OR INJURY (Accident) OR PREGNANCY(LMP)

15. IF PATIENT HAS HAD SAME OR SIMILAR ILLNESS. GIVE FIRST DATE MM ‖ DD ‖ YY

16. DATES PATIENT UNABLE TO WORK IN CURRENT OCCUPATION MM ‖ DD ‖ YY   MM ‖ DD ‖ YY
FROM ___ TO ___

17. NAME OF REFERRING PHYSICIAN OR OTHER SOURCE

17a. I.D. NUMBER OF REFERRING PHYSICIAN

18. HOSPITALIZATION DATES RELATED TO CURRENT SERVICES MM ‖ DD ‖ YY   MM ‖ DD ‖ YY
FROM ___ TO ___

19. RESERVED FOR LOCAL USE

20. OUTSIDE LAB? ☐ YES ☐ NO $ CHARGES

21. DIAGNOSIS OR NATURE OF ILLNESS OR INJURY. (RELATE ITEMS 1,2,3 OR 4 TO ITEM 24E BY LINE)

1. ‖___. ___   3. ‖___. ___
2. ‖___. ___   4. ‖___. ___

22. MEDICAID RESUBMISSION CODE   ORIGINAL REF. NO.

23. PRIOR AUTHORIZATION NUMBER

24. A					B	C	D	E	F	G	H	I	J	K
DATE(S) OF SERVICE From — To					Place of Service	Type of Service	PROCEDURES, SERVICES, OR SUPPLIES (Explain Unusual Circumstances) CPT/HCPCS MODIFIER	DIAGNOSIS CODE	$ CHARGES	DAYS OR UNITS	EPSDT Family Plan	EMG	COB	RESERVED FOR LOCAL USE
MM	DD	YY	MM	DD	YY									
1														
2														
3														
4														
5														
6														

25. FEDERAL TAX I.D. NUMBER SSN☐ EIN☐

26. PATIENT'S ACCOUNT NO.

27. ACCEPT ASSIGNMENT? (For govt. claims, see back) ☐ YES ☐ NO

28. TOTAL CHARGE $

29. AMOUNT PAID $

30. BALANCE DUE $

31. SIGNATURE OF PHYSICIAN OR SUPPLIER INCLUDING DEGREES OR CREDENTIALS (I certify that the statements on the reverse apply to this bill and are made a part thereof.)

SIGNED _____ DATE _____

32. NAME AND ADDRESS OF FACILITY WHERE SERVICES WERE RENDERED (If other than home or office)

33. PHYSICIAN'S, SUPPLIER'S BILLING NAME, ADDRESS, ZIP CODE & PHONE #

PIN# _____ GRP# _____

(APPROVED BY AMA COUNCIL ON MEDICAL SERVICE 8/88)

PLEASE PRINT OR TYPE

APPROVED OMB-0938-0008 FORM HCFA-1500 (12-90), FORM RRB-1500,
APPROVED OMB-1215-0055 FORM OWCP-1500, APPROVED OMB-0720-0001 (CHAMPUS)

PATIENT AND INSURED INFORMATION

PHYSICIAN OR SUPPLIER INFORMATION

Figure 12-1. CMS-1500 claim form.

BILLING

Two types of bills are used to collect payment for medical services—those sent to the insurer and those sent to the patient—or the patient must be charged. The bill to the insurance carrier is submitted by filling out a claim form. The bill to the patient summarizes the charges and payments and lets him or her know how much is owed.

Even though patients are asked to pay for medical care when they receive it, extenuating circumstances often make paying the bill immediately an unrealistic expectation. Sometimes, it is a matter of not knowing how much of the charge, if any, the patient's insurance will pay. Established patients who are known and have a history of paying promptly when billed may be expected to continue to pay promptly, but, sometimes, the patient may be temporarily unable to pay. In each of these situations, periodic billing by mail becomes necessary.

When the patient is admitted into the hospital or receives services in the emergency room, pharmaceutical items or hospital items are not billed directly to patients. This is different in the retail pharmacy. The pharmacist or technician should send a claim form to a third party, and the patient should be charged for the co-payment.

SUMMARY

An understanding of financial issues, accounting, and various types of insurance coverage is essential for pharmacists and pharmacy technicians because the practice of pharmacy is a business and the costs of medical care and drug prescriptions are increasing. Customers and patients without insurance may not be able to afford to purchase their prescriptions and durable medical equipment. Thus, a pharmacy technician must understand the challenges involved in the role of insurance in the management of the pharmacy. He or she must be able to explain insurance procedures to the patient and know how to make contact with appropriate representatives to determine eligibility and answer questions about coverage.

CRITICAL THINKING

1. Describe the cost of drug delivery systems and personnel.
2. Compare private health insurance with government plans.

REVIEW QUESTIONS

1. Which of the following is another method of calculating products prices besides the professional fee and the markup method?
   A. Cost and productivity
   B. Sliding scale
   C. Third-party payer
   D. Claim form

2. Which of the following was a pioneer of nonprofit prepaid group practice beginning in California?
   A. Workers' compensation
   B. Health maintenance organization
   C. Preferred provider organization
   D. The Kaiser Foundation

3. An example of indirect cost includes which of the following?
   A. Prescription labels
   B. Medication containers
   C. Manager's salary
   D. Patient education materials

4. Which of the following statements is true about Medicare Part C plans?
   A. The patient will not need coverage under Part A and Part B.
   B. These plans do not receive a fixed amount of money from Medicare to spend on their Medicare members.
   C. These plans are designed for low-income and disabled people.
   D. These plans cover the expenses of the families of veterans with total and service-connected disabilities.

5. The ingredient cost of a drug was $3.00 and the fees were $6.45, the prescription price would be $9.45. If the ingredient costs were $57.25, the price would be which of the following?
   A. $47.80
   B. $50.70
   C. $60.25
   D. $66.70

Continues

6. Administrative control of drug cost is implemented through reductions in which of the following?
   A. Selecting trade name drugs that are approved by the FDA
   B. Inventory management
   C. Negotiating with the FDA to provide cheaper drugs
   D. Selecting small vendors

7. The Blue Shield® plan, a part of Blue Cross®-Blue Shield®, covers which of the following benefits?
   A. Home care
   B. Hospital
   C. Vision care
   D. Ambulatory care

8. TRICARE is a comprehensive health benefits program offering three types of plans for which of the following groups?
   A. Poor
   B. Military
   C. Disabled
   D. Children only

9. The pharmacy management team should maximize leverage of drug and human resource costs by developing effective strategies that include
   A. computerizing the pharmacy to reduce the cost of human resources.
   B. providing automation of distribution tasks.
   C. hiring pharmacists instead of technicians to prevent medication errors.
   D. reducing services in community.

10. A specific amount of money, which must be paid yearly before the policy benefits begin, is called
    A. a premium.
    B. a time limit.
    C. a deductible.
    D. a beneficiary.

11. An example of private health insurance is
    A. Blue Cross®-Blue Shield®.
    B. Medicaid.
    C. Medicare.
    D. CHAMPVA.

12. Which of the following is perhaps the most challenging part of pharmaceutical care today?
    A. Research for new diseases
    B. Continuing education for pharmacists and technicians
    C. Balancing effectiveness and cost
    D. Medication errors

13. The cost of the coverage that the insurance policy contains is known as the
    A. proscenium.
    B. premium.
    C. preauthorization.
    D. privatization.

14. The largest single medical benefits program in the United States is which of the following?
    A. Medicaid
    B. Workers' compensation
    C. Health maintenance organizations
    D. Medicare

15. Which of the following is the goal of reducing drug acquisition costs?
    A. Quality drugs at the lowest possible price
    B. Quality of health care at the lowest possible price
    C. Urging physicians to order less expensive drugs
    D. Urging the pharmacist to use automation of distribution tasks instead of technicians

13   Safety in the Workplace

OBJECTIVES

Upon completion of this chapter, the reader should be able to

1. Explain the Occupational Safety and Health Administration (OSHA).
2. Specify potentially infectious bodily fluids.
3. Describe the exposure control plan.
4. Summarize standard precautions.
5. Differentiate disinfection, sanitization, and sterilization procedures.
6. Describe an autoclave and the indication for its use.
7. Explain a laminar airflow hood.
8. Differentiate between vertical and horizontal laminar airflow hoods.
9. List four responsibilities of employees for compliance with OSHA regulations.

GLOSSARY

autoclave A sterilizing machine. An autoclave uses a combination of heat, steam, and pressure to sterilize equipment.

biohazard symbol An image or object that serves as an alert that there is a risk to organisms, such as ionizing radiation or harmful bacteria or viruses.

carcinogenic A substance that causes cancer.

caustic A substance that eats away at something.

chemical sterilization A method of cleaning equipment used for instruments that cannot be exposed to the high temperatures of steam sterilization.

disinfection Destruction of pathogens by physical or chemical means.

dry heat sterilization A method of sterilization that uses heated dry air at a temperature of 320 to 356°F (160 to 180°C) for 90 minutes to 3 hours.

exposure control plan A written procedure for the treatment of persons exposed to biohazardous or similar chemically harmful materials.

fire safety plan A written procedure that includes fire extinguisher locations, fire alarm pull-box locations, sprinkler system location, exit signs, and clear directions to the quickest and safest exit of a building during an emergency.

gas sterilization The use of a gas such as ethylene oxide to sterilize medical equipment.

hazard communication plan Application of warning labels for all hazardous chemicals.

laminar airflow hood A system of circulating filtered air in parallel-flowing planes in hospitals or other health care facilities. The system reduces the risk of airborne contamination and exposure to chemical pollutants in surgical theaters, food preparation areas, hospital pharmacies, and laboratories.

GLOSSARY continued

material safety data sheet (MSDS) Written or printed material concerning a hazardous chemical that includes information on the chemical's identity and physical and chemical characteristics.

medical asepsis Complete destruction of organisms after they leave the body.

sanitization A process of cleansing to remove undesirable debris.

standard precautions A set of guidelines for infection control.

sterilization Complete destruction of all forms of microbial life.

surgical asepsis The complete destruction of organisms before they enter the body.

teratogenic A substance that causes developmental malformation.

OVERVIEW

Safety issues are present in any place, and common sense precautions need to be taken in the workplace, particularly in the pharmacy. The purpose of environmental protection measures is to minimize the risk of occupational injury by isolating or removing any physical or mechanical health hazard in any workplace. In 1970, the federal government passed the Occupational Safety and Health Act, the first national health and safety law, with the goal of ensuring safe and healthful working conditions for all workers in the United States. The Act established the Occupational Safety and Health Administration (OSHA) in the Department of Labor. OSHA establishes safety regulations for employers and monitors compliance.

OCCUPATIONAL SAFETY AND HEALTH ADMINISTRATION STANDARDS

OSHA provides for research, information, education, and training in the field of occupational safety and health and authorized enforcement of OSHA standards. OSHA also establishes standards requiring employers to provide their workers with workplaces free from recognized hazards that could cause serious injury or death. In addition, employees must abide by all safety and health standards that apply to their jobs (see Table 13-1).

OSHA regulates all workplace environments by enforcing protocols for the proper removal of hazards and for fire safety and emergency plans. Two specific functions related to the pharmacy, specifically the hospital pharmacy, are protection of employees from exposure to disease and protection from exposure to chemicals. Chemical materials may be flammable, **caustic**, poisonous, **carcinogenic**, and/or **teratogenic**. Employees can be exposed to these dangers through inhalation, direct absorption through the skin, ingestion, entry through a mucous membrane, or entry through a break in the skin. Information and training on safe work practices must be provided to all workers.

The general health of the employee must be protected, and many standards require plans such as an infection control plan, training of employees, availability of personal protective equipment, provision of vaccinations such as hepatitis B, and medical intervention after exposure incidents and monitoring of injuries with detailed records. OSHA has the right to inspect private and public work sites to be sure all protocols and guidelines are being followed.

TABLE 13-1. Safety Guidelines for the Pharmacy Technician

- Observe warning labels on biohazard containers and equipment.
- Minimize splashing, spraying, and splattering of drops of potentially infectious materials. Splattering of blood onto skin or mucous membranes is a proven mode of transmission of hepatitis B virus.
- Bandage any breaks or lesions on your hands before gloving.
- If exposed body surfaces, such as the eyes, come in contact with body fluids, flush with water and/or scrub with soap and water as soon as possible.
- Do not recap, bend, or break contaminated needles and other sharps.
- Use hemostats to attach and remove scalpel blades from handles.
- Do not use mouth pipetting or suck blood through tubing.
- Decontaminate contaminated test materials before reprocessing or place in impervious bags and dispose of according to policy.
- Do not keep food and drink in refrigerators, freezers, shelves, or cabinets or on countertops where blood or other potentially hazardous chemical materials could be present.

Training of Employees

Because of the importance of safety in the workplace, the employer must provide special training sessions during working hours at no cost to employees. Training must be provided at the initial time of employment and then annually if there are new procedures. Training material must be appropriate for the literacy and education level of the employee. It must be interactive and permit questions and answers.

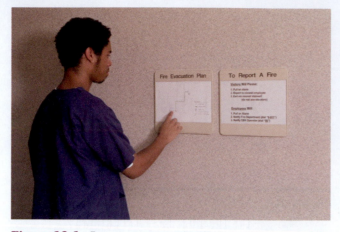

Figure 13-1. Escape routes must be clearly posted as part of the fire safety plan of a facility.

Fire Safety Plan

An OSHA-compliant **fire safety plan** must include written procedures. Exits must be marked and escape routes published (see Figure 13-1). Fire extinguishers and fire alarm pull boxes must be present, and the employer must provide fire prevention training, conduct fire drills, and test the fire alarm and sprinkler systems.

Hazard Communication Plan

A **hazard communication plan** protects the rights of employees to know what types of hazardous chemicals are present in the workplace and what health risks are associated with those chemicals. All hazardous chemicals must have warning labels as shown in Figure 13-2.

OSHA requires pharmacies to have a **material safety data sheet (MSDS)** for each hazardous chemical material used. A pharmacy can use sheets provided by the local OSHA area office or by the manufacturer of the hazardous chemical. The pharmacy technician must be familiar with the MSDS information and ensure the implementation of proper protective measures for exposure to hazardous materials. Each MSDS contains basic information about the specific chemical or product. This includes the trade name, chemical name and synonyms, chemical family, manufacturer's name and address, telephone number for emergencies, hazardous ingredients, physical data, fire and explosion data, and health hazard and protection information (see Figure 13-3).

Containers with chemicals should be tightly sealed and properly labeled. A hazard identification system was developed by the National Fire Protection Association that provides an identification coding method. This consists of four small, colored, diamond-shaped symbols grouped into a larger diamond shape. The top diamond is red and indicates a flammability hazard. The diamond on the left is blue and indicates hazards to health. The bottom diamond is white

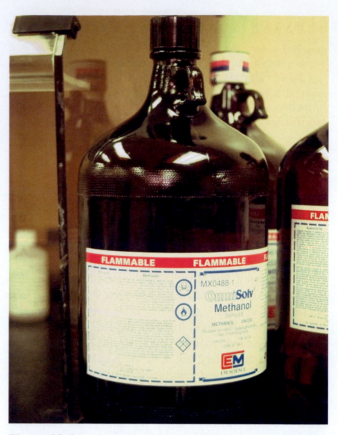

Figure 13-2. Chemicals used in the workplace must be clearly and accurately labeled.

and provides special hazard information, including radioactivity, special biohazards, and other dangerous situations. Finally, the diamond on the right is yellow and indicates reactivity/stability hazards. The system indicates the severity of the hazard by using numbers from 0 to 4 imprinted in the diamonds, with 4 meaning "extremely hazardous" and 0 meaning "no hazard" (see Figure 13-4).

Exposure Control Plan

The **exposure control plan** is designed to minimize risk of exposure to infectious material and blood-borne disease. The plan must be written and updated as necessary. OSHA also has regulations for or provides information about hazards associated with radioactive materials (see Figure 13-5).

Immunizations

OSHA regulations require that all health care workers be immunized against hepatitis B, because they are at risk for exposure to blood-borne pathogens. This vaccine must be available free of charge to all who are at risk for occupational exposure to blood-borne pathogens, whether they are full-time or part-time workers, within 10 days of starting employment. Employees may decline the immunization but

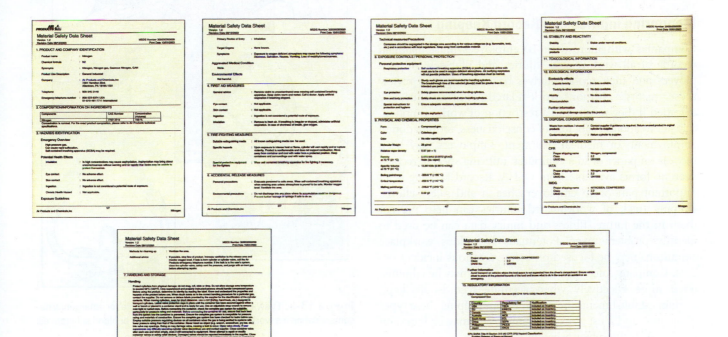

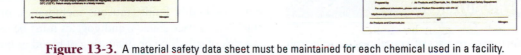

Figure 13-3. A material safety data sheet must be maintained for each chemical used in a facility.

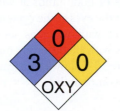

Figure 13-4. The National Fire Protection Association hazard identification symbol.

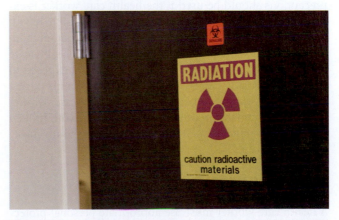

Figure 13-5. Radioactive hazards must be clearly marked using this symbol.

must sign a declination form that is kept on file as a record of worker refusal. However, the employee may still receive the vaccine at a future date free of charge. For more information about the hepatitis B vaccination, see Chapter 28.

Monitoring Injuries and Record Keeping

Companies with more than 10 employees must maintain records of all work-related injuries and illnesses. All employees and their representatives have the right to review these records. Minor, work-related injuries must be recorded if they resulted in a restriction of work or motion, transfer to another job, loss of consciousness, termination of employment, or medical treatment. Employers may keep records on paper or in a computer, utilizing specific record-keeping forms available from OSHA. Record keeping is an important part of an employer's health and safety efforts. Keeping track of work-related injuries can help prevent them in the future. Illness and injury data can be used to identify problem areas. Potentially hazardous workplace conditions may be focused on before a serious incident occurs. Company safety and health programs may be administered more effectively when accurate records are kept. Certain establishments are exempt from keeping these types of records, and a list of exempt employers may be found on OSHA's Web site (www.osha.gov).

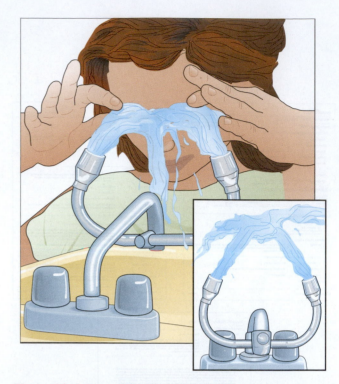

Figure 13-6. Eyewash stations must be available for emergency decontamination if a worker is exposed to chemicals or blood substances.

STANDARD PRECAUTIONS

Standard precautions are a set of guidelines for infection control requiring the employer and employee to assume that all human blood and specified human body fluids are infectious for human immunodeficiency virus (HIV), hepatitis B virus, and other blood-borne pathogens. Standard precautions should be used if the health care worker is exposed to blood, other body fluids containing visible blood, semen, vaginal secretions, cerebrospinal fluid, pleural fluid, synovial fluid, and any other body fluids. A health care worker should also use standard precautions if exposed to urine, feces, nasal secretions, sputum, breast milk, tears, saliva, and vomitus. In addition, a health care worker should use standard precautions when dealing with broken skin and the mucous membranes inside the mouth, nose, and body cavities.

Use of Personal Protective Equipment

A health care worker must use appropriate personal protective equipment, such as gloves, gowns, masks, laboratory coats, face shields, and goggles, to protect himself or herself from exposure to pathogens (disease-causing microorganisms). This equipment is used to place a barrier between the employee and blood or bodily fluids along with other methods of compliance to prevent exposure that can contaminate

skin, mucous membranes, or nonintact skin. Gloves must be worn when there is a possibility of hand contact with blood or bodily fluids, mucous membranes, or nonintact skin. Masks, face shields, and goggles must be used if there is a risk of splashing or splattering of blood or bodily fluids. Gowns, laboratory coats, or scrubs must be worn to protect against exposure and must be left at the work site in an area set aside for their storage. Eyewash stations are required in each facility by law for emergencies. If an employee is exposed to chemicals or body fluids at work, he or she must be able to flush out the eyes at the eyewash station and flush mucous membranes with water as soon as possible after contact of the eyes with blood or chemical substances (see Figure 13-6). Figure 13-7 shows a pharmacy technician who is ready for sterile compounding.

Disposal of Hazardous Materials

Any materials that have come into contact with blood or body fluids are treated as hazardous waste. Various containers are used to collect hazardous material. Waste containers are labeled with the **biohazard symbol** to ensure that all employees are aware of the contents (see Figure 13-8). Plastic bags are used for gloves, paper towels, dressings, and other soft material; rigid containers are used for sharps such as needles, glass slides, scalpel blades, or disposable syringes (see Figure 13-9A). Most facilities contract with a company that specializes in removal and disposal of hazardous waste. Cleaning staff should be instructed not to empty hazardous

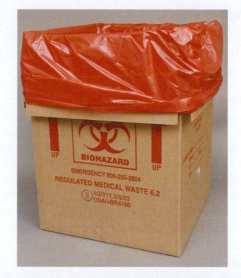

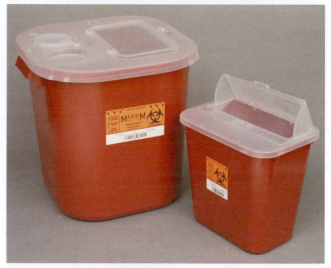

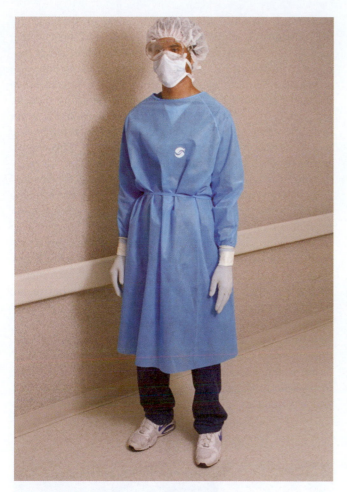

Figure 13-7. Proper personal protective equipment must be worn at all times.

Figure 13-9. Hazardous materials must only be disposed of in the containers properly labeled with the biohazard symbol. Any sharp items must be disposed of in a hard plastic "sharps" container.

ASEPTIC TECHNIQUE

The most effective way to eliminate transmission of disease from one host to another is through asepsis, which means "being completely sterile (free from microorganisms)." There are two types of asepsis: medical asepsis and surgical asepsis.

Medical Asepsis

Medical asepsis is the removal of pathogens to reduce transfer of microorganisms by cleaning any body part or surface that has been exposed to them. Medical asepsis benefits both the patient and the health care worker by preventing exposure to pathogens from other patients, from each other, or from other staff. Medical asepsis is also called *clean technique.*

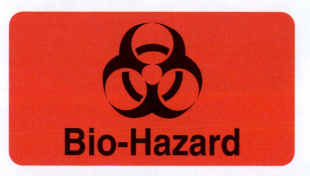

Figure 13-8. Biohazard symbols alert the pharmacy technician to hazardous materials.

waste containers. When health care workers change hazardous waste bags, they must wear gloves, masks, and protective eyewear; close the bags securely; and put the bag inside a second hazardous waste bag (double bag) if there is any chance of leakage.

Hand Hygiene

The single most important means of preventing the spread of infection is frequent and effective hand hygiene by all health care workers. Hands must be washed, using the correct technique. An extended scrub is not needed each time hands are washed, but the first scrub in the morning should be extensive, lasting 2 to 4 minutes, unless the hands are excessively contaminated. A good antimicrobial soap with chlorhexidine, such as Hibiclens®, which has antiseptic residual action that will last several hours, should be used. Even with this technique, the hands are still not sterile, because skin cannot be sterilized. Normal flora (nonpathogens) remain, but most pathogens have been removed. Proper handwashing depends on two factors: running water and friction. The water should be warm, because water that is too cold or too hot will cause the skin to become chapped. Friction involves the firm rubbing of all surfaces of the hands and wrists. Figure 13-10A through 13-10D shows the steps of handwashing that a technician should use.

Cleaning and Sanitizing

Equipment and instruments need to be cleaned promptly and carefully after every use to remove visible residue before proceeding with the steps of disinfection or sterilization. Microorganisms may hide under residue and survive the disinfection or sterilization process if residue is not removed. **Sanitization** is the cleansing process that decreases the number of microorganisms to a safe level as dictated in public health guidelines. This cleansing process removes debris such as blood and other body fluids from instruments or equipment. Blood and debris must be removed so that when instruments are later disinfected or sterilized, chemicals (disinfection) or steam, heat, or gases (sterilization) can penetrate to all surfaces of the instruments. Items that cannot be cleaned at once are usually rinsed with cold water and placed in a soaking solution to prevent anyone from touching them and to prevent the residue from hardening. When instruments are sanitized, the soaking solution is drained off, and each instrument is rinsed in cold, running water. The sharp instruments should be separated from the others because other metal instruments may damage the cutting edges, and the sharp instruments may damage the other instruments or injure someone. All the sharp instruments are cleaned at one time, to avoid the dangers of injury. Instruments are rinsed in hot water. The items should be hand-dried with a towel to prevent spotting. Sanitization is a very important step, and it cannot be overlooked or done carelessly. The use

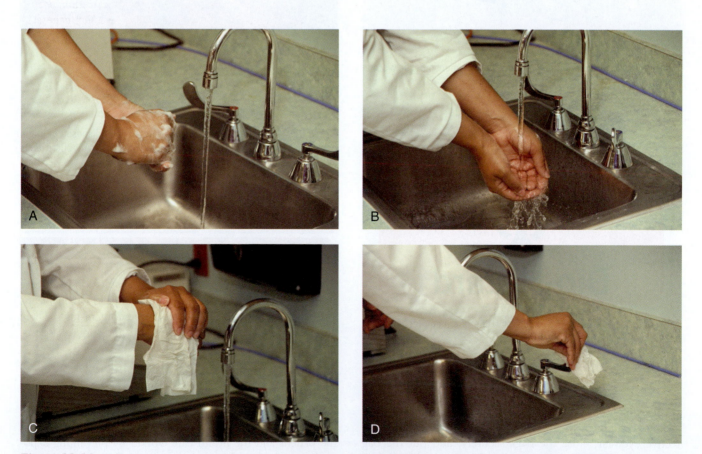

Figure 13-10. A. Firmly rub hands together using a cleansing agent. B. Rinse hands thoroughly, allowing water to run off the fingertips. C. Dry hands using a clean towel. D. Turn off the whater using the towel not your bare hands.

of *disposable* instruments when working with human blood or giving injections minimizes the need for sanitization, disinfection, and sterilization. All instruments and items must be sanitized after each use.

Disinfection

Disinfection is the ability to kill microorganisms on the surface of various items. Disinfection can be accomplished by use of a chemical disinfectant or by boiling. Boiling is used for items that enter body cavities such as the mouth or anus, which are not sterile. Disinfection is also used for items that are sensitive to heat such as glass thermometers or rubber materials. Large equipment and counter surfaces that cannot fit into an autoclave for sterilization should be disinfected by use of chemical disinfectants. Boiling kills many microorganisms but does not kill bacterial spores. Directions for proper use are provided on labels of disinfectant solutions, including the proper length of time to soak items. Many pharmacies use commercial solutions or prepare solutions containing household bleach. A 1:10 solution of household bleach (1 part bleach to 10 parts water) provides disinfection. Small spills of blood or body fluids on counter surfaces can be cleaned with bleach solution and paper towels (see Figure 13-11).

Surgical Asepsis

Surgical asepsis is the destruction of all microorganisms, pathogenic and nonpathogenic, on an object or instrument. Therefore, all equipment used is sterile. The goal of surgical asepsis is to prevent any microorganisms from entering the patient's body through an open wound, especially during

surgery. It is used when sterility of supplies and the immediate environment is required. Any item that will come into contact with the sterile field (the area in which the sterile procedure will be performed or where sterile supplies will be maintained during the procedure) must be sterilized using physical or chemical agents. Once the surfaces are sterilized, every precaution must be taken to prevent contamination of the sterile areas from a nonsterile surface or from airborne contamination.

Living tissue surfaces such as skin cannot be sterilized, but can be rendered as free of pathogens as possible with the use of a sterile covering. One example is the use of surgical handwashing technique before sterile gloves are applied. Another example is the use of a **laminar airflow hood** in the pharmacy whenever a sterile working environment is needed; this will be discussed later in this chapter. Surgical asepsis requires sterile handwashing (surgical scrub), sterile gloves, special handling procedures, and sterilization of materials. Most dangerous microorganisms are destroyed at a temperature of 122 to 140°F (50 to 60°C).

Sterilization

Sterilization is the process of killing or destroying all microorganisms and their pathogenic products. Methods of sterilization include the application of steam under pressure, dry heat, gas, chemicals, and radiation. Sterilization can be achieved through the use of an **autoclave**, which generates steam under pressure (see Figure 13-12). When moist heat of 270°F (or 132°C) under pressure of 30 pounds is applied to instruments, all organisms will be killed in 20 minutes. Autoclaving is one of the most effective methods for destruction of all types of microorganisms. The autoclave must be cleaned after each load.

Dry heat sterilization is another method of sterilization that uses heated dry air at a temperature of 160 to 180°C (320 to 356°F) for 90 minutes to 3 hours. The gas ethylene oxide is used for items that are sensitive to heat; this method of sterilization is called **gas sterilization**. It requires special

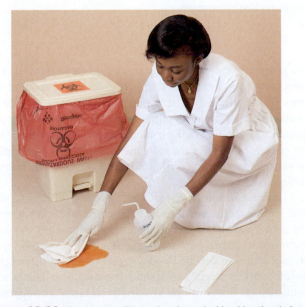

Figure 13-11. Blood and spills can be cleaned with a bleach solution.

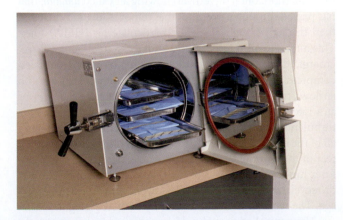

Figure 13-12. The autoclave is one of the most effective methods used to clean and sterilize equipment.

equipment and aeration of materials after application of the gas. The gas is highly flammable and toxic. Gas sterilization is commonly used in hospitals that have room-sized gas sterilization chambers. Many prepackaged products for intravenous infusion and bandages are sterilized using this method. **Chemical sterilization** is used for instruments, and chemicals can be applied topically to the body for disinfection. Iodine, household bleach, Mercurochrome®, and alcohol are examples of disinfectants that can be used in this manner.

LAMINAR AIRFLOW HOODS

A laminar airflow hood is a piece of equipment designed for the handling of materials whenever a sterile working environment is required (see Figure 13-13). This device uses a system of circulating filtered air in parallel flow planes. Because room air may be highly contaminated, the system reduces the risk of bacterial contamination or exposure to chemical pollutants in surgical theaters, hospital pharmacies, laboratories, and food preparation areas. Sneezing, for example, produces up to 200,000 aerosol droplets, which can attach to dust particles and stay in the air for weeks! Laminar airflow hoods are very effective for providing a clean area, if they are operating properly.

There are two types of laminar airflow hoods: vertical and horizontal (see Figure 13-14A and 13-14B). A horizontal airflow hood should be used for preparation of numerous types of parenteral medications and sterile product mixtures. A vertical airflow hood is used for all chemotherapeutic agents, because of the direction of the airflow and the specifications of the hood. It can also be used to mix nonchemotherapeutic agents. However, chemotherapeutic agents should not be mixed in a horizontal airflow hood. The horizontal hoods used in hospital pharmacies must be inspected each year by an authorized inspector to ensure the effectiveness of the filtering system. Laminar airflow hoods basically have a box-like structure, with the top and sides made of Plexiglas, a transparent acrylic material. The work area is bathed by positive pressure (horizontal or vertical) flowing air called *laminar,* that has passed through a pre-filter that removes lint and dust and then through a high efficiency particulate air (HEPA) filter. This filter, the most important part of the system, removes microorganisms and small particles of matter from room air, compressing and redistributing the now ultra clean air into airflow streams that are parallel to each other. The air moves at a rate of 90 to 120 linear feet per minute, with very little turbulence, at a uniform velocity. This process removes nearly all of the bacteria from the air. The HEPA filter is located at the rear of the work area, with a removable, perforated metal diffuser further toward the front. HEPA filters cannot be cleaned or recycled and must be replaced every 3 to 5 years on average. The work area is illuminated by fluorescent lights.

The controlled area should be a limited-access area sufficiently separated from other pharmacy operations to minimize

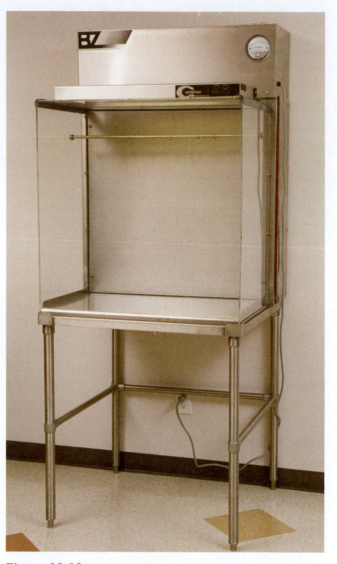

Figure 13-13. Laminar airflow hoods are designed to provide a sterile working environment.

the potential for contamination that could result from the unnecessary flow of materials and personnel into and out of the area. The controlled air is a buffer from outside air that is needed because strong air currents from briefly opened doors, personnel walking past the laminar airflow workbench, or the air stream from the heating/ventilating/and air conditioning system can easily exceed the velocity of air from the laminar airflow workbench.

Laminar airflow hoods should be left on 24 hours a day and require regular maintenance. If turned off for any reason, the unit should be turned on for at least 30 minutes and then thoroughly cleaned before reusing. Also, all items to be used in procedures under the hood should be cleaned thoroughly before work is begun, as should the operator's hands and arms. Excess dust must be avoided at all costs. The operator should remove any jewelry from the hands and wrists. Technicians should use gowns with knit cuffs and rubber

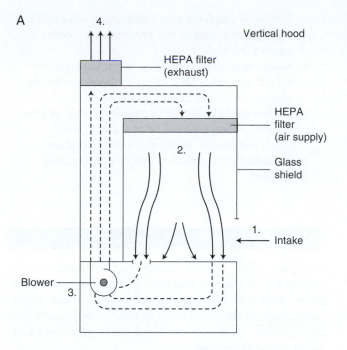

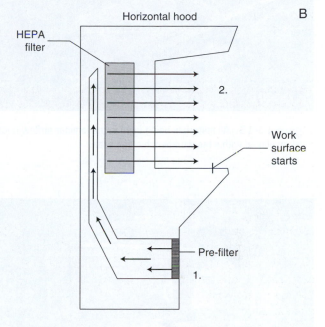

1. Room air enters the laminar airflow. This makes up about 30% of the air in the hood.

2. HEPA-filtered air enters and makes up 70% of the air in the hood.

3. Air from the work area is drawn down into the base and pulled back through the unit.

4. Air is exhausted after being filtered through carbon or HEPA filters.

1. Room air enters, is filtered and drawn up to the top of the hood, where it is filtered through a HEPA filter.

2. Filtered air is directed out over the work surface.

Figure 13-14. A. Vertical hood. B. Horizontal hood.

gloves while doing work inside laminar airflow hoods. Masks are recommended because most personnel talk or may cough or sneeze. Personnel who have a sensitivity to latex should use powder-free, low-latex protein gloves, or, if the allergy is severe, latex-free (synthetic) gloves are recommended. This minimizes the shedding of skin flora into the work area. Conventional laboratory coats are not sufficient, because their open cuffs allow entrapment of contaminated air between the technician's wrist and forearms and inside the sleeves. It is important for operators to keep their hands within the cleaned area of the hood as much as possible and not touch hair, face, or clothing. Only materials essential for preparing the sterile product should be placed in the laminar airflow workbench or barrier isolator (see Figure 13-15). The surface of ampules, vials, and container closures (e.g., vial stoppers), should be disinfected by swabbing or spraying with alcohol before placement in the workbench. All aseptic procedures should be performed at least 6 inches inside the front edge of the laminar airflow workbench, in a clear path of unidirectional airflow between the HEPA filter and work materials (e.g., needles or closures). The operator should avoid spraying or squirting solutions onto the HEPA filter, always aiming away from the filter when opening ampules or adjusting syringes. In a horizontal hood, items should be placed away from the sides and HEPA filter, and nothing should touch the filter. Large objects should never be placed near the back of the hood, because they will contaminate everything downstream from them and disrupt the flow pattern of air. Work areas should be cleaned after each use. Before and after a series of intravenous admixtures are prepared (the preparation of sterile products) or anytime something is spilled, the work surface of the laminar airflow hood should be thoroughly cleaned with alcohol. A long side-to-side motion should be used, starting at the back of the hood and then working forward (see Figure 13-16). The acrylic plastic sides should also be cleaned periodically with solutions that can be used on them and by following the directions closely. Disinfectants should be alternated periodically to prevent development of resistant microorganisms. The laminar airflow hood should be serviced and certified every 6 months. Active work surfaces in the controlled area (e.g., carts, compounding devices, and counter surfaces) should be

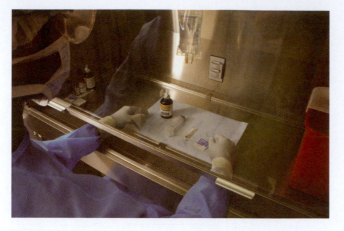

Figure 13-15. All materials being used in the laminar airflow hood must be placed within the workbench clean area.

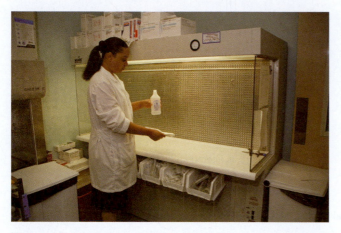

Figure 13-16. Laminar airflow hoods must be properly cleaned after use.

disinfected. Refrigerators, freezers, shelves, and other areas where pharmacy-prepared sterile products are stored should be kept clean. The floors of the controlled area should be nonporous and washable to enable regular disinfection.

EMPLOYEE RESPONSIBILITIES

Although OSHA does not cite employees for violations of their responsibilities, each employee shall comply with all occupational safety and health standards and all rules, regulations, and orders issued under the Act that are applicable. Employee responsibilities and rights in a state that has its own occupational safety and health programs are generally the same as those for workers in states using federal OSHA regulations. An employee should do the following:

- Read the OSHA poster at the job site.
- Comply with all applicable OSHA standards.

- Follow all employer safety and health rules and regulations, and wear or use prescribed protective equipment while working.
- Report hazardous conditions to the supervisor.
- Report any job-related injury or illness to the employer and seek treatment promptly.
- Cooperate with the OSHA compliance officer conducting an inspection if he or she inquires about safety and health conditions in the workplace.
- Exercise rights under the Act in a responsible manner.

SUMMARY

Workplace safety is a responsibility of the employer and employee. It is a shared responsibility that protects the employer from noncompliance penalties and, more importantly, protects the employee's health. Patient health and safety are also protected by sound safety practices in the health care environment.

The Occupational Health and Safety Administration (OSHA) is the federal agency that is responsible for workplace safety rules and the enforcement of those rules. In health care, OSHA's primary concern is protection of employees from biological and chemical hazards. OSHA requires health care employers to have a written exposure control plan that outlines protective measures against bloodborne pathogen transmission to employees. OSHA also requires employers to have a written chemical hygiene plan that outlines chemicals present in the workplace and safe handling and disposal procedures for those chemicals.

The health care employee has the responsibility to abide by the employer's safety policies and procedures. The best-written exposure control plans and chemical hygiene plans are ineffective unless employees understand and follow the written plans. Employee training and mandatory compliance with safety procedures are essential for an effective workplace safety program.

When employers and employees are attuned to workplace safety, the patient is also protected. Closely followed procedures for disinfection, sterilization, and aseptic technique assure that patients are not exposed to harmful biological agents in the health care setting.

CRITICAL THINKING

1. Describe the importance of safety precautions in the pharmacy setting. How do these needs differ in the hospital and ritual pharmacy?
2. What vaccinations must a pharmacy technician maintain to protect himself or herself while on the job? Are there pros and cons to these vaccines? Would you choose to obtain the vaccines or opt not to get the vaccine? Why or why not?

REVIEW QUESTIONS

1. For each hazardous chemical material, the pharmacy should provide a material safety data sheet (MSDS) from which of the following places?
   A. Office Depot
   B. Post office
   C. Manufacturer
   D. Government authority

2. Standard precautions should be followed if the pharmacy technician is exposed to which of the following?
   A. Radioactive substances
   B. Chemical materials
   C. Dangerous gases
   D. Human body fluids

3. The Occupational and Safety and Health Act established _____.
   A. Department of Labor
   B. OSHA
   C. JCAHO
   D. HIPAA

4. Employers must provide safety training to employees
   A. upon hiring them.
   B. upon firing them.
   C. if they are expectant mothers.
   D. at least once a month.

5. Exits must be marked and escape routes published on a(n) _____.
   A. exposure control plan.
   B. hazard communication plan.
   C. fire safety plan.
   D. OSHA poster.

6. OSHA requires that employers with more than 10 employees
   A. maintain vacation records.
   B. must record injuries that happen to their employees at home.
   C. keep records only if they feel it necessary.
   D. maintain records of all work-related injuries and illnesses.

7. Standard precautions are a set of guidelines for infection control requiring the employer and employee to assume that all human blood and specified human body fluids are
   A. radioactive.
   B. infectious for HIV, hepatitis B, and other blood-borne pathogens.
   C. viral.
   D. disease-causing.

8. Any materials that have come into contact with blood or body fluids are treated as
   A. sterile.
   B. aseptic.
   C. hazardous waste.
   D. disposable.

9. When health care workers change hazardous waste bags, they must wear
   A. shoes.
   B. gowns.
   C. gloves.
   D. protective collars.

10. The most effective way to eliminate transmission of disease from one host to another is through
    A. asepsis.
    B. cleanliness.
    C. friction.
    D. protective clothing.

11. The single most important means of preventing the spread of infection is frequent and effective
    A. steam cleaning.
    B. chemical rinsing.
    C. hand hygiene.
    D. pressure sterilization.

12. Disinfection is the ability to kill _____ on the surface of various items.
    A. insects
    B. worms
    C. mites
    D. microorganisms

13. The goal of surgical asepsis is to prevent
    A. reoccurring viruses.
    B. microorganisms from entering the patient's body.
    C. the need for excessive handwashing.
    D. sterilization of the patient.

14. A device that generates steam under pressure to sterilize medical instruments, is called a(n)
    A. soaking tub.
    B. autoclave.
    C. subclave.
    D. laminar airflow hood.

15. Because of the direction of the airflow, a _____ is used for the preparation of all chemotherapeutic agents.
    A. vertical airflow hood
    B. horizontal airflow hood
    C. both
    D. neither of these answers is appropriate

14

Computer Applications in Drug-Use Control

OBJECTIVES

Upon completion of this chapter, the reader should be able to

1. Explain the basic four parts of a computer system.
2. Explain the terms *data* and *file*.
3. Discuss the various types of input and output devices.
4. Explain the types of tasks that robotic machinery can accomplish.
5. Describe how physicians may handle order entry for inpatients and to describe some of the equipment available.
6. Describe how personal digital assistants (PDAs) may be used for working with outpatients and their information.
7. Discuss requirements for hospital and community pharmacy applications.
8. Communicate what the future holds for pharmacy information systems.
9. Discuss five areas in which pharmacy information systems support pharmacists and pharmacy technicians' efforts.

GLOSSARY

automated touch-tone response system A system in which the patient can call in an order or refill a prescription and the system routes the refill orders to the proper pharmacy and assigns each order a place in the order-fulfillment sequence.

central processing unit (CPU) The part of the computer that does the computations.

computer A piece of programmable equipment that stores, retrieves, and processes data.

data The raw facts the computer can manipulate.

file A set of data or a program that has been given a name.

hardware The parts of the computer that you can touch.

input devices Any piece of equipment that allows data to be entered into the computer system.

memory The ability of the computer to store and retrieve data.

modem A device used to transfer information from one computer to another.

output devices Any piece of equipment that allows data to exit the computer system.

personal digital assistant (PDA) A hand-held device that runs on its own battery power so that it may be used anywhere.

programs A set of electronic instructions that tell the computer what to do.

software A set of electronic instructions that tell the computer what to do.

touch screen A monitor with a touch-sensitive surface, on which the touch of a finger makes a selection as a mouse pointer does.

users The individuals who work with computers regularly.

OVERVIEW

Computers have revolutionized the world of pharmacy. Computer applications have been developed in both retail pharmacy and segments of hospital pharmacy, which include drug distribution, administration, clinical practice, and ambulatory care. A great deal of attention has been given to the administrative applications, because programs have the most impact on the financial health of the pharmacy. Developing computer systems to aid in drug distribution has also been the focus of program development, because this has been targeted as the primary problem in pharmacy practice. Today, computers are the main component of pharmacy practice. If computers are used properly, then they can significantly decrease the cost of any operation that involves the processing of information; therefore, it is essential for pharmacy technicians to be computer literate. In addition, the pharmacy technician must be aware of procedures to prevent compromise of confidential pharmacy records.

The overall goal of the use of better computer applications in the pharmacy is to reduce errors, and, therefore, to prevent harm to patients. Computers can help accomplish these goals by

- Allowing patient information to be kept up-to-date and easily accessible
- Allowing drug information to be up-to-date and easily accessible
- Establishing closed-drug formulary systems to limit choices to the essential and most effective drugs
- Establishing standardized methods of communicating drug orders automatically to reduce errors
- Allowing correction of confusing drug names, labeling, and packaging
- Establishing methods of clearly labeling all drug containers to the point of their administration
- Establishing standards for intravenous (IV) solutions, drug concentrations, doses, and administration times

COMPUTER COMPONENTS

A **computer** is a piece of programmable equipment that stores, retrieves, and processes data. Computers can be used for commercial, financial, billing, shipping and receiving, inventory control, and similar functions. Computers gather and analyze data from which tables, graphics, models, and designs can be created. They can also be used to create multimedia demonstrations, animated graphics, illustrations, printed materials, and instructional materials. A computer system consists of four parts: hardware, software, data, and users (see Figure 14-1). A pharmacy technician should be able to recognize the components and uses of a computer.

Hardware

The term **hardware** refers to the part of the computer you can touch. It consists of interconnected electronic devices that control everything the computer does. The hardware can be broken down into four types of physical components: the processor (the central processing unit, or CPU), memory, storage, and input/output devices (Figure 14-2).

Pharmacists are advised to purchase a system with sufficient capacity for their current and future needs. Although the costs of hardware are decreasing, processing power and storage capacity continue to double about every 2 years. Reliable technical advice about hardware options should be sought so that the pharmacy can obtain the optimal hardware for staff needs. In the pharmacy, hardware-related technology has progressed at great speed. Most pharmacy-focused hardware, such as servers and workstations, allow connection of computer components via local area networks (LANs) to the World Wide Web, as well as easy expansion of the system. Multiple workstations and printers are just some of the components that may be easily added as the pharmacy staff grows. Printed manuals, on-site training, and specialized training classes may be provided to ensure that all the features of the hardware are used.

Central Processing Unit

The **central processing unit (CPU)**, or processor, is the part of the computer that actually does the computations. This part of the computer houses the arithmetical and logical formulas that perform the operations of the computer programs. Some computers have more than one processor, allowing them to do multiprocessing. Processor control units retrieve and decode instructions and are the components that run the operation of the computer. This portion of the computer allows information to be passed within the processing components of the computer and between programs. The CPU is the "brains" of the computer.

Memory

The main storage component of the computer is called **memory**. Random access memory (RAM) is the basic type of internal memory. RAM is able to access any information stored anywhere within the system. Different types of RAM differ in how information is stored and for how long it is stored. The amount of RAM that is necessary is a function of how the computer is to be used. If it will be necessary to run several different programs at one time or support many people working at the same time on a network, then greater RAM capacity will be required. As RAM amounts increase, speed and accuracy of the system increase.

Storage

External storage (also called "auxiliary storage") consists of any storage other than the main memory. This includes hard drives and removable media such as zip disks, floppy disks,

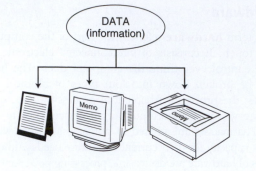

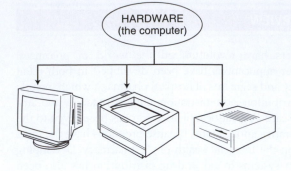

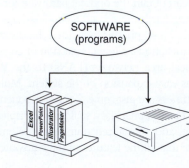

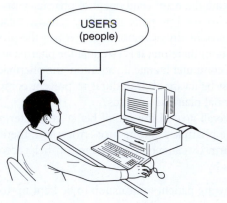

Figure 14-1. Components of a computer.

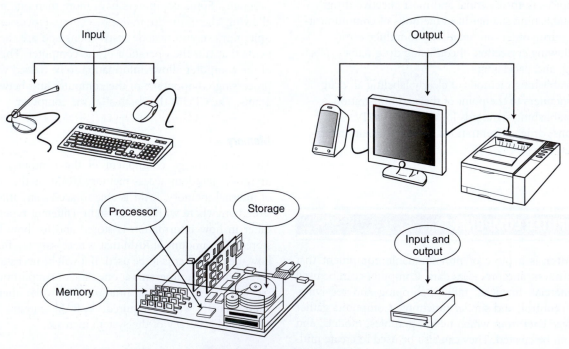

Figure 14-2. Hardware devices.

and optical media. USB connectors allow many different computer components and devices to be interconnected. Tape drives are usually used for backup of a system's files regularly.

Electronic medical record systems provide better control over distinct patient identification, correct information, and identifying codes to help locate a specific record among large numbers of other patient records. Electronic systems are more accurate, and offer much quicker search capabilities than previous, paper-based storage systems. Paper files must be continually updated to ensure that information is current and accurate, which is a considerably more cumbersome task than updating electronic information. For example, when updated insurance information is provided to an electronic storage medium, that information is automatically passed to the billing department of a medical facility so that the information is consistent and current, without the need for duplicate data entry. Medication changes on patients' charts trigger automatic updates of lists of medications in all related electronic files. Paper medical records are located by flipping pages until the desired item is found. Electronic medical records may be located by entering short keywords or phrases, and near-instant recovery of the desired item is possible. Progress notes, as previously handled in a paper-based office, were produced by dictation or transcribing from the physician, direct handwriting of notes, or completing of forms. With a full-function electronic medical records system, progress notes are automatically created as the visit is occurring. Storage in an electronic medium uses less space than in a paper-based system, because of the advent of compact disc technology, zip disks, and other storage formats. Volumes of information that previously may have filled an entire storage room can now be contained on a series of discs or diskettes that may be kept on a single shelving unit. Electronic charts are never lost, out of order, or misfiled in the wrong section of a filing system. They are always exactly where they should be, and they may be accessed from any point in a health care facility that has access to medical records.

Input and Output Devices

Input devices bring information into a computer. These consist of the keyboard, mouse, touch screen, scanner, and modem. In the pharmacy setting, computers are also often linked with robotic machinery that can handle dispensing, labeling, counting, and packaging tasks. Input devices move data into the system either in small bits of information at a time (serial input device, for example, a modem), in small groupings of information at a time (parallel input device, for example, some types of printers), or in large blocks of information at a time (block input device, for example, floppy disks). **Output devices** bring information out of a computer and include monitors and printers.

Keyboard The most common device used to input information into the computer is the keyboard, which resembles a typewriter. Alphabetic characters, numeric characters,

symbols, and punctuation marks can be entered via the keyboard. The keyboard is a series of switches monitored by a microprocessor that initiates a specific response to a change in the state of each switch, or "key." Figure 14-3 shows a basic keyboard.

The most common keyboards have between 82 and 108 keys, although laptop computers often have custom keyboards that differ slightly from standard desktop computers. A typical keyboard, however, has four basic types of keys:

- Typing keys (also called alphabetic keys)
- Numeric keypad
- Function keys
- Control keys

The typing keys contain letters generally laid out in the same style as that of their predecessor, the typewriter. The name for this arrangement of letters is "QWERTY," named after the first six letters in the layout. Another, less popular type of letter layout is known as "DVORAK," which places the most commonly used letters in the most convenient arrangement. The numeric keypad was created as the need for quicker data entry occurred. Because a large part of business data was numbers, this set of 17 keys was added to the standard keyboard layout in the same configuration used by adding machines and calculators. In 1986, the "function" and "control" keys were added in a line across the top of the keyboard. These keys can be assigned specific commands by the current application or the operating system. Control keys provide cursor and screen control. Four keys arranged in an inverted "T" formation between the typing keys and numeric keyboard allow the computer operator to move the cursor on the monitor in small increments in various directions. The control keys allow larger movements to be made and include the following keys:

- Home and End keys
- Insert and Delete keys
- Page Up and Page Down keys
- Control (Ctrl), Alternate (Alt), and Escape (Esc) keys

The popular operating systems include a few system-specific keys that their competitors do not offer, but these are not very important to the overall focus of this text. Underneath the keyboard is a key matrix, which is a grid of circuits. Pressing a key bridges a gap in the circuit for that key, allowing a tiny amount of current to flow through, and instructing the processor which key has been pressed. The key matrix corresponds to a character map in the ROM and is the "bridge" that the processor needs to understand the operator's keystrokes. Keyboards are usually connected to computers with 4-, 5-, or 6-pin connectors at the end of a 6-foot-long cable. These cables carry the data traveling between the keyboard and computer, as well as a small amount of power, which enables the keystrokes to be transmitted.

Monitor A monitor, also known as a "display," is a device that resembles a television screen and is used by the computer to display information. Monitors come in a range of

The Computer Keyboard

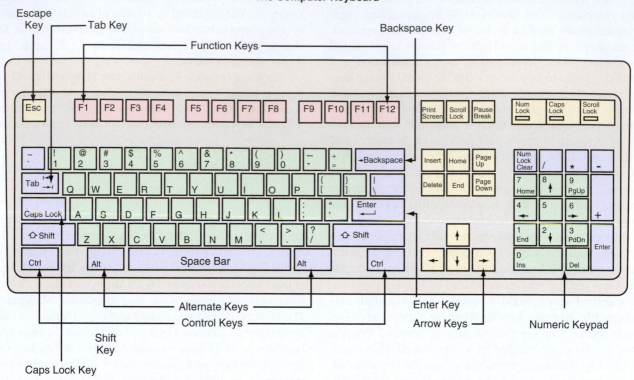

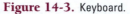

Figure 14-3. Keyboard.

sizes and currently may have convex or flat screens. Also, various new options exist, including liquid-crystal display screens, which offer greater clarity and less eye strain to the user. The monitor is the most-used output device on a computer. It provides instant feedback by showing you text and graphic images. The pharmacy should purchase a monitor with the maximum resolution, dot pitch, refresh rate, color depth, and most economical amount of power consumption that is affordable. The display unit includes a projection surface commonly called the "screen." Popular screen sizes are 15 to 21 inches, although more sizes are becoming available. Displays use tiny dots of light called "pixels" to make up the various graphical components on their screens. The size of the display affects the resolution: The same pixel resolution will be sharper on a small monitor and fuzzier on a large monitor, because the pixels are spread out over the larger number of screen inches.

Mouse A mouse is a device that enables the user to move a pointer on the monitor to make selections or to place information. The mouse provides a better way to move graphics and windows, which allow access to and processing of information more quickly. This particular piece of hardware is very inexpensive and takes up little space. A mouse translates your hand motions into signals that the computer can use. A new type of mouse, the optical mouse, is becoming the preferred device for pointing and clicking. It works via a

tiny camera that can take 1500 pictures/second. Optical mice have the following benefits over wheeled mice:

- No moving parts, less wear, and lower chance of failure
- No way for dirt to enter the mouse and harm the sensors
- Increased tracking resolution for a smoother response
- No special surface, such as a mouse pad, required

Touch Screen A **touch screen** is a monitor with a touch-sensitive surface, on which the touch of a finger makes a selection as a mouse pointer does. Many of the computer programs that interface with robotic dispensing machinery offer touch screens as an integral part of their system. These screens enable the pharmacy technician to enter the required information and commands for the robotics machinery much more quickly. Studies have shown that people younger than age 35 years are more familiar with using touch screens to access information. Companies are currently improving and simplifying their touch screen programs so that users of all ages will be more inclined to try them and, further, to become proficient in their use. The most often accessed topics via touch screen programs are "good eating," "exercise," and "alcohol," showing that users want to know more about healthy lifestyles and are comfortable searching for information themselves. One of the newest touch screen systems offers a split screen capability, which can double the amount of prescriptions filled. Flat panel touch screen monitors take up less counter space than full-sized monitors, and installation (along with training) only takes 2 days to complete. Under this system, each new prescription is assigned a bar code and then bar-coded labels are printed. The image of the original written prescription is retained in the system so that, at the end of the process, the pharmacist can verify the filled prescription package with the original prescription order. All the pharmacy staff's inputs and responses to the system's prompts are handled via the touch screen display.

Scanner A scanner is a device that can convert printed matter and images to information that can be interpreted by the computer. The most common of these devices resemble small photocopying units with a horizontal glass panel and a hinged cover that keeps any documents placed onto the glass free from outside sources of light, which would degrade the scanned image's quality. Linear laser scanners are capable of decoding two-dimensional bar codes and pharmacy applications and may even be used to verify driver license information. These scanners use various types of laser, holographic, and vision-based technologies and may come in hand-held, in-counter, and fixed projection varieties—flatbed scanners are not the only type available. Staff members may rely on the new types of scanners to reduce patient drug administration errors by cross-referencing the bar codes on the medicine packages with the patient information.

Modem A **modem** is a device used to transfer information from one computer to another using telephone lines and servers. Modems allow the user to access the Internet (which is an invaluable research and informational tool), and to use e-mail (offering quicker communications between users at different locations and reduced cost of postage and shipping). The word *modem* is a blend of two words: modulator and demodulator. The sending modem modulates the data into a signal that is compatible with the phone line, and the receiving modem demodulates the signal back into digital data. Wireless modems convert digital data into radio signals and back again. The first modems had working speeds that were very slow compared with those of today, starting at approximately 300 bits/second, with the average modem on a telephone line achieving speeds up to 8 megabits/second.

Printer A printer is a device used to produce a paper copy of information to be sent to pharmacies, vendors, insurance companies, and others. Full-color printers are now readily available, enabling very detailed reproductions of graphics and photographs. The most popular form of printer today is the laser printer. The primary principle at work in a laser printer is static electricity, an electrical charge built up on an insulated object. The computer uses various languages to communicate with the printer, which culminates in the printed image in the form of dots, called a bitmap. In most laser printers, print-job data are saved in a separate memory under the power of a printer controller. This lets the controller put different printing jobs into a print queue so that it can work on them one at a time. Inside the printer, the laser system consists of a laser, a movable mirror, and a lens. In this way, laser printers operate in a way that is similar, but not identical, to photocopiers. Laser printers are preferred over inkjet and other types of printers because of their speed, precision, and economy. Laser printers are more expensive, but toner for them is inexpensive and lasts a lot longer than the ink cartridges that are required for inkjet printers.

Software

The term **software** refers to sets of electronic instructions that tell the hardware what to do. These sets of instructions are also known as **programs**, and each of them has a specific purpose, such as entering, editing, and formatting data. Computer software can be classified into operating systems and applications. Both are built from the same elements, with electronic instructions to the processor. Information management is a vital part of the modern pharmacy. Specialized pharmacy software has been created to help eliminate repetitive data entry, simplify tracking of patient consultation and outcomes, and storage of patient and facility records in one convenient place. Information from other programs may be imported, exported, and transferred between users. Generating reports and forms has never been easier. Historical reports about outcomes and drug use may be more easily prepared than ever before, as can professional reports for physicians, facility managers, patients, and pharmacy managers. Some of the best software programs designed for pharmacy use offer digital video surveillance (DVS) solutions, which are integrated with their cash register systems. These DVS systems allow owners and authorized personnel to view all transactions, either live or digitally recorded, at any register via a Web browser, allowing the pharmacist to be linked to anywhere in the world. Other software allows the performance of drug regimen reviews, meeting of Centers for Medicare & Medicaid Services and Joint Commission on Accreditation of Healthcare Organization guidelines, and performance of disease management. Cross-referencing of drug information is easily done by using software that allows one to build an information library. These can include special manufacturer instructions, administration guidelines, and therapy monitoring notes. Multiple methods to monitor outcomes, including statistical monitoring of medication counts and drug utilization reviews, may be handled efficiently and easily. For home infusion pharmacies, there are software packages that allow full integration, including the following:

- Patient intake, order entry, profiling, distribution, clinical support, operations, reporting, and financial support

- Electronic and paper billing with user-defined templates
- Intravenous drug/infusion ordering, as well as oral and injectable drugs, supplies, equipment, and nursing services
- Clinical features for care plans, progress notes, laboratory results, and outcomes
- Health Insurance Portability and Accountability Act (HIPAA) code sets and insurance claim processing, billing formats, and privacy and security features
- Windows interface making data entry and retrieval fast and easy
- Server database platforms that provide stability, security, and scalability
- Online access to historical data libraries and multi-site support

In the retail and hospital pharmacy settings, various software packages are available. Most of them meet all Omnibus Budget Reconciliation Act (OBRA) requirements, offer family linking (which eliminates redundant data entry), and allow up to four claims at a time for third parties to provide judgment on claims. Extensive pricing capabilities, unlimited patient comments and allergy notes, doctor call labels, and laser labeling are commonplace features as well. By adding to basic programs, users can interface with nearly all popular automated dispensing systems, work with voice response interfaces, use integrated signature captures, and view pill images. Multisite pharmacy systems include multiple site dispensing, centralized inventory management, site-to-site transfer of inventory, and integration with central patient health management organization (HMO) data files. Institutional and long-term care pharmacy software offers unit-dose, modified unit-dose, blister pack (plastic packaging for which the medication is surrounded by a plastic "blister" or bubble that allows the patient to push the medication through a thin piece of protective material for easy use), and conventional dispensing. Medication acquisition requisition forms (MARs) and physician order sheets are easily prepared, and multisite inventory ordering and control are offered. For pharmacy accounting, all of the following are easily managed:

- Accounts payable and receivable
- Payroll
- General ledger and financial reporting

Operating Systems

The best manufacturers of pharmacy hardware today offer operating systems (such as Windows 2000) that are popularly used, so that the pharmacy staff does not have to deal with clumsy, hard-to-use operating systems. Interfaces are straightforward and user-friendly. They also offer the ability for multitasking, so that prescriptions may be continually filled while the user is using the word processor functions or the Internet. When choosing an operating system, pharmacists should consider the functions that their computers will be required to perform. Systems vary widely and can do anything from basic data management, word processing, and accounting to electronic point-of-sale and labeling. Pharmacists should make sure that the system they choose has sufficient processor speed, memory (RAM), and storage capacity for the functions it will be performing. Independent expert advice should be sought before committing to purchase, especially when it comes to operating system choice. Pharmacists should keep abreast of new developments, such as new Internet capabilities and the National Health Service Net (NHSNet). The NHSNet is a private Intranet for the staff and contractors of the National Health Service. It is secure for sending and receiving patient-identifiable data between NHS sites.

Applications

Currently many diverse computer-application packages are available, including some that can capture and track everything that goes on in the pharmacy. Reports can then be generated to help streamline the flow of daily activity. Computerized machines now count pills and tablets at very high speeds. Prescription tracking software frees up the pharmacy technician to deal with patients in a more professional and effective manner. Interactive voice response systems are being used more often in the pharmacy today. Customers can phone in their prescription refill orders via an **automated touch-tone response system**. These systems route refill orders to the proper pharmacy and assign each order a place in the order sequence. This greatly reduces the amount of time pharmacy staff must spend on the phone. Some programs offer completely automated dispensing, which merges robotics, software, and drug-counting technology. Other similar systems offer the ability to fill about 90 prescriptions per hour, including multiple prescriptions for multiple customers simultaneously.

Data

Data are the raw facts the computer can manipulate. Data can consist of letters, numbers, sounds, or images. A computer **file** is simply a set of data or program instructions that has been given a name. A file containing data is often called a document, examples of which are addresses, medical records, insurance carriers, and transactions.

Users

The last part of the computer system is the people who use the computers, usually called **users** (see Figure 14-4). In the pharmacy setting, computers are used to synchronize workflow, orchestrate patient care, improve operational efficiency, and raise patient satisfaction. Once received at the pharmacy, a typical prescription order is entered into the computer system. The best systems check their data with the

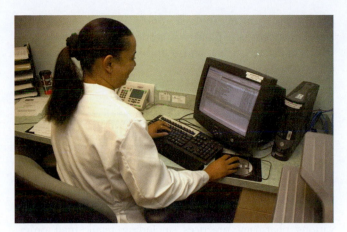

Figure 14-4. The computer is a valuable tool to the pharmacy technician.

order for potentially adverse interactions with other medicines the patient is receiving or for patient's allergies. The pharmacist should then review the order and substitute generic drugs if appropriate. Point-of-sale systems integrate data that are collected to increase security and to maintain better inventory control, strategic merchandising, and up-to-date pricing. Pharmacy data management provides insurance companies with better data, making it easier to process claims, produce customized reports, and manage cash flow. Up to now, it routinely took a month or longer for new customer data to be integrated and processed through the insurance company system. Data can now be organized into databases that offer ready access to everyone who needs to add new patients, modify information about patients, and adjust insurance plan benefits. For military clients, the Department of Defense has developed the Pharmacy Data Transaction Service, which provides common patient drug profiles for all its beneficiaries worldwide, allowing prescriptions to be reviewed against all previous prescriptions filled at any point of service in the Military Health System. This includes military treatment facilities, retail network pharmacies, and the National Mail Order Pharmacy.

PHYSICIAN ORDER ENTRY FOR INPATIENTS

Physicians must have access to available clinical information to make optimal patient care decisions. Hospitals have highly sophisticated diagnostic capabilities, but providers often do not have access to the results. For inpatients, physicians routinely maintain individual patient lists with names, hospital identifiers, room numbers, and pertinent clinical information. The most popular systems used today for order entry have been designed specifically for hospital and institutional pharmacies. For drug dispensing, most of them offer single-screen order entry; automatic screening for drug interactions, allergies, food, and therapeutic duplication;

label printing for packing and distribution; preparation of pick/fill lists; on-screen patient profiles; customized forms for each patient; electronic bedside charting interfaces; and automatic stop orders. For unit-dose distribution, the system supports flexible cart exchanges, assembly line distribution, interfacing with all popular dispensing machinery, physician order entry interfaces, and the ability to also handle traditional and floor dose distribution. General questions to consider when a physician order-entry system is implemented include the following:

- Is the system designed correctly, and does it prevent access by outsiders?
- Does it integrate with any existing systems, and what new elements must the users learn to use it effectively?
- Does the system allow for off-site order entry or entry from personal digital assistants?
- Does it store and allow access to patient information from previous hospital admissions and clinic visits, and is it a well-standardized system?
- It is easily upgradable, and what is its method of password use or identification requirements for users?
- Can it manage the formulary, and how does it deal with multiple formularies?
- What order-entry interfaces are available, and does it allow for the inputting of notes?
- Does it reduce errors by not allowing abbreviations, mnemonics, and incomplete information to be entered?
- Does it check for interactions, contraindications, and high costs that may be avoided by less-expensive alternatives; and does it alert the user to dangerous situations?
- Can medical procedure orders be integrated into the system?
- Does it alert the user of new, discontinued, or changed orders or changed administrations?

USE OF PERSONAL DIGITAL ASSISTANTS WITH OUTPATIENTS

A **personal digital assistant (PDA)** is a hand-held device that runs on its own battery power so that it may be used anywhere. PDAs are usually not much larger than the user's palm and resemble hand-held video games. Information may be typed into the PDA via a small keyboard, or it may be written into it on a flat screen that can decode handwriting into recognizable characters. The data then may be stored on an internal chip, similar to the way computer systems operate. Information may also be loaded into a PDA from another device via a cable that transfers data back and forth, as long as the proper interfacing software has previously been installed into the PDA. Probably the simplest definition of a PDA is as follows: a small, portable device that can store and then transfer information (including text and graphics) into larger computer-related systems and devices for use in complicated patient treatments.

Physicians can enter notes into a patient's online chart and get up-to-date information on prescription drugs— right from the patient's bedside, instantly and securely. With the ready availability of PDAs, many physicians now keep patient lists in electronic formats. Technology is readily available to allow pharmaceutical settings to interface with a physician's PDA. To provide patient privacy, PDAs offer data encryption, password protection, and disabling infrared messaging. PDAs allow doctors and other people in the outpatient setting to be able to share information from various devices, including telephones, pagers, and computers. Electronic signatures may be captured, procedure room waiting lists checked, contacts of all medical personnel kept and managed, and appointments scheduled. PDAs are used in high-volume retail pharmacies and hospital pharmacy networks. For patient records, they offer registration interfaces; on-screen patient profiles; prescription histories; early and late refill notification; drug interaction, allergy, or disease state information; and multiple third-party membership or billing dates. For drug dispensing, PDAs offer single-screen order entry, automatic drug interaction screening, diagnosing, therapeutic duplication preventatives, customized labels and receipts, updating of patient records, updating of drug inventories and pricing, order status tracking, and automated dispensing. Software used by PDAs can handle many different functions, including the following:

- 10-year risk assessment
- Calculations for emergency medication dosing, blood alcohol, creatinine clearance, dieting, osmolality, total parenteral nutrition, chemotherapeutic dosing regimens, arterial oxygen, acid-base balance, urine, and mean arterial pressure
- Conversions between conventional and international units, including temperature conversions and dosing equivalency tables
- Diabetic and drug table databases and drug comparisons

THE HOSPITAL PHARMACY APPLICATION

To operate a hospital pharmacy, it is necessary to gain approval from the board of pharmacy via a formal application form. Hospital pharmacy applications usually take approximately 90 days from the time the application is complete until it has been completely processed by the board of pharmacy. Applications for operating a hospital pharmacy require a processing fee of more than $300 and can be made by a corporation, limited-liability company, partnership, or an individual. Hospital pharmacy applications require

copies of a financial affidavit, wholesale credit agreement, lease agreement, any pharmacy certifications that exist, hospital acute care license, and if applicable, a Department of Corporations license.

THE COMMUNITY PHARMACY APPLICATION

The board of pharmacy also handles the registration of community pharmacies, and a application form similar to that for a hospital pharmacy must be submitted to gain their approval. A community pharmacy application may pertain to various pharmacy practices, including retail, mail order, home health care, skilled nursing facilities, nuclear, and board and care settings. Six of every 10 pharmacists provide care to patients in a community setting. Community pharmacists talk to people when they are healthy or sick, giving advice and information. Pharmacists serve their communities also by referring patients to other sources of care and are depended on as sources of health care information of the highest caliber. The community pharmacy application itself may be submitted by individuals, partnerships, corporations, not-for-profit corporations, or government-owned entities. Items that must be made available to the board of pharmacy for review, in consideration of approving the application, are articles of incorporation, partnership agreements, seller's certificates, wholesale agreements, financial affidavits, stock certificates, corporate by-laws, and lease agreements.

THE FUTURE OF PHARMACY INFORMATION SYSTEMS

In the last quarter century, pharmacy has expanded its role within the health care delivery system. Pharmacists now can focus much more on various patient-oriented services, rather than just focusing on preparing and dispensing medications. Change is a constant thing in the development of today's pharmacy information systems. New technology, governmental policies, and consumer demands all create the need for improved information systems. Pharmacy information systems support pharmacists and pharmacy technicians' efforts in five major areas:

1. The management of prescribed medicines
2. The management of long-term conditions
3. The management of common ailments
4. The promotion and support of healthy lifestyles
5. Advice and support for other health care professionals

Improved communication between pharmacy staff and their clientele is vital to the continued growth and success of the industry of pharmacy and for the continual well-being of all patients. It is best that, wherever possible, machinery be used to count, pour, label, and seal drugs and drug-related products, freeing the pharmacist to concentrate more on the patients. Rising volumes of prescriptions, lower profit margins, and growing demand for pharmacists to give better clinical and patient care are pushing the industry of pharmacy toward allowing pharmacy technicians to assume larger roles than ever before. The growing capabilities of computers in the pharmacy setting also require that training be a constant and expanding part of the overall picture. Suppliers should provide adequate training in system use during implementation of their system as well as afterward. Pharmacists should provide regular training updates and appropriate resources for all current and future staff members. Facilities for migrating existing data should be available to ensure continuous patient records for future reference. Ongoing support packages offered by the suppliers of system components are important and should be used. As pharmacy practice relies more on its computer system, it is necessary for the supplier to ensure high availability of the system during the entire week and a very quick response to any system problems. Future technologies and those being improved upon from previous versions of similar technologies include the following:

- Custom screen setups for touch screen systems, with specialized icons
- One-touch "hot keys" or "shortcut keys" for complex tasks
- Full color scanning capabilities
- Instant credit card authorizations
- Real time processing

One of the most important events driving upcoming advances in computer technologies is the Food and Drug Administration (FDA)'s insistence on development of bar codes for every drug, biological specimen, blood sample, and so on. The FDA is aware that by utilization of bar coding to keep all medical items and paperwork organized, the possibility of serious errors is greatly reduced. The automation of this type of system is much more reliable than double-checking performed by humans, because the machinery involved is not prone to stress, fatigue, or distractions.

Another area of medicine in which the future offers promising developments is the area of telemedicine. Telemedicine is the use of telecommunications for medical diagnosis and patient care. Telecommunications technology is used to provide medical services to sites that are far away from the medical care provider. Telemedicine may be conducted by using any of the following:

- Standard telephone service
- High-speed computers linked via modems, phone lines, direct-connection lines, fiber optics, and satellites
- Other sophisticated peripheral equipment and software

Collaborative arrangements are essential for the future of telemedicine, so that payment arrangements, staff credentialing, liability, and licensure issues related to potential crossing of state lines are all addressed.

CONFIDENTIALITY ISSUES IN A COMPUTERIZED SYSTEM

Patient details should always be collected, stored, and displayed with the utmost regard for confidentiality. Ethically, patients' privacy must be protected at all times. Violation of these ethical principles may result in harm to patients and their families, as well as legal action against the pharmacy and its staff. Patient details that must be protected in most situations include the following:

- Name, address, and zip code
- Telephone number, area code, fax number, and e-mail address
- Date of birth, sex, and race
- National Health Service number
- Name of residential or nursing home, if appropriate
- General practitioner's name
- Details of dispensed medications, including name, form, strength, quantity, quantity units, dosage regimen, and date of dispensing

Physicians have always had the responsibility of keeping their patients' information confidential. The Code of Medical Ethics states that patient information must be confidential to ensure that patients will feel free to fully disclose all points about their health. Correct diagnosis and treatment hinge upon complete and honest disclosure. Medical professionals' legal obligations are defined by the U.S. Constitution, by federal and state laws and regulations, and by the courts. The major challenge today is that confidentiality of patient information must be honored and respected, although technology has permitted access to larger amounts of it than ever before. A breach of confidentiality is a disclosure to a third party without the patient's consent or court approval of the disclosure.

SUMMARY

Almost all pharmacies (hospital or retail) are computerized in the United States today. Computerization offers a systemic method of order entry, patient profile development, label production, allergy and sensitivity detection, verification of dosage, and interaction of drugs and food. The pharmacy technician becomes involved in all aspects of computerization in the pharmacy setting. The processes of dispensing, record keeping, pricing, creating new prescriptions, and refilling prescriptions are faster and easier than ever before. Computers offer the ability to have a direct link between the pharmacy and the physician's office, increasing formulary compliance, simplifying pharmaceutical administration, reducing dispensing or other errors related to illegible handwritten prescriptions, and ultimately, increasing patient satisfaction. Access to computer systems is limited by passwords and other security measures, offering better patient confidentiality. Patient data are better protected, and their integrity is ensured through the systemic use of computerization. The future of the pharmacy profession is assured with the use of computerization, which is integral to both the pharmacy management and patient satisfaction that can be provided.

CRITICAL THINKING

1. Research a particular computer application commonly used in pharmacies. What are the pros and cons of this system?

2. The pharmacy you work in is upgrading to a new computer system. What are the requirements of a computer system in the pharmacy? What factors should be taken into account? Name three key features and benefits the system should have and why these are necessary.

3. Describe the challenges of maintaining confidentiality of patients in the computer age.

REVIEW QUESTIONS

1. The main component of pharmacy practice is
   A. administration.
   B. distribution.
   C. computers.
   D. information processing.

2. A computer system consists of four parts: hardware, software, data, and _____.
   A. users
   B. devices
   C. memory
   D. storage

3. The term _____ refers to the part of the computer you can touch.
   A. *software*
   B. *file*
   C. *hardware*
   D. *record*

4. Many automated dispensing systems offer the ability to fill about _____ prescriptions per hour.
   A. 9
   B. 50
   C. 90
   D. 100

5. The most common device used to input information into the computer is the _____.
   A. keyboard
   B. mouse
   C. touch screen
   D. scanner

6. Which device is used to transfer information from one computer to another using telephone lines and servers?
   A. Modem
   B. Mouse
   C. Monitor
   D. Scanner

7. Which type of system offers electronic bedside charting interfaces, automatic stop orders, and customized MAR forms for each patient?
   A. Outpatient order entry
   B. IVARs
   C. Inpatient order entry
   D. LANs

8. The abbreviation *PDA* stands for
   A. physician/doctor/administration.
   B. personal digital assistant.
   C. professional digital assistant.
   D. pharmaceutical-doctoral assistant.

9. PDAs allow the sharing of information from various devices, including
   A. telephones.
   B. computers.
   C. pagers.
   D. all of the above.

10. Outpatient systems offer all of the following, except
    A. early and late refill notification.
    B. drug interaction or allergy information.
    C. the ability to pay insurance claims directly.
    D. diagnosing.

Continues

11. Hospital pharmacy applications require copies of
   A. a financial affidavit.
   B. a seller's pharmacy certification.
   C. an FDA license.
   D. A and B.

12. Of every 10 pharmacists, how many provide care to patients in a community setting?
   A. 2
   B. 4
   C. 6
   D. 7

13. Who approves an application for a community pharmacy?
   A. Food and Drug Administration
   B. Board of toxicology
   C. Board of nursing
   D. Board of pharmacy

14. It is best that, wherever possible, _____ count, pour, label, and seal drugs and drug-related products.
   A. pharmacy technicians
   B. machinery
   C. pharmacists
   D. pharmacy administrators

15. The future of pharmacy is assured with the use of _____, which is integral to both the pharmacy management and patient satisfaction that can be provided.
   A. inexpensive drug formulation
   B. additional pharmacy personnel
   C. trained pharmacy technicians
   D. computerization

15

Communications

OBJECTIVES

Upon completion of this chapter, the reader should be able to

1. Describe defense mechanisms.
2. Name five examples of defense mechanisms.
3. State the various methods of communication.
4. Discuss professional relations.
5. Explain some of the barriers to effective communication.
6. Define negative communication.
7. Explain the communication process.
8. Differentiate between verbal and nonverbal communication.

GLOSSARY

apathy A lack of feeling, emotion, interest, or concern.

autonomy The right of an individual to make informed decisions for his or her own good.

channels Spoken words, written messages, and body language.

communication The sharing of information, ideas, thoughts, and feelings.

compensation An unconscious mechanism by which an individual tries to make up for fancied or real deficiencies.

consumer The person coming to you for the filling of prescriptions or the purchase of over-the-counter remedies for a wide variety of situations.

decode Translation of a message by the receiver into what is perceived to be said.

defense mechanisms Tools an individual uses when required to deal with uncomfortable or threatening situations.

denial A psychological defense mechanism in which confrontation with a personal problem or with reality is avoided by denying the existence of the problem or reality.

displacement The transfer of impulses from one expression to another, such as from fighting to talking.

expressive aphasia Inability of an individual to form language and express his or her thoughts accurately even though thought processes are intact.

external noise Physical noise such as typing or traffic that interferes with hearing a message.

internal noise An individual's beliefs or prejudices that interfere with decoding a message.

prejudice A preformed and unsubstantiated judgment or opinion about an individual or a group, either favorable or unfavorable.

professionalism Behavior based on a body of knowledge and ethical standards to serve the public.

projection A defense mechanism by which a repressed complex in the individual is denied and conceived as belonging to another person, such as when faults that the person tends to commit are perceived in or attributed to others.

rationalization A psychoanalytic defense mechanism through which irrational behavior, motives, or feelings are made to appear reasonable.

receptive aphasia A physical limitation after certain neurological injuries, which leaves the person incapable of understanding all that is said.

regression An unconscious defense mechanism involving a return to earlier patterns of adaptation.

repression A defense mechanism of keeping out and ejecting or banishing from consciousness an unacceptable idea or impulse.

sarcasm Hostile and cruel language intended to hurt someone.

sexual harassment Intentional, clearly understood statements or intentional, clearly understood action that causes another to feel that his or her job is at risk if the sexual advances are rejected.

sublimation An unconscious defense mechanism in which unacceptable instinctual drives and wishes are modified into more personally and socially acceptable channels.

OVERVIEW

The pharmacy technician may work in very diverse practice settings such as hospitals, community pharmacies, clinics, health maintenance organizations, home health care organizations, retirement centers, and nursing homes. It is essential that pharmacy technicians are able to communicate effectively with patients, their caregivers, and other health care providers. An individual's success as a pharmacy technician begins and ends with the ability to communicate both professionally and courteously. It starts at the time of first contact with a potential employer and influences every aspect of the technician's career. Maintaining good relationships with co-workers and successfully developing rapport with clients depend on the pharmacy technician's ability to present himself or herself as competent, caring, knowledgeable, and presentable. It encompasses appearance as well as verbal and nonverbal communication. It takes place face to face, via telephone or fax, on the Internet, or through written documentation. First impressions have an enormous impact on those we meet and generally influence the course of any relationship, personal or professional. One would not feel comfortable trusting a dentist with poor oral hygiene or an ophthalmologist with dirty, broken glasses, or a surgeon with dirty hands and would doubt the teachings of an English professor who mispronounced even the simplest of words. Similarly, a patient meeting the pharmacy technician for the first time has certain expectations. An individual's presentation ultimately reflects back on his or her employer.

COMMUNICATION PROCESS

The communication process consists of the communication cycle, which involves two or more individuals participating in an exchange of information. The cycle involves the sender, or source, communicating a message to the receiver through a chosen channel of communication, to which the receiver responds with feedback (see Figure 15-1).

The communication cycle includes five basic elements:

- The sender or source
- The message
- The channel or mode of communication
- The receiver
- Feedback

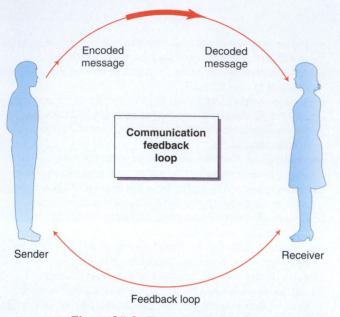

Figure 15-1. The communication loop.

Sender

The sender is the person who sends a message through a variety of different **channels**. Channels can be spoken words, written messages, or body language. The sender encodes the message, which simply means that he or she chooses a specific way of expression using words or other channels.

Message

The message must contain all necessary information (complete). The message must not contain any unnecessary information (concise). It must be free from obscurity and ambiguity (clear). The message must be organized and logical (cohesive), and the message must be respectful and considerate of others (courteous).

Channel

A channel is a path that a message takes from the sender to the receiver. It may be downward (from superiors to employees), upward (from employees to superiors), or horizontal (used between people on similar levels of responsibility).

Receiver

The receiver **decodes** the message according to his or her understanding of what is being communicated. However, there are times that the receiver understands the message incorrectly. This is often because of noise, which is anything that interferes with the message being sent. There are two kinds of noise: external and internal. **External noise** is literal noise, such as a radio or a jackhammer on the street

outside. **Internal noise** includes the receiver's own thoughts, prejudices, and opinions.

Feedback

Feedback can be verbal expressions or body language, expressing the fact that the receiver understood the message he or she received. When you communicate information to a patient or ask customers a question, always look for feedback. For example, when a technician dispenses a prescription and the patient needs consultation, the technician can ask the patient if he or she can wait until the pharmacist finishes a phone call so that he can answer their questions. The technician should look for a response. If the patient responds positively, the pharmacy technician then knows that the patient will wait for the pharmacist to be able to talk with him or her directly.

The basic guidelines for giving feedback are as follows:

- Be clear
- Have a positive emphasis—feedback is intended to help, not hurt
- Be specific—avoid generalized comments. Notice when the person uses terms such as "always" or "never" and ask him or her to be more specific
- Focus—highlight the person's behavior
- Refer—to behavior that might be changed
- Be descriptive—avoid evaluations
- Own your feedback—use "I" statements
- Be very careful with your advice—the person usually needs to understand how his or her actions can be improved in the future

Feedback is sometimes called *criticism*, but this term negatively affects the perceptions of what feedback really is. Feedback is a way to let people know whether they are effectively communicating their message to you. It helps everyone to become more effective communicators. Feedback is not designed to harm the person who is receiving it, only to help him or her to become a better communicator and also to become more effective in actions on a daily basis. The following types of negative or "closed" styles of receiving feedback should be avoided:

- Defensive—defends personal actions and objects to the feedback that is being given.
- Attacking—verbally attacks the person giving feedback
- Denial—refutes the accuracy or fairness of the feedback
- Disrespectful—devalues the speaker and the feedback provided
- Closed—ignores the feedback and is not interested in it
- Inactive listening—makes no attempt to understand the feedback
- Rationalizing—finds explanations that remove personal responsibility

- Patronizing—listens, but shows little interest.
- Superficial—listens and agrees without intending to use the feedback to make any changes

The positive or "open" style of receiving feedback includes the following:

- Open—listens without interruptions or objections
- Responsive—listens without "turning the tables"
- Accepting—accepts the feedback without denying it
- Respectful—recognizes the feedback's value as well as the value of the giver of the feedback
- Engaged—interacts well with the speaker and asks for clarifications
- Active listening—listens carefully and tries to understand
- Thoughtful—tries to understand the personal behaviors that influenced the feedback being given
- Interested—shows genuine interest in getting feedback
- Sincere—really wants to make personal changes if they are appropriate

It is a good idea for the receiver to take notes about feedback received, especially in a group situation. One will not be able to remember everything spoken about, especially if there are numerous points. It is wise to have a written record to review to be able to act on every point covered.

To give feedback well, one should strive to be supportive, direct, sensitive, considerate, descriptive, specific, thoughtful, and helpful and try to give the feedback at a healthy time. For example, after the patient received and understood the message, you should ask him or her a question as feedback. One should avoid attacks, giving indirect feedback, being insensitive, disrespectful, or judgmental, giving feedback that is too generalized, and completely avoid being impulsive or selfish so that the receiver does not feel that the feedback was initiated only for personal reasons. Also, avoid poor timing because it can cause the receiver to be ill-prepared to receive the feedback from the outset. For example, if you make an effort to develop good interpersonal skills, it will not be difficult to communicate with most individuals. You will, however, encounter patients in special circumstances which may cause them to be anxious or angry, and this will affect your interactions with them. Start with the most important things first. Be as brief as possible, and do not overly focus on small points because the receiver may then feel that the feedback is "nitpicking" or unfair.

Giving feedback about feedback is also a good practice. The receiver of the feedback should be given a chance to express his or her views about what was said and to discuss what he or she thought about the feedback (e.g., it was embarrassing, too general, repetitive, shallow, or too critical). This interaction can quickly show whether the receiver was disappointed with the quality of the feedback received and help to solve any existing difficulties that otherwise might go unaddressed.

In giving feedback, be honest but not brutal. In receiving feedback, try to use it to change what can be changed, and ask more questions about the rest—there is no reason to feel overwhelmed by a lot of feedback and then not act on it. Giving and receiving feedback is a continual learning process for both the speaker and receiver.

VERBAL COMMUNICATION

The goal of all communication is understanding. **Communication** is the sharing of information, ideas, thoughts, and feelings. It involves not just the spoken word, but also what is transported through inflection, vocal quality, facial expression, body posture, and other behavioral responses. Whether or not a person complies with the medical regimen set down by his or her physician depends on a full understanding of the reasons behind the treatment prescribed. The communication between a client and the pharmacy technician may determine the treatment outcome (see Figure 15-2). If a patient comprehends why it is important to take a medication in the exact manner in which it is prescribed, he or she is much more likely to comply. Many times individuals will alter the dose or duration of medications based on how they feel if they are unaware of the reasons behind the specific directions. If pharmacy technicians understand their role in treatment, they also understand the crucial position they hold and will gain and maintain knowledge through education and communication with all persons involved.

Verbal communication consists of much more than just words. Tone, inflection, and level of pitch determine the meaning of the message we are sending even more than the words we choose. Phrasing, which refers to the style of speaking and the words we use to express ourselves, communicates to the receiver its own message. Choice of words is no more important than the way we pronounce them or the way we present them in determining how another understands us. Proper diction and enunciation are required

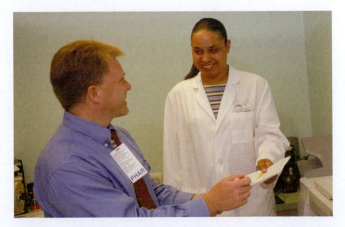

Figure 15-2. Communication is not just words. Facial expression, posture, and behavior all play a role in the message that is sent.

for speaking clearly and accurately. Quality communication requires much more than the giving of information. It includes the full scope of skills of listening, comprehending, imparting that information to others, obtaining feedback to validate that the information was received accurately and fully, and documenting the fact that each step in the process of communication was followed.

WRITTEN COMMUNICATION

Excellent written communication skills are also important in the pharmacy setting. The pharmacy technician should be concerned about his or her writing. Inaccurate or confusing writing in the pharmacy setting not only irritates others but also may lead to harmful patient care. The pharmacy technician will often be responsible for many kinds of writing, including memos, e-mail messages, ordering supplies, and record keeping. Written communication can reinforce or back up oral instructions or explanations of possible side effects of medications and can clarify misunderstandings to others.

NONVERBAL COMMUNICATION

By far, most of our communicative transmissions are nonverbal. We express ourselves both consciously and unconsciously through what is known as body language. Body language involves eye contact, facial expressions, hand gestures, grooming, dress, space, tone of voice, posture, touch, and much more.

Eye Contact

Certain aspects of body language are universal, such as smiles or frowns, and others are culture specific. Maintaining good eye contact is the most important nonverbal communication skill. It imparts to the receiver the impression that one is indeed interested in and paying attention to him or her. Anyone coming to a pharmacy rightly believes that he or she automatically deserves the undivided attention of the pharmacy technician for the duration of the transaction. With direct eye contact the pharmacy technician is conveying to the client that he or she is indeed receiving undivided attention. Conversely, the pharmacy technician needs to be aware of the possible adverse affect that eye contact can create when interacting with individuals coming from different cultures who believe that looking directly at someone's face is rude and invasive. By being sensitive and attentive, the pharmacy technician should be able to modify his or her approach accordingly. Eye contact is not comparable to staring, which is impolite

and invasive. Staring is rarely, if ever, eye-to-eye contact and is often perceived as communicating a judgmental and negative message, if not an openly aggressive one.

Facial Expressions

Often, when individuals become patients, they experience feelings of embarrassment, self-consciousness, decreased self-esteem, and fear of being dehumanized by medical professionals. Facial expressions that accompany direct eye contact can either reinforce or dispel a patient's preconceived fears. The pharmacy technician can and must demonstrate professional interest in the individual as well as care and concern. Shocked, judgmental, disapproving, or disbelieving attitudes are almost exclusively conveyed nonverbally through facial expressions and body language in general, and under no circumstance are they appropriate behavioral attitudes to be demonstrated in the professional setting.

Hand Gestures

The way one holds or moves the arms and hands (and the rest of the body) can project strong nonverbal messages. Primarily, the hands are used to emphasize important aspects of the words being said by the sender.

Grooming and Dress

Appearance is an integral part of nonverbal communication. It influences the way others view us and can present a conflicting message or even a totally incorrect message. When we see someone who is dressed or groomed in a way that is very different from our own style, we tend to assume that personalities are opposite. This is not always true. Although we should not judge people by the way they dress or how they are groomed, it is difficult not to form opinions based on what is seen.

Spacial Awareness

Another aspect of nonverbal communication that requires cultural awareness is perceived territory. Generally speaking, Anglo-Saxon Americans tend to require more personal space than persons of other cultures and feel most comfortable at arms length in all but intimate relations. In some other cultures, too much separation between interacting individuals is viewed as insulting or dismissive. As with direct eye contact, an awareness of the client's response to the approach taken will assist in modifying and improving interactions.

Tone of Voice

Use of the correct tone of voice in all situations with patients and customers cannot be emphasized enough. All people respond more favorably when spoken to in a tone that makes them feel respected, cared for, and understood. Your voice should convey an attitude of helpfulness and respect. You should reflect positive feelings about your job, patients, and skills. The sound of your voice should always remain calm, confident, and respectful. Pharmacy technicians should be aware of their vocal tone and never sound sarcastic, impatient, bored, parental, bullying, weak, or hesitant.

Posture

Posture is the position of the body with respect to the surrounding space. A posture is determined and maintained by coordination of the various muscles that move the limbs by the sense of balance. During communication, posture can usually be described as open or closed.

Open Posture

Open posture signifies a feeling of receptiveness and friendliness. An open posture position consists of the arms lying comfortably at the sides or in the lap. One should face the person to whom one is speaking and lean forward to indicate interest in what is being said. All of these actions signify that one is listening and demonstrate positive forms of communication.

Closed Posture

A closed posture conveys the opposite—a feeling of not being totally receptive to what is being said. It can also signal that someone is angry or upset. A person in a closed posture may hold the arms rigidly or fold them across the chest. This person may lean back in a chair, away from the other person or may turn away to avoid eye contact. Slouching is a kind of closed posture that can convey fatigue or lack of caring.

Physical Contact

Touching can be an extremely powerful tool for the medical professional when utilized appropriately and therapeutically. The boundary between appropriate and inappropriate touching is well defined and inviolable without grave repercussions. On the other hand, one must also be aware of the proper use of appropriate touching in the workplace. Touching another without his or her permission is never acceptable, and it is essential that the pharmacy technician understand the different forms of consent that may be offered or denied other than verbally. Occasionally the technician might be required to demonstrate the proper use or application of a prescribed treatment. It is, however, important to ask permission or explain the necessity of any procedure that requires a hands-on approach before acting. The mere act of asking permission imparts respect and facilitates cooperation. It also creates an atmosphere of safety and comfort.

COMMUNICATION WITH OTHERS

The first priority when communicating with another is to have one's message received accurately. One way of accomplishing this is to show consistency between verbal and nonverbal communication. Do nonverbal characteristics emphasize the words spoken or misrepresent them? If a person is smiling or, worse, happy when offering condolences, the communication sent is inconsistent. Rarely is the verbal message received over the more believable nonverbal message. Another method used to determine whether or not your message has been received accurately is to ask the other individual to provide feedback. Ask questions that encourage specific details relating to the information given. The answers received will determine whether or not further explanation is required. The second and equally important concern is to ensure that one has accurately received the message sent. Provide feedback by restating the message heard, thereby providing opportunity for clarification or validation. A pharmacy technician will be instructing the client about the prescribed use of medications. This includes many details such as dose, amount, route of administration, frequency, and duration of use. It is essential that the client understand accurately because misunderstandings could have lethal consequences. Providing accurate written instructions is an added reinforcement of the verbal instructions, not a substitute for them.

METHODS OF COMMUNICATION

One-on-one, face-to-face communication will be the method the pharmacy technician will be engaged in the most, although there are numerous other modes he or she will be required to use during the course of a workday. In the pharmacy these might include telephones, computers, e-mail, networking through the Internet, telecommunication conferences, pagers, and voice mail. The pharmacy technician will also be required to provide written documentation. Each method of communication has its own specific characteristics; however, it is important to remember that all require courtesy, clarity, and accuracy of information both given and received.

Telephones and Telephone Skills

The pharmacy technician will be required to conduct much of the pharmacy's daily business over the telephone. The manner in which he or she answers the phone sets the tone for the rest of the conversation (see Figure 15-3). The tone of voice should be pleasant yet professional. Properly identify the place of business and yourself by name followed by an offer of assistance. Remember that only half of the introductions have been made. Allow the caller time to complete the introductory phase of the communication including the

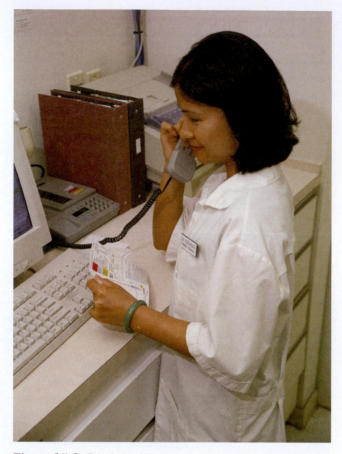

Figure 15-3. Telephone skills are important and should demonstrate professionalism.

Gulf View Associates

MESSAGE

TO _____

DATE _____ TIME _____

WHILE YOU WERE OUT

M _____
OF _____
PHONE _____

Telephoned	Will Call Again
Please Phone	Returned Your Call
Came To See You	IMPORTANT

MESSAGE _____
_____
_____
_____

TAKEN BY _____

Figure 15-4. A message pad used to facilitate proper message taking.

purpose of the call before placing him or her on hold. This will reflect positively on you, your employer, and your place of business. When placing a telephone call, introduce yourself and your place of employment followed by a short statement of the purpose of the call. Be prepared before initiating the telephone call to ensure that you communicate precisely, accurately, and cohesively.

Proper Taking of Telephone Messages

Proper written message taking is essential when the technician answers the telephone. Several calls may be answered before there is an opportunity to relay a message or carry out a promise of action. Numerous types of message pads are available today to facilitate proper message taking (see Figure 15-4). Never use small scraps of paper for messages; they are too easily lost. Bear in mind that the message book should be kept indefinitely in the pharmacy, because it could be used as evidence in a court of law.

At least seven items are needed to take a telephone message correctly:

1. The name of the person to whom the call is directed
2. The name of the person calling
3. The caller's daytime and/or evening telephone number
4. The reason for the call
5. The action to be taken
6. The date and time of the call
7. The initials of the person taking the call

The nature of the message will determine whether it should be reported immediately. The person who completes the call must sign and date the message. The message procedure is not complete until the necessary action has been taken.

Fax Machines

The use of fax machines has greatly increased the efficiency of day-to-day operations in the pharmacy. Connected to a normal phone line, a fax machine allows transmittal of documents to the fax machines of other people instantly. Advances in technology have created systems wherein fax machines can correspond with computer programs as well as other fax machines. Doctors regularly fax written information to pharmacies, helping to avoid errors in communication caused by not hearing or not understanding information spoken over the phone or phone calls that are interrupted by static and other noise. One key to reducing medication errors is to provide real-time decision support and timely notification of inappropriate medication orders to the health care providers responsible for patient care. Pharmacy technicians should be very familiar with the use of fax machines, because they are used every day in the pharmacy.

Computers

Computers are another tool for communication and are covered more thoroughly in Chapter 14. The pharmacy technician should learn how to use the particular machines available with accuracy and efficiency. Today, the Internet affects all types of business communications. It is used to do research, work with customers, handle voice and video conferences, and communicate via e-mail.

E-Mail

Electronic mail has become a very popular method of communication in the medical community, as in every sphere of society. The inexpensiveness and ease-of-use of e-mail makes it the preferred method of communication compared with regular mail delivery. Some important do's and don'ts to consider when using e-mail are the following:

- Use normal upper and lower case letters. Avoid using all capital letters because this is used for emphasizing certain words; using all capitals is considered "shouting."
- Do not assume your intentions will be understood, because people cannot see your face or body language.
- Do not send insulting remarks via e-mail; this is referred to as "flaming."
- Double check e-mails by rereading them, and never send an e-mail in anger.
- Remember that e-mail can be easily forwarded without the sender's knowledge and is not necessarily a private communication between two people.
- Include part of the original e-mail you are responding to.
- Make sure you are identified clearly in the "From" line of the e-mail or within the e-mail itself.
- Turn off the "HTML encoding" in the "preferences" section of the e-mail program; it is better to have the "Plain text" option turned on.

Delete all e-mail messages that you received for which the sender cannot be identified. It is all right to ignore e-mails that are not critical to your work, as you would a letter or phone message. Send short, informal e-mail messages. Never open e-mail attachments unless you were previously told from a reliable source that they were being sent. Keep your e-mail address book up to date so that all important contacts are easily accessible. Do not get involved in sending "chain" e-mails. Remember that e-mail messages are written documents, so never put something in an e-mail that you would not write onto company letterhead for mailing!

Networking through the Internet

The Internet offers users the ability to network with many people from all over the world. To network effectively through the Internet, you should establish the following practices:

- Have your computer and networking tools with you at all times. Laptop computers have made quick accessibility from any location a reality.
- Have an agenda in mind, but address the needs of your networking contacts first.
- Be open-minded in adding new networking contacts. You never know who can help you, or how they can help you in the future.
- Manage your time effectively.
- Ask for referrals.
- Make notes about each conversation and place these notes in an easily accessible computer location.
- Follow-up on all leads you are given, and stay in touch with the contacts who referred you.
- Ask for information and advice.
- Stay positive and upbeat at all times.

Telecommunication Conferences

The use of teleconferences over the phone or via computers has grown greatly in the past few years. For example, a pharmacist in Florida may converse with medical centers, hospitals, or other pharmacies out of state to discuss problems, solutions, costs, or medications, in a group setting. This allows many different people to share differing knowledge of important and complicated subjects in a forum that is easy to use and offers very efficient use of time to accomplish tasks and goals. Occasionally pharmacy technicians will be included in teleconferences, and it is important for them to be aware of the basic etiquette and manner of utilizing these new technologies to their best potential.

Pager and Voice Mail

A new phenomenon in the pharmacy setting is the use of customer paging systems. After customers put in their prescription orders at the pharmacy, they are given a paging device and allowed to circulate around the store while their order is prepared. When it is ready, their pager signals them to return to the pharmacy counter, where they can then pick up their prescription. Another popular type of technology used in pharmacies is the voice mail message system. Refills may be called in by leaving a voice mail message for what is needed from the pharmacy. This system utilizes touchtone phones to make selections and enter data via a computer that controls the message system. Patients can enter their prescription numbers, name, Social Security number, name of the prescription medication they need to be refilled, and other information. Most of their refills are then processed and ready for pickup within 24 hours.

Written Documentation

State boards of pharmacy require pharmacy records to be kept for 2 years. It is important to keep track of all dispensed medications, manufacturer data, lot numbers, and patient records to ensure proper management and business practices. A competent plan for records management on a day-to-day basis can save a pharmacy a lot of time and trouble in the future. This is especially true if legal issues arise. The pharmacy can protect itself greatly by having a good record of activities to prove proper business management and good patient service.

TYPES OF CUSTOMERS

In a pharmacy, customers are not only clients with a prescription. Customers are also the physicians who write the prescriptions, the nurses who call in the prescriptions, and others, such as pharmaceutical representatives.

Consumers

In the community pharmacy setting, the **consumer** is the person coming to the pharmacy for the filling of prescriptions or the purchase of over-the-counter remedies for a wide variety of situations. Above all, the consumer is seeking information. The pharmacy technician will be called upon to answer many questions. It is important for the technician to remember that he or she cannot be expected to know all things, and the most valuable technician will know when to refer questions or concerns directly to the pharmacist.

Physicians

Physicians are the pharmacist's livelihood. Most contact with them will be via the telephone. It is important for the pharmacy technician to be respectful, pleasant, and courteous when taking their calls.

Nurses

Often the nurse working with a physician will be the person calling in a prescription. He or she should be treated with respect.

Pharmaceutical Representatives

Pharmaceutical sales is a widely growing segment of the business of pharmacy. Pharmaceutical representatives regularly contact physicians in their coverage area to secure use of the products and companies they represent for the physicians' patients. Thus, these individuals must have current information on new medicines, research, and technologies that relate to drugs and usage of drug products.

PROFESSIONALISM

Professionalism is behavior based on a body of knowledge and ethical standards to serve the public. Pharmacy technicians must maintain professional behavior, show respect, and exhibit a positive attitude in all of their dealings with customers and other medical personnel.

The most important characteristics a good pharmacy technician can display are honesty, reliability, dependability, integrity, and organization. The pharmacist and other personnel must be able to rely on the technician to maintain professional behavior at all times. They must be able to trust that the technician will behave ethically and maintain confidentiality regardless of the presence or absence of direct supervision.

Autonomy

The principle of **autonomy** establishes a patient's right to self-determination. He or she can choose what will be done to his or her body. This right is considered paramount even if a health professional may judge a patient's decision as being damaging to his or her health. One area of importance is patient respect in situations involving death with dignity and euthanasia. Health professionals should respect the wishes of all patients uncritically, enhancing their sense of self-worth and focusing on the active involvement of competent patients. Informed consent must be given to the health professional by the patient before any procedure is undertaken.

Honesty

The honesty principle states that patients have the right to the truth about their medical condition, the course of their disease, treatments recommended, and alternative treatments available.

Attitude

Pharmacy technicians must be warm and caring and display a genuine interest in helping people. They must be able to perform their duties effectively and efficiently while keeping in mind that their first priority is to the patient met in the hospital or the client coming to the neighborhood pharmacy.

Confidentiality

Confidentiality assures patients that information about their medical conditions and treatment will not be given to third parties without permission. Confidentiality is essential for preserving the human dignity of the patient. Patients are expected to reveal the most personal details of their existence to virtual strangers. They must be able to trust that this information will not be shared with others not involved in their medical care.

Faithfulness

The right of patients to have health professionals provide services that promote the patient's interest rather than those that serve a competing or conflicting interest is faithfulness. A pharmacist or technician who encourages the use of vitamins the patient does not need may be promoting his or her financial well-being at the expense of that of the patient. Ethically, the responsibility of a health professional is, first and foremost, the welfare of the patient.

Appearance

Pharmacy technicians are professionals and should not only act professional but also dress professionally. Cleanliness and neatness say more about an individual than dressing in the latest fad and instill good impressions in others.

Sexual Harassment

Sexual harassment occurs whenever any person makes intentional, clearly understood statements or takes intentional, clearly understood action that causes another to feel that his or her job is at risk if the sexual advances are rejected. Harassment may be physical or verbal, expressed in gestures or images, or written or spoken. It can occur at any level within the hierarchy of the work environment and can result in personal distress. The legal implications can be extremely distressing and debilitating for all concerned.

BARRIERS TO COMMUNICATION

The number of barriers to good communication in any situation is great, but they present especially challenging dilemmas in the pharmaceutical setting. The potential for life-threatening mistakes make it essential that communication is accurate and timely. Work conditions may be crowded and noisy. The physical environment may not allow for privacy and ease of confidentiality. Personal characteristics and concerns of clients and co-workers alike can interfere with the smooth communication in the workplace. Time constraints add pressure and may increase stress. The general administrative philosophy also plays a part in setting the tone of working relationships.

Environmental (Physical Impairment)

A pleasant environment is one in which, among other things, acoustics are sufficient to carry on a conversation without having to raise one's voice. Also, an environment in which good rapport can be established and the confidentiality assured is essential for any pharmacy. If a patient does not feel that all communication is treated with care, concern, courtesy, and, above all else, confidentiality, that patient will at best be less than direct and honest. This not only prolongs the time

needed to properly understand and accurately meet the needs of the individual, but it also could easily lead to misinformation and inaccurate treatment. At worst, the patient's health and, in fact, life, are placed in jeopardy. Another result of an uncomfortable or unpleasant atmosphere could be the loss of that patient's continuing his or her relationship with the pharmacy. The client loses good continuity of care, the pharmacist loses business, and eventually his or her reputation suffers. The pharmacy technician who is aware of the relationship between excellent medical care and an environment conducive to good communication will be seen as a valuable asset.

Non-English-Speaking People

Language barriers occur when an individual neither speaks nor comprehends an adequate amount of English. This presents unique challenges for the pharmacy technician. Communication can often be facilitated by the use of proper English and elimination of complex words or phrases. Use of demonstrative gestures may also help. The availability of preprinted instructions in a variety of languages is a valuable aid.

Hearing Impairment

The client's role in the communication process is multifaceted. Barriers to good communication on the client's part can be of a physical or psychological nature. The important role of the pharmacy technician is to observe early on whether or not the client has any limitations that might interfere with good communications. There are a number of physical abnormalities that could limit the client's ability to participate fully and/or accurately in the communication process. Is the person hearing correctly under all circumstances? A client may hear perfectly well in a small room with only one other person communicating but may be unable to accurately hear in a room full of background noise. Is the client capable of hearing lower tones well but cannot follow the conversation of someone with a high, soft voice? On the other hand, the client might be fully hearing impaired and communicate only through sign language or an interpreter or by reading lips. Another situation the pharmacy technician might face is a client whose hearing is unimpaired, but who has another form of physical impairment that makes communication challenging. **Receptive aphasia** is a physical limitation that occurs after certain neurological injuries and leaves the person incapable of understanding all that is said. Another client might exhibit **expressive aphasia**, a condition in which he or she cannot form language and express his or her thoughts accurately even though thought processes are intact.

Prejudice

Personal and social bias, which brings about discrimination, is called **prejudice**. The word *discrimination* is used to describe unfair treatment of a person because of race, gender, religious affiliation, handicap, or any other reason. Discrimination is unethical, immoral, and socially wrong. Sometimes it is even illegal, and it also prevents effective communication.

NEGATIVE COMMUNICATION

The pharmacy technician should be aware of the negative impression he or she can have on others. Some examples of negative communication include the following:

- Speaking too softly or indistinctly
- Appearing bored or disinterested
- Appearing impatient (e.g., drumming fingers or clicking a pen)
- Interrupting
- Ignoring common courtesies such as saying "please" and "thank you"
- Speaking too quickly or sharply
- Confronting or being loud and aggressive
- Using negative body language (e.g., chomping gum or slouching)
- Appearing judgmental (e.g., frowning or crossing one's arms)
- Avoiding eye contact or staring

DEFENSE MECHANISMS

The human body may react to anxiety or stress in many different ways. **Defense mechanisms** are tools an individual uses when required to deal with uncomfortable or threatening situations. These are often subconscious reactions designed for emotional protection. They help us to deal with whatever difficult event has triggered such a response. There are many types of defense mechanisms, and pharmacy technicians should be familiar with them to better communicate with patients and others they come into contact with in the course of their duties. Commonly employed defense mechanisms include the following.

Regression

Responding to a perceived threat or conflict in an immature way is called **regression**. The individual calls upon coping skills learned early in life to avoid or escape conflict in the present. Examples include making excuses for not doing a certain thing or saying that it cannot be done, instead of the truth—which is that the person does not want to do it.

Projection

Shifting one's own unacceptable feelings onto another person is called **projection**. An example is when a man who has competitive or hostile feelings about another says that the other person "does not like him."

Repression

Repression is characterized by pushing uncomfortable thoughts or conflicts out of consciousness to avoid the discomfort of confrontation. Examples include blocking a problem out of the mind and changing the subject when it is mentioned.

Rationalization

Giving reasonable justification to explain unreasonable behavior is called **rationalization**. An example is when you buy something you want because you are convinced that a similar item you already own will not be of value much longer.

Compensation

Exaggerating one acceptable characteristic to make up for an unacceptable one is called **compensation**. A person who compensates makes up for one behavior by stressing another. Compensation is not always a negative response, but it is often used as an excuse for not accomplishing what should be accomplished. An example is a person with a deficiency in one area who becomes extremely proficient in a different area.

Sublimation

Sublimation is redirecting a socially unacceptable impulse into a socially acceptable act. An example is using work or hobbies to divert your thoughts from a problem you do not want to address.

Displacement

Displacement is giving one's own negative feelings to someone or something else unrelated to the situation. When faced with situations that are uncomfortable and potentially volatile, the pharmacy technician should remain calm, observant, willing to try different approaches, flexible, and patient. The technician should not hesitate to request assistance from a supervisor or employer if needed. An example of displacement behavior is when a person who has been angered at work goes home and punishes his or her child for a behavior that is usually tolerated.

Apathy

A lack of feeling, emotion, interest, or concern is called **apathy**. An apathetic person shows indifference to what is happening or a pretense of not caring about a situation. Apathy is sometimes a sign of depression. An example is when an individual does not do regular menial tasks that should be done because he or she has no interest in the outcome of being responsible for them.

Sarcasm

In most cases, the use of **sarcasm** is hostile and cruel; however, some individuals use it constantly, thinking that it is quite witty. On the contrary, it often makes bitter enemies of its victims. An example is when an individual makes fun of co-workers' behavior or mistakes to improve his or her standing in the office, even though it only causes them continuing embarrassment.

Denial

Denial is a psychological defense mechanism in which confrontation with a personal problem or with reality is avoided by denying the existence of the problem or reality. An example is a parent who reacts with hostility to someone who discusses his or her child's affliction, saying that the person is overreacting or misinformed even though the child's condition is a medical certainty.

DEALING WITH CONFLICT

Conflict may develop in the pharmacy over many issues including pricing, prescriptions, and the perceptions of patients or customers. Conflict can be dealt with in many ways. The first way to assure good communication is for pharmacy technicians to be open and willing to listen to the people they talk to about health problems and medication requirements. Second, pharmacy technicians should avoid confrontational terms and keep the focus of their discussions on the good of the patient. They should never enter into any discussion that is beyond their scope of training and always refer customers directly to the pharmacist or back to their physician if needed. The most important thing for pharmacy technicians to remember is to remain professional at all times. If a situation starts to get out of hand, it is best to alert the pharmacist so the proper decision can be made regarding the customer's complaint or problem.

ELIMINATING BARRIERS TO COMMUNICATION

The elimination of barriers to good communication requires the realization that they exist, the identification of the specific nature of the barriers, and the willingness to take appropriate action to eliminate them. This is the responsibility of every member of the working team. Good working relationships can compensate for any barrier created by the actual physical space occupied by the pharmacy. Working conditions will improve with recognition of the barriers present and with the staff working together as a team. This will result in increased quality of services and increased client satisfaction, which will be evidenced by increased revenues.

Time

In the world we live in today few of us have too much time on our hands. The pharmacist cannot and usually will not tolerate unnecessary delays in the routine workings of his or her place of business. The pharmacy technician must prioritize his or her time with extreme care to complete each task efficiently before the next is due to begin. Every worker must operate under similar time constraints. Most clients have only limited available time as well. For any facility to function within the designated time constraints of all, good communication is the essential key.

SUMMARY

How you present yourself will determine the course your career will take. The pharmacy technician who pays attention to how others perceive him or her and who acts, speaks, and dresses accordingly will have greater job satisfaction and security. Verbal communication depends on words and sound, whereas nonverbal communication consists of messages that are conveyed to another without the use of words. Eye contact, facial expressions, and hand gestures are some of the many ways we use body language to communicate. Some of the barriers to communication include physical impairment, language differences, and prejudice. Defense mechanisms are psychological methods of dealing with stressful situations and include regression, projection, repression, rationalization, compensation, sublimation, displacement, and several others.

CRITICAL THINKING

1. Think about a situation in which you have dealt with someone who left you feeling angry or disappointed. What was it about the encounter that made you feel this way? What could have improved the outcome of the encounter?
2. Now think about an encounter in which you have dealt with someone who left you feeling satisfied and happy. What was it about this encounter that made you feel this way?
3. Explain why professionalism is important to the pharmacy technician. Visit pharmacies in your area and observe the pharmacists and technicians working there. What characteristics do they exemplify?

REVIEW QUESTIONS

1. An individual's success as a pharmacy technician begins and ends with the ability to
   A. work in very diverse practice settings.
   B. communicate both professionally and courteously.
   C. become certified.
   D. explain the value of listening.

2. The communication cycle includes the sender, the message, the channel, the receiver, and _____.
   A. documentation
   B. first impressions
   C. presentation
   D. feedback

3. The goal of all communication is
   A. completeness.
   B. cohesiveness.
   C. body language.
   D. understanding.

4. Pharmacy technicians must have excellent oral, nonverbal, and _____ communication skills.
   A. phrasing
   B. written
   C. prescribing
   D. receiving

5. The pharmacy technician can and must demonstrate _____ to patients, as well as care and concern.
   A. professional interest
   B. body language
   C. hand gestures
   D. spacial awareness

6. The type of communication you, as a pharmacy technician, will be engaged in the most is
   A. written.
   B. face-to-face.
   C. telephone.
   D. e-mail.

7. When answering the pharmacy's phone, you should properly identify
   A. the hours of operation.
   B. the place of business and yourself by name.
   C. the caller's name first.
   D. whether the pharmacy is having a sale on certain medications.

8. Which of the following is NOT one of the seven items you should write down when taking a telephone message properly?
   A. The name of the person to whom the call is directed
   B. The caller's daytime and/or evening telephone number
   C. The caller's social security number
   D. The date and time of the call

9. As a pharmacy technician, it is important to know when to
   A. close the store for the day.
   B. take your breaks during the day.
   C. exhibit a positive attitude.
   D. refer questions or concerns directly to the pharmacist.

10. One of the most important characteristics a good pharmacy technician can display is
    A. knowing the prices of over-the-counter medications.
    B. being at least an hour early into work.
    C. integrity.
    D. giving prescription advice and opinions to customers.

11. The principle of _____ establishes a patient's right to self-determination.
    A. ethics
    B. autonomy
    C. confidentiality
    D. faithfulness

12. Sexual harassment may be verbal, written, or
    A. physical.
    B. intentional.
    C. legal.
    D. illegal.

13. Personal and social bias, which brings about discrimination, is called
    A. prejudice.
    B. unfairness.
    C. negative.
    D. confrontational.

14. _____ are tools an individual uses when required to deal with uncomfortable or threatening situations.
    A. Social wrongs
    B. Negative communicators
    C. Defense mechanisms
    D. Conscious reactions

15. _____ is a psychological defense mechanism in which confrontation with a personal problem, or with reality, is avoided by not admitting the existence of the problem or reality.
    A. Sublimation
    B. Displacement
    C. Hostility
    D. Denial

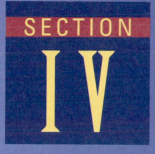

Mathematics Review

16

Basic Mathematics

OUTLINE

Overview
Arabic Numbers and Roman Numerals
Fractions
  Classification of Fractions
  Changing Improper Fractions into Whole or Mixed Numbers
  Changing Mixed Numbers to Improper Fractions
  Comparing Fractions
  Lowest Common Denominator
  Adding Fractions
  Subtracting Fractions
  Multiplying Fractions
  Dividing Fractions

Decimals
  Changing Common Fractions to Decimals
  Multiplying Decimals
  Dividing Decimals
  Adding Decimals
  Subtracting Decimals
  Rounding Decimals
Ratios
  Proportions
  Percentages

OBJECTIVES

Upon completion of this chapter, the reader should be able to

1. Explain the difference between Arabic numbers and Roman numerals.
2. Change an improper fraction to a mixed number.
3. Add fractions having the same denominator.
4. Subtract fractions having the same denominator.

5. Multiply fractions and mixed numbers.
6. Divide fractions and mixed numbers.
7. Multiply, divide, add, and subtract decimals.
8. Define ratios, proportions, and percentages.

GLOSSARY

Arabic numbers Standard numerical numbers.

common fraction Equal parts of a whole.

complex fraction The numerator or the denominator or both as a whole number, proper fraction, or mixed number. The value may be less than, greater than, or equal to 1.

decimal A numerator that is expressed in numerals with a decimal point placed so that it designates the value of the denominator, and the denominator, which is understood to be 10 or some power of 10; also called decimal fraction.

decimal fraction A numerator that is expressed in numerals, with a decimal point placed so that it designates the value of the denominator, and the denominator, which is understood to be 10 or some power of 10; also called decimal.

denominator The number the whole is divided into.

divisor The number performing the division.

extremes The two outside terms in a ratio.

fraction An expression of division with a number that is the portion or part of a whole.

improper fraction The numerator is greater than or equal to the denominator.

means The two inside terms in a ratio.

mixed fraction A whole number and a proper fraction that are combined. The value of the mixed number is always greater than 1.

multiplicand The number to be multiplied by another.

multiplier A number by which another is multiplied.

numerator The portion of the whole being considered.

percent A fraction whose numerator is expressed and whose denominator is understood to be 100.

product The answer from multiplying two or more quantities together.

GLOSSARY continued

proper fraction The numerator is smaller than the denominator and designates less than one whole unit.

proportion The relationship between two equal ratios.

quotient The answer to a division problem.

ratio A mathematical expression that compares two numbers by division.

OVERVIEW

The first technical operation that pharmacy technicians must learn is the manipulation of measures of volume, balance, and weights. In this learning process, familiarity with the various systems of weights and measures and their relationships and a mastery of basic mathematics are necessary. Pharmacy technicians must learn basic mathematics to be able to calculate the dosage of drugs by weight, measures of volume, and balances. He or she must also be able to convert from one system to another. To become skilled in math, the pharmacy technician needs extensive practice in solving various types of mathematics problems such as adding, subtracting, multiplying, and dividing whole numbers. The technician should also have a working knowledge of fractions, decimals, ratios, and percentages and basic problem-solving skills. This chapter summarizes these important mathematical operations to support various dosage calculations in the pharmacy.

ARABIC NUMBERS AND ROMAN NUMERALS

The system of Roman numerals uses letters to represent number values. Unlike the Arabic system that is commonly used for counting, the Roman system has no symbol for zero. Roman numerals are used less commonly than Arabic numbers in dosage calculation. Still, some physicians and practitioners use this system in prescriptions. The pharmacy technician needs to understand Roman numerals to interpret physicians' orders and drug dosages precisely. In pharmacy settings, the technician usually sees and uses only the Roman numerals that represent the values 1 through 30.

Roman numerals can be written as either uppercase or lowercase letters. In medical usage, "iv," which represents the number 4, is generally written in lowercase to differentiate it from "IV," which is the abbreviation for intravenous.

The building blocks of the Roman system include the letters I, V, X, L, C, D, and M. Only I, V, and X are required to show the values 1 through 30:

I = i = 1
V = v = 5

X = x = 10
L = l = 50
C = c = 100
D = d = 500
M = m = 1000

Most of the medications administered or ordered should be measured by amounts expressed in **Arabic numbers**. The familiar system of whole numbers (0 through 9), fractions (e.g., $\frac{1}{5}$), and decimals (e.g., 0.7) is used widely in the United States and internationally. Table 16-1 shows some examples of Arabic numbers and Roman numerals.

FRACTIONS

Pharmacy technicians need to understand fractions to be able to interpret and act on practitioners' orders, read prescriptions, and understand patient records and information in the pharmacy literature. Fractions are used in apothecary and household measures for dosage calculations. A **fraction**

TABLE 16-1. Examples of Arabic Numbers and Roman Numerals

ARABIC NUMBER	ROMAN NUMERAL
½	$\overline{ss}$
1	I
2	II
3	III
4	IV
5	V
6	VI
7	VII
8	VIII
9	IX
10	X
20	XX
30	XXX
50	L
100	C
500	D
1000	M

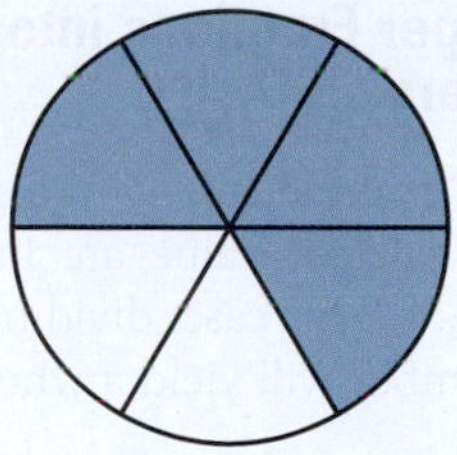

Figure 16-1. Fractions.

is an expression of division with a number that is the portion or part of a whole amount. A fraction has two parts (these fractions are known as common fractions). The bottom is referred to as the **denominator**, which represents the whole. It can never equal zero. The **numerator** is the top part of the fraction and represents parts of the whole. See Figure 16-1, which is a diagram representing fractions of a whole. Four parts shaded out of six parts represents:

$$\frac{\text{Numerator (4 parts)}}{\text{Denominator (6 parts)}} = \frac{4}{6}$$

The fraction $2/3$ is read as "two-thirds." It means two parts out of the three parts that make up the whole. The fraction bar also means "divided by." Thus, $2/3$ can be read as "two divided by three" or $2 \div 3$. This definition is important when one changes fractions to decimals.

Classification of Fractions

There are two types of fractions: common fractions and decimal fractions. A **common fraction** usually represents equal parts of a whole. It consists of two numbers and a fraction bar and is shown in the form:

$$\frac{\text{Numerator}}{\text{Denominator}}$$

for example, $1/4$, $2/5$, and $9/10$. A **decimal fraction** is commonly referred to simply as a decimal (e.g., 0.5). Decimal fractions will be discussed later in the chapter.

There are four types of common fractions: proper, improper, mixed, and complex.

Proper Fractions

A **proper fraction** has a numerator that is smaller than the denominator and designates less than one whole unit. Whenever the numerator is less than the denominator, the value of the fraction must be less than 1 (see Figure 16-2).

Example

$$\frac{3}{5} = \frac{\text{Numerator}}{\text{Denominator}} = <1$$

Other examples of proper fractions are $3/4$, $1/9$, $32/45$, and $94/1000$.

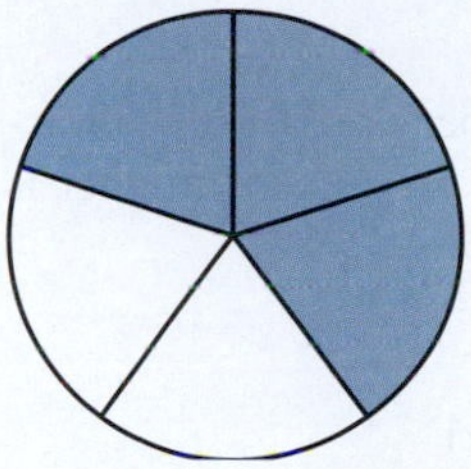

Figure 16-2. Proper fractions.

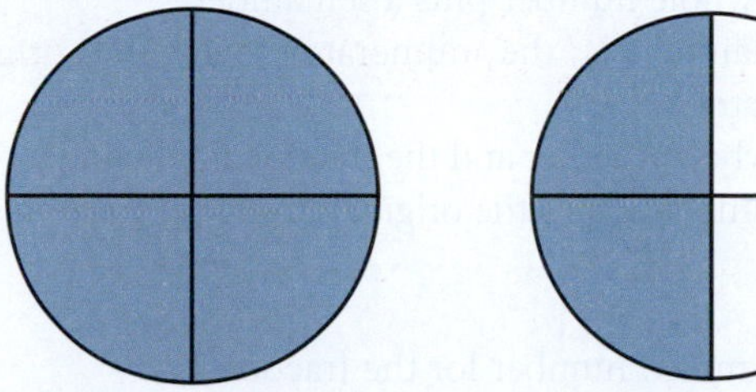

Figure 16-3. Improper fractions.

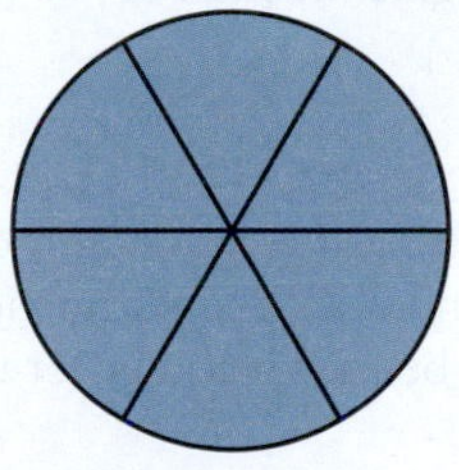

Figure 16-4. When the numerator and denominator are the same the value of the fraction is equal to 1.

Improper Fractions

An **improper fraction** has a numerator that is greater than or equal to the denominator. The value of an improper fraction is greater than or equal to 1 (see Figure 16-3).

Example

$$\frac{6}{4} = >1$$

More examples of improper fractions are $35/30$, $28/23$, and $155/10$.

Whenever the numerator and denominator are equal, the value of the improper fraction is always equal to 1 (see Figure 16-4).

Example

$$\frac{6}{6} = 1$$

More examples of improper fractions that equal 1 are $3/3$, $16/16$, and $8/8$.

Mixed Fractions

A **mixed fraction** has a whole number and a proper fraction that are combined. The value of the mixed number is always greater than 1 (see Figure 16-5).

> **Example**
>
> $$1\frac{3}{5} = 1 + \frac{3}{5} = >1$$

To convert an improper fraction to a mixed number, follow the rule:

1. Divide the numerator by the denominator. The result will be a whole number plus a remainder.
2. The remainder is the numerator over the original denominator.
3. Mix the whole number and the fractional remainder. This mixed number equals the original improper fraction.

> **Example**
>
> Find the mixed number for the fraction $^{16}/_5$.
> Divide the numerator by the denominator: 16 divided by 5.
> The result is $3\frac{1}{5}$.
> To check, convert 3 into 15/5. Then add it to $^1/_5$, which leaves the original fraction of $^{16}/_5$.

Complex Fractions

A **complex fraction** has the numerator or the denominator or both as a whole number, proper fraction, or mixed number. The value may be less than, greater than, or equal to 1.

> **Examples**
>
> $$\frac{^3/_5}{^1/_2} = >1$$
>
> $$\frac{^3/_5}{2} = <1$$
>
> $$\frac{1^3/_5}{^1/_5} = >1$$
>
> $$\frac{^1/_2}{^2/_4} = 1$$

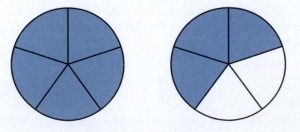

Figure 16-5. Mixed fractions.

Changing Improper Fractions into Whole or Mixed Numbers

Fractions that have a numerator with a greater value and a denominator with a lesser value are known as improper fractions, such as $^4/_2$. In this case, dividing the bottom number into the top number will yield a whole number.

> **Example**
>
> $$\frac{4}{2} = 4 \div 2 = 2 \text{ (whole number)}$$

However, in some cases, the numbers do not divide equally. Therefore, a mixed number is the result, such as $3^1/_5$.

> **Example**
>
> $$\frac{15}{4} = 15 \div 4 = 3\frac{3}{4} \text{ (mixed number)}$$

Because the closest whole number less than 15 that 4 will divide into is 12, 3 is the whole number (4 multiplied by 3 equals 12). Now, 15 minus 12 is the remainder, which equals 3. Therefore, 3 out of 4 is the remainder. This fraction is already expressed in lowest terms.

Changing Mixed Numbers to Improper Fractions

To convert a mixed number to an improper fraction first, the whole number is multiplied by the bottom number (denominator) of the fraction. Next, the top number (numerator) is added to the product of the previous step. The result is the answer of the numerator calculation, and the denominator remains the same as in the original improper fraction.

> **Example**
>
> $$3\frac{2}{5} = \frac{5 \times 3 + 2}{5} = \frac{17}{5}$$
>
> **Example**
>
> $$6\frac{3}{7} = \frac{7 \times 6 + 3}{7} = \frac{45}{7}$$

Comparing Fractions

When calculating some drug dosages, it is helpful for the technician to know whether the value of one fraction is greater than or less than the value of another fraction. The size of a fraction can be determined by comparing the numerators when the denominators are the same or comparing the denominators if the numerators are the same. If the numerators are the same, the fraction with the smaller denominator has the greater value (see Figure 16-6).

> **Example**
>
> Compare $^1/_2$ and $^1/_3$.
> Numerators are both 1.
> Denominator 2 is less than 3.
> Therefore, $^1/_2$ has the greater value.

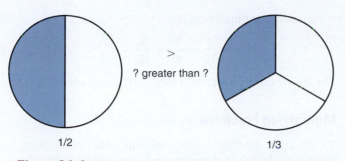

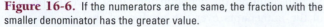

? greater than ?

1/2   1/3

Figure 16-6. If the numerators are the same, the fraction with the smaller denominator has the greater value.

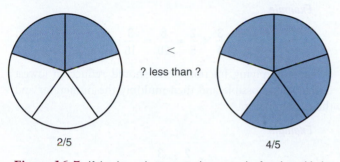

? less than ?

2/5   4/5

Figure 16-7. If the denominators are the same, the fraction with the smaller numerator has the lesser value.

On the contrary, if the denominators are both the same, the fraction with the smaller numerator has the lesser value (see Figure 16-7).

Example

Compare $^2/_5$ and $^4/_5$.
Denominators are both 5.
Numerator 2 is less than 4.
Therefore, $^2/_5$ has a lesser value.

Lowest Common Denominator

The smallest whole number that can be divided evenly by all denominators is known as the lowest common denominator. This is used when one adds and subtracts fractions. It is important to notice whether one of the denominators is evenly divisible by each of the other denominators. This denominator will be determined to be the lowest common denominator.

Example

Find the lowest common denominator of $^1/_3$ and $^2/_{15}$.
In this problem, 15 is evenly divisible by 3.
Therefore, 15 is the lowest common denominator.

Example

Find the lowest common denominator of $^3/_7$ and $^3/_{14}$ and $^1/_{28}$.
In this problem, 28 is evenly divisible by 7 and 14.
Therefore, 28 is the lowest common denominator.
To determine a fraction equivalent to a fraction with the lowest common denominator, first use the lowest common denominator to divide the denominator of the fraction to be changed. Next, multiply this number by the numerator of the fraction to be changed. Finally, use the **product** as the numerator over the lowest common denominator.

Example

$$\frac{4}{5} = \frac{?}{20} \quad 20 \div 5 = 4 \quad 4 \times 4 = 16 \quad \frac{4}{5} = \frac{16}{20}$$

Example

$$\frac{3}{8} = \frac{?}{32} \quad 32 \div 8 = 4 \quad 4 \times 3 = 12 \quad \frac{3}{8} = \frac{12}{32}$$

To determine a fraction equivalent to a mixed number with the lowest common denominator, an improper fraction must first be determined from the mixed number. Next, divide the lowest common denominator by the denominator of the fraction. Then, multiply this answer by the numerator of the improper fraction. Finally, use the product as the numerator over the lowest common denominator.

Example

$$1\frac{2}{3} = \frac{?}{15} \quad \text{change } 1\frac{2}{3} \text{ to an improper fraction}$$

$$\frac{3 \times 1 + 2}{3} = \frac{5}{3} \quad \text{your equation is now}$$

$$\frac{5}{3} = \frac{?}{15} \quad 15 \div 3 = 5 \quad 5 \times 5 = 25 \quad \frac{5}{3} = \frac{25}{15} \text{ or } 1\frac{2}{3} = \frac{25}{15}$$

Example

$$2\frac{1}{4} = \frac{?}{12} \quad 4 \times 2 + 1 = 9 \quad 3 \times 9 = 27 \quad \frac{9}{4} = \frac{27}{12}$$

$$\text{or } \frac{21}{4} = \frac{27}{12} \quad \frac{9}{4} = \frac{?}{12} \quad 12 \div 4 = 3$$

Sometimes the lowest common denominator is not included in the denominators of the problem. In this case, one must determine the lowest common denominator by the method of trial and error. However, there are two suggestions that may help in determining the common denominator. One suggestion is to multiply the two denominators together and determine the lowest common denominator for that case. If this fails, another suggestion is to multiply the denominators by 2, 3, or 4.

Example

$$5\frac{1}{3} \text{ and } \frac{2}{5}$$

Multiply the two denominators:

$$5 \times 3 = 15 \quad 5\frac{1}{3} = \frac{?}{15} \quad \frac{5 \times 3 + 1}{3} = \frac{16}{3}$$

$$\frac{16}{3} = \frac{?}{15} \quad 15 \div 3 = 5 \quad 5 \times 16 = 80 \quad 5\frac{1}{3} = \frac{80}{15}$$

$$\frac{2}{5} = \frac{?}{15} \quad 15 \div 5 = 3 \quad 3 \times 2 = 6 \quad \frac{2}{5} = \frac{6}{15}$$

Example

$$\frac{2}{3} \text{ and } \frac{1}{6} \text{ and } \frac{5}{12}$$

Example

Multiply the denominator 6 by 2:

$$6 \times 2 = 12 \quad \frac{2}{3} = \frac{?}{12} \quad 12 \div 3 = 4 \quad 4 \times 2 = 8 \quad \frac{2}{3} = \frac{8}{12}$$

$$\frac{1}{6} \times \frac{?}{12} \quad 12 \div 6 = 2 \quad 2 \times 1 = 2 \quad \frac{1}{6} = \frac{2}{12} \quad \frac{5}{12}$$

Adding Fractions

To add two fractions, it is necessary to find the lowest common denominator first. Next, add the numerators together and keep the value of the common denominator the same. Finally, reduce the resulting value to its lowest terms.

Example

Add $\frac{1}{6}$ and $\frac{4}{12}$.

To obtain a common denominator of 12, it is necessary to multiply the numerator and denominator of $\frac{1}{6}$ by 2. (*Note:* Both the numerator and denominator must be multiplied so that the value of the fraction remains constant.)

$$\frac{1}{6} \times \frac{2}{2} = \frac{2}{12}$$

Now we have a common denominator and are able to simply add the numerators. Be sure to reduce the final answer. To reduce a fraction, find the largest number that may be divided into both the numerator and the denominator and then divide them by that number.

$$\frac{2}{12} + \frac{4}{12} = \frac{6}{12} = \frac{1}{2}$$

$\frac{6}{12}$ is reduced to lowest terms, which is $\frac{1}{2}$. (The largest number which may be divided into both the numerator and the denominator, is 6.) So, $\frac{6}{12}$ (after both the numerator and denominator are divided by 6) becomes $\frac{1}{2}$.

Subtracting Fractions

The first step in subtracting fractions is to find a common denominator, then subtract the numerator, and, finally, obtain the result by keeping the denominator the same and taking the difference of the numerator. After that, reduce to lowest terms to obtain the final answer.

Example

Subtract $\frac{1}{2}$ from $\frac{8}{10}$.

Find a common denominator.

Multiplying the numerator and denominator by 5 will produce 10 as the common denominator:

$$\frac{1}{2} \times \frac{5}{5} = \frac{5}{10}$$

Subtract the numerator:

$$\frac{8}{10} - \frac{5}{10} = \frac{3}{10}$$

The answer cannot be reduced further. The final answer is $\frac{3}{10}$.

Multiplying Fractions

To multiply fractions, first, multiply the numerators. Second, multiply the denominators, then place the product of the numerators over the product of the denominators, and finally, reduce to lowest terms.

Example

$$\frac{3}{4} \times \frac{2}{5} = \frac{6}{20} = \frac{3}{10}$$

When multiplying fractions, one should reduce to lowest terms when possible and then multiply the numerator and the denominator.

Example

$$\frac{2}{4} \times \frac{3}{4}$$

Reduce $\frac{2}{4}$ to $\frac{1}{2}$, then multiply:

$$\frac{1}{2} \times \frac{3}{4} = \frac{3}{8}$$

Dividing Fractions

To divide fractions, first invert (or turn upside down) the divisor. Second, multiply the two fractions, and then reduce to lowest terms. In addition, when dividing fractions, one must reduce all possible fractions before performing the operations.

Example

$$\frac{3}{4} \div \frac{2}{3} = \frac{3}{4} \times \frac{3}{2} = \frac{9}{8}$$

Example

$$\frac{3}{4} \div \frac{8}{9} = \frac{3}{4} \times \frac{9}{8} = \frac{27}{32}$$

Example

$$\frac{32}{12} \div \frac{2}{3}$$

Reduce:

$$\frac{32}{12} = \frac{8}{3} \quad \frac{8}{3} \times \frac{3}{2} = \frac{24}{6} = \frac{4}{1} = 4$$

■ DECIMALS

Decimal fractions or decimals are used with the metric system, which is the system most often used in the calculation of drug dosages. It is very important for the pharmacy

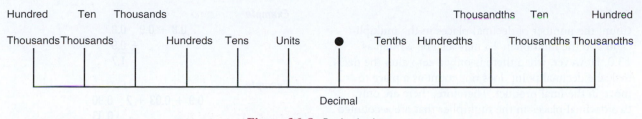

Figure 16-8. Decimal values.

TABLE 16-2.	Fractions and Their Related Decimal Fractions

FRACTION	DECIMAL FRACTION	DESCRIPTION
$^4/_{10}$	0.4	Because 10 has **1** zero, the decimal point of 4 is moved to the left **once.**
$^{17}/_{100}$	0.17	Because 100 has **2** zeros, the decimal point of 17 is moved to the left **twice.**
$^{334}/_{1000}$	0.334	Because 1000 has **3** zeros, the decimal point of 334 is moved to the left **three** places.

technician to be able to manipulate decimals easily and accurately. Each decimal fraction consists of a numerator that is expressed in numerals, a decimal point placed so that it designates the value of the denominator, and the denominator, which is understood to be 10 or some power of 10. In writing a decimal fraction, always place a zero to the left of the decimal point, so that the decimal point can readily be seen. Table 16-2 shows some examples.

For reading and writing decimals, observe Figure 16-8, which shows that all whole numbers are to the left of the decimal point and all fractions are to the right.

The technician should remember when dealing with decimal fractions (such as one-tenth) to always place a zero in front of the decimal, e.g., 0.1. This prevents one from mistaking the decimal one-tenth for the whole number 1. It is of vital importance that decimal calculations be double-checked before using them for drug dosages. An example of the dangers of not carefully checking the existence of a decimal point for an unfamiliar drug is the following. A dose of 0.30 mg of morphine may be administered for pain. However, if a doctor wrote the order for .30 mg without placing a zero before the decimal point, and the health care worker did not see the decimal point in the .30 mg order or know about the lethal levels of morphine, 30 mg could be administered by error, and the patient would probably die. This situation has a great potential for disaster because a 30 mg dose of morphine can kill a healthy person within

5 minutes by slowing breathing to the point that the brain would not receive enough oxygen to live.

Changing Common Fractions to Decimals

To obtain a decimal from a common fraction, divide the numerator by the denominator, and place a decimal point in the proper position on the answer line.

Examples

$$\frac{3}{5} = 5\overline{)3.0}^{\,0.6}$$

$$\frac{1}{4} = 4\overline{)1.00}^{\,0.25}$$

Multiplying Decimals

To multiply decimals, first, find the product as usual. Second, count the number of decimal places in both the **multiplicand** and the **multiplier**. Third, mark off the total number of decimal places in the product, and insert a decimal point.

Example

Multiply 2.05 × 0.3.
Step 1

> 2.05 **(multiplicand)**
> × 0.2 **(multiplier)**
> 0410 **(product)**

Step 2
Count the number of decimal places in the multiplicand and the multiplier

> 2.0<u>5</u>
> × 0.<u>2</u> = Total of three decimal places

Step 3
Mark off three decimal places in product.

> New decimal = 0.410

Example

Multiply 13 × 0.34.
Step 1

> 13 **(multiplicand)**
> × 0.34 **(multiplier)**
> 0442 **(product)**

Step 2

Count the number of decimal places in the multiplicand and the multiplier; 13 may also be written as 13.0. However, when there is only a zero after the decimal, the decimal point does not count as a place to move in the final product. Therefore, there are only two decimal places in the multiplier that are accounted for in the final answer: 4.42.

Dividing Decimals

To divide a decimal by a whole number, first, write the problem as usual. Second, place a decimal point in the quotient line directly above the decimal in the dividend and then find the quotient. Division is written using several symbols, such as $1 \div 2$ or $\frac{1}{2}$. The **divisor** (the number performing the division) is on the right of the first symbol, the left of the second symbol, and the bottom of the third symbol. The answer to a division problem is called the **quotient**. The divisor must be a whole number (a number with no decimal point), and the decimal point must be correctly placed in the answer. When a decimal number is being divided by a whole number, the decimal point is placed directly above the decimal point in the dividend (number being divided). When a number is being divided by a decimal number, the decimal point in the divisor must be moved to the right as many places as needed to make the divisor a whole number. The decimal point in the dividend must be moved the same number of places to the right. The decimal point in the quotient is placed directly above the new position of the decimal point in the dividend.

Example

$$3.25 \div 0.5 = \frac{3.25}{0.5} = \frac{dividend}{divisor}$$

To divide decimal numbers, convert the divisor to a whole number. Move the decimal point in the dividend the same number of places to the right:

$$3\overline{2.5} = 5$$

Place the decimal point in the quotient directly above its new position in the dividend:

5 divided into 32.5

Perform the calculation:

5 divided into 32.5 = 6.5

Adding Decimals

To add decimals, write the decimals in a column, placing the decimal points directly under each other. Then, add as in the addition of whole numbers, and place the decimal point in the sum directly under the decimal points in the addends.

Example

$$\begin{array}{r} 0.8 \\ + 0.9 \\ \hline 1.7 \end{array}$$

0.8 + 0.9

Example

$$\begin{array}{r} 0.90 \\ 0.03 \\ + 2.00 \\ \hline 2.93 \end{array}$$

0.9 + 0.03 + 2

Subtracting Decimals

To subtract decimals, write the decimals in columns, keeping the decimal points under each other. Then, subtract as with whole numbers (zeros may be added after the decimal without changing the value), and place the decimal point in the remainder, directly under the decimal point in the subtrahend and minuend. In addition, if a certain number is shorter, it may be easier to add zeros to the digits on the right side of the decimal to make all numbers equally long.

Example

$$\begin{array}{r} 0.800 \\ -0.423 \\ \hline 0.377 \end{array}$$

0.80 − 0.423

Example

$$\begin{array}{r} 0.700 \\ -0.239 \\ \hline 0.461 \end{array}$$

0.7 − 0.239

Rounding Decimals

To round a decimal, it is necessary to obtain an answer one decimal place after the desired place. Therefore, if the last digit is less than 5, the answer remains the same. However, if the last digit is 5 or greater, the prior digit must increase by one number. Finally, the last digit that indicates rounding up or remaining the same must be dropped.

Examples

Round 4.6 to the nearest whole number. Consider the tenths column. Because 6 is greater than 5, the answer is 5 and 0.6 is discarded.

Round 3.57 to the nearest tenth. Because the hundredths column includes 7 and this number is greater than 5, the answer is 3.6, and the 7 is dropped.

Round 2.896 to the nearest hundredth. Because the last digit is 6, and this number is greater than 5, the answer is 2.90, and the 6 is dropped.

RATIOS

A **ratio** is a mathematical expression that compares two numbers by division. It is used to indicate the relationship of one part of a quantity to the whole. When written, the two quantities are separated by a colon (:). The use of the colon is a traditional way to write the division sign within a ratio, which is expressed as "3 is to 7."

Example

$^3/_7$ may be expressed as a ratio: 3:7

Example

1:150 may be expressed as a fraction: $^1/_{150}$

Proportions

A **proportion** shows the relationship between two equal ratios. A proportion may be expressed as

$$4:8 :: 1:2$$

or

$$4:8 = 1:2$$

where, in the first case, (::) is read as "so as." Thus, 4 is to 8 so as 1 is to 2. These ratios are equal because multiplying 1 and 2 by 4 will result in 4 and 8, respectively. In a proportion, the terms have names. The **extremes** are the two outside terms, and the **means** are the two inside terms. This relationship is shown in Figure 16-9. In a proportion, the product of means is equal to the product of extremes.

To convert a proportion into fractions, use the techniques of cross multiplying or dividing.

Example

$$1:4 :: 3:12$$

Convert to fractions: $^1/_4$ and $^3/_{12}$.
Cross multiply first the numerator of the fraction on the left by the denominator of the fraction on the right:

$$1 \times 12$$

and then the denominator of the fraction on the left by the numerator of the fraction on the right:

$$4 \times 3$$

In this formula, the answer is

$\dfrac{12}{12}$, which reduces to 1.

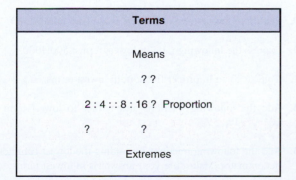

Figure 16-9. The means and the extremes.

It is evident that the term $^4/_2 :: ^{16}/_8$ is a proportion because 4 multiplied by 8 is 32 and 2 multiplied by 16 is also 32. Most of the time we know only three terms of a proportion. The term we do not know is the *unknown*, and in this book, it is labeled *X*. To solve for unknown proportion terms, first multiply the extremes and then multiply the means. Set their products equal. Then, divide both sides of the equation by the number to the left of *X*.

Example

$$2:4 = X:10$$
$$4X = 2 \times 10$$
$$4X = 20$$
$$X = \frac{20}{4} = 5$$

Example

$$\frac{1}{2}:X = 1:8$$
$$1X = (8 \times \frac{1}{2})$$
$$1X = 4$$
$$X = \frac{4}{1} = 4$$

Percentages

The term **percent** and its symbol % mean hundredths. A percent is a fraction whose numerator is expressed and whose denominator is understood to be 100. It can be changed to a decimal by moving the decimal point two places to the left to signify hundredths or to a fraction by expressing the denominator as 100.

Example

$$7\% \text{ means } \frac{7}{100} \text{ or } 0.07$$

Example

$$\frac{1}{5}\% \text{ means } \frac{^1/_5}{100} \text{ or } 0.002$$
$$\frac{1}{5} \times \frac{1}{100} = \frac{1}{500} = 0.002$$

When the percentage is unknown, you can use the formula of *X*.

Example

What percent of 10 ounces is 3 ounces? You are looking for a percentage in this case:

$$3 = X \times 10$$
$$3 = 10X \text{ or } 10X = 3$$
$$10X \text{ divided by } 10 = 3 \text{ divided by } 10$$
$$X = \frac{3}{10} \text{ or } X = 30\%$$

CRITICAL THINKING

1. When a numerator is equal to the denominator, this fraction is known as _____.
2. When the technician is dealing with decimal fractions, what should he do?

REVIEW QUESTIONS

1. Which of the following defines how to multiply fractions?
   A. Find the least common denominator and then add.
   B. Multiply numerators by numerators and denominators by denominators.
   C. Multiply numerators by denominators and denominators by numerators.
   D. Don't worry about how; just use a calculator.

2. Rate per hundred means
   A. variation.
   B. decimal.
   C. density.
   D. percentage.

3. Which of the following Arabic numerals is expressed by the letter "C" in the Roman system?
   A. 100
   B. 1000
   C. 10
   D. 5

4. When dividing two fractions, it is necessary to
   A. divide the numerators first and then divide the denominators.
   B. invert the divisor and then multiply.
   C. divide the denominators and then divide the numerators.
   D. none of the above.

5. To add or subtract two fractions, one must
   A. add/subtract the numerator and denominator.
   B. keep the numerator the same and add/subtract the denominators.
   C. invert one fraction and then add/subtract.
   D. find a common denominator first.

6. The Roman numeral that stands for 29 is which of the following?
   A. XXIX
   B. IIIX
   C. XXVIII
   D. IXXX

7. The mixed fraction for $6\frac{2}{3}$ is which of the following?
   A. $\frac{11}{3}$
   B. $\frac{20}{6}$
   C. $\frac{20}{3}$
   D. $\frac{55}{3}$

8. If you were to multiply the fractions $\frac{6}{7}$ and $\frac{3}{5}$, which of the following would be the answer?
   A. $\frac{30}{21}$ (or $1\frac{3}{7}$)
   B. $\frac{18}{35}$
   C. $\frac{42}{15}$ (or $2\frac{4}{5}$)
   D. $\frac{21}{30}$

9. If you divided $\frac{1}{4}$ by $\frac{2}{16}$, what would the answer be?
   A. 2
   B. 4
   C. $\frac{2}{64}$ (or $\frac{1}{32}$)
   D. $3\frac{1}{4}$

10. $12 = X:8$. What does X stand for?
    A. 96
    B. 3.00
    C. 2.65
    D. 3.33

11. Find the sum of these whole numbers: $910 + 3 + 125$.

12. Subtract 2,289 from 4,547. What is the answer?

13. Multiply $9,004 \times 73$. What is the answer?

14. Divide 74,943 by 271. Round the answer to the nearest tenth.

15. Round 2,987 to the nearest 1,000.

16. Find the average of the following numbers: 90, 80, 60, 15, and 40.

17. Find the equivalent fraction: $\frac{1}{3} = \frac{8}{?}$

18. Reduce to lowest terms: $\frac{5}{255}$.

19. Reduce to lowest terms but keep as a mixed number: $4\frac{22}{30}$.

20. Express the following ratio in lowest terms: 500:4000.

21. Convert to an improper fraction, in lowest terms: $\frac{23}{18}$.

22. Add the following fractions and reduce to lowest terms: $101\frac{3}{4}$, $33\frac{1}{2}$, $5\frac{1}{4}$.

23. Add the following fractions by finding the lowest common denominator. Make sure your answer is in lowest terms: $\frac{1}{6}$ and $\frac{4}{18}$.

Continues

24. Add the following mixed fractions and reduce to lowest terms: $4\frac{3}{4}$, $1\frac{1}{16}$, $3\frac{2}{32}$.

25. Add the following and reduce to lowest terms: $\frac{1}{9} + \frac{7}{8}$.

26. Subtract the following and reduce to lowest terms: $101\frac{3}{51}$ minus $55\frac{4}{17}$.

27. Place the following fractions in order from largest to smallest: $\frac{7}{8}$, $\frac{2}{16}$, $\frac{3}{4}$, $\frac{1}{2}$.

28. Subtract the following and reduce to lowest terms: $500\frac{4}{5}$ minus $150\frac{2}{9}$.

29. Multiply the following and reduce to lowest terms: $\frac{4}{5} \times \frac{1}{20}$.

30. Multiply the following and reduce to lowest terms: $\frac{11}{50} \times 20$.

31. Multiply the following and reduce to lowest terms: $\frac{9}{10} \times \frac{1}{3} \times \frac{8}{13}$.

32. Change this mixed number into an improper fraction: $10\frac{1}{3}$.

33. Multiply and reduce to lowest terms: $1\frac{1}{2} \times 2\frac{1}{3}$.

34. Divide the following and reduce to lowest terms: $1\frac{9}{12}$ divided by $\frac{1}{12}$.

35. Round to the nearest hundredth: 4.719.

36. Arrange the following decimal numbers from largest to smallest: 0.04, 0.0040, 0.4, 0.044.

37. Add the following numbers: $35.01 + 76.02 + 0.0998$.

38. Subtract the following numbers: 0.07×0.007.

39. Multiply the following numbers: 94.13×32.09.

40. Divide 2603.72 by 34.

41. Divide 12.24 by 4.

42. Multiply and round to the nearest whole number: $23.850 \times 1{,}000$.

43. Divide and round to the nearest thousandth: 10.275×100.

44. Convert 100.46 to a fraction, and reduce to lowest terms.

45. Convert $\frac{3}{18}$ into a decimal, and round to the nearest hundredth.

46. In the following ratio, find the value of X: $1:X = 5:200$

47. Solve for X in the following ratio: $20:40 = X:15$

48. Solve for X in the following ratio: 1 tablet:0.1 mg = X tablets:0.15 mg.

49. $30:120 = ?:12$.

50. $X:625 = 1:5$.

51. $128:1 = X:5$.

52. Convert $44\frac{1}{2}\%$ to a decimal.

53. Convert 0.076 to a percent.

54. 15 is what percent of 300?

55. $87\frac{1}{2}\%$ of 120 is what number?

56. A surgical instrument is listed at $189.90 but sold for a discounted price, which is 40% less. What is the amount in dollars of the discount? What is the discounted sale price?

57. 8 is what percent of 40?

58. What percent is 4 tablets of a prescription written for 36 tablets? Round to the nearest tenth of a percent.

59. Express 8:125 as a percent.

60. 33 is what percent of 44?

61. Convert $\frac{4}{6}$ into a percent. Round to the nearest tenth of a percent.

17

Measurement Systems

OBJECTIVES

Upon completion of this chapter, the reader should be able to

1. Explain the rules of the metric system and the basic units of weight, volume, and length.
2. Describe common equivalents in the metric system.
3. Discuss the apothecary system.
4. Explain the household system.
5. Convert metric measures to their equivalents in metric.
6. Name the metric equivalents that are used in the medical profession.
7. Define common prefixes used in the metric system.

GLOSSARY

apothecary system An old English system of measurement.

avoirdupois An old English system of weights.

dram A unit of weight in the apothecary system; 1 dram equals 60 grains.

grain The basic unit of weight in the apothecary system.

gram The basic unit for weight in the metric system.

household system System of measurement used in most homes; this is not an accurate system of measurement for medications.

international units A standardized amount of medication required to produce a certain effect.

liter The basic unit for volume in the metric system.

meter The basic unit for length in the metric system.

metric system Worldwide standard system of measurement.

milliequivalent A unit of measure based upon the chemical combining power of a substance.

milliunit One thousandth of a unit.

minim The basic unit of volume in the apothecary system.

ounce A unit of weight in the apothecary system; 1 ounce equals 8 drams.

unit The amount of medication required to produce a certain effect.

OVERVIEW

Administration of the medications prescribed for the patient must be accurate and the amounts must be correct. Pharmacy technicians must have a comprehensive knowledge of the weights and measures used in drug administration for prescribed amounts. Three systems are used for measuring medication and solutions: **metric system**, **apothecary system**, and **household system**. It is necessary for the pharmacy technician to know each system and be able to convert from one system to another. Most medications and measurements used in the health care field are calibrated and calculated by the metric system. Thus, knowledge of the metric system is very important, because dosage units are calculated in metric measurements. Although some medications are still prescribed in apothecary and household terms, health care workers will find that the majority of medication calculation and administration skills involve accurate use of the metric system. Measurement of weight, volume, and length of the prescription and administration of drugs is done with three parameters in mind. Weight is the most utilized parameter. It is essential as a dosage unit. The metric weight units, such as milligrams and grams, are the most accurate. Measurement of volume is the next most important parameter. Volume is the parameter used for liquids. Volume also includes two additional parameters for dosage calculations: quantity and concentration. The most commonly used metric volume unit for dosage calculations is the milliliter. Today, household and apothecary measures such as teaspoons and ounces are used less commonly. Length is the least utilized parameter for dosage calculations.

THE METRIC SYSTEM

The metric system of measure was introduced in 1799 in France. Its use in the United States was legalized in 1866. By an Act of Congress in 1893, it became our legal standard of measure, and all other systems refer to it for official comparison. It is now the standard for scientific and industrial use and measurements and is used in approximately 90% of the world's developed countries. Today, the metric system is the system of choice when one deals with the weights and measures involved in the calculation of drug dosages. Its accuracy and simplicity are related to its basis on the decimal system, which is based on units of 10. The use of decimals can eliminate errors in measuring medications. The three basic units of the metric system are the following:

1. **Gram**: the basic unit for weight
2. **Liter**: the basic unit for volume
3. **Meter**: the basic unit for length

TABLE 17-1. Metric Prefixes

METRIC PREFIX		VALUE
micro	=	One millionth of a unit (0.000001) or $1/_{1,000,000}$ of the base unit
milli	=	One thousandth of a unit (0.001) or $1/_{1,000}$ of the base unit
centi	=	One hundredth of a unit (0.01) or $1/_{100}$ of the base unit
ceci	=	One tenth of a unit (0.1) or $1/_{10}$ of the base unit
deka	=	Ten units (10)
hecto	=	One hundred units (100)
kilo	=	One thousand units (1,000)

TABLE 17-2. International Metric System Abbreviations

WEIGHT	VOLUME	LENGTH
gram (basic unit), g	liter (basic unit), L	meter (basic unit), m
milligram, mg	milliliter, mL	centimeter, cm
microgram, mcg	cubic centimeter, cc	millimeter, mm
kilogram, kg	deciliter, dL	kilometer, km

Parts of these basic units are named by adding a prefix. Each prefix has a numerical value, which is shown in Table 17-1. It is essential for individuals who deal with measurement, calculation, and administration of drugs to be familiar with prefixes that are commonly used in the metric system.

It is also important that pharmacy technicians be familiar with common metric abbreviations, which are shown in Table 17-2.

A system for international standardization of metric units was established throughout the world in 1960 with the introduction of the International System, or SI (from the French Système International). Table 17-3 shows SI standardized abbreviations.

Gram

The gram is the basic unit of weight in the metric system. A gram equals approximately the weight of 1 cubic centimeter (cc) or 1 milliliter (mL) of water. One gram is equal to approximately 15 grains (gr) or 0.035 ounce (oz). Some medications are ordered as fractions of grams. A milligram (mg) is 1000 times smaller than a gram; medications may be ordered in milligrams. The kilogram is a very large unit that is not used for measuring medications. A kilogram is 1000 times larger than a gram. It is used to determine a patient's weight. Table 17-4 shows values equivalent to a gram.

TABLE 17-3. The International System of Standardized Abbreviations

METRIC SYSTEM	UNIT	ABBREVIATION	EQUIVALENTS
Weight	**gram** (basic unit)	g	1 g = 1000 mg
	milligram	mg	1 mg = 1000 mcg = 0.001 g
	microgram	mcg	1 mcg = 0.001 mg = 0.000001 g
	kilogram	kg	1 kg = 1000 g
Volume	**liter** (basic unit)	L or l	1 L = 1000 mL
	milliliter	mL or ml	1 ml = 1 cc = 0.001 L
	cubic centimeter	cc	1 cc = 1 mL = 0.001 L
Length	**meter** (basic unit)	m	1 m = 100 cm = 1000 mm
	centimeter	cm	1 cm = 0.01 m = 10 mm
	millimeter	mm	1 mm = 0.001 m = 0.1 cm

TABLE 17-4. Value of the Gram

GRAM	EQUIVALENTS
1 g	1,000,000 mcg
	1,000 mg
	100 cg
	$\frac{1}{1,000}$ kg

TABLE 17-5. Approximate Equivalent Measures for Weight

METRIC	APOTHECARY
60 mg	1 gr
30 mg	$\frac{1}{2}$ gr
15 mg	$\frac{1}{4}$ gr
1 mg	$\frac{1}{60}$ gr
1 g (1000 mg)	15 gr
0.5 g	$8\frac{1}{3}$ gr
1 kg	2.2 lb

Example

How many milligrams are there in 0.65 g?

Solution:

Multiply 0.65 g by 1000 to determine that there are 650 mg in 0.65 g. The rule for converting between decimals and percents can be expanded to include multiplying and dividing by 10, 100, or 1000 by moving the decimal point to the left or right for the same number of places as there are zeros. Multiplication by 1000 can be accomplished by simply moving the decimal point three places to the right, so 0.65 g equals 650 mg.

Conversion of weight in the metric system to the apothecary system was explained earlier, when we learned that 1 gr is equivalent to either 60 or 65 mg.

$$1 \text{ gr} = 60 \text{ mg or } 1 \text{ gr} = 65 \text{ mg}$$

The relationship between grains and milligrams or grams is more complex (see Table 17-5).

Example

How many kg does a 62-lb child weigh?

1st fraction: 62 lb/X kg

Remember that 1 kg = 2.2 lb

2nd fraction: 2.2 lb/1 kg

Write the proportion:

$$\frac{62 \text{ lb}}{X \text{ kg}} = \frac{2.2 \text{ lb}}{1 \text{ kg}}$$

Cross-multiply to solve:

$$62 \times 1 = 2.2X$$

$$62 = 2.2X$$

$$X = \frac{6.2}{2.2} = 28.18$$

Liter

The liter is the basic unit of volume used to measure liquids in the metric system. It is equal to 1000 cubic centimeters of water. One cubic centimeter is considered equivalent to 1 milliliter (mL); thus, 1 liter (L) = 1000 mL or cc. The cubic centimeter is the amount of space that 1 mL of liquid occupies. One liter is equal to 1.056 quarts, which is 0.26 of a gallon or 2.1 pints. Table 17-6 summarizes metric volumes.

Example

How many liters are there in 350 mL?

Solution

Divide 350 mL by 1000. The division by 1000 can be accomplished by simply moving the decimal point three places to the left so 0.35 L equals 350 mL.

TABLE 17-6. Metric Volumes	
VOLUME	**LITER**
1 kiloliter (kL)	1000.000 L
1 hectoliter (hL)	100.000 L
1 dekaliter (daL)	10.000 L
1 liter (L)	1.000 L
1 deciliter (dL)	0.100 L
1 centiliter (cL)	0.010 L
1 milliliter (mL)	0.001 L

TABLE 17-7. Approximate Equivalent Measures of Volume		
METRIC	**HOUSEHOLD**	**APOTHECARY**
1 mL	15 drops (gtt)	—
4 mL	1 tsp	1 dr
15 mL	1 tbsp	3 or 4 dr
30 mL	2 tbsp	1 oz
240 mL	1 cup	8 oz
480 mL	2 cups = 1 pt	16 oz
960 mL	2 pt = 1 qt	32 oz

Meter

The meter is used for linear (length) measurement. Linear measurements (e.g., meter and centimeter) are commonly used to measure the height of an individual and to determine growth patterns and are not used in the calculation of doses. Therefore, only the units of weight and volume are discussed in this chapter.

HOUSEHOLD MEASUREMENTS

Household measurements are not accurate enough for health care professionals to use in the calculation of drug dosages in the hospital or pharmacy. However, the household system is still in use for doses given primarily at home, as indicated by the name. It is perfectly safe to use for measurements in cooking but should be avoided for administration of medications. The household system is the least accurate of the three systems of measure. Capacities of utensils such as teaspoons, tablespoons, and cups vary from one house to another. The basic units of volume in the household system, in increasing size, are the drop, teaspoon, tablespoon, ounce, cup, pint, quart, and gallon. Of these, the four smallest measures are most commonly used for medications.

When one discusses medications specifically, the word *ounce* generally implies volume, which is represented as *fluid ounces*. In other contexts, ounce may represent a unit of weight, as does the term *pound*. Sixty drops are equivalent to a teaspoon. There are 3 teaspoons (tsp) in 1 tablespoon (tbsp). There are 2 tbsp to 1 oz; 6 oz are equal to an average teacup, and 8 oz are equal to an average cup or glass. Because spoons, cups, and glasses come in all sizes and shapes one can understand why this system is not completely accurate. Table 17-7 shows a list of approximate equivalents among the metric, household, and apothecary measurement systems.

APOTHECARY SYSTEM

The apothecary system is also called the wine measure or U.S. liquid measure system. This system is a very old English system. It has slowly been replaced by the metric system. A few units of measure in this system are used for medication

administration. In the following paragraphs, some basic units for weight and volume in the apothecary system are discussed.

Weight

The basic unit for weight is the **grain**. The abbreviation for grain is gr. **Dram** is also a unit of weight; 1 dr is equal to 60 gr. The dram is usually abbreviated as dr. An **ounce** is larger than a dram; 1 oz is equal to 8 dr. The ounce is usually abbreviated as oz.

Example

How many grains are there in 5 dr?

Solution:

Remember that 1 dr is equal to 60 gr, so multiply the 5 dr by 60. Therefore, 300 gr equals 5 dr.

Example

How many fluid ounces are in 48 fluid drams?

Solution

You know that 1 fluid ounce is equal to 8 fluid drams. Divide 48 fluid drams by 8. The answer is that 48 fluid drams equals 6 fluid ounces.

Volume

The basic unit for volume is the **minim**. The abbreviation for minim is a lower-case letter "m." A minim is extremely small, perhaps the size of 1 drop. Volume can also be measured by drams and ounces. In summary, the units of the apothecary system are as follows:

Weight: grain (gr)
Volume: minim (m)
                     dram (dr)
                     ounce (oz)

AVOIRDUPOIS WEIGHT

Avoirdupois is the English system of weights in which there are 7000 gr, 256 dr, or 16 oz to 1 lb, which equals 453.59 g.

UNITS OF MEASURE USED FOR MEDICATIONS

The quantity of medicine prescribed may also be expressed as four other measurements: international units, units, milliunits, and milliequivalents. Arabic numbers with the appropriate sign are used to indicate an amount. For instance, vitamins and chemicals are measured in international units to establish potency of such items. Likewise, the amount of medication to produce a standardized desired effect is expressed in units. However, some medications, such as penicillin, heparin, and insulin, are assigned a specific numeral amount in conjunction with the kind of unit to indicate a separate meaning.

International Units

A **unit** is the amount of medication required to produce a certain effect. The size of a unit varies for each drug. Some medications, such as vitamins, are measured in standardized units called **international units** (IU). These units represent the amount of medication needed to produce a certain effect, but they are standardized by international agreement. As with milliequivalents, you do not need to convert from units to other measures. Medications that are ordered in units will also be labeled in units. Insulin, heparin, and penicillin are measured in USP units.

Milliunits

A **milliunit** (mU) represents one thousandth (1/1000) of a unit (U), thus, 1 U is equal to 1000 mU. The drug oxytocin (Pitocin®) is measured in milliunits.

Milliequivalents

Some drugs are measured in **milliequivalents** (mEq), which is a unit of measure based on the chemical combining power of a substance. One thousandth (1/1000) of the same amount of a chemical is known as a milliequivalent. The concentrations of serum electrolytes, such as calcium, potassium, sodium, and magnesium, are measured in milliequivalents. Because of the electrical activity of ions, it is impossible to use weight units (e.g., milligrams or grams) to measure quantities of electrolytes. An equivalent (Eq) represents 1000 mEq and is the weight of a substance that combines with or replaces 1 g (atomic weight of hydrogen). Sodium bicarbonate and potassium chloride are examples of drugs that are measured in milliequivalents. You do not need to learn to convert from milliequivalents to another system of measurement.

Example

Heparin 7500 U is ordered, and heparin 10,000 U/mL is the stock drug.

Example

Potassium chloride 10 mEq is ordered, and potassium chloride 20 mEq/15 mL is the stock drug.

Example

Oxytocin (Pitocin®) 2 mU (0.002 U) intravenous per minute is ordered and Pitocin 10 U/mL to be added to a 1000 mL intravenous solution is available.

Note that the international unit, unit, and milliequivalent are measures that require no conversion because the drugs ordered using these units are prepared and given in the same system.

CONVERTING WITHIN AND BETWEEN SYSTEMS

When the pharmacy technician calculates dosages, he or she must often convert between the metric, apothecary, and household systems of measurement. Therefore, the technician will need to know how the measure of a quantity in one system compares to its measure in another system. For example, the relationships between milliliters and liters and between teaspoons and tablespoons were discussed. In pharmacy and medicine, use of the metric system currently predominates over that of the other commonly used systems. Most prescriptions and medication orders are written in the metric system, and labeling on most prefabricated pharmaceutical products has drug strengths and dosages described in metric units, replacing to a great extent the use of other common systems of measurement. Medications are usually ordered in a unit of weight measurement such as grams or grains. Pharmacy technicians must be able to convert and calculate the correct dosage of drugs. The technician can convert between units of measurement within the same system or convert units of measurement from one system to another. He or she must also interpret the order and administer the correct number of tablets, capsules, tablespoons, milligrams, or milliliters.

Conversion of Weights

Remember that 1000 mg = 1 g and 1000 micrograms (mcg) = 1 mg. To convert grams to milligrams, you should always multiply by 1000 or move the decimal point three places to the right.

Example

$$2 \text{ g} = 2000. \text{ mg}$$
$$0.2 \text{ g} = 200. \text{ mg}$$
$$0.02 \text{ g} = 020. \text{ mg}$$

To convert milligrams to grams, divide by 1000 or move the decimal point three places to the left.

Example

$$250 \text{ mg} = 0.250 \text{ g}$$
$$50 \text{ mg} = 0.050 \text{ g}$$
$$5 \text{ mg} = 0.005 \text{ g}$$

To convert milligrams to micrograms, multiply by 1000 or move the decimal point three places to the right.

Example

$$3 \text{ mg} = 3000. \text{ mcg}$$
$$0.5 \text{ mg} = 500. \text{ mcg}$$
$$0.08 \text{ mg} = 080. \text{ mcg}$$

To convert micrograms to milligrams, divide by 1000 or move the decimal point three places to the left.

Example

$$1500 \text{ mcg} = 1.500 \text{ mg}$$
$$600 \text{ mcg} = 0.600 \text{ mg}$$
$$20 \text{ mcg} = 0.020 \text{ mg}$$

The microgram, milligram, and gram are the most commonly used measurements for medication administration. Tablets and capsules are most often supplied in milligrams. Antibiotics can be provided in grams, milligrams, or units. For small dosages or for very powerful drugs in pediatric and critical care patients, micrograms are used.

Conversion of Liquids

To convert and calculate the correct dosage of liquid medications, remember the units of the metric system for volume.

Example

Convert 0.02 L to mL.

Equivalent: 1 L = 1000 mL.

Conversion factor is 1000.

Multiply by 1000:

$$0.02 \text{ L} = 0.02 \times 1000 = 20 \text{ mL}$$

or move the decimal point 3 places to the right:

$$0.02 \text{ L} = 0.020. = 20 \text{ mL}$$

To convert milliliters to liters, one must divide. Remember that the equivalent of 1 L = 1000 mL and then divide the number of milliliters by 1000.

Example

Convert 3000 mL to L.

Equivalent: 1 L = 1000 mL.

Conversion factor is 1000.

Divide by 1000:

$$3000 \text{ mL} = 3000 \div 1000 = 3 \text{ L}$$

Or move the decimal point 3 places to the left:

$$3000 \text{ mL} = 3.000 = 3 \text{ L}$$

Conversion of Length

Remember that 2.54 cm = 1 inch and 25.4 mm = 1 inch. To convert centimeters to inches, or millimeters to inches, see the following examples.

Example

Convert 75.4 cm to inches.

$$\frac{75.4 \text{ cm}}{2.54} = 29.685 \text{ inches}$$

Convert 80 mm to inches.

$$\frac{80 \text{ mm}}{25.44} = 3.145 \text{ inches}$$

■ CRITICAL THINKING

An infant suffering from otitis media is given 5 mL of an antibiotic every 8 hours for 10 days. Her mother is using a household measuring device to measure the dose of antibiotic.
1. Which household device should the mother use?
2. How much antibiotic should the infant take considering the device that the physician recommends?

REVIEW QUESTIONS

1. A gram is a metric unit that measures _____.

2. How many mL equal a liter? _____.

3. 1 g is equal to _____ mcg.

4. 1 mL is equal to _____ cc.

5. A liter is a metric unit that measures _____.

6. 1 kg = _____ g.

7. 10 cm = _____ mm.

8. A meter is a metric unit that measures _____.

9. 10 kg = _____ g.

10. 1 mm = _____ m.

11. 2 cc = _____ L.

12. 3 g = _____ mg.

13. 11 mg = _____ mcg.

14. 5 L = _____ mL.

Continues

15. 9 g = _____ kg.

16. 760 mcg = _____ mg.

17. 2500 mL = _____ L.

18. 8.5 g = _____ mg.

19. 36 kg = _____ g.

20. 3.5 L = _____ mL.

21. If 1 medium size glass = 8 oz, how many ounces do 2.5 medium size glasses equal?

22. 4 tbsp = _____ tsp.

23. 6 oz = _____ tbsp.

24. 3 tsp = _____ drops.

25. 220 drops = _____ tsp.

26. 7 tsp = _____ tbsp.

27. 5 tbsp = _____ oz.

28. 4 oz = _____ tbsp.

29. 5 tbsp = _____ tsp.

30. 2½ cups = _____ oz.

31. 1½ tsp = _____ drops.

32. 10 tsp = _____ tbsp.

33. 7 tbsp = _____ oz.

34. 100 drops = _____ tsp.

35. 22 oz = _____ cups.

36. 34 oz = _____ medium size glasses.

37. 22 tsp = _____ tbsp.

38. 6 glasses = _____ oz.

39. 4 tbsp = _____ tsp.

40. 3 cups = _____ oz.

41. 3 dr = _____ gr.

42. 4 pt = _____ fluid oz.

43. 5 fluid oz = _____ fluid dr.

44. 40 gr = _____ d.

45. 90 fluid oz = _____ pt.

46. 3 fluid dr = _____ fluid oz.

47. 4 qt = _____ pt.

48. 3 pt = _____ fluid oz.

49. 340 gr = _____ dr.

50. 4 fluid dr = _____ fluid oz.

51. gr viiss = _____.

52. 1 fluid oz = _____ dr.

53. 3.5 gr = _____ g.

54. 4.5 fl oz = _____ pt.

55. 12 fl dr = _____ fl oz.

56. 15 gr = _____ dr.

57. 20 pt = _____ fl oz.

58. 5.5 pt = _____ qt.

59. 12 qt = _____ pt.

60. 16 oz = _____ pt.

61. 1 cc = _____ mL.

62. _____ mg = 26 mcg.

63. 19.5 kg = _____ g.

64. _____ g = 0.3 kg.

65. 0.07 mg = _____ mcg.

66. 14 cm = _____ m.

67. _____ L = 250 cc.

68. _____ mg = 0.6 g.

69. _____ mg = 36 g.

70. 7500 mL = _____ L.

71. 12.5 mg = _____ mcg.

72. 24 dm = _____ cm.

Continues

73. 12.76 kg = _____ g.

74. 23.5 cm = _____ mm.

75. 800 cm = _____ m.

76. 1000 mL = _____ L.

77. 12,500 cm = _____ m.

78. 0.125 g = _____ mg.

79. 45,250 mg = _____ g.

80. 1000 mcg = _____ g.

81. 5524 g = _____ kg.

82. 1.25 m = _____ cm.

83. 0.09 L = _____ mL.

84. 0.1 g = _____ mg.

85. 8500 mcg = _____ mg.

86. 0.75 g = _____ mg.

87. _____ kg = 54.6 g.

88. 0.014 g = _____ mcg.

89. 10 mcg = _____ g.

90. _____ mg = 0.015 g.

91. 0.008 mcg = _____ mg.

92. 25 cm = _____ m.

93. _____ cc = 65 L.

94. 30 mg = gr _____.

95. 75 mg = gr _____.

96. gr $\frac{1}{6}$ = _____ mg.

97. 15 g = gr _____.

98. gr _____ = 0.30 mg.

99. gr iiiss = _____ mg.

100. gr xv = _____ mg = _____ g.

101. 0.015 g = gr _____ = _____ mg.

102. _____ mg = _____ mcg = gr 1/4.

103. gr iss = _____ mg = _____ g.

104. gr viiiss = _____ mg = _____ g.

105. 1 tbsp = _____ mL.

106. 20 mL = _____ tsp.

107. $2\frac{3}{5}$ qt = _____ mL.

108. 1 tsp = _____ cc.

109. 15 tsp = _____ mL.

110. 60 mL = _____ tbsp.

111. gr $\frac{1}{2}$ = _____ mg.

112. $12\frac{1}{2}$ tsp = _____ cc.

113. $2\frac{1}{3}$ qt = _____ mL.

114. 35 cc = _____ tsp.

115. gr viii = _____ mg.

116. 0.3 mg = gr _____.

117. gr v = _____ mg.

118. gr $\frac{1}{150}$ = _____ mg.

119. gr viii = _____ mg.

120. 14 m = _____ cm.

121. 5 tsp = _____ cc.

122. 600 mg = gr _____.

123. 5 tbsp = _____ mL.

124. 20 cc = _____ tsp.

125. gr xv = _____ mg.

126. $4\frac{2}{3}$ qt = _____ mL.

127. 0.1 mg = gr _____.

128. 4.5 L = _____ qt.

129. $1\frac{1}{3}$ cups = _____ mL.

130. 120 mL = _____ tsp.

Continues

131. $3\frac{2}{3}$ cups = _____ mL.

132. The order is for 30 mg. On hand are 10 mg tablets. You give _____.

133. The order is for 1500 mg. On hand are 500 mg tablets. You give _____.

134. The order is for 10 mg. On hand are vials containing 20 mg/mL. You give _____.

135. The order is for 1.5 mg. On hand are vials containing 3.0 mg/mL. You give _____.

136. The order is for 0.15 g. On hand are 25 mg tablets. You give _____.

137. The order is for 1 g. On hand are vials containing 50 mg/2 mL. You give _____.

138. The order is for 0.5 g. On hand are 300 mg caplets. You give _____.

139. The order is for 0.06 g. On hand are 15 mg tablets. You give _____.

140. The order is for 1.5 g. On hand are 1000 mg tablets. You give_____.

141. The order is for 1.5 g. On hand are 750 mg tablets. You give _____.

142. The order is for 25 mg PO. On hand are 10 mg tablets. You give _____.

143. The order is for gr iss. On hand are 50 mg caplets. You give _____.

144. The order is for 50 mg PO. On hand are 20 mg tablets. You give _____.

145. The order is for 12.5 mg PO after meals. On hand are 25 mg tablets. You give _____.

146. The order is for 120 mg PO. On hand are tablets with gr ss per tablet. You give _____.

147. 300 mg = gr _____.

148. 0.3 mg = gr _____.

149. The order is for 1.25 mg. On hand are vials containing 0.25 mg/5 mL. You give _____.

150. The order is for 200 mg PO q4h. On hand are vials containing 125 mg/ 5 mL. You give _____.

151. The order is for 50 mg PO. On hand are vials containing 12.5mg in each 5 mL. You give _____.

152. The order is for gr v PO. On hand are 0.15 g tablets. You give _____.

153. The order is for 30 mg of phenobarbital. On hand are 15 mg tablets. You give _____.

154. The pharmacy technician works 8 hours a day for 20 days in a month. How many total hours does she work per month?

155. Round 7872 to the nearest ten.

156. $\frac{5}{9} - \frac{1}{3}$ = _____.

157. 200 divided by $\frac{2}{5}$ = _____.

158. $\frac{1}{200}$ divided by $\frac{1}{4}$ = _____.

159. Round 10.295 to the nearest tenth.

160. 4.6×0.68 = _____.

Calculation of Dosages

OBJECTIVES

Upon completion of this chapter, the reader should be able to

1. Recognize the appropriate equipment used for medication preparation and administration.
2. Determine the amount of drug needed for a specified time.
3. Understand and select a dosage formula, such as a basic formula, ratio and proportion, fraction equation, or dimensional analysis, for solving drug dosage problems.
4. Calculate the number of tablets or capsules that are contained in prescribed dosages.
5. Calculate doses for oral and liquid medications using the formula method.
6. Read and measure doses on a syringe.
7. Read medication labels on parenteral medications.
8. Identify appropriate syringes to administer calculated doses.
9. Convert all units of measurement to the same system and size units.
10. Measure insulin in a matching insulin syringe.

GLOSSARY

conversion factor Used to determine equivalents of specific units of measure.

dosage strength The amount of medication per unit of measure.

drop rate The number of drops an intravenous infusion is administered at over a specific period of time.

drug label factor The form of the drug dose with its equivalent in unit.

form The structure and composition of a drug.

meniscus The dip in fluid level when an oral liquid medication is dispensed.

nomogram A quick reference for calculating pediatric doses.

supply dosage Refers to both the dosage strength and the form of the drug: the number of measured units per tablet of the concentration of a drug.

total volume The quantity contained in a package.

OVERVIEW

One of the most important functions of pharmacy service is to ensure that patients get the intended drug in the correct amount. The correct dosage of a medication may depend on the patient's age, weight, or state of health or on what other drugs the patient may be taking. Often, the pharmacist or technician will receive an order for a medication in a dosage that is different from that of the medications in stock. The difference may be in the system of measurement, the strength, or the form of the drug. There are formulas and mathematical tables of conversion for calculating the correct dosage of medication to be administered. It is helpful to look at how the correct calculation is arrived at, one step at a time. Learning to correctly calculate drug dosages is an extremely important skill, because it can often be the difference between life and death for a patient. Calculating incorrect dosages could lead to undertreatment and result in the patient's condition not improving or worsening. An overdose can cause the patient serious harm.

The ability to calculate drug dosages is a skill that should not be taken lightly. In fact, all health care professionals who deal with the preparation and/or administration of medications should aim for 100% success in performing this task. Recall the Seven Rights of Medication Administration discussed in Chapter 5:

- Right patient
- Right route
- Right drug
- Right technique
- Right dose
- Right documentation
- Right time

The use of calculators is recommended for complex calculations of dosages to ensure accuracy and save time. Basic math skills are needed to use the calculator properly.

READING MEDICATION LABELS

Medication labels give information on the dose contained in the package. For the patient's safety, a pharmacy technician must be able to identify and interpret the information on a medication label. He or she must read the label carefully and understand essential information. The technician must recognize the generic name, trade name, dosage strength, form, supply dosage, total volume, route of administration, directions for mixing, and cautions. It is essential for the technician to cross-check the names of all medications, whether just the generic name or both the trade and generic names are indicated on the label, to accurately identify a drug. The amount of the medication per unit of measure (the amount per tablet, capsule, milligram, or milliliter) is called the **dosage strength**.

Example

The medication may be read as 125 mg/2 mL (125 mg in 2 mL), whereas in tablets or capsules, the amount of medication may be stated as 25 mg/tablet (25 mg in 1 tablet) or 500 mg/capsule (500 mg in 1 capsule).

The form of medication specifies the type of preparation available, such as tablets, capsules, suppositories, liquids, or ointments. Labels may also use abbreviations or words that explain the form of the drug. Examples are LA (long-acting), SR (sustained release), CR (controlled release), DS (double strength), and XL (extra long-acting).

The route of administration describes how the medication is to be administered, for example, oral (PO), intramuscular (IM), intravenously (IV), or topical. The label also indicates the total volume for injection or oral liquids. **Total volume** refers to the quantity contained in a package, bottle, or vial. It is important to recognize the difference between the amount per milliliter and the total volume to avoid any errors.

Example

A bottle may contain 50 capsules; however, the dosage strength is the number of milligrams per capsule. On its label, a syrup shows 240 mL (the total volume), but the dosage strength is 15 mg/mL.

Sometimes medication comes in a powdered form; the directions for how to mix or reconstitute it and with which solution are found on the label. The reconstitution must be performed exactly as the label directs. Medication labels also contain information such as expiration date, which indicates the last date a drug should be used. Other information can be seen on the back or side of a label, such as storage information, lot numbers, the name of the drug manufacturer,

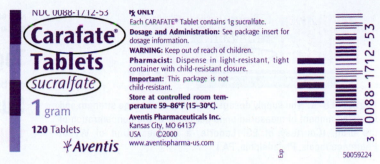

Figure 18-1. The established generic name of a drug appears directly underneath its trade name. (Courtesy of Aventis Pharmaceuticals.)

and a National Drug Code (NDC) number. The labels in Figures 18-1 through 18-9 show generic name, brand name, dosage strength, form, total volume, administration route, directions for mixing, cautions, name of the manufacturer, and control numbers.

Generic Names

The established generic (also called *nonproprietary*) name of a drug appears directly underneath its trade, brand, or proprietary name (see Figure 18-1). Generic names are sometimes printed inside parentheses and must be identified on all drug labels by law. Generic equivalents of many trade-name drugs are regularly ordered by prescribers as substitutes. On these products, only the generic name appears. It is advisable for the pharmacy technician to always carefully cross-check names of all medications to avoid inaccurate dispensing to patients.

Trade Names

Manufacturers' names for their medications are called trade, brand, or proprietary names. These names are usually the most prominently printed names on drug labels and may appear in larger and/or bold type. They are often followed by the ® sign, indicating that both the name of the drug and its formulation are registered.

Dosage Strength

Dosage strength of a drug refers to its dosage *weight*, the amount of the drug provided in a specific unit of measurement (see Figure 18-2). Milligrams are common dosage measurements. Some drugs have two different but equivalent dosage strengths, such as "milligrams per tablet" and "units per tablet." This allows either type of measurement to be used by prescribers.

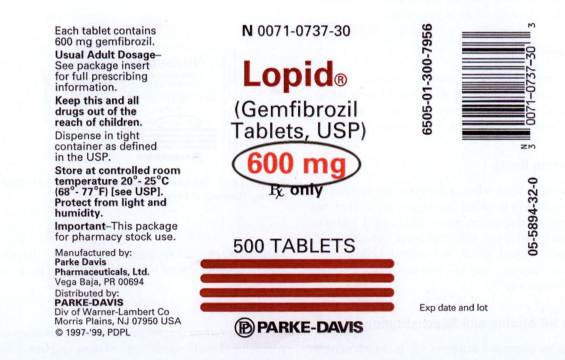

Figure 18-2. Dosage strength refers to the weight of a drug or the amount of drug provided in a specific unit of measurement. (Courtesy of Pfizer Inc.)

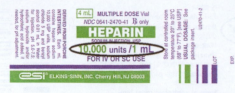

Figure 18-3. The supply dosage refers to both dosage strength and form: the amount of measured units per tablet or the concentration of the drug. (Courtesy of ESI Lederle, a Business Unit of Wyeth Pharmaceuticals, Philadelphia, PA.)

Form

The **form** of a drug identifies its *structure and composition.* Solid dosage forms include tablets and capsules. Powders and granules can be directly combined with food and beverages. Some must be reconstituted (liquefied) and measured precisely, either in milliliters, drops, or ounces. These forms may be clear solutions (crystalloids) or suspensions (in which the liquid contains solid particles that separate from the solution in its container). Medicines to be injected may be available in a solution or in a dry powder form that is then reconstituted. After reconstitution, they are measured in cubic centimeters or milliliters. There are many other different forms of medications, including patches for transdermal administration, creams, and suppositories.

Supply Dosage

Supply dosage is a term that refers to both *dosage strength* and *form.* For solid-form medications, supply dosage is read as "*X* measured units per tablet" (see Figure 18-3). For liquid medications, it is the same as the medication's concentration, such as "*X* measured units per milliliter."

Total Volume

Total volume refers to the *full quantity* contained in a vial, bottle, or package (see Figure 18-4). For solid medications, it is the total number of individual items (e.g., capsules or tablets). For liquids, it is the total fluid volume.

Administration Route

The administration route refers to the site of the body or the *method of drug delivery* intended (see Figure 18-5). There are many different administration routes (also called routes of administration), including oral, sublingual, enteral, injection, otic, optic, topical, rectal, and vaginal. Unless otherwise instructed, capsules, caplets, and tablets are intended for oral administration.

Directions for Mixing and Reconstituting

Certain drugs are dispensed in a *powder form*, which must be reconstituted before use (see Figure 18-6). Often, an initial concentrate of a powdered drug is prepared by mixing it with

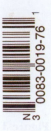

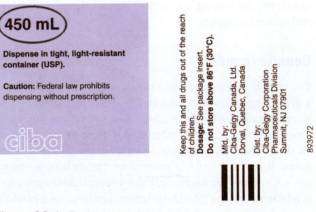

IMPORTANT: Shake well before using.

Each 5 mL contains 100 mg carbamazepine USP.

Figure 18-4. Total volume refers to the full quantity of the drug contained within a particular package. (Courtesy of Novartis Pharmaceuticals Corporation.)

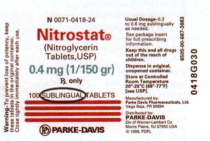

Figure 18-5. The administration route refers to the method of drug delivery. (Courtesy of Pfizer Inc.)

sterile water or some specified agent, and then the solution is shaken vigorously until no large visible particles are seen.

Cautions

Often manufacturers print cautions or special alerts onto the packaging of medications. Some of these cautions or alerts are "refrigerate at all times," "protect from light," or "keep in a dry place" (see Figure 18-7). Suspensions that are reconstituted

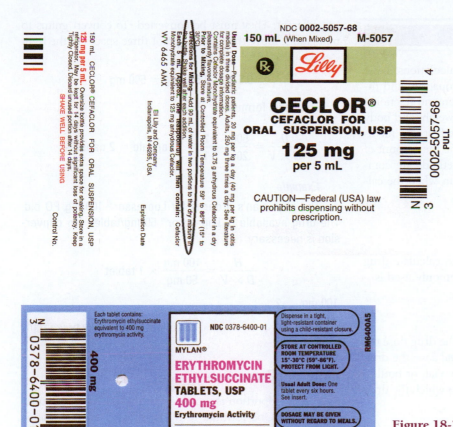

Figure 18-6. Directions for remixing a concentrated (powered) form of a drug. (Courtesy of Eli Lilly and Company.)

Figure 18-7. Cautions on the label alert the user to conditions that may alter the effect of the drug. (Courtesy of Mylan Pharmaceuticals Inc.)

may be dispensed already prepared for the patient to use, or there may be instructions to "shake well before using." All instructions given as cautions and alerts should be followed carefully.

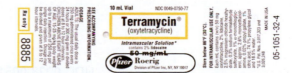

Figure 18-8. The manufacturer's name and address. (Courtesy of Pfizer Inc.)

Name of the Manufacturer

The manufacturer's name is present on all drug labels and usually contains the company's logo as well as its location (city, state, and zip code) (see Figure 18-8).

Control Numbers

By federal law, all medications must be identified with control numbers, sometimes called lot numbers (see Figure 18-9). For drug recalls, these numbers identify a particular group of medication packages that must be removed from store shelves. Using these numbers to remove groups of medications that may have been damaged or tampered with has helped to avoid the harming of large numbers of people.

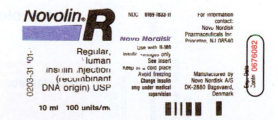

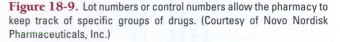

Figure 18-9. Lot numbers or control numbers allow the pharmacy to keep track of specific groups of drugs. (Courtesy of Novo Nordisk Pharmaceuticals, Inc.)

National Drug Code

Every prescription medication must have a unique identifying number according to federal law. This number, with

the letters "NDC" followed by three specific groups of numbers, is to appear on every manufacturer's label. For example, the NDC number for Procanbid® (probenecid) is NDC 61570-069-60.

METHODS OF CALCULATION

There are four methods for drug dosage calculations: basic formula, ratio and proportion, fractional equation, and dimensional analysis. The ratio and proportion and fractional equation methods are similar. When body weight and body surface area calculations are used, one of the first four methods for calculation is necessary to determine the amount of drug needed from the container. These methods are commonly used by the pharmacist or technician when the calculation of drug doses is required.

Basic Formula

The basic formula method is often used to calculate drug dosage. The basic formula that is most commonly used is

$$\frac{D}{H \times V} = \text{Amount to give}$$

In this equation, D stands for *desired dose*: the drug dose ordered by the prescriber. H stands for *on-hand dose*: the drug dose on the label of the container (ampule, vial, or bottle). V stands for *vehicle*: the form and amount in which the drug is supplied (capsule, tablet, or liquid).

Example

The physician's order is for ampicillin 0.5 g, PO, tid. The drug available is ampicillin 250 mg.

Both the dosage of the drug ordered and the dosage available are in the metric system; however, the units of measurement are different. They must be converted. To convert grams to milligrams, move the decimal point three spaces to the right (see Chapter 16):

$$0.5 \text{ g} = 0.500 \text{ mg} = 500 \text{ mg}$$

The basic formula is

$$\frac{D}{H \times V} = \frac{500}{200} = \frac{2}{1} \times 1 \text{ capsule} = 2 \text{ capsules}$$

Example

The physician's order is for Lopressor® 100 mg PO bid. The drug available is Lopressor® 50 mg/tablet. No conversion is necessary.

$$\frac{H}{D \times V} = \frac{100 \text{ mg}}{50 \text{ mg}} \times 1 \text{ tablet}$$

$$\frac{100 \text{ mg}}{50 \text{ mg}} = \frac{2}{1} \times 1 \text{ tablet} = 2 \times 1 =$$
$$2 \text{ tablets given orally twice daily}$$

Ratio and Proportion

Ratio and proportion is the oldest method used for calculating dosage. One formula uses ratios based on the *dose on hand and the dose desired*. The formula is as follows:

$$H:V :: D:X$$

In this formula, H stands for *on-hand dose*, V stands for *vehicle*, D stands for *desired dose*, and X stands for *amount to give*.

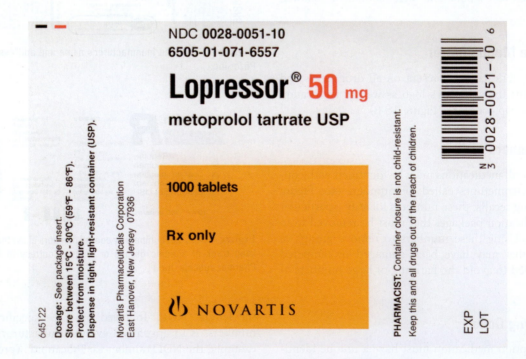

Courtesy of Novartis Pharmaceuticals Corporation.

H and *V* are the known quantities. *D* and *X* are the desired dose and the unknown amount to give:

$$H{:}V :: D{:}X$$

V and *D* are called the *means*, and *H* and *X* are called the *extremes*. Multiply the means and then the extremes and solve for *X*.

Example

Amoxicillin 500 mg PO qid (dose desired) is prescribed by the physician; the dose on hand is 250 mg/5 mL. The formula is as follows:

$$\frac{250 \text{ mg (dose on hand)}}{5 \text{ mL (dose on hand)}} = \frac{500 \text{ mg (dose desired)}}{X \text{ (dose desired)}}$$

Cross-multiply:

$$250X = 5 \times 500$$

$$X = 5 \times \frac{500}{250}$$

$$X = 10 \text{ mL}$$

Example

The ratio formula can be used in calculating dosages. For example, the prescriber orders heparin 10,000 units SC; the dose on hand is 40,000 units/mL.

$$\frac{40,000 \text{ units}}{1 \text{ mL}} = \frac{10,000 \text{ units}}{X}$$

Units cancel out:

$$40,000X = 10,000$$

$$X = \frac{10,000}{40,000}$$

$$X = \frac{1}{4}$$

$$X = 0.25 \text{ mL}$$

Fractional Equation

The fractional equation method is similar to the ratio and proportion method, except that the calculation is written as a fraction.

$$\frac{H}{V} = \frac{D}{X}$$

H stands for the *dosage on hand*, *V* stands for *vehicle*, *D* stands for *desired dosage*, and *X* stands for the *unknown amount to give*. Cross-multiply and then solve for *X*.

Example

The physician's order is for kanamycin (Kantrex®) 1 g PO qid × 3 days. The drug available is Kantrex® 500 mg.

Step 1: Convert grams to milligrams:

$$1.0 \text{ g} = 1.000 \text{ mg} = 1000 \text{ mg}$$

Step 2:

$$\frac{H}{V} = \frac{D}{X} = \frac{500 \text{ mg}}{1 \text{ capsule}} = \frac{1000}{X}$$

$$500X = 1000$$

$$X = 2$$

1 g of kanamycin = 2 capsules. Therefore, 2 capsules should be given.

Example

The physician's order is for Motrin® 600 mg PO bid. The drug available is Motrin® 300 mg tablets.

Step 1: There is no need to convert.

Step 2:

$$\frac{H}{V} = \frac{D}{X} = \frac{300 \text{ mg}}{1 \text{ tablet}} = \frac{600 \text{ mg}}{X}$$

$$300X = 600$$

$$X = \frac{600}{300} = 2$$

Therefore, 2 tablets should be given.

Dimensional Analysis

The dimensional analysis method (the label factor method) is used for calculating dosages with three factors, which include the following:

1. **Drug label factor**. The form of the drug dose (V) with its equivalence in unit (H).

   Example: 1 tablet = 250 mg

2. **Conversion factor**. This can help if the following factor conversions are memorized:

Metric Equivalents	Metric Apothecary Equivalents
1 kg = 1000 g	1 g = 15 gr
1 g = 1000 mg	1000 mg = 15 gr
1 mg = 1000 mcg	1 gr = 60 mg

3. **Drug order factor**. The three factors *D*, *H*, and *V* are set up in an equation that helps to cancel the units, giving the right answer in the right units for delivery.

$$V = V \text{(vehicle)} \times C \text{(H)} \times \frac{D \text{ (desired)}}{H \text{ (on hand)}} \times C \text{ (D)} \times 1$$

(drug label)   (conversion factor)   (drug order)

Example

An IM medication order is for 1500 mg. The solution strength available is 500 mg/mL. How many mL must be prepared to get this dosage?

This is a very straightforward calculation, and you can quickly determine that you must give 3 mL. Here is how the dosage would be calculated using dimensional analysis.

Step 1: Identify the unit of measure being calculated. In parenteral dosages this will always be mL. Always enter the unit being calculated to the left of the equation, followed by an equal (=) sign. In this problem you are calculating mL:

$$mL =$$

There are two very important reasons for identifying the unit being calculated first:

1. It eliminates any confusion over exactly which measure is being calculated.
2. It dictates how the first ration factor is entered in the equation.

The unit being calculated is mL. Locate the complete factor which contains mL. This is provided by the dosage strength available: 500 mg = 1 mL. This becomes the starting factor, and it is entered with 1 mL as the numerator, to match the mL unit being calculated; 500 mg becomes the denominator.

$$mL = \frac{1 \text{ mL}}{500 \text{ mg}}$$

starting factor

Notice that the units of measure are entered with each quantity: 1 mL and 500 mg (not 1 and 500). This is mandatory, because the units of measure are used to check the completed equation for correct factor/ratio entry.

All additional factors are entered so that each successive numerator matches the unit of measure in the previous denominator. The denominator in the starting factor is mg, so the second numerator must be mg. The medication order is for 1500 mg. Enter 1500 mg as the second numerator/factor.

$$mL = \frac{1 \text{ mL}}{500 \text{ mg}} \times 1500 \text{ mg}$$

All the pertinent factors/dosages have now been entered for this problem, and its dimensional analysis equation is complete.

Step 2: Cancel the alternate denominator/numerator measurement units to be sure they match, which indicates that the factors were correctly entered in the equation. The mg are cancelled (but not their quantities: 500 and 1500), leaving only mL, the unit being calculated, remaining in the equation. The numerator of the starting factor never cancels; it remains in the equation to identify the unit of measure being calculated.

$$mL = \frac{1 \text{ mL}}{500 \text{ mg}} \times 1500 \text{ mg}$$

The math can now be done.

$$mL = \frac{1 \text{ mL}}{500 \text{ mg}} \times 1500 \text{ mg} = 3 \text{ mL}$$

The answer obtained, 3 mL, is the same as that calculated mentally, so you can now feel secure that dimensional analysis really works, and it works exactly the same way for *every* calculation. There are no complicated rules to be memorized.

Example

A dosage of 50,000 U is ordered to be added to an intravenous solution. The strength available is 10,000 U/1.5 mL. Calculate how many mL will contain this dosage.

Write the mL being calculated to the left of the equation followed by an equal sign.

$$mL =$$

Look back at the problem and locate the factor that contains mL: 10,000 U/1.5 mL. Enter this as the starting factor, with 1.5 mL as the numerator, to match the mL being calculated. The 10,000 U becomes the denominator.

$$mL = \frac{1.5 \text{ mL}}{10,000 \text{ U}}$$

The starting factor denominator is U. Match this in the next numerator with the 50,000 U ordered.

$$mL = \frac{1.5 \text{ mL}}{10,000 \text{ U}} \times 50,000 \text{ U}$$

The DA equation is complete for this problem. Cancel the alternate denominator/numerator units of measure (U) to be sure your entries are correct. Do the math.

$$mL = \frac{1.5 \text{ mL}}{10,000 \text{ U}} \times 50,000 \text{ U} = 7.5 \text{ mL}$$

It will require a 7.5 mL volume of the 10,000 U/mL solution to prepare the 50,000 U ordered for this intravenous additive.

CALCULATION OF ORAL MEDICATIONS

A variety of forms of drugs are commonly administered orally. These include tablets, capsules, powders, and liquids. Oral medications are referred to as "PO" (per os [by mouth]) drugs. They are absorbed by the gastrointestinal tract, mainly from the small intestine.

The advantages of oral drug administration include the facts that the drugs are more convenient to use and cheaper. Disadvantages of oral drug administration are as follows:

- Varied absorption rate
- Irritation of the gastric mucosa
- Retention or inactivation of the drugs in the body (liver diseases)
- Destruction of drugs by digestive enzymes
- Aspiration of drugs into the lungs
- Discoloration of tooth enamel

Measuring Tablets or Capsules

Tablets and capsules are solid medications that are supplied in different strengths or dosages. Their dosages can be expressed in apothecary or metric measures, for example, grains or milligrams.

Conversion Factors

Converting drug measures from one system to another and from one unit to another to determine the dosage to be administered can result in discrepancies, depending on the conversion factor used.

Example

The label for Tylenol® may indicate 325 mg (5 gr). This is based on the equivalent 65 mg = 1 gr. On the other hand, the label for aspirin may indicate 300 mg (5 gr). Here the equivalent 60 mg = 1 gr was used. Both of the equivalents are correct. *Remember that equivalents are not exact.* Use the common equivalents when making conversions, for example, 60 mg = 1 gr.

Rule of 10% Variation

If the precise number of tablets or capsules is determined and administering the amount calculated is unrealistic or impossible, always use the following rule to avoid an error in administration: *No more than 10% variation should exist between the dose ordered and the dose administered.*

Example

One may determine that a patient should receive 0.9 tablet or 0.9 capsule. Administration of such an amount accurately would be impossible. In this case, 1 tablet or 1 capsule could be safely administered.

Administration of Capsules

Capsules are not scored and cannot be divided. They are administered in whole amounts only. Never crush or open a timed-release capsule or empty its contents into a liquid or food.

Other Units of Measure

In the calculation of oral doses, measures other than apothecary or metric may be encountered. For example, with electrolytes such as potassium, the number of milliequivalents (mEq) per tablet will be indicated. Another measure that may be seen for oral antibiotics or vitamins is units (U). For example, the label for vitamin E capsules will indicate 400 U per capsule. Unit and milliequivalent measurements are specific to the drugs they are being used for. There is no conversion between these and apothecary or metric measures.

Measurement of Oral Liquids

Liquid medications include elixirs, syrups, tinctures, and suspensions. Certain liquid drugs are irritating to the stomach mucosa and must be well diluted before administration. An example is potassium chloride (KCl). Tincture medications are always diluted. Any liquid medication that may

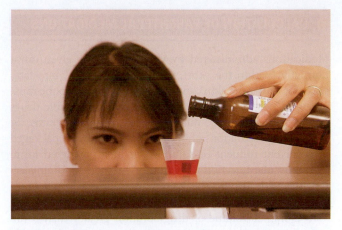

Figure 18-10. Oral medications must be measured at eye level for accuracy.

cause discoloration of the teeth should be diluted and taken through a drinking straw. In general, liquid cough medicines are not diluted. Liquid medications contain a specific amount of drug in a given amount of solution.

When a liquid medication is measured, hold the transparent measuring device at eye level. The liquid curve in the center is called the **meniscus**. All liquid medication is measured at the meniscus level (see Figure 18-10).

For medications in liquid form, calculate the volume of the liquid that contains the ordered dosage of the medication. The label of drugs bottled may indicate the amount of drug per 1 mL or per multiple milliliters of solution, for example, 20 mg/5 mL, 250 mg/5 mL, or 1.4 g/30 mL. Liquid drugs must be calculated with the formula:

$$\frac{D}{H} \times V = X$$

In this formula, D represents the desired dosage or the dosage ordered. H represents the dosage you have on hand per a quantity. V represents the volume of the drug.

Example

A prescription is written to give 4 mL of ampicillin with a dosage strength of 125 mg/5 mL. The following formula is used:

$$\frac{D}{H} \times V = \frac{100 \text{ mg}}{125 \text{ mg}} \times 5 \text{ mL} = X$$

$$\frac{4}{5} \times 5 \text{ mL} = \frac{20}{5 \text{ mL}} = 4 \text{ mL}$$

Example

A prescription is written to give 100 mg of ampicillin. The medication is available with a dosage strength of 250 mg/5 mL. The following formula is used:

$$\frac{D}{H} \times V = \frac{100 \text{ mg}}{250 \text{ mg}} \times 5 \text{ mL} = X$$

$$\frac{2}{5} \times 5 \text{ mL} = \frac{10}{5} = 2 \text{ mL}$$

CALCULATION OF PARENTERAL MEDICATIONS

Medications administered by injection can be given intradermally (within the skin), subcutaneously (SC, into fatty tissue or under the skin), intramuscularly (IM, into the muscle), and intravenously (IV, into the vein). Injectable drugs are ordered in grams, milligrams, micrograms, grains, or units. The preparations of injectable drugs may be packaged in a solvent (diluent or solution) or in a powdered form. Intramuscular injection is a common method of administering injectable drugs. The volume of solution for an intramuscular injection is 0.5 to 3.0 mL, with the average being 1 to 2 mL. A volume of drug solution greater than 3 mL causes increased muscle tissue displacement and possible tissue damage. Occasionally, 5 mL of certain drugs, such as magnesium sulfate or immunoglobulin (given after exposure to rabies), may be injected in a large muscle, such as the dorsogluteal. Dosages greater than 3 mL are usually divided and given at two different sites. Drug solutions for injection are commercially premixed and stored in vials and ampules for immediate use. At times there may be enough drug solution left in a vial for another dose, and the vial may be saved. The balance of a drug solution in an ampule is always discarded after the ampule has been opened and used. For calculating intramuscular dosage, the following example can be used:

Example

An order is given for gentamicin 60 mg IM. The available dosage strength of gentamicin is 80 mg/2 mL in a vial. The following formula is used:

$$\frac{D}{H} \times V = \frac{60}{80} \times 2 = \frac{120}{80} = 1.5 \text{ mL}$$

or

$$H:V :: D:X$$

$$80 \text{ mg}:2 \text{ mL} :: 60 \text{ mg}:X \text{ mL}$$

$$80X = 120$$

$$X = \frac{120}{80} = 1.5 \text{ mL}$$

Example

The physician's order is for atropine 0.2 mg SC stat. The drug is available at a dosage of 400 mcg/mL (0.4 mg/mL). The following formula is used:

$$\frac{D}{H} \times V = \frac{0.2 \text{ mg}}{0.4 \text{ mg}} \times 1 \text{ mL} = \frac{0.2}{0.4} \times 1 = 0.5 \text{ mL}$$

Injectable Medications

Injectable drugs are packaged in ampules or vials (discussed in Chapter 5). The medication is in either liquid or powder form in ampules or vials. Because drugs in solution deteriorate rapidly, they are packaged in dry form and diluent is added before administration. If the medication is in powdered form, mixing directions and dose equivalents such as milligrams (mg) per milliliter (mL) are usually given; if not, check the drug information insert. After the dry form of the drug is reconstituted with sterile water, bacteriostatic water, or saline, the medication is used immediately or must be refrigerated. Usually, the reconstituted drug in the vial is used within 48 hours to 1 week.

STANDARDIZED UNITS OF DRUG DOSAGES

Several drugs that are obtained from animal sources can be standardized in units according to their strengths rather than on weight measures such as milligrams and grams. Some hormones such as insulin are too complex to be completely purified to obtain the exact weight of the drug per unit of volume. Therefore, insulin and many other drugs are measured in units for parenteral administration. The labels of such medications indicate how many units are needed per milliliter.

Insulin Calculations

Insulin is ordered and measured in USP units. Most types of insulins are manufactured in concentrations of 100 U/mL. Insulin should be administered with an insulin syringe, which is calculated to correspond with the U-100 insulin. Insulin bottles and syringes are color-coded. The U-100 insulin bottle and the U-100 syringe are color-coded orange.

A new insulin, called 70/30 insulin, is now available for use with U-100 syringes (Figure 18-11). The 70/30 insulin concentration means there is 70% NPH insulin and 30% regular insulin in each unit. Therefore, if the physician orders 10 units of 70/30 insulin, the patient would receive 7 U of NPH insulin (70% or 0.7 × 10 U = 7 U) and 3 U of regular insulin (30% or 0.3 × 10 U = 3 U).

Insulin orders must be written clearly and contain specific information to prevent errors. The order for insulin should include the brand name, supply dosage, number of units to be given, and the route and time or frequency of administration. The two types of insulin used most often are the rapid-acting regular insulin and the intermediate-acting NPH insulin.

Example

An order is given for Humulin R Regular U-100® 14 U SC stat or for Iletin 11 NPH U-100® 24 U SC ½ hour after breakfast.

Insulin is supplied in 10 mL vials labeled with the number of units per milliliter; thus, U-100 insulin means there are 100 U/mL. In the past, insulin was administered in U-40 and U-80 dosage forms. Today, however, the U-100 form has almost totally replaced the weaker strength forms. The smaller volume required per dose decreases local reactions at the injection site, as well as simplifying

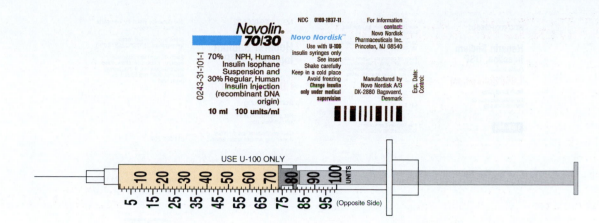

Figure 18-11. Standard dosing of insulin. (A. Courtesy of Novo Nordisk Pharmaceuticals, Inc.)

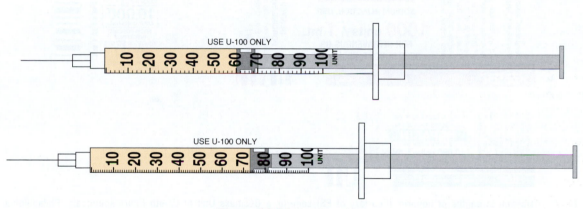

Figure 18-12. Insulin syringe.

mathematical calculations. The simplest and most accurate method to measure insulin is within an insulin syringe. The insulin syringe is calibrated in units, and the desired dose may be read directly on the syringe. U-100 insulin should be measured only in a U-100 insulin syringe. It is important to note that for U-100 insulin, 100 units = 1 mL. Two types of insulin syringes are available: Lo-Dose and 1 mL size. Figure 18-12 shows both sides of a standard U-100 syringe with Novalin®. The standard U-100 syringe has a dual scale with even numbers on one side and odd numbers on the other side.

If an insulin syringe is not available, a tuberculin syringe may be used, and the unit dosage may be converted to the equivalent number of cubic centimeters, using the proportion method.

Example

Give 40 U of insulin, using U-100 insulin and a tuberculin syringe. The amount administered is calculated as follows:

$$\frac{40}{100} \times 1 \text{ mL} = 0.4 \text{ mL}$$

Heparin Calculations

Heparin is a potent anticoagulant that prevents clot formation and blood coagulation. Heparin dosages are expressed in USP units (U). The therapeutic range for heparin is determined individually by monitoring the patient's partial thromboplastin time. However, the normal adult heparin dosage is 20,000 to 40,000 U every 24 hours. Heparin can be administered IV or SC. When administered IV, heparin is ordered in units per hour or milliliters per hour. Usually, heparin is ordered on the basis of units per hour or per day for intravenous administration. Heparin is available in single-dose and multidose vials, as well as in commercially prepared intravenous solutions. Because heparin is available in different strengths, it is important to read labels carefully when it must be administered. Heparin sodium for injection is available in several strengths (e.g., 100, 5,000, and 20,000 U/mL). Heparin lock fluid solution (which is used for flushing) is available in 10 and 100 U/mL. The pharmacy technician must remember that heparin sodium for injection and heparin lock solution are different drugs and can never be used interchangeably. Figure 18-13 shows the various heparin dosage strengths.

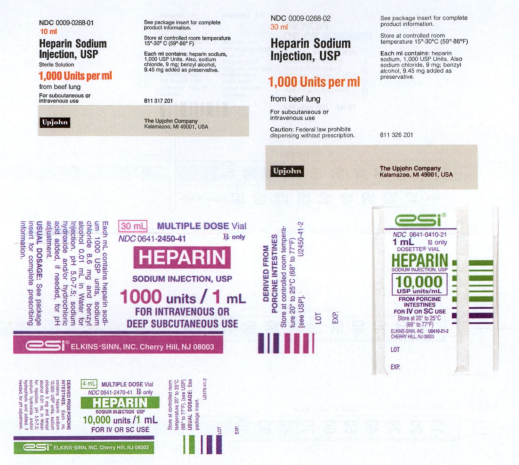

Figure 18-13. Dosage strengths of heparin. (Courtesy of ESI Lederle, a Business Unit of Wyeth Pharmaceuticals, Philadelphia, PA, and Pharmacia Corporation, Peapack, NJ.)

Heparin is administered using an electronic infusion device, and the patient requires continuous monitoring. Heparin is derived from animal sources. It is often given intravenously to produce a rapid effect and then is given in deep subcutaneous injections in larger and more infrequent doses.

Example

A physician's order is for heparin 7,500 U SC. Heparin is available in a dosage of 10,000 U/mL (see Figure 18-3). The amount administered is calculated as follows:

$$10,000 \text{ U} = 1 \text{ mL} = 7,500 \text{ U}:X \text{ mL}$$

$$10,000X = 7,500$$

$$X = \frac{7,500}{10,000}$$

$$X = 0.75 \text{ mL}$$

Example

A physician's order is for D5W (5% dextrose in water) 1000 mL containing 20,000 U of heparin, which is to be infused at 30 mL/hr. The dose of heparin the patient is to receive per hour is

$$20,000 \text{ U}:1,000 \text{ mL} = X \text{ U}:30 \text{ mL}$$

$$1,000X = 20,000 \times 30$$

$$\frac{1,000X}{1,000} = \frac{60,000}{1,000} = 600 \text{ U/hr}$$

Antibiotic Calculations

The dosages of many antibiotics are still standardized in units. These may be prepared for injection in the form of a liquid containing a specified number of units per cubic centimeter. Antibiotics are also available in the form of a dry powder in a vial that must first be diluted with water or another diluent. The powder should be diluted so that the desired dose is in 1 or 2 cc (mL) amounts if the dose is to be given IM. If it is to be given IV, a larger amount of diluent may be used.

Example

A vial of powdered penicillin G contains 1,000,000 units. The amount of diluent to be added to obtain a solution containing 100,000 U/mL is

$$100,000:1 \text{ mL} = 1,000,000:X \text{ mL}$$

$$100,000X = 1,000,000 \times 1$$

$$X = \frac{1,000,000}{100,000}$$

$$X = 10 \text{ mL}$$

INTRAVENOUS SOLUTIONS, EQUIPMENT, AND CALCULATIONS

The term *intravenous* literally means "within a vein." Intravenous infusion is the slow introduction of a substance such as a solution, whole blood, plasma, or antibiotics into a vein. Intravenous solutions fall into four functional categories: replacement fluids, maintenance fluids, therapeutic fluids, and agents to keep the vein open. If the patient is dehydrated and unable to eat or drink or if he or she has lost blood, replacement fluids are ordered. Maintenance fluids help patients maintain normal electrolyte and fluid balances. Therapeutic fluids deliver medication to the patient. Some intravenous lines provide access to the vein for emergency situations. Fluids prescribed to keep the vein open include 5% dextrose in water. Intravenous fluids and drugs may be administered by two methods: intermittent and continuous infusion. Intermittent infusion, such as intravenous piggyback and intravenous push infusions are used for intravenous administration of drugs and supplemental fluids. Continuous intravenous infusions are used to replace fluid or to help in maintaining fluid levels and electrolyte balance and serve as vehicles for drug administration. Saline or heparin locks are used to maintain venous access without continuous fluid infusion. Thus, the pharmacy technician must learn how to effectively calculate infusion rates and monitor the administration of these agents. Table 18-1 shows common abbreviations for components of intravenous infusions.

Calculation of Intravenous Heparin Flow Rate

Units per hour of heparin can be calculated by using the ratio and proportion method. Use the following formula to calculate intravenous heparin flow in mL/hr:

$$\frac{DI}{H} \times Q = R$$

TABLE 18-1. Common IV Component Abbreviations

SOLUTION COMPONENT	ABBREVIATION
Dextrose	D
Lactated Ringer's	LR
Normal saline	NS
Saline	S
Ringer's lactate	RL
Water	W

$$\frac{D \text{ (U/hr desired)}}{H \text{ (U available)}} \times Q \text{ (mL available)} = R \text{ (mL/hr)}$$

or the ratio of supply dosage is equivalent to ratio of desired dosage rate:

$$\text{Supply, U/mL} = \frac{\text{Desired U/hr}}{X \text{ mL/hr}}$$

This rule also applies to other drugs ordered in mU/hr, mg/hr, mcg/hr, g/hr, or mEq/hr.

Example

An order is given for D5W 500 mL with heparin 25,000 U IV at 1,000 U/hr. What is the flow rate in mL/hr?

$$\frac{D}{H} \times Q = \frac{1,000 \text{ U/hr}}{25,000 \text{ U}} \times 500 \text{ mL} = R \text{ (mL/hr)}$$

The units (U) cancel out to leave mL/hr in the $\frac{D}{H} \times Q = R$ formula.

$$\frac{1000 \text{ U/hr}}{25,000 \text{ U}} \times 500 \text{ mL} = \frac{1000}{50} = 20 \text{ mL/hr}$$

Or use the ratio and proportion method to calculate the flow rate that will administer 1000 U/hr in mL/hr.

$$\frac{25,000 \text{ U}}{500 \text{ mL}} = \frac{1000 \text{ U/hr}}{X \text{ mL/hr}}$$

$$25,000X = 500,000$$

$$X = \frac{500,000}{25,000} = 20 \text{ mL/hr}$$

Example

An order is given for D5W 250 mL with heparin 25,000 IV at 750 U/hr. Calculate the flow rate in mL/hr.

$$\frac{D}{H} \times Q = \frac{750 \text{ U/hr}}{25,000} \times 250 \text{ mL} = 750 = 7.5 \text{ mL/hr}$$

or use the ratio and proportion method:

$$\frac{25,000 \text{ U}}{250 \text{ mL}} = \frac{750 \text{ U/hr}}{X \text{ mL/hr}}$$

$$25,000X = 187,500$$

$$X = \frac{187,500}{25,000} = 7.5 \text{ mL/hr}$$

Intravenous Solution Concentrations

Solutions may have different concentrations of dextrose (glucose) or 5% dextrose in lactated Ringer's or saline (sodium chloride) solution. For example, 5% dextrose contains 5 g of dextrose per 100 mL. Figure 18-14A and 18-4B shows a label for a 5% dextrose solution and a 5% dextrose in lactated Ringer's solution.

Normal saline is 0.9% saline; it contains 900 mg or 0.9 g of sodium chloride per 100 mL (see Figure 18-14C).

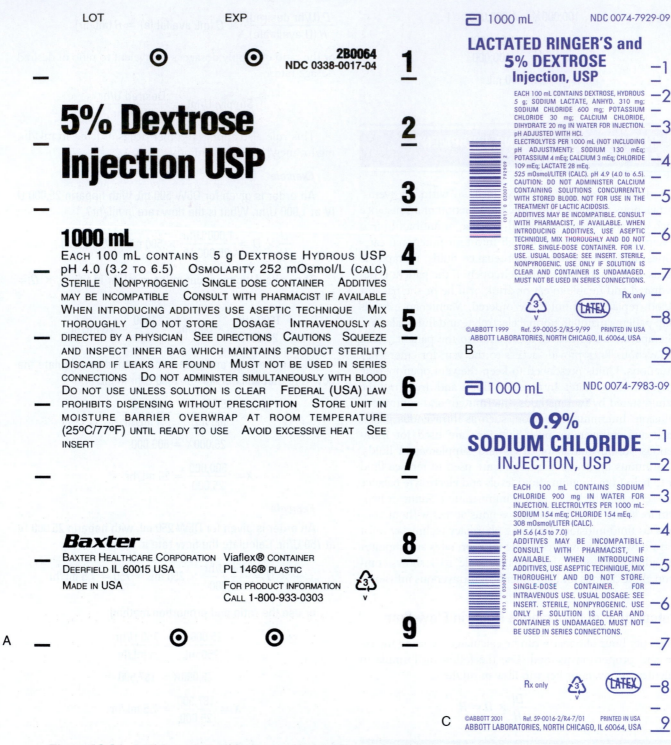

LOT   EXP

2B0064
NDC 0338-0017-04

1

2

5% Dextrose Injection USP

3

1000 mL

4

EACH 100 mL CONTAINS   5 g DEXTROSE HYDROUS USP
pH 4.0 (3.2 TO 6.5)   OSMOLARITY 252 mOsmol/L (CALC)
STERILE NONPYROGENIC SINGLE DOSE CONTAINER ADDITIVES
MAY BE INCOMPATIBLE CONSULT WITH PHARMACIST IF AVAILABLE
WHEN INTRODUCING ADDITIVES USE ASEPTIC TECHNIQUE MIX
THOROUGHLY DO NOT STORE DOSAGE INTRAVENOUSLY AS
DIRECTED BY A PHYSICIAN SEE DIRECTIONS CAUTIONS SQUEEZE
AND INSPECT INNER BAG WHICH MAINTAINS PRODUCT STERILITY
DISCARD IF LEAKS ARE FOUND   MUST NOT BE USED IN SERIES
CONNECTIONS DO NOT ADMINISTER SIMULTANEOUSLY WITH BLOOD
DO NOT USE UNLESS SOLUTION IS CLEAR   FEDERAL (USA) LAW
PROHIBITS DISPENSING WITHOUT PRESCRIPTION STORE UNIT IN
MOISTURE BARRIER OVERWRAP AT ROOM TEMPERATURE
(25ºC/77ºF) UNTIL READY TO USE AVOID EXCESSIVE HEAT SEE
INSERT

5

6

7

Baxter
BAXTER HEALTHCARE CORPORATION Viaflex® CONTAINER
DEERFIELD IL 60015 USA   PL 146® PLASTIC
MADE IN USA   FOR PRODUCT INFORMATION
                CALL 1-800-933-0303

8

A

9

1000 mL   NDC 0074-7929-09

LACTATED RINGER'S and 5% DEXTROSE
Injection, USP

−1

−2

EACH 100 mL CONTAINS DEXTROSE, HYDROUS 5 g; SODIUM LACTATE, ANHYD. 310 mg; SODIUM CHLORIDE 600 mg; POTASSIUM CHLORIDE 30 mg; CALCIUM CHLORIDE, DIHYDRATE 20 mg IN WATER FOR INJECTION. pH ADJUSTED WITH HCl.
ELECTROLYTES PER 1000 mL (NOT INCLUDING pH ADJUSTMENT): SODIUM 130 mEq; POTASSIUM 4 mEq; CALCIUM 3 mEq; CHLORIDE 109 mEq; LACTATE 28 mEq.
525 mOsmol/LITER (CALC). pH 4.9 (4.0 to 6.5). CAUTION: DO NOT ADMINISTER CALCIUM CONTAINING SOLUTIONS CONCURRENTLY WITH STORED BLOOD. NOT FOR USE IN THE TREATMENT OF LACTIC ACIDOSIS.
ADDITIVES MAY BE INCOMPATIBLE. CONSULT WITH PHARMACIST, IF AVAILABLE. WHEN INTRODUCING ADDITIVES, USE ASEPTIC TECHNIQUE, MIX THOROUGHLY AND DO NOT STORE. SINGLE-DOSE CONTAINER. FOR I.V. USE. USUAL DOSAGE: SEE INSERT. STERILE, NONPYROGENIC. USE ONLY IF SOLUTION IS CLEAR AND CONTAINER IS UNDAMAGED. MUST NOT BE USED IN SERIES CONNECTIONS.

−3

−4

−5

−6

−7

Rx only

©ABBOTT 1999   Ref. 59-0005-2/R5-9/99   PRINTED IN USA
ABBOTT LABORATORIES, NORTH CHICAGO, IL 60064, USA

B

−8

9

1000 mL   NDC 0074-7983-09

0.9%
SODIUM CHLORIDE
INJECTION, USP

−1

−2

EACH 100 mL CONTAINS SODIUM CHLORIDE 900 mg IN WATER FOR INJECTION. ELECTROLYTES PER 1000 mL: SODIUM 154 mEq; CHLORIDE 154 mEq. 308 mOsmol/LITER (CALC).
pH 5.6 (4.5 to 7.0)
ADDITIVES MAY BE INCOMPATIBLE. CONSULT WITH PHARMACIST, IF AVAILABLE. WHEN INTRODUCING ADDITIVES, USE ASEPTIC TECHNIQUE, MIX THOROUGHLY AND DO NOT STORE. SINGLE-DOSE CONTAINER. FOR INTRAVENOUS USE. USUAL DOSAGE: SEE INSERT. STERILE, NONPYROGENIC. USE ONLY IF SOLUTION IS CLEAR AND CONTAINER IS UNDAMAGED. MUST NOT BE USED IN SERIES CONNECTIONS.

−3

−4

−5

−6

−7

Rx only

©ABBOTT 2001   Ref. 59-0016-2/R4-7/01   PRINTED IN USA
ABBOTT LABORATORIES, NORTH CHICAGO, IL 60064, USA

C

−8

9

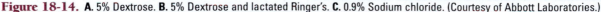

Figure 18-14. A. 5% Dextrose. **B.** 5% Dextrose and lactated Ringer's. **C.** 0.9% Sodium chloride. (Courtesy of Abbott Laboratories.)

Equipment for Intravenous Infusion

Equipment used to administer intravenous medications is available in several forms. Administration is either completely manual or electronic.

The primary intravenous line may consist of a bag or bottle of solution and tubing. Bags for intravenous infusion come in different sizes. The solution of fluid to be infused is often 500 or 1000 cc (mL). The tubing, which is the primary line, usually includes a drip chamber, roller clamp, and in-

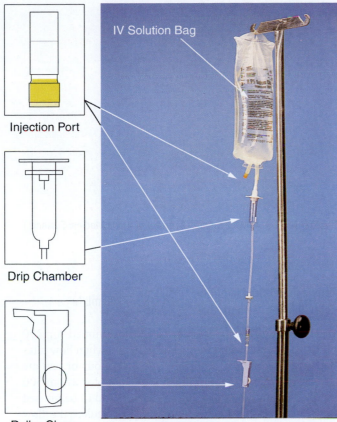

Injection Port

Drip Chamber

Roller Clamp

Figure 18-15. Standard gravity flow intravenous system.

IV Solution Bag

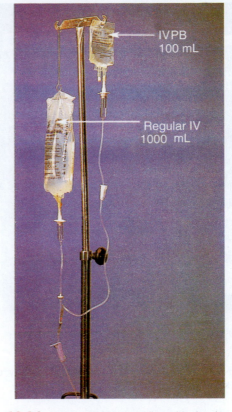

IVPB
100 mL

Regular IV
1000 mL

Figure 18-16. Standard intravenous line with piggyback (PB IV).

jection ports (see Figure 18-15). The nurse can either regulate the rate manually by using the roller clamp or place the tubing in an electronic infusion pump.

The secondary intravenous tubing is used when medications are administered by "piggybacking" into the primary line (see Figure 18-16). This type of tubing generally is shorter and also contains a drip chamber and roller clamp. The benefit of this technique is that it gives access to the primary intravenous catheter without having to start another line.

To measure the flow rate, the drip chamber must be squeezed until it is half full, making it easier to appropriately count the number of drops falling into the chamber. The roller clamp is used to adjust the speed of the infusion either up or down, as needed. The injection port is available to inject medications into the primary line or to attach a second intravenous line. Two sizes of tubing are available: macrodrop and microdrop. Macrodrop tubing is used for fluids infused at a higher rate, for example, infusions that are set at 80 mL/hr or higher. Microdrop tubing is used for slower infusions for which accuracy of dosage delivery is essential, such as in critical care or pediatric settings.

Monitoring the Intravenous Infusion

The infusion of intravenous fluids is monitored in many different ways. Most times, for manual monitoring, the bag containing the intravenous solution is hung 36 inches above the patient's heart so that gravity will draw the fluid into the patient. When the infusion is monitored, the roller clamp is used to adjust the rate of delivery.

Electronically Regulated Intravenous Infusions

Another method of monitoring is the use of an electronic infusion pump, which applies a set amount of pressure so that a set volume is infused over a set time period. Manufacturers supply special volumetric tubing that must be used with their infusion devices. This special tubing ensures accurate and consistent intravenous infusions. Each device can be set for a specific flow rate and will set off an alarm if this rate is interrupted. There are three types of controllers, including infusion pumps and a syringe pump (see Figures 18-17, 18-18, and 18-19).

The flow rate is generally programmed into the device in milliliters per hour. The pumps do not rely on gravity, but rather on pressure that the pump creates to force the solution through the tubing and into the patient's vascular system. Most electronic pumps are armed with sensors that sound when the bag of solution is empty or if the rate cannot be properly maintained. Despite advances in technology,

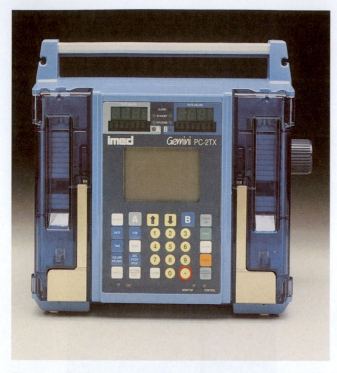

Figure 18-17. Volumetric infusion pump. (Courtesy of Alaris Medical Systems.)

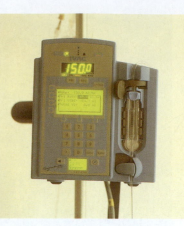

Figure 18-18. Infusion pump. (Courtesy of Alaris Medical Systems.)

$$\frac{\text{Total amount ordered (mL)}}{\text{Total number of hours (hr)}} = \frac{500 \text{ mL}}{2 \text{ hr}} = 250 \text{ mL/hr}$$

Therefore, the infusion device is programmed for 250 mL/hr. Another formula is especially helpful when flow rates that have a prescribed infusion time of $\frac{1}{2}$ hour or less are calculated. For example, J.P. Ellen is a patient for whom 500 mg of an IV antibiotic in a *100 mL* bag of fluid to be infused over *30 minutes* has been prescribed. To calculate the flow rate for this patient, use the following formula (remember that 60 minutes = 1 hr):

$$\frac{\text{Total milliliters ordered}}{\text{Total hours ordered}} = \frac{X \text{ (mL)}}{1 \text{ hr}} = \frac{100 \text{ mL}}{30 \text{ min}} = \frac{X \text{ mL}}{60 \text{ min}}$$

Cross-multiply to get

$$30X = 6{,}000$$

and divide both sides by 30 to get

$$X = 200 \text{ mL/hr}$$

Thus, the electronic infusion pump should be set at 200 mL/hr for the 100 mL bag of fluid to be infused over 30 minutes.

Manually Calculating Drop Rates

The pharmacy technician may, depending on the setting, have to calculate a **drop rate** of an intravenous fluid and then manually regulate the equipment to control the speed at which the fluid is being infused. To calculate the drop rate, the technician must determine how many drops (abbreviated as gtt) per minute should be infused over a prescribed time period. The number of drops per minute depends on the type of intravenous tubing used. Two types of tubing are available: standard (or macrodrop) and microdrop. Standard tubing has a drop factor of 10, 15, or 20 gtt/mL, whereas microdrop tubing has a drop factor of 60 gtt/mL. The drop factor is generally found on the outside packaging of the tubing and indicates the number of drops

there is still no substitute for a vigilant health care provider to ensure that the right patient is receiving the right medication, at the right time, and at the right infusion rate.

Calculation of Intravenous Flow Rates

A flow rate is the speed at which intravenous fluids are infused into a patient. Allowing the patient to receive a prescribed fluid too fast or too slow can result in adverse reactions. The ability of the pharmacy technician to correctly and efficiently calculate flow rates of intravenous fluids is critical to the well-being of the patient. Flow rates are generally prescribed or written as 125 mL/hr or 500 mL/2 hr, meaning that the fluids should be infused into the patient at a rate of 125 mL over a period of 1 hour or at a rate of 500 mL over a period of 2 hours, respectively. Flow rates can be regulated either by the use of an electronic pump or by manually adjusting the intravenous equipment to achieve the prescribed flow rate. When an electronic pump is used, the flow rate is calculated in milliliters per hour and can be arrived at by using the following formula:

$$\frac{\text{Total amount ordered (mL)}}{\text{Total number of hours (hr)}} = \text{mL/hr}$$

After the flow rate is successfully calculated, the rate is then programmed into an electronic infusion device. For example, Jane Doe is a patient for whom a *500 mL* bag of intravenous fluids to be infused over *2 hours* has been prescribed. To calculate the flow rate, use the preceding formula:

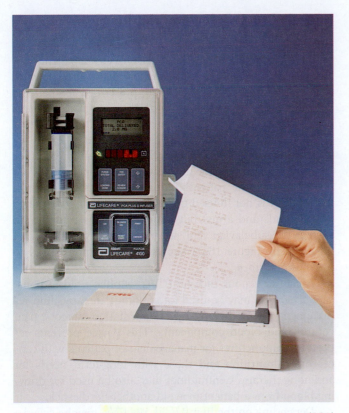

Figure 18-19. Abbott Lifecare patient-controlled anesthesia (PCA) pump. (Courtesy of Abbott Laboratories.)

per milliliter a particular intravenous tubing set will deliver. Figure 18-20 shows the size and number of drops in 1 mL for each drop factor. Notice that as the number of drops per milliliter gets smaller, the actual drop size becomes larger.

The following formula is used to calculate flow rates in drops per minute:

$$\frac{V \text{ (total volume to be infused in mL)}}{T \text{ (total time in minutes)}} \times$$

$$C \text{ (drop factor in gtt/mL)} = R \text{ (rate of flow in gtt/min)}$$

or the formula can also be written as

$$\frac{V}{T} \times C = R$$

Example

John Brown is to receive *200 cc* of intravenous fluids over *2 hours*. Macrodrop tubing has been selected, which has a drop factor of *20 gtt/min*. The job of the technician is to calculate how many drops per minute are needed so that all 200 cc is infused over 30 minutes.

Step 1: Convert 2 hours into minutes (reminder: 1 hour = 60 minutes):

$$2 \times 60 = 120 \text{ min}$$

Step 2: Set up the problem using the formula $\frac{V}{T} \times C = R$:

$$\frac{200}{120} \times 20 = 33.3 \text{ gtt/min}$$

Note that the number of drops per minute needs to be rounded to the nearest whole number. In this example, round down to get 33 gtt/min.

Step 3: Set the drop rate by adjusting the roller clamp and counting the amount of drops per minute that fall into the drip chamber.

Example

The order is for 0.9% NS 500 mL with U-200 regular insulin infused at 10 U/hr. The drop factor is 60. Answer the following questions:

Amount of drug/mL: _____
How many mL/hr? _____
How many mL/min? _____
How many gtt/min? _____

1. First, determine the amount of drug in each milliliter. This may be done by using a proportion:

$$\frac{500 \text{ mL NS}}{200 \text{ U insulin}} = \frac{1 \text{ mL NS}}{X \text{ U insulin}}$$

$$500X = 200$$

$$X = \frac{200}{500}$$

$$X = 0.4$$
$$X = 0.4 \text{ U insulin/mL}$$

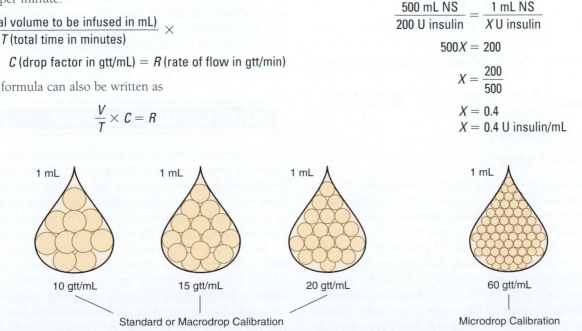

Figure 18-20. Comparison of drop size in macrodrop and microdrop infusions.

2. Second, determine the flow in mL/hr:

$$\frac{0.4 \text{ U insulin}}{1 \text{ mL}} = \frac{10 \text{ U insulin}}{X \text{ mL}}$$

$$\frac{0.4}{1} = \frac{10}{X}$$

$$0.4X = 10$$

$$X = \frac{10}{0.4}$$

$$X = 25$$

$$X = 25 \text{ mL/hr}$$

3. Third, determine the flow in mL/min:

$$\frac{25 \text{ mL}}{60 \text{ min}} = \frac{X}{1 \text{ min}}$$

$$\frac{25}{60} = \frac{X}{1}$$

$$60X = 25$$

$$X = \frac{25}{60}$$

$$X = 0.416$$

$$X = 0.42 \text{ mL/min}$$

4. Finally, determine gtt/min:

$$\frac{60 \text{ gtt}}{1 \text{ mL}} = \frac{X \text{ gtt}}{0.42 \text{ mL}}$$

$$\frac{60}{1} = \frac{X}{0.42}$$

$$X = 25.2$$

$$I = 25.2 \text{ gtt/min}$$

5. Alternatively, use the following shortcut to determine gtt/min

$$X \text{ (gtt/min)} = \frac{25 \text{ (volume per hour)}}{60 \text{ (minutes per hour)}} \times \frac{60 \text{ (drop factor)}}{1}$$

$$X = 25/60 \, (\, 60/1$$

$$X = 25 \text{ gtt/min}$$

Many people may see the ability to adequately calculate and manually adjust drop rates to be outdated because of the improved technology available with electronic infusion pumps, which can be easily programmed. However, the opposite is true. It is important for pharmacy technicians to know the math behind what electronic pumps do because an electronic pump may not be available. In addition, emergency situations require immediate attention, and the ability to correctly determine intravenous infusion drop rates without the aid of an infusion pump is an invaluable skill.

Dosing of Total Parenteral Nutrition

Total parenteral nutrition (TPN), also called hyperalimentation, is an intravenous infusion that provides a patient with all of his or her daily nutritional requirements in the form of a liquid infusion. TPN is generally prescribed for patients who, because of their disease process or surgical intervention, are unable to eat. It includes fluids such as dextrose, electrolytes, amino acids, trace elements, and vitamins. In some cases, other substances such as fat, insulin, or other drugs can be added to the infusion. The contents of TPN are determined by the patient's individual nutritional requirements. TPN is not infused through a peripheral vein (veins in the hands and arms) but rather through a central vein such as the subclavian vein, superior vena cava, or internal jugular vein. Figure 18-21 shows veins commonly used to place central lines.

A central venous catheter (CVC) is often used in home care. The CVC may be used for antibiotic therapy, fluid replacement, chemotherapy, hyperalimentation, narcotic pain control, and blood components. This device prevents repeated venipunctures for management of patients with cancer or malnutrition and those with long-term needs for antibiotic therapy. Central lines may also be used for drawing blood from a patient to avoid another needlestick. Depending on the brand used, the CVC may be called a Hickman, Broviac, or Groshong. The line is placed by a physician using sterile technique and local or general anesthesia. A subclavian catheter is placed for short-term use of fewer than 60 days. Tunneled catheters such as a Hickman catheter are placed for long-term use of 1 to 2 years.

Central lines are used to deliver TPN because its higher concentration of agents, such as concentrated dextrose solutions, could potentially damage peripheral veins. In addition, central lines, once established, can be left in place long term, whereas peripheral lines are inserted for short-term use. The contents of TPN can be changed on a daily basis as the physical and caloric needs of the patient change.

PEDIATRIC DOSAGE CALCULATIONS

Several rules are used to calculate dosages for infants and children's dosages such as Young's rule, Clark's rule, and Fried's rule, but these rules give only approximate dosages. Even when pediatric drug dosages are calculated on the basis of body surface area, weight, and age of the child, they are based on a proportion of the usual adult dose (approximate).

Because of their age, weight, height, and physical condition, children are more sensitive to medications than are adults. Therefore, children are not able to tolerate adult doses of drugs. Dosage must be measured accurately according to the age and weight of infants and children. When you calculate drug dosages, do not consider a child to be a small adult. The average child does not metabolize drugs the

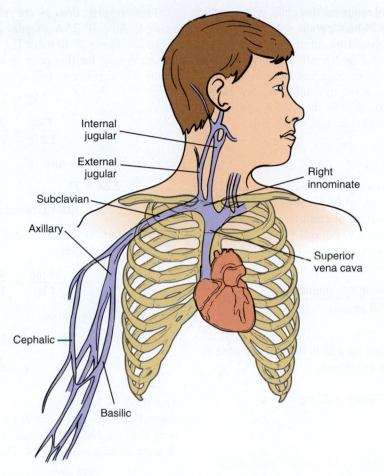

Figure 18-21. Common veins used for placement of central venous catheters.

way an adult does. For instance, many organ systems in infants and toddlers are immature. Responses to medications are significantly different in children from those in adults. Several methods are used for calculating dosage for this group of patients. The dosage form per kilogram or pound of body weight is more accurate than dosage calculated by age. The body surface area method is another way to measure the dosage for children. Charts are available to determine the body surface area in square meters, according to height and weight. The amount of medication to be given in 24 hours is calculated and then divided into an equal number of doses. The number of doses is determined by the recommended frequency of administration.

Example

The order is for ampicillin 125 mg PO qid for a child weighing 26.44 lb. On hand is ampicillin suspension 125 mg/5 mL. The recommended daily PO dose for a child is 20 to 40 mg/kg/day in divided dosages every 8 hours.

1. Change the child's weight to kg. Remember there are 2.2 lb in each kg.

$$\frac{2.2 \text{ lb}}{26.44 \text{ lb}} \times \frac{1 \text{ kg}}{X \text{ kg}}$$

$$\frac{2.2}{1} = \frac{26.44}{X}$$

$$2.2X = 26.44$$

$$X = \frac{26.44}{2.2}$$

$X = 12.01$ kg (which you then round down to 12 kg)

2. Write a proportion(s) using the recommended dosage and child's weight as your known values to determine the safe recommended dosage or range for this child.

$$20 \text{ mg} \times 1 \text{ kg} = X \text{ mg} \times 12 \text{ kg}$$

$$20 \times 1 = X \times 12 \text{ kg}$$

$$X = 20 \times 12$$

$$X = 240 \text{ mg}$$

$$40 \text{ mg} \times 1 \text{ kg} = X \text{ mg} \times 12 \text{ kg}$$

$$21 \times 1 = X \times 12$$

$$X = 40 \times 12$$

$$X = 480 \text{ mg}$$

The safe recommended range for this child, who weighs 12 kg, is 240 to 480 mg in a 24-hour period.

Many drugs are not advised for administration to children because of their potential for harmful side effects in the growing child or because they have not been sufficiently tested in children to give a recommended dosage range. Three formulas are used to calculate dosage for infants and children: Clark's rule, Young's rule, and Fried's rule.

Clark's Rule

Clark's rule is based on the weight of the child. This system is much more accurate than other pediatric methods, because the size and body weight of children of any age can vary greatly. Clark's rule uses 150 pounds (70 kg) as the average adult weight and assumes that the child's dose is proportionately less.

$$\text{Pediatric dose} = \frac{\text{Child's weight in pounds}}{150 \text{ pounds}} \times \text{Adult dose}$$

Example

Find the dose of cortisone for a 30-lb infant (adult dose = 100 mg). The calculation is as follows:

$$\frac{30}{150} \times 100 \text{ mg} = 20 \text{ mg}$$

Young's Rule

Young's rule is used for children older than 1 year of age.

$$\text{Pediatric dose} = \frac{\text{Child's age in years}}{\text{Child's age in years} + 12} \times \text{Adult dose}$$

Example

Find the dose of acetaminophen for a 4-year-old child (adult dose = 1000 mg). The calculation is as follows:

$$\frac{4 \text{ (years)}}{4 \text{ (years)} + 12} \times 1000 \text{ mg} = \frac{4000}{16} = 250 \text{ mg}$$

Note that Young's rule is not valid after 12 years of age. If the child is small enough to warrant a reduced dose after 12 years of age, the reduction should be calculated on the basis of Clark's rule.

Fried's Rule

Fried's rule is a method of estimating the dose of medication for infants younger than 1 year of age.

$$\frac{\text{Age in months}}{150} \times \text{average adult dose} = \text{child's dose}$$

Example

Find the dose of phenobarbital for a 15-month-old infant (adult dose = 400 mg). The calculation is as follows:

$$\frac{15}{150} \times 400 \text{ mg} = 40 \text{ mg}$$

Pediatric drug dosages are calculated in three steps. For example, Amoxil® 25 mg/kg/day given every 12 hours is being ordered for a 24-lb baby. The first step in calculating the correct dosage for this baby is to convert pounds to kilograms. The conversion rule is

$$1 \text{ kg} = 2.2 \text{ lb}$$

$$\frac{1 \text{ kg}}{2.2 \text{ lb}} = \frac{X \text{ kg}}{24 \text{ lb}}$$

Cross-multiply this ratio:

$$2.2X = 24$$

$$X = 10.9 \text{ kg (round up to 11.0 kg)}$$

The next step is to calculate the drug dosage based on 25 mg/kg of body weight:

$$\frac{25 \text{ mg}}{1 \text{ kg}} = \frac{X \text{ mg}}{11 \text{ kg}}$$

Cross-multiply this ratio:

$$X \text{ mg} = 275$$

$$X = \frac{275 \text{ mg}}{24 \text{ hr}}$$

The third and final step is to calculate out how much Amoxil® this patient receives per dose. Remember, the patient is to receive a dose once every 12 hours or 2 divided doses in one 24-hour period. The calculation is as follows:

$$\frac{275 \text{ mg}}{2} = 137.5 \text{ mg per dose}$$

Amoxil® is available in 250 mg/5 mL dosages so the exact number of milliliters to give the patient per dose needs to be calculated:

$$\frac{250 \text{ mg}}{5 \text{ mL}} = \frac{137.5 \text{ mg}}{X \text{ mL}}$$

Cross-multiply this ratio:

$$250 X = 687.5$$

$$\frac{687.5}{250 X}$$

$$X = 2.75 \text{ mL}$$

Therefore, the patient would receive 2.75 mL of Amoxil® every 12 hours.

Calculating drug dosages for the pediatric patient is not as time-consuming as it initially appears. After a technician has practiced doing several dosage calculations, he or she will soon become proficient.

West's Nomogram

West's nomogram uses a calculation of the body surface area (BSA) of infants and young children to determine the pediatric dose. Many physicians use the **nomogram** as a quick reference for pediatric doses (see Figure 18-22).

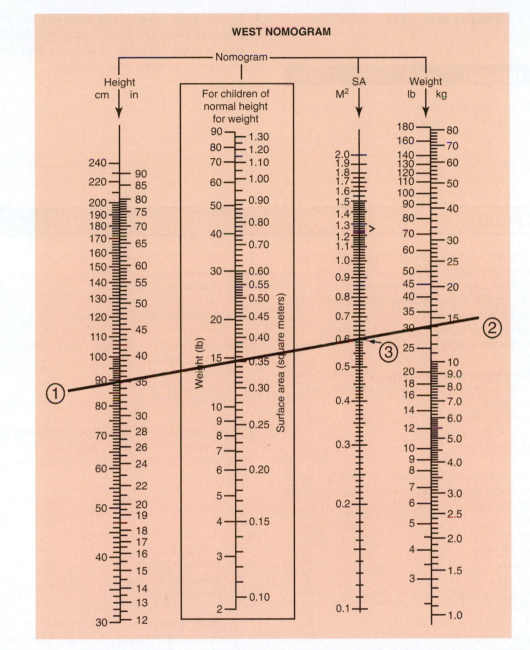

WEST NOMOGRAM

Figure 18-22. The West nomogram. (From Behrman RE, Kliegman RM, Jenson HB (Eds): *Nelson Textbook of Pediatrics,* 16th ed. Philadelphia: WB Saunders, 2000. Reprinted with permission.)

The nomogram is used to calculate BSA in square meters (or m²).

$$\text{Pediatric dose} = \frac{\text{Body surface area (BSA) of child in m}^2}{1.7 \text{ m}^2 \text{ (average adult BSA)}} \times$$

Adult dose

BSA is also important for determination of medication doses for burn victims and for patients undergoing open heart surgery, chemotherapy, and radiation therapy. The calculation of the dose to administer by BSA and nomogram is as follows.

1. Calculate the patient's BSA.
2. Calculate the desired dose.

Dosage ordered × BSA = desired dose

3. Confirm whether or not the desired dose is safe. If it is unsafe, consult the physician who wrote the order.
4. Calculate the amount to administer, using fraction equation, ratio and proportion, or the formula method.

Example

The child's BSA is 0.65 m². The recommended dosage is 0.4 mg/m². Determine the child's dose.

$$\text{Pediatric dose} = \frac{0.65 \text{ m}^2}{1.7 \text{ m}^2} \times 0.4 \text{ mg/m}^2 = 0.65 \times \frac{0.4}{1.7} = \frac{0.260}{1.7}$$

Pediatric dose = 0.15

CRITICAL THINKING

1. Insulin may be administered in U-40, U-80, and U-100 dosage forms. U-100 insulin is equivalent to
   A. 1 mL.
   B. 5 mL.
   C. 10 mL.

2. In case of severe pathologic hypersecretory conditions, a physician may order Zantac® up to 6 g /day. If the patient is to be given 1.5 g/day divided into four doses, what is the amount to administer per dose?

REVIEW QUESTIONS

1. One of the most important functions of pharmacy service is to ensure that patients get
   A. the intended drug in the correct amount.
   B. an order of medication in a dosage that is different from stocked medications.
   C. formulas and mathematical tables of conversion.
   D. appropriate equipment.

2. There are four methods for drug dosage calculations: basic formula, ratio and proportion, fractional equation, and
   A. right technique.
   B. complex calculations.
   C. dimensional analysis.
   D. individualized dosing.

3. In the basic formula used to calculate drug dosage, the D stands for *desired dose* and the V stands for *vehicle*. What does the H stand for?
   A. Heparin
   B. Hepatic level
   C. On-hand dose
   D. Handy dose

4. Which is the oldest method used for calculating dosage?
   A. Conversion
   B. Basic formula
   C. Means and extremes
   D. Ratio and proportion

5. Which dose calculation method is also known as the *label factor method*?
   A. Drug dose
   B. Apothecary equivalent
   C. Ratio and proportion
   D. Dimensional analysis

6. A generic name is also known as a _____ name.
   A. nonproprietary
   B. proprietary
   C. brand
   D. genetic

7. The form of a drug identifies its
   A. solid particles.
   B. structure and composition.
   C. full quantity.
   D. suspension and constitution.

8. By federal law, all medications must be identified with
   A. control numbers.
   B. drug recalls.
   C. powdered forms.
   D. alerts.

9. No more than _____ variation should exist between the dose ordered and the dose administered.
   A. 0.9%
   B. 5%
   C. 10%
   D. 15%

10. Insulin is ordered and measured in
    A. NPH units.
    B. cubic centimeters.
    C. milligrams.
    D. USP units.

11. A patient is supposed to receive 30 mL of a medication. There is no measuring cup available. What is an equivalent dose?
    A. 2 tsp
    B. 4 tsp
    C. 6 tsp
    D. 10 tsp

12. A standard U-100 insulin syringe can hold up to
    A. 10 U.
    B. 1.0 U.
    C. 100 U.
    D. 10.01 U.

Continues

13. 0.08 g = _____mg.
   A. 8
   B. 80
   C. 800
   D. ⅛

14. 0.008 L = _____ mL.
   A. 4
   B. 8
   C. 80
   D. 0.08

15. An oral medication comes in a bottle labeled 5 U/cc. The dose to be administered is 25 U. Which of the following is the correct dose?
   A. 25 mL
   B. 25 cc
   C. 5 cc
   D. 0.25 mL

16. The dose of a liquid medication for oral administration is ¾ oz. Which of the following is the correct equivalent dose?
   A. 20 mL
   B. 25 mL
   C. 7.5 dr
   D. 1.5 tbsp

17. To convert grams to milligrams, you should move the decimal point
   A. four spaces to the right.
   B. two spaces to the right.
   C. three spaces to the left.
   D. three spaces to the right.

18. If an order is for Lopressor® 100 mg PO bid, but the pharmacy only has 50 mg tablets on hand, how many tablets per day should this patient receive in total?
   A. 2
   B. 10
   C. 4
   D. 5

19. Amoxicillin 500 mg PO qid is prescribed, but the dose on hand is 250 mg/5 mL. Which of the following dosages is correct?
   A. 5 g
   B. 5 mL
   C. 10 mL
   D. 15 mL

20. Kanamycin 1 g is prescribed, but the amount on hand is 500 mg. How many capsules should be given?
   A. 1 capsule
   B. 2 capsules
   C. 3 capsules
   D. 4 capsules

21. Motrin® 750 mg has been ordered, but the only available tablets are 300 mg each. How many tablets, if scored, should the patient take?
   A. 3
   B. 4
   C. 2½
   D. 3½

22. An order is given for gentamicin 60 mg IM. The available dosage strength of gentamicin is 80 mg/2 mL in a vial. Using the formula $^D/_H \times V$, determine how many milliliters should be given to the patient?
   A. 0.015 mL
   B. 0.15 mL
   C. 1.5 mL
   D. 15 mL

23. The physician's order is for atropine 0.2 mg, but the drug is available at a dosage of 400 mcg/mL (which is 0.4 mg/mL). Using the formula $^D/_H \times V$, determine how many milliliters should be given to the patient?
   A. 0.2 mL
   B. 0.4 mL
   C. 1 mL
   D. 0.5 mL

24. If 10,000 U = 1 mL, how many mL does 7,500 U equal?
   A. 0.075 mL
   B. 0.75 mL
   C. 7.5 mL
   D. 0.175 mL

25. A physician's order is for D5W 1000 mL containing 20,000 U of heparin, which is to be infused at 30 mL/hr. How much heparin is the patient to receive per hour?
   A. 60,000 U/hr
   B. 6,000 U/hr
   C. 600 U/hr
   D. 60 U/hr

26. A vial of powdered penicillin G contains 1 million units. The amount of diluent to be added to obtain a solution that contains 100,000 U/mL is
   A. 1 mL.
   B. 10 mL.
   C. 100 mL.
   D. 1 L.

27. An order of D5W 500 mL with heparin 25,000 U IV at 1,000 U/hr is received. What is the flow rate, in mL/hr? Use the formula $^D/_H \times Q$.
   A. 500 mL/hr
   B. 50 mL/hr
   C. 200 mL/hr
   D. 20 mL/hr

Continues

28. An order has been received for D5W 250 mL with heparin 25,000 U IV at 750 U/hr. Calculate the flow rate in mL/hr.
    A. 750 mL/hr
    B. 75 mL/hr
    C. 15 mL/hr
    D. 150 mL/hr

29. A patient must have 500 mL of intravenous fluids infused over 2 hours. Calculate the flow rate by using the formula (total amount ordered in mL)/(total number of hours).
    A. 500 mL/hr
    B. 250 mL/hr
    C. 25 mL/hr
    D. 50 mL/hr

30. A patient must have 500 mg of an IV antibiotic in a 100 mL bag infused over 30 minutes. Calculate the flow rate, remembering that 60 minutes = 1 hour.
    A. 20 mL/hr
    B. 200 mL/hr
    C. 30 mL hr
    D. 300 mL/hr

31. A patient must receive 200 cc of intravenous fluids over 2 hours. The macrodrop tubing which will be used has a drop factor of 20 gtt/min. How many drops per minute are needed to infuse the entire 200 cc over 30 minutes? Remember to convert the 2 hours into minutes to help solve this problem.
    A. 33.3 gtt/min
    B. 66.6 gtt/min
    C. 99.9 gtt/min
    D. 120 gtt/min

32. 0.9% NS, 500 mL, with 200 U of regular insulin must be infused at 10 U/hr. The drop factor is 60. After figuring the amount of drug per milliliter, determine how many mL will be infused in 1 hour.
    A. 42 mL/hr
    B. 25 mL/hr
    C. 52 mL/hr
    D. 2.5 mL/hr

33. Ampicillin 125 mg PO qid is prescribed for a child who weighs 26.44 pounds. Available is an ampicillin suspension 125 mg/5 mL. The recommended daily PO dose for a child is 20 to 40 mg/kg/day in divided dosages every 8 hours. Remembering to change the child's weight to kilograms (there are 2.2 lb in 1 kg), determine the recommended safe dosage range, in mg.
    A. 24 to 48 mg
    B. 240 to 480 mg
    C. 12 to 24 mg
    D. 120 to 240 mg

34. Clark's rule, which is the *weight of the child/150 × the average adult dose*, should be used to determine the child's dose in the following scenario. How much cortisone should be given to a 30-lb infant if the adult dose is 100 mg?
    A. 20 mg
    B. 2 mg
    C. 3 mg
    D. 30 mg

35. Young's rule uses the formula *child's age divided by age plus 12, multiplied by the average adult dose* to calculate pediatric doses. If a child patient is 6 years old, and the average adult dose is 100 mg, what is the pediatric dose for this child?
    A. 6 mg
    B. 18 mg
    C. 33.3 mg
    D. 24 mg

36. Using Fried's rule, find the dose of phenobarbital for a 15-month-old infant. Fried's rule is *age in months/150 × average adult dose*. The average adult dose in this scenario is 400 mg.
    A. 15 mg
    B. 150 mg
    C. 45 mg
    D. 40 mg

37. West's nomogram is used to calculate pediatric doses on the basis of body surface area (BSA). If a certain child's BSA is 0.65 m² and the recommended dosage is 0.4 mg/m², determine the child's dose for this patient.
    A. 1.5 mg
    B. 0.15 mg
    C. 0.015 mg
    D. 150 mg

38. If 1 kg equals approximately 2.2 lb, how many pounds are equivalent to 50 kg?
    A. 110 lb
    B. 1.1 lb
    C. 111 lb
    D. 100 lb

39. If 1 lb equals 0.45 kg, how many kg are in 69 lb?
    A. 50.13 kg
    B. 31.05 kg
    C. 35.01 kg
    D. 53 kg

40. In the U-100 insulin syringe, 100 U = _____ mL.
    A. 1
    B. 10
    C. 100
    D. 0.1

Continues

41. Calculate one dose of the following: Demerol® syrup 75 mg PO q4h prn pain. On hand is Demerol® syrup 50 mg/5 mL. One dose equals how many mL?
    A. 75 mL
    B. 7.5 mL
    C. 0.75 mL
    D. 750 mL

42. The order is for Trilisate® liquid 750 mg PO tid. On hand is a supply of Trilisate® liquid 250 mg/2.5 mL. What is one dose, in mL?
    A. 2.57 mL
    B. 7.25 mL
    C. 7.5 mL
    D. 75 mL

43. Maalox Plus® is available in 30 mL containers. The order is for 30 mL PO 30 min pc and hs. How many containers will be needed for a 24-hour period?
    A. 1
    B. 2
    C. 3
    D. 4

44. The order is for Orinase® 250 mg PO bid. On hand is Orinase® 0.5 g tablets. How many tablets, which are scored in half, are correct for one dose?
    A. ½
    B. 1
    C. 1½
    D. 2

45. The order is for V-Cillin K® 300,000 U PO qid. On hand is V-Cillin K® 200,000 U/5 mL. What is one dose, in mL?
    A. 7 mL
    B. 17 mL
    C. 7.5 mL
    D. 7.75 mL

46. Coumadin® is ordered as follows: 7.5 mg PO qd. On hand are 2.5 mg tablets of Coumadin®. How many tablets constitute one dose?
    A. 1 tablet
    B. 2 tablets
    C. 3 tablets
    D. 4 tablets

47. There are 60 U of U-100 insulin per _____ mL.
    A. 6
    B. 0.6
    C. 60
    D. 0.06

48. If Demerol® 20 mg IM q3-4h prn pain is ordered, how much Demerol® should be administered in a 24-hour period?
    A. 20 to 60 mg/day
    B. 100 to 200 mg/day
    C. 120 to 160 mg/day
    D. 240 to 320 mg/day

49. The order is for Garamycin® 40 mg IM q8h. On hand is Garamycin® 80 mg/2 mL. How many mL constitute one dose?
    A. 1 mL
    B. 2 mL
    C. 3 mL
    D. 10 mL

50. The order is for neostigmine 0.5 mg IM tid. On hand is neostigmine 1:2000. How many mL constitute one dose?
    A. 0.1 mL
    B. ½ mL
    C. 1 mL
    D. 2 mL

51. A dose of 225 mcg is equal to
    A. 225 mg.
    B. 2.25 mg.
    C. 22.5 mg.
    D. 0.225 mg.

52. Ampicillin 500 mg IM q4h is ordered, and ampicillin 500 mg is on hand. If the ampicillin is reconstituted with 1.8 mL diluent for a concentration of 250 mg/mL, what does one dose consist of, in mL?
    A. 20 mL
    B. 22 mL
    C. 2 mL
    D. 1 mL

53. Cefepime 500 mg IM q12h is ordered, and 1 g of cefepime is on hand. If cefepime is reconstituted with 2.4 mL diluent for an approximate volume of 3.6 mL at a concentration of 280 mg/mL, what does one dose consist of, in mL?
    A. 18 mL
    B. 1.8 mL
    C. 24 mL
    D. 3.18 mL

54. Ticar® 4 g IV q6h is ordered. On hand is Ticar® 200 mg/mL. The recommended adult dosage is 200 to 300 mg/kg/day q4-6h. The patient weights 150 lb. By converting the patient's weight to kilograms (1 lb = 0.45 kg), determine the amount to be given IV every 6 hours, in mL.
    A. 2 mL
    B. 12 mL
    C. 20 mL
    D. 120 mL

Continues

55. Lanoxin® 0.15 mg PO q12h is ordered for a child who weighs 31.8 kg. If the recommended dosage is 7 mcg/kg/day, how much should be given to this child over the course of 24 hours?
   A. 22 mg/day
   B. 1.22 mg/day
   C. 0.22 mg/day
   D. 2.2 mg/day

56. 12 lb = _____ kg.
   A. 5.1
   B. 1.5
   C. 5
   D. 5.4

57. If D5W 1000 mL is ordered, how much dextrose is contained in this mixture?
   A. 5 g
   B. 5 mg
   C. 50 g
   D. 50 mg

58. If D51/4 NS 500 mL is ordered, how much sodium chloride is contained in the mixture?
   A. 25 g
   B. 1.5 g
   C. 2.15 g
   D. 1.125 g

59. If the total amount ordered is 1000 mL, and this must be infused over 3 hours, approximately how many mL will be infused in just 30 minutes?
   A. 111.1 mL
   B. 166.6 mL
   C. 133.3 mL
   D. 333.3 mL

60. NS IV 3000 mL is to be infused over 24 hours, and the drop factor is 15 gtt/min. How many drops per minute will be required to accomplish this infusion?
   A. 3 gtt/min
   B. 13 gtt/min
   C. 30 gtt/min
   D. 31 gtt/min

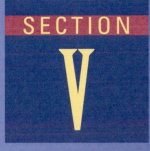

Drug Classification

Biopharmaceutics

19

OUTLINE

OBJECTIVES

Upon completion of this chapter, the reader should be able to

1. Describe the mechanisms of drug action and define pharmacokinetic and pharmacodynamic.
2. Explain drug half-life.
3. Describe the process of filtration, secretion, and reabsorption for renal excretion of drugs.
4. Define the cytochrome P-450 enzyme pathways.
5. Describe factors affecting drug action.
6. Explain therapeutic index.
7. Differentiate side effects and adverse effects.
8. Define idiosyncratic and anaphylactic reactions.

GLOSSARY

absorption The movement of a drug from its site of administration into the bloodstream.

agonist The drug that produces a functional change in a cell.

amide A chemical compound formed from an organic acid by the substitution of an amino (NR_2) group for the hydroxyl of a carboxyl (COOH) group.

bioavailability Measurement of the rate of absorption and total amount of drug that reach the systemic circulation.

biotransformation The conversion of a drug within the body; also known as metabolism.

conjugation The biosynthetic process of combining a chemical compound with a highly polar and water-soluble natural substance to yield a water-soluble, usually inactive, product.

distribution The process by which blood leaves the bloodstream and enters the tissues of the body.

diffusion Particles in a fluid move from an area of higher concentration to an area of lower concentration, resulting in a even distribution of the particles in the fluid.

ester A class of chemical compounds formed by the bonding of an alcohol and one or more organic acids. Fats are esters, produced by the bonding of fatty acids with the alcohol glycerol.

filtration The movement of water and dissolved substances from the glomerulus to the Bowman's capsule.

first-pass effect The drug reaches the liver where it is partially metabolized before being sent to the body.

glomerular filtration rate (GFR) The rate of filtration in the kidney.

half-life The time it takes for the plasma concentration to be reduced by 50%.

hydrolysis The process of adding a water molecule to split a molecule into smaller portions.

idiosyncratic reaction Experience of a unique, strange, or unpredicted reaction to a drug.

metabolism The conversion of a drug within the body; also known as biotransformation.

oxidation The process by which oxygen combines with another chemical; the removal of hydrogen or the loss of electrons.

GLOSSARY continued

pharmacodynamics The study of the biochemical and physiological effects of drugs.

pharmacokinetics The study of the absorption, distribution, metabolism, and excretion of drugs.

placebo Sugar pill.

reabsorption The movement of water and selected substances from the tubules to the peritubular capillaries.

receptor The cell that a drug has an affinity to.

specific affinity The attraction a drug has for particular cells.

tolerance Reduced responsiveness of a drug because of adaptation to it.

tubular secretion The active secretion of substances such as potassium from the peritubular capillaries into the tubules.

OVERVIEW

The biochemical and physiological properties of drugs, as well as their mechanisms of action, differ widely. In clinical applications, however, drugs must penetrate, be absorbed by, and be distributed among the body tissues. The usual route of drug administration and mode of termination of their use should also be considered. Certain general principles help explain these differences. These principles have both pharmaceutic and therapeutic implications. For action, a drug must be absorbed, transported to the target tissue or organ, and then it must penetrate into the cell membranes and their organelles and alter the ongoing processes. The drug may be distributed to a number of tissues, bound or stored and metabolized to inactive or active products. Then it must be excreted.

PHARMACOKINETICS

Pharmacokinetics is the study of the action of drugs within the body, including the mechanisms of absorption, distribution, metabolism, and excretion. It also encompasses the onset of action, duration of effect, biotransformation, and effects and route of excretion of the metabolites of the drug.

Drug Absorption

The movement of a drug from its site of administration into the bloodstream is **absorption**. In general, the process may be achieved through diffusion or active transport, and the barriers to that movement are largely lipid in nature. In many cases, a drug must be transported across one or more biological membranes to reach the blood circulation. The most common and important mode of traversal of drugs through membranes is **diffusion**. This process depends upon the lipid solubility of the drug. Agents that are relatively lipid soluble diffuse more rapidly than less lipid-soluble drugs. Diffusion is the process in which particles in a fluid move from an area of higher concentration to an area of lower concentration, resulting in an even distribution of the particles in the fluid. This mechanism requires little or no energy.

Generally, absorption takes place through the digestive system unless an agent is administered directly into the bloodstream by injection into the veins, arteries, muscles, or other sites for administration by injection. The digestive system is the most convenient, economical, and common route of administration and generally safe for most drugs. Lipid-soluble drugs and weak acids may be absorbed directly from the stomach. Weak bases are not normally absorbed from this site. The small intestine is the primary site of absorption because of the very large surface area across which drugs may diffuse. Acids are normally absorbed more extensively from the intestine than from the stomach, even though the intestine has a higher pH.

Factors Influencing Absorption

The gastrointestinal tract absorption of drugs may be influenced by many factors. These factors include physiochemical properties, acidity of the stomach, presence of food in the stomach, dosage, and routes of administration.

Physiochemical Properties The rate of absorption of a drug may be affected greatly by the rate at which the drug is made available to the biological fluid at the site of administration. Intrinsic physiochemical properties, such as solubility and the thermodynamics of dissolution, are only some of the factors that affect the rate of dissolution of a drug from a solid form.

Acidity of the Stomach Drugs with an acidic pH, such as aspirin, are easily absorbed in the acid environment of the stomach, whereas alkaline medications are more readily absorbed in the alkaline environment of the small intestine. Milk products and antacids tend to change the pH of the stomach. Therefore, some drugs are not absorbed properly. The infant who is consuming formula or milk may need to be given medications on an empty stomach because regular feedings will change the stomach acid level.

Presence of Food in Stomach The presence of food in the stomach or intestine can have a profound influence on the rate and extent of drug absorption. Food in the stomach decreases the absorption rate of medications, whereas an empty stomach increases the rate. Sometimes the drug must be effective quickly, requiring the stomach to be empty. If the medication causes irritation of the stomach, food should be eaten to serve as a buffer and decrease irritation.

Routes of Administration Drugs can be administered under the tongue (sublingual), inner lining of the cheeks (buccal), or within the rectum (rectal). These routes are logical because they protect drugs from chemical decomposition that might occur in the stomach or liver. Drugs given orally are usually absorbed in the upper gastrointestinal tract and are immediately exposed to metabolism by the liver enzymes before reaching the systemic circulation. This exposure is called the **first-pass effect**: the drug reaches the liver, where it is partly metabolized before being sent to the body for systemic effects. Therefore, medications that are metabolized too rapidly in the liver cannot be given orally. Some examples of drugs that exhibit first-pass metabolism include acetylsalicylic acid, alprenolol, dopamine, imipramine, lidocaine, morphine, propranolol, and verapamil. The choice of the administration route is crucial in determining the suitability of a drug for each patient. When the drug is injected directly into the bloodstream (vein or artery) and distributes throughout the body, it acts rapidly and the process of absorption is bypassed. The time for this injection is typically short compared with the times for other pharmacokinetic processes that are ignored. The drug may be injected deeply into a skeletal muscle. The rate of absorption depends on the vascularity of the muscle site and the lipid solubility of the drug. If it is injected beneath the skin, drug absorption is less rapid, because the subcutaneous region is less vascular than the muscle tissues. Topical drugs may be absorbed through several layers of skin for local absorption. Nitroglycerin commonly is applied to the skin in the form of an ointment or transdermal patches; it is absorbed rapidly and provides sustained blood levels. Drugs administered in high concentrations tend to be more rapidly absorbed than those administered in low concentrations. Sometimes, a drug may be initially administered in large doses that temporarily exceed the body's capacity to absorb them.

Drug Distribution

The process by which drug molecules leave the bloodstream and enter the tissues of the body is called **distribution**. When a drug reaches the bloodstream it is ready to travel through blood, lymphatics, and other fluids to its site of action. To reach sites beyond the major organs, a drug may have to pass over the lipid membranes. Lipid solubility is important for effective distribution in this case. The initial rate of distribution of a drug is heavily dependent on the blood flow to various organs. Lipid-soluble drugs enter the central nervous system rapidly. Because of the nature of the blood-brain barrier, ionized drugs are poorly distrib-

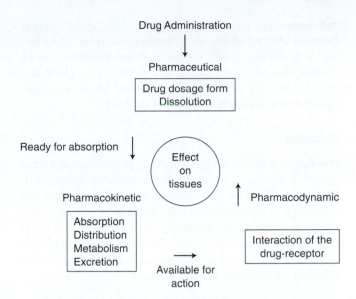

Figure 19-1. The effect of drug administration on drug action.

uted to their desired site because they must pass through this barrier. The clinician must always consider the possibility that drugs administered to the mother may cross the placenta and reach the fetus. Drugs are often bound to plasma proteins, particularly albumin. Albumin is the principal protein of plasma in terms of drug binding. If these drugs are bound to albumin, they are known as inactive drugs, whereas those that are unbound are called pharmacologically active drugs. If binding is extensive and firm, it will have a considerable impact upon the distribution and excretion of the drug in the body. Obviously, a drug that is bound to a protein cannot be filtered by the kidneys, and in general, is pharmacologically inert. Only the unbound form can pass among the various compartments of the body. Drug administration and its effect on drug action are shown in Figure 19-1.

Drug Metabolism

The overwhelming majority of drugs undergo **metabolism** after they enter the body. In most cases, biotransformation can terminate the pharmacological action of the drug and increase removal of the drug from the body. Most drugs are acted upon by enzymes in the body and are converted to metabolic derivatives during metabolism. The process of conversion is called **biotransformation**. The liver is the major site of biotransformation. Many biotransformations in the liver occur in the smooth endoplasmic reticulum of the hepatocytes. Numerous enzymes, which biotransform many drugs, are present in the endoplasmic reticulum. These drug-metabolizing enzymes are often called microsomal enzymes. One of these enzymes is cytochrome P-450, which has a very important role in drug metabolism. The reaction products that are produced by the action of these enzymes are known as metabolites. The majority of these metabolites are inactive and toxic. Drug metabolism influences drug action, such as duration of drug effects, drug interactions, drug activation, and drug toxicity or side effects. Biotransformations may be divided into four main categories: (1) oxidation, (2) reduction, (3) hydrolysis, and (4) conjugation. These occur primarily in the microsomal system of the liver.

Oxidation

Oxidation is the process in which oxygen content of a compound is increased, including the removal of hydrogen or the loss of electrons. Oxidation is more common than any other type of biotransformation. Oxidation that occurs primarily in the liver microsomal system includes side-chain hydroxylation and deamination. Examples are the oxidation of alcohols by alcohol dehydrogenase and the oxidation of aldehyde by aldehyde dehydrogenase.

Reduction

Reductions are relatively uncommon. They occur mainly in liver microsomes, but they occasionally take place in other tissues. Examples are the reduction of nitro and nitroso groups (as in chloramphenicol, nitroglycerin, and organic nitrites) and of certain aldehydes to corresponding alcohols.

Hydrolysis

Hydrolysis is the processing of adding a water molecule to split a molecule into smaller portions. Hydrolysis, which occurs during digestion, breaks down large molecules into smaller ones. It is a common biotransformation among **esters** and **amides**. Esterases are located in many structures besides the microsomes. For example, cholinesterases are found in plasma, erythrocytes (red blood cells), the liver, and nerve terminals. Procaine esterases are found in plasma.

Conjugation

A large number of drugs or their metabolites are conjugated. **Conjugation** is the biosynthetic process of combining a chemical compound with a highly polar and water-soluble natural substance to yield a water-soluble, usually inactive, product. Formation of glucuronide conjugate represents one of the major degradative processes involved in drug detoxification and inactivation. Glucuronic acid is the most common partner to the drug in conjugation. Although most conjugations occur in the liver, some occur in the kidney or in other tissues. All drug conjugation reactions are catalyzed by specialized enzymes present in multiple forms.

Drug Excretion

Drugs may be excreted from the body by many routes, including urine, feces (unabsorbed drugs and those secreted in the bile), saliva, sweat, milk, lungs (alcohols and anesthetics), and tears. Any route may be important for a given drug, but the kidney is the major site of excretion for most drugs. Unchanged drugs or drug metabolites can be eliminated by the kidneys. Drugs and their metabolites may undergo three processes during renal excretion: (1) filtration, (2) secretion, and (3) reabsorption.

Filtration

Urine formation begins in the glomerulus and Bowman's capsule in the kidneys. **Filtration** causes water and dissolved substances to move from the glomerulus into Bowman's capsule. Filtration occurs when the pressure on one side of a membrane is greater than the pressure on the opposite side. Substances with small molecules such as water, sodium, potassium, chloride, glucose, uric acid, and creatinine move through the wall of the glomerulus very easily. These substances are filtered in proportion to their plasma concentration. In other words, if the concentration of a particular substance or drug in the plasma is high, many of these substances are filtered (see Figure 19-2). Approximately one fifth of the plasma reaching the kidney is filtered. The rate of filtration is referred to as the **glomerular filtration rate (GFR)** and is normally 125 to 130 mL/min.

Secretion

Although most water and dissolved substances enter the tubules because of filtration across the glomerulus, a second process moves very small amounts of substances from the blood into the tubules. This is called **tubular secretion**. It involves the active secretion of substances such as potassium ions (K^+), hydrogen ions (H^+), uric acid, the ammonium ion, and drugs from the peritubular capillaries into the tubules. Secretion occurs primarily in the proximal convoluted tubule. This is an active process mediated by two carrier systems, one specific for organic acids and one specific for organic bases. Therefore, the pH of the urine may affect the rate of drug excretion by changing the chemical form of a drug to one that can be more readily excreted or to one that can be reabsorbed. Penicillins or barbiturates are weak acids and are available as sodium or potassium salts. These agents can be better excreted if the urine pH is less acid. On the other hand, any drug that is available as a sulfate, hydrochloride, or nitrate salt, such as atropine or morphine, can be excreted better if the urine is more acidic. By altering the pH of urine, increased elimination of certain drugs can be facilitated, thus preventing prolonged action or overdosage of a toxic compound. Another technique to alter the rate of excretion of a drug is to produce a competitive blocking effect. For example, probenecid may be used to block the renal excretion of penicillin. This prolongs the effect of the antibiotic by maintenance of a higher therapeutic plasma level. Secretions of drugs are active transport systems. They require energy and may become saturated.

Reabsorption

Reabsorption may occur throughout the tubules of the nephrons. It causes water and selected substances to move from the tubules into the peritubular capillaries. The mechanism

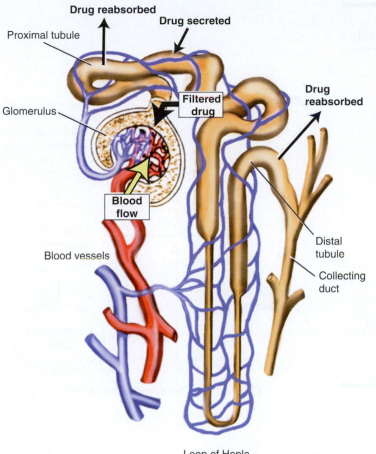

Figure 19-2. Renal excretion of drugs. Note sites where drugs are secreted and reabsorbed.

is passive diffusion; therefore, only the un-ionized form of a drug is reabsorbed. Reabsorption depends on the lipid solubility of a drug. For example, the kidneys selectively reabsorb substances such as glucose, proteins, and sodium, which they have already secreted into the renal tubules. These reabsorbed substances return to the blood.

PHARMACODYNAMICS

Pharmacodynamics is the study of the biochemical and physiological effects of drugs. It is also defined as the study of the mechanisms of action of drugs. A basic understanding of the factors that control drug concentration at the site of action is important for the optimal use of drugs. This is the area of study referred to as pharmacokinetics, as discussed earlier. Blood represents the fluid most commonly sampled to characterize the pharmacokinetics of drugs. The drugs must dissolve before being absorbed. They must pass across many lipoid barriers and some metabolizing systems before reaching the site of action. Table 19-1 shows the factors that may influence onset, duration, and intensity of drug effects.

Usually there are links between pharmacokinetics and pharmacodynamics that demonstrate the relationship between drug dose and blood or other biological fluid concentrations. The pharmacological response by itself does not provide information about some very important determinants of that response, for example, dose or drug concentration in plasma or at the site of action. Pharmacokinetic and pharmacodynamics can determine the dose-effect relationship (see Figure 19-3).

Drug Action

Drugs produce their effects by altering the normal function of the cells and tissues of the body. Correct cells are chosen because a particular drug has a **specific affinity** for a particular cell. The specific cell recipient is called a **receptor**, and the drug that has the affinity for it and produces a functional change in the cell is known as the **agonist**. Not all drugs that bind to specific cells cause a functional change in the cell. These drugs act as antagonists to the natural process and work by blocking a sequence of biochemical events. Some drugs may act by affecting the enzyme functions of the body. When drugs are metabolized in the liver, they produce antimetabolites. Various factors are important in determining the correct drugs for a patient, such as age, sex, body weight, diurnal body rhythms, the presence of illnesses, psychological factors, tolerance, drug toxicity, drug interactions, and idiosyncratic reactions.

TABLE 19-1.	Factors That Influence Onset, Duration, and Intensity of Drug Effects	
FACTORS	**DRUG EFFECTS**
Absorption	Gastrointestinal
	Sublingual
	Percutaneous
	Subcutaneous
	Intramuscular
	Pulmonary and nasal
	Ocular
Metabolism	Activation
	Deactivation
	Polarization
Excretion	Urinary
	Biliary (excretion)
	Pulmonary
	Salivary
Reabsorption	Renal, tubular
	Enterohepatic
Site of action	Enzyme systems or "receptors" in specific organs
Observed response	Therapeutic
	Toxic

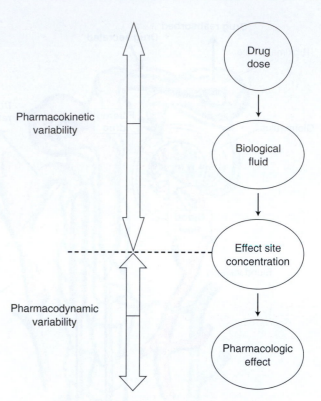

Figure 19-3. The dose-effect relationship.

Drug Half-Life

The **half-life** of a drug is the time it takes for the plasma concentration to be reduced by 50%. This is one of the most common methods used to explain drug actions. The half-life of each drug may be different; for example, a drug with a short half-life, such as 2 or 3 hours, will need to be administered more often than one with a long half-life, such as 8 hours. Another method of describing drug action is a graphic depiction of the plasma concentration of the drug versus time (see Figure 19-4).

Age

Newborns and elderly individuals show the greatest effects of a drug. Because of their ages, they are more sensitive to medications that affect the central nervous system and are at risk for development of toxic drug levels. Drug dosages for these two groups must be carefully calculated and treatment usually starts with very small doses.

Sex

Men and women respond to drugs differently. Some medications pose a risk in pregnant women because of damage to the developing fetus. In addition, certain drugs may have side effects that can stimulate uterine contractions, causing premature labor and delivery. Drugs administered intramuscularly are absorbed faster by men. They remain in women's tissues longer than in men's tissues because of higher body fat content.

Body Weight

Basically, the same dosage has less effect in a patient who weighs more and a greater effect in an individual who weighs less. Pediatric medications are designed for the body weight or body surface area of children. If adult medications are used for children, the correct dosage must be calculated and adjusted for the child's body weight.

Diurnal Body Rhythms

Diurnal (during the day) body rhythms play an important part in the effects of some drugs. For example, sedatives given in the morning will not be as effective as those administered before bedtime. On the other hand, the preferred time for corticosteroid administration is in the morning, because this best mimics the body's natural pattern of corticosteroid production and elimination.

Presence of Illnesses

Patients with liver or kidney disease may respond to drugs differently, because the body is not able to detoxify and excrete chemicals properly.

Psychological Factors

Psychological factors involve how patients feel about the drug(s) prescribed for them and the different ways they respond to them. If an individual believes in the therapy,

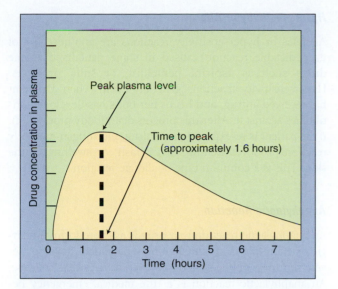

Figure 19-4. Plot of drug concentration in plasma versus time after a single oral administration of a drug.

even a **placebo** (sugar pill or sterile water thought to be a drug) may help to bring relief. Some patients cooperate in following the directions for a specific drug, and a patient's mental attitude can reduce or increase an expected response to a drug.

Tolerance

Tolerance is the phenomenon of reduced responsiveness to a drug. The body becomes so adapted to the presence of the drug that it cannot function properly without it.

Drug Toxicity

Almost all drugs are capable of producing toxic effects. There is a range between the therapeutic dose of a drug and its toxic dose. This range is measured by the therapeutic index, which is used to explain the safety of a drug. The therapeutic index is expressed in the form of a ratio:

$$\text{Therapeutic index (TI)} = \frac{LD_{50}}{ED_{50}}$$

where LD_{50} is the lethal dose of a drug that will kill 50% of animals tested and ED_{50} is the effective dose that produces a specific therapeutic effect in 50% of animals tested. The greater the therapeutic index, the safer a drug is likely to be.

There are four general mechanisms by which drugs can change the physiology of the body's cells or tissues. They include the following:

1. Nonspecific chemical or physical interactions
2. Alterations in the level of the activity of enzymes
3. Action as antimetabolites
4. Interaction with receptors

The final effect of a drug may be removed from its site of action.

Drug Interactions

Drug interactions are defined as effects of medications taken together. When two or more drugs are prescribed together, one of the following results is generally seen:

1. The drugs have no effects on each other's action.
2. The drugs increase each other's effect.
3. The drugs decrease each other's effect.

Any of these results may also be affected by the ingestion of food. Most drugs do not interact with other drugs or food, but when such interactions do occur, some may be life-threatening. Plasma protein binding can be a source of drug interaction if several drugs compete for binding sites on protein molecules. Drug interactions may result in elevated concentrations of drugs by displacement of protein-bound drugs or by reduced rates of drug disposition that result in toxic drug concentrations (see Figure 19-5).

Some drug interactions are wanted, and the medications are prescribed together to produce the desired effect. Other interactions are unintended and unwanted, producing possible dangers for the patient. Drug interactions may also cause more rapid drug disappearance, with plasma concentrations decreasing to below minimum effective values. Drug interactions often take place during the process of metabolism in the liver and result from the cytochrome P-450 enzyme pathways each person inherits. Actions of many drugs may be altered by the cytochrome P-450 system when they are taken with other drugs. Examples include many antidepressants,

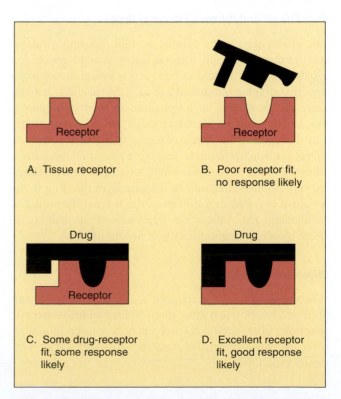

Figure 19-5. Drug-receptor interaction. Binding with specific receptors occurs only when the drug and its receptors have a compatible chemical shape.

cimetidine, ciprofloxacin, codeine, isoniazid, ketoconazole, morphine, phenobarbital, phenytoin, rifampin, tolbutamide, and warfarin. Some medications are given together because the drug interactions are helpful. For example, probenecid is given with penicillin to increase the absorption of penicillin. Other drug interactions may cause adverse effects. For example, some antibiotics make birth control pills less effective. Multiple-drug therapy should never be used without convincing evidence that each drug is beneficial beyond the possible detriments of combined administration or without proof that a therapeutically equivocal combination is definitely harmless.

Drug Bioavailability

Bioavailability is a term that indicates measurement of both the rate of drug absorption and total amount of drug that reaches the systemic blood circulation from an administered dosage form. The route of drug administration is essential for this measurement. If a drug is administered by intravenous injection, all of the dose enters the blood circulation. This is not true for drugs administered by other routes, especially for drugs given orally. Solid drugs such as tablets and capsules must dissolve. Thus, route of administration is a major source of difference in drug bioavailability. Poor solubility or incomplete absorption of a drug in the gastrointestinal tract and rapid metabolism of a drug during its first pass through the liver are other factors that influence bioavailability.

Side Effects and Adverse Effects of Drugs

Side effects are usually defined as mild, but annoying, responses to a medication. Adverse reactions or adverse effects usually are characterized as more severe symptoms or problems that develop because of a drug. Adverse effects may require the patient to be hospitalized or may even pose a threat to the patient's life. Certain side effects such as nausea may disappear if the dosage of a drug is reduced. Some side effects such as drowsiness may go away after the patient takes the medication for a while. Occasionally, side effects are very problematic, and the dispensing of the drug to the patient is stopped or a different drug is used. Examples of problematic side effects are hyperactivity or inability to sleep, bleeding, nephrotoxicity, or hepatotoxicity.

Idiosyncratic Reactions

When a patient has experienced a unique, strange, or unpredicted reaction to a drug, this is termed an **idiosyncratic reaction**. Idiosyncratic reactions may be caused by underlying enzyme deficiencies resulting from genetic or hormonal variation.

Hypersensitivity or Allergy

Allergies or hypersensitivity reactions are another type of unpredictable reaction caused in some patients by some drugs such as aspirin, penicillin, or sulfa products. Hypersensitivity reactions generally occur when a patient has received a drug, and his or her body has developed antibodies against it. After this process of antibody production, if the patient is re-exposed to the drug, the antigen-antibody reaction produces itching, hives, rash, or swelling of the skin. This is a common type of allergic reaction.

Anaphylactic Reaction

An anaphylactic reaction to a drug is a severe form of allergic reaction that is life threatening. The patient develops severe shortness of breath and may even have cardiac collapse. An anaphylactic reaction is a true medical emergency because the patient may exhibit paralysis of the diaphragm, swelling of the oropharynx, and an inability to breathe.

SUMMARY

A biological response is induced within a living organism when a drug is ingested. In this chapter absorption, distribution, metabolism, and excretion of drugs are reviewed in addition to biochemical and physiological effects of drugs. The mechanisms of drug action depend on several factors that affect pharmaceutical, pharmacokinetic, and pharmacodynamic phases. In addition, drugs may induce side effects or adverse reactions. An adverse drug effect is more serious than a side effect and is unintended, undesirable, and often unpredictable. Drug interaction is another major consideration. Multiple-drug therapy should never be used without a convincing indication that each drug is beneficial and less or not harmful when used in combination with other drugs.

CRITICAL THINKING

1. Explain why you would not give the same dose of drug to a child as to an adult. What processes are involved? How do these processes differ in children and adults? How are they the same?
2. Research some common drugs and the interactions they have either with other drugs, food, or drink. Why do these interactions occur?
3. Choose a common drug and trace its route through the body. How might your findings change if your patient was elderly? How might they change if your patient was an infant?

REVIEW QUESTIONS

1. For action to occur, a drug must be _____, transported to tissues or organs, and penetrate cell membranes.
   A. filtered
   B. secreted
   C. absorbed
   D. therapeutic

2. The study of the action of drugs within the body is known as
   A. metabolism.
   B. pharmacokinetics.
   C. pharmacology.
   D. diffusion.

3. The most common and important mode of travel of drugs through membranes is
   A. absorption.
   B. transportation.
   C. diffusion.
   D. solubility.

4. Idiosyncratic reactions may be caused by which of the following factors?
   A. Genetics
   B. Obesity
   C. Gender
   D. Age

5. The process by which drug molecules leave the bloodstream and enter the tissues of the body is called
   A. solubility.
   B. distribution.
   C. suitability.
   D. concentration.

6. The process of converting drugs to metabolic derivatives during metabolism is known as
   A. ionization.
   B. binding.
   C. excretion.
   D. biotransformation.

7. The major site of excretion for most drugs is the
   A. spleen.
   B. sweat glands.
   C. gallbladder.
   D. kidney(s).

8. A second process that moves very small amounts of substances such as potassium and hydrogen from the blood into the renal tubules is known as
   A. tubular secretion.
   B. pH alteration.
   C. increased elimination.
   D. blocking effect.

9. _____ is the study of the biochemical and physiological effects of drugs.
   A. Duration
   B. Acidosis
   C. Pharmacodynamics
   D. Pharmacokinetics

10. A drug that has a specific affinity for a particular cell receptor is known as the
    A. antagonist.
    B. agonist.
    C. blocker.
    D. biochemical event.

11. The _____ of a drug is the time it takes for the plasma concentration to be reduced by 50%.
    A. fluid concentration
    B. pharmacological response
    C. half-life
    D. half-action

12. Newborns and _____ show the greatest effects of a drug's effectiveness.
    A. fetuses
    B. women
    C. men
    D. elderly individuals

13. Sedatives given in the morning will not be as effective as those administered before bedtime because of
    A. diurnal (during the day) body rhythms.
    B. nocturnal (during the night) body rhythms.
    C. corticosteroids.
    D. placebos.

14. The phenomenon of reduced responsiveness to a drug is known as
    A. adaptation.
    B. toxicity.
    C. tolerance.
    D. therapeutic index.

15. When a patient has experienced a unique, strange, or unpredicted reaction to a drug, this reaction is called
    A. hormonal.
    B. idiosyncratic.
    C. hypersensitive.
    D. biological.

20 Antimicrobial Agents

OBJECTIVES

Upon completion of this chapter, the reader should be able to

1. Describe various mechanisms of action of antimicrobial therapy.
2. Explain the indications and contraindications of antibiotics.
3. Describe the major side effects of antimicrobial agents.
4. Understand the importance of drug interactions.
5. Explain the mechanisms of action for penicillins, cephalosporins, aminoglycosides, tetracyclines, macrolides, and quinolones.

6. Compare the effectiveness of penicillins with cephalosporins.
7. Explain the four commonly used antifungal agents.
8. Describe why antiviral drug treatments are limited compared with other antibacterial agents.
9. Name common drugs used for the malarial parasite.

GLOSSARY

agent An entity capable of causing disease.

airborne transmission Contaminated droplets or dust particles suspended in the air are transferred to a susceptible host.

antibiotics Substances that have the ability to destroy or interfere with the development of a living organism.

bacteremia Bacteria present in the circulatory system.

biological agents Living organisms that invade the host.

broad-spectrum antibiotic Antibiotics that are used for the treatment of diseases caused by multiple organisms.

broad-spectrum penicillins Drugs that have a wider antibacterial spectrum.

chemical agents Substances that can interact with the body.

compromised host A person whose normal defense mechanisms are impaired and is therefore more susceptible to a disease.

contact transmission The physical transfer of an agent from an infected person to an uninfected person.

fomites Objects contaminated with an infectious agent but are symptom free.

fungi Microorganisms that grow in single cells or in colonies.

Gram stain A sequential procedure involving crystal violet and iodine solutions followed by alcohol that allows rapid identification of organisms as gram-positive or gram-negative types.

gram-negative Microorganisms that stain red or pink with Gram stain.

gram-positive Microorganisms that stain blue or purple with Gram stain.

mode of transmission The process that bridges the gap between the portal of exit of the infectious agent and the portal of entry of the susceptible host.

narrow-spectrum antibiotics Antibiotics that are effective against only a few organisms.

physical agent Factors in the environment that interact with the body.

portal of entry The route by which an infectious agent enters the host.

portal of exit The route by which an infectious agent leaves the reservoir to be transferred to a susceptible host.

reservoir The place where an agent can survive.

sepsis A syndrome involving multiple system organ involvement that is the result of microorganisms or their toxins in the blood.

septicemia A systemic infection caused by multiplication of microorganisms in the blood circulation.

spores A resistant stage of bacteria that can withstand an unfavorable environment.

susceptible host A person who lacks resistance to an agent and is vulnerable to contracting a disease.

vector-borne transmission An agent is transferred to a susceptible host by animate means.

vehicle transmission An inanimate material (solid object, liquid, or air) that serves as a transmission agent for pathogens.

OVERVIEW

Pathogenic microorganisms may cause a wide spectrum of illnesses. They produce infections of different organs or systems of the body, such as upper respiratory tract infections, meningitis, pneumonia, tuberculosis, and urinary tract infections. The invasion of pathogenic microorganisms that cause infection may be classified primarily as either local or systemic. A localized infection may involve the skin or internal organs and sometimes can progress to a systemic infection. A systemic infection can affect the whole body rather than a specific area of the body. Often viable bacteria may be present in the circulatory system. This is called **bacteremia**. A systemic infection caused by microorganism multiplication in the blood circulation is called **septicemia**. The term **sepsis** is used for a syndrome involving multiple system organ involvement that is a result of microorganisms or their toxins circulating through the bloodstream.

CHAIN OF INFECTION

The chain of infection describes the elements of an infectious process. It is an interactive process that involves the agent, host, and environment. This process must include several essential elements or "links in the chain" for the transmission of microorganisms to occur. Figure 20-1 identifies the six essential links.

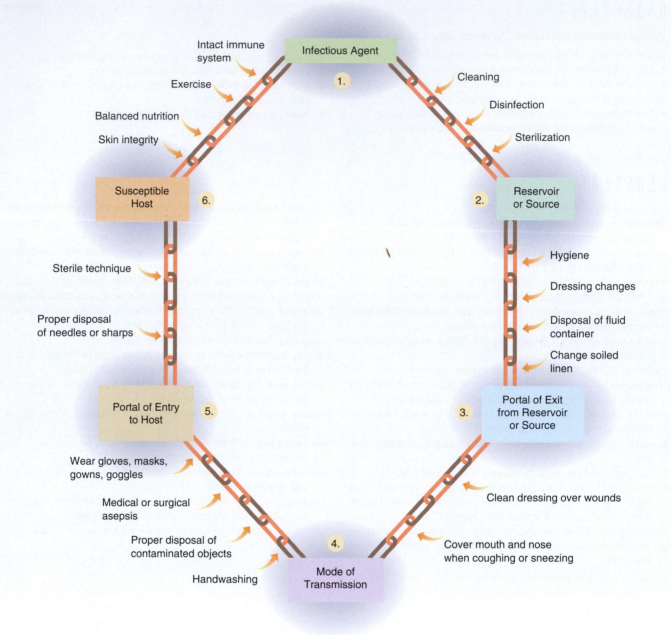

Figure 20-1. The chain of infection.

Without the transmission of microorganisms, the infectious process cannot occur. Knowledge about the chain of infection facilitates control or prevention of disease by breaking the links in the chain. This is achieved by altering one or more of the interactive links of agent, host, or environment.

Agent

An **agent** is an entity that is capable of causing disease. Agents that cause disease include the following:

Biological agents: Living organisms that invade the host, such as bacteria, virus, fungi, protozoa, and rickettsia

Chemical agents: Substances that can interact with the body such as pesticides, food additives, medications, and industrial chemicals

Physical agents: Factors in the environment such as heat, light, noise, and radiation

In the chain of infection, the main concern is biological (infectious) agents and their effect on the host.

Reservoir

The **reservoir** is a place where the agent can survive. Colonization and reproduction take place while the agent is in the reservoir. A reservoir that promotes growth of pathogens must contain the proper nutrients (such as oxygen and organic matter), have the proper temperature, contain moisture, have a compatible pH level, and have the proper amount of light exposure. The most common reservoirs are humans, animals, environment, and **fomites**. Fomites are objects contaminated with an infectious agent such as instruments or dressings. Humans and animals can have symptoms caused by the infectious agents or can be strictly carriers of this agent. Carriers have the infectious agent but are symptom free. The agent can be spread to others in both instances.

Portal of Exit

The **portal of exit** is the route by which an infectious agent leaves the reservoir to be transferred to a susceptible host. The agent leaves the reservoir through body secretions, such as sputum, semen, vaginal secretions, urine, saliva, feces, blood, and draining wounds.

Mode of Transmission

The **mode of transmission** is the process that bridges the gap between the portal of exit from the infectious agent from the reservoir and the portal of entry into the susceptible "new" host. Most infectious agents have a usual mode of transmission; however, some microorganisms may be transmitted by more than one mode (see Table 20-1).

Contact transmission involves the physical transfer of an agent from an infected person to an uninfected person. Contact with the infected person through contaminated secretions is called indirect contact (see Figure 20-2).

Examples of diseases that are caused by direct contact are sexually transmitted diseases, colds, and flu. **Airborne transmission** occurs when a susceptible person contracts a disease through contact with contaminated droplets or dust particles that are suspended in the air (see Figure 20-3).

The longer the particle is suspended, the greater the chance it will find an available port of entry in the human host. An example of an organism that relies on air-borne transmission is measles. Spores of anthrax are also transmitted in an air-borne powder form.

Vehicle transmission occurs when an agent is transferred to a susceptible host by contaminated inanimate objects such as water, food, meat, drugs, and blood (see Figure 20-4). An example is salmonellosis transmitted through contaminated food.

Vector-borne transmission occurs when an agent is transferred to a susceptible host by animate means such as mosquitoes, fleas, ticks, lice, and other animals (see Figure 20-5). Lyme disease is an example.

TABLE 20-1. Modes of Transmission

MODE	EXAMPLES
Contact	Direct contact with infected person
	Touching
	Bathing
	Rubbing
	Toileting (urine and feces)
	Secretions from client
	Indirect contact with fomites
	Clothing
	Bed linens
	Dressings
	Health care equipment
	Instruments used in treatments
	Specimen containers used for laboratory analysis
	Personal belongings
	Personal care equipment
	Diagnostic equipment
Air-borne	Inhaling microorganisms carried by moisture or dust particles in air
	Coughing
	Talking
	Sneezing
Vehicle	Contact with contaminated inanimate objects
	Water
	Blood
	Drugs
	Food
	Urine
Vector-borne	Contact with contaminated animate hosts
	Animals
	Insects

Portal of Entry

A **portal of entry** is the route by which an infectious agent enters the host. Portals of entry include the following:

Integumentary system: Through a break in the skin or mucous membrane

Respiratory tract: By inhaling contaminated droplets

Genitourinary tract: Through contamination with infected vaginal secretions or semen

Gastrointestinal tract: By ingesting contaminated food or water

Circulatory system: Through the bite of insects or rodents

Transplacental: Through transfer of a microorganism from mother to fetus via the placenta and umbilical cord

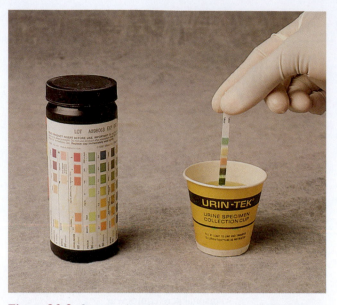

Figure 20-2. Care must be taken in the handling of bodily fluids to prevent the transfer of infectious agents through contact with secretions.

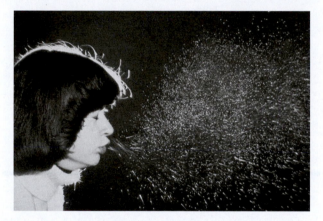

Figure 20-3. The width of the area that droplet nuclei from a sneeze can encompass. (Courtesy of Lester V. Bergman/Corbis.)

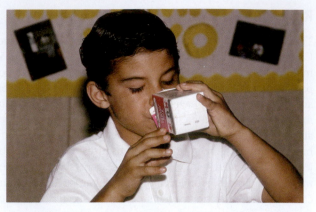

Figure 20-4. Vehicle transmission can occur through contaminated food such as milk.

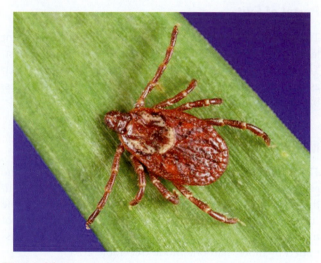

Figure 20-5. Lyme disease is caused by the bite of a deer tick. (From the Centers for Disease Control and Prevention Public Health Image Library.)

Host

A host is a simple or complex organism that can be affected by an agent. As the term is used here, a host is an individual who is at risk of contracting an infectious disease. A **susceptible host** is a person who lacks resistance to an agent and is vulnerable to a disease. A **compromised host** is a person whose normal defense mechanisms are impaired and who is therefore more susceptible to infection. The following characteristics of the host influence the susceptibility to and severity of infections.

Age: As a person ages, immunity declines.

Concurrent disease: The existence of other diseases indicates susceptibility.

Stress: A person experiencing a compromised emotional state has lower defense mechanisms.

Immunization/vaccination status: Certain people are not fully immunized.

Lifestyle: Practices such as having multiple sex partners, sharing needles, or tobacco/drug use can alter defenses.

Occupation: Some jobs involve increased exposure to pathogenic sources such as needles or chemical agents.

Nutritional status: People who maintain targeted weight for height and body frame are less prone to illness.

Heredity: Some people are naturally more susceptible to infections than others.

MICROORGANISMS

Microorganisms are divided into several groups: bacteria, viruses, fungi, protozoa, and rickettsia. Bacteria are classified according to their shape, such as cocci, bacilli, and spirilla.

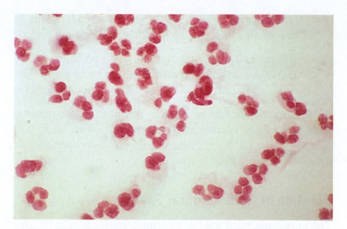

Figure 20-6. Gram-negative specimen showing urethritis. (From the Centers for Disease Control and Prevention Public Health Image Library.)

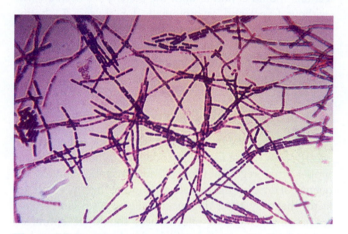

Figure 20-7. Gram-positive specimen showing *Bacillus anthracis.* (Courtesy of the Centers for Disease Control and Prevention Public Health Image Library.)

They are also classified into two groups on the basis of their capacity to be stained. Gram stains can identify specific types of bacteria. A **Gram stain** is a sequential procedure involving staining with crystal violet and iodine solutions followed by alcohol, which allows the rapid classification of organisms into two groups: gram-positive or gram-negative. The culture procedures identify specific organisms, but they require 24 to 48 hours for completion. Gram staining is performed on all specimens except blood cultures. The Gram stain helps to identify the cause of the infection immediately. By determining whether the causative agent is gram-positive or gram-negative, the test allows a better choice of drug therapy, particularly when an anti-infective regimen must begin without delay. **Gram-negative** microorganisms stain red or rose-pink (see Figure 20-6). **Gram-positive** microorganisms stain blue or purple (see Figure 20-7). **Fungi** may also be identified by Gram staining. Culture and sensitivity tests can be performed to determine which antibiotics should be prescribed.

Bacteria

Bacteria are small, one-celled microorganisms that lack a true nucleus or mechanism to provide metabolism. Bacteria need an environment that will provide food for survival. Although most bacteria multiply by simple cell division, some forms of bacteria produce **spores**, a resistant stage that can withstand an unfavorable environment. When proper environmental conditions return, spores germinate and form new cells. Spores are resistant to heat, drying, and disinfectants. Pathogenic bacteria cause a wide range of illnesses including diarrhea, pneumonia, sinusitis, urinary tract infections, and gonorrhea.

Viruses

Viruses are organisms that can live only inside cells. They cannot get nourishment or reproduce outside the cell. Viruses contain a core of DNA or RNA surrounded by a protein coating. Some viruses have the ability to create an additional coating called an envelope. This envelope protects the virus from attack by the immune system. Viruses damage the cell they inhabit by blocking normal protein synthesis and by using the cell's mechanism for metabolism to reproduce themselves. The same viral infection may cause different symptoms in different individuals. Some viruses will immediately trigger a disease response, whereas others may remain latent for many years. Viral infections include the common cold, influenza, measles, hepatitis, and genital herpes and infections caused by human immunodeficiency virus (HIV) and the West Nile virus.

Fungi

Fungi grow in single cells (e.g., yeast) or in colonies (e.g., molds). Fungi obtain food from living organisms or organic matter. Fungi cause disease mainly in individuals who are immunologically impaired. Fungi can cause infections of the hair, skin, nails, and mucous membranes. Athlete's foot is an infection caused by fungi.

Protozoa

Protozoa are single-celled parasitic organisms with the ability to move. Most protozoa obtain their food from dead or decaying organic matter. Infection is spread through ingestion of contaminated food or water or through insect bites. Common protozoal infections are malaria, gastroenteritis, and vaginal infections.

Rickettsia

Rickettsia are intercellular parasites that need to be in living cells to reproduce. Infection from rickettsia is spread through the bites of fleas, ticks, mites, and lice. Common examples of these infections are Lyme disease, Rocky Mountain spotted fever, and typhus.

PRINCIPLES OF ANTI-INFECTIVE THERAPY

Anti-infective agents are used to treat infection by destroying or suppressing the causative microorganisms. The goal is to suppress the causative agent sufficiently so that the body's own defense can eliminate it. Anti-infective drugs derived from natural substances are called **antibiotics**. Those produced from synthetic substances are called antimicrobials. During the last few years, efforts were made to change antibiotic usage policy, rendering prescribing practices clinically stronger, but less costly. There is now an emphasis on rapid conversion from parenteral to oral therapy for a variety of infectious processes. Major research is being done to understand the underlying principles associated with the interaction of antibiotics, host, and pathogens. A new area of research with HIV-infected patients is the study of medication compliance to assess adherence with prophylaxic and primary antiretroviral therapies. Other clinical studies with in vitro and in vivo therapies are being conducted.

Selection of Agents

An anti-infective agent should be chosen on the basis of its pharmacologic properties and spectrum of activity as well as on various patient factors:

1. *Pharmacologic properties:* These include the drug's ability to reach the infection site and to attain a desired level in the target tissue. Investigations into these properties of fluoroquinolones indicate that bacterial killing is concentration dependent as opposed to time dependent. *In vivo* studies have confirmed that the total daily dose and not the frequency of administration was significantly associated with bactericidal activity against *Escherichia coli,* staphylococcal bacteria, and *Pseudomonas aeruginosa.*
2. *Spectrum of activity:* To treat an infectious disease successfully, an anti-microbial agent must be effective against the causative pathogen. The effectiveness of an anti-infective drug can be confirmed by a sensitivity test. Clinical resistance to an antimicrobial agent occurs when the minimum inhibitory concentration of the drug for a particular strain of bacteria exceeds that which is capable of being achieved safely *in vivo.* Resistance to an antimicrobial can arise by mutation in the gene that determines sensitivity/resistance to the agent or by acquisition of an extrachromosomal DNA (plasmid) carrying a resistance gene.
3. *Patient factors:* Various patient factors determine what type of antimicrobial agent should be administered. These factors include immunity of patients, age, presence of a foreign body, adverse drug reactions, pregnancy and lactation, and underlying disease. Choosing an antimicrobial agent that does not offer enough protection is a common problem. Some commonly used drugs such as aminoglycosides and vancomycin are poorly absorbed and can be used to treat gastrointestinal (GI)l infections

without systemic effects. Other patient considerations in the use of anti-infective agents include the following:

- Diminished renal function in elderly persons
- Partially developed hepatic function in neonates
- Circulation problems such as those seen with diabetes

Antimicrobials can be used as prophylaxis for patients with meningitis or tuberculosis; patients who have had surgery to the GI tract, urinary tract, or dental regions; or those with rheumatoid fever.

Duration of Antimicrobial Therapy

The most important goal of anti-infective therapy is to continue it for a sufficient duration. Infections are generally characterized as acute or chronic. Although infection can be present without fever, treatment for acute uncomplicated infections should continue until the patient has been afebrile (without fever) and asymptomatic for at least 72 hours. However, all antibiotics should be taken for the prescribed amount of time. Treatment for chronic infection such as osteomyelitis or endocarditis may require a longer duration of treatment, for example, 4 to 6 weeks.

Lack of Therapeutic Effectiveness

Several factors may be associated with a lack of therapeutic effectiveness. These factors include misdiagnosis and an improper drug regimen (dosage, administration route, frequency of dose, or inadequate duration of therapy). Another factor that may affect therapeutic effectiveness is microbial resistance. Therapeutic effectiveness should be optimized and resistance to antimicrobials should be minimized to protect public health. The main objectives are as follows:

- Support development of a scientific knowledge base that provides the basis for judicious therapeutic use of antimicrobials.
- Support educational efforts that promote judicious therapeutic use of antimicrobials.
- Preserve the therapeutic effectiveness of antimicrobials.
- Ensure current and future availability of antimicrobials.

Antibiotic Spectrum

Effectiveness of antibiotics against different microorganisms may be divided into two groups: broad-spectrum and narrow-spectrum. **Broad-spectrum antibiotics** are effective against a wide variety of both gram-positive and gram-negative pathogenic microorganisms. **Narrow-spectrum antibiotics** are effective against a few gram-positive or gram-negative pathogens.

Route of Administration

The intravenous (IV) or intramuscular (IM) routes are preferred to guarantee good serum and tissue levels at the time of infusion; however, the oral route is often used.

These are used to treat infections caused by bacteria. The major categories for antibacterial agents include aminoglycosides, cephalosporins, macrolides, penicillins, sulfonamides, tetracyclines, fluoroquinolones, and other miscellaneous agents.

Aminoglycosides

Aminoglycosides are used primarily for infections caused by gram-negative enterobacteria. The toxic potential of these drugs limits their use. Since their introduction into clinical use 50 years ago, aminoglycosides continue to play an important role for the treatment of severe infections. Traditionally, aminoglycosides have been administered in multiple daily doses. However, physicians are becoming increasingly aware that pulse dosing may be the preferred method of administration of these agents. Pulse dosing involves achieving a high aminoglycoside peak to maximize the drug's effectiveness and allowing a drug-free interval of 3 to 5 hours to minimize toxicity and perhaps reverse adaptive postexposure resistance. For example, the single dose for gentamicin and tobramycin is 5 mg/kg of actual body weight (ABW) unless the patient is more than 20% heavier than the ideal body weight (IBW). For obese patients, dosing weight should be calculated by using the following equation:

Creatinine clearance (C_{Cr}) > 60 = dosing interval of 24 hours

or

Creatinine clearance (C_{Cr}) = 40 to 59 = dosing interval of 36 hours

The calculated dose is diluted in 100 mL of normal saline and infused over 1 hour. Doses as high as 7 mg/kg have been used, but there is no evidence that doses greater than 5 mg/kg offer any advantage. Major aminoglycosides are shown in Table 20-2.

Aminoglycosides such as gentamicin, tobramycin, and amikacin cause drug interactions with medications commonly prescribed for patients with acquired immunodeficiency syndrome (AIDS). These drugs as well as other aminoglycosides may also cause ototoxicity when used in combination with different medications. *In vitro* mixing of an aminoglycoside with penicillins or cephalosporins may result in significant mutual inactivation.

Mechanism of Action

Aminoglycosides are bactericidal; they inhibit bacterial protein synthesis. Their mechanism of action is not fully known.

Therapeutic Uses

Aminoglycosides are prescribed for a variety of disorders and infectious diseases.

1. *Streptomycin:* This drug can be used to treat tularemia, acute brucellosis, bacterial endocarditis, tuberculosis, and plague.
2. *Amikacin, gentamicin, netilmicin, and tobramycin:* These drugs are prescribed for serious infections caused by gram-negative bacteria such as *Enterobacter* and *Klebsiella,* bacteremia, meningitis, and peritonitis.
3. *Neomycin:* This drug is used for preoperative bowel sterilization and hepatic coma and in topical form for burns.

Adverse Effects

Aminoglycosides can cause serious adverse effects such as ototoxicity and nephrotoxicity. Neomycin is the most nephrotoxic aminoglycoside, and streptomycin is the least

TABLE 20-2. Major Aminoglycosides

GENERIC NAME	TRADE NAME	ROUTE OF ADMINISTRATION	COMMON DOSAGE RANGE
Amikacin	Amikin®	IV, IM	15 mg/kg/day in 2–3 divided doses
Clindamycin	Cleocin®	Oral, IM, IV, topical	500 mg–2 g/day in 3–4 divided doses; 500 mg IV q6h
			Oral 8–20 mg/kg/day in 3–4 equal doses
			Parenteral 15–40 mg/kg/day in 3–4 equal doses
Gentamicin	Garamycin®	IV, IM	3–5 mg/kg/day (standard dose)
			6–7 mg/kg/day (once daily)
Kanamycin	Kantrex®	Oral, IM, IV	15 mg/kg each 8–12 hours
Neomycin sulfate	Mycifradin®	Oral, topical	50–100 mg/kg/day (oral)
			10–15 mg/day (topical)
Netilmicin	Netromycin®	IV, IM	3–6 mg/kg/day
Streptomycin		IM	0.5–1 g each 12–24 hours
Tobramycin	Nebcin®	IV, IV, ophthalmic	3–5 mg/kg/day (standard dose)
Vancomycin	Vancocin®	Oral, IV	6–7 mg/kg/day (once daily)

TABLE 20-3. Classification of Cephalosporins

GENERIC NAME	TRADE NAME	ROUTE OF ADMINISTRATION	COMMON DOSAGE RANGE
First Generation			
Cephalothin	Cephalonia®	IV	50 mg–2 g
Cephradine	Velosef®	Oral, IM, IV	250 mg
Cephapirin	Cefadyl®	Oral	25 mg–4 g
Cephalexin	Keflex®	Oral	25 mg–1 g
Cefadroxil	Duricef®	Oral	500 mg–1 g
Cefazolin	Ancef®, Zolicef®, Kefzol®	IM, IV	250 mg–1 g
Second Generation			
Cefoxitin	Mefoxin®	IV	2 g
Cefaclor	Ceclor®	Oral	125–500 mg
Cefuroxime	Ceftin®	Oral	125–500 mg
Cefonicid	Monocid®	IM, IV	50 mg–12 g
Third Generation			
Cefotaxime moxalactam	Claforan®	IV	75 mg–4 g
Cefixime	Suprax®	Oral	100–400 mg
Ceftriaxone	Rocephin®	IV	1–2 g
Cefprozil	Cefzil®	Oral	250–500 mg
Cefoperazone	Cefobid®	IM, IV	1–6 g
Fourth Generation			
Cefepime	Maxipime®	IM, IV	500 mg–2 g

nephrotoxic. Gentamicin and tobramycin are nephrotoxic to the same degree.

Drug Interactions

Amikacin and other nephrotoxic drugs do not interact well with cyclosporine A or tacrolimus.

Cephalosporins

These agents are also known as β-lactam antibiotics. Cephalosporins are semisynthetic antibiotics structurally and pharmacologically related to penicillins. They are usually bactericidal in action. The antibacterial activity of the cephalosporins results from inhibition of mucopeptide synthesis in the bacterial cell wall. The cephalosporins are classified into four different "generations" (see Table 20-3).

First-generation cephalosporins are effective against most gram-positive organisms and some gram-negative organisms. They are used mainly for *Klebsiella* infections and penicillin- and sulfonamide-resistant urinary tract infections. Cephalothin, cephapirin, and cefazolin are used parenterally; the others can be administered orally.

Second-generation cephalosporins extend the spectrum of the first-generation cephalosporins to include *Haemophilus influenzae* and some *Proteus* strains. Second-generation cephalosporins are used primarily for the treatment of urinary tract, bone, and soft tissue infections and prophylactically with various surgical procedures. All are administered parenterally except for cefaclor and cefuroxime, which may be given orally.

Third-generation cephalosporins have even broader gram-negative activity and less gram-positive activity than do second-generation agents. Cefotaxime moxalactam is a third-generation cephalosporin that is effective against *H. influenzae*, *Neisseria gonorrhoeae*, and enterobacteria. All are administered parenterally. Third-generation agents are used primarily for serious gram-negative bacterial infections, alone or in combination with aminoglycosides. Cefixime and cefprozil are given orally.

Fourth-generation cephalosporins have the greatest action against gram-negative organisms among the four generations and minimal action against gram-positive organisms.

Mechanism of Action

The mechanism of action of cephalosporins is to prevent bacterial cell wall synthesis because they bind to enzymes called penicillin-binding proteins. These enzymes are essential for the synthesis of the bacterial cell wall.

Therapeutic Uses

Cephalosporins are used to treat community-acquired and hospital-acquired infections of the skin, soft tissue, urinary tract, and respiratory tract. First-generation agents given parenterally are used for surgical wound prophylaxis. The cephamycin group is useful for mixed aerobic/anaerobic infections of the skin and soft tissues, intra-abdominal and gynecologic infections, and surgical prophylaxis.

Adverse Effects

All cephalosporins except cefoperazone are eliminated by the kidneys. Doses must be adjusted for patients with renal impairment. Cephalosporins can cause hypersensitivity reactions similar to those with penicillin. The most common adverse effects include nausea, vomiting, diarrhea, and nephrotoxicity. Adverse effects of cephalosporins include hypoprothrombinemia and bleeding, alcohol intolerance, hypersensitivity reactions, and thrombophlebitis.

Drug Interactions

Cephalosporins have drug interactions with alcohol, diarrhea medications, birth control pills, anticoagulants, blood viscosity-reducing medicines, and antiseizure medicines. Cephalosporins are contraindicated for use with alcohol, alcohol-containing medications, aminoglycosides, anticoagulants, carbenicillin by injection, dipyridamole, divalproex, heparin, pentoxifylline, plicamycin, sulfinpyrazone, ticarcillin, thrombolytic agents, valproic acid, potent diuretics, iron-iron supplements, and probenecid.

Macrolides

The macrolides include erythromycin, azithromycin, clarithromycin, dirithromycin, and troleandomycin. Erythromycin is produced by *Streptomyces erythreus*. Macrolides are bacteriostatic at normal doses and bactericidal at higher doses. They are also used as alternative agents when the patient is allergic to penicillin. Table 20-4 shows common macrolides.

Erythromycin can be administered topically, ophthalmically, orally, and by IV or IM injection. It is a relatively safe antibiotic typically used for community-acquired pneumonias and upper respiratory tract, genitourinary tract, and soft tissue infections caused by susceptible organisms. GI intolerance for clarithromycin is less than that for erythromycin and adverse effects are relatively minor. Its effects are similar to those of erythromycin, except that it is more effective against

Mycobacterium avium complex and also has activity against *Mycobacterium leprae* and *Toxoplasma gondii*. Azithromycin is absorbed rapidly and is recommended by the Centers for Disease Control and Prevention specifically as an alternative to doxycycline in patients with uncomplicated urethral, endocervical, rectal, or epididymal chlamydial infections.

Mechanism of Action

Erythromycins may be bactericidal (bringing death to bacteria) or bacteriostatic (tending to restrain the development or reproduction of bacteria). They inhibit bacterial protein synthesis. Erythromycins generally penetrate the cell walls of gram-positive bacteria more readily than those of gram-negative bacteria.

Therapeutic Uses

Erythromycins are the drug of choice for the treatment of *M. pneumoniae*, *Campylobacter* infections, Legionnaires' disease, chlamydial infections, and pertussis. In patients with penicillin allergy, erythromycins are the best alternatives for the treatment of gonorrhea, syphilis, and pneumococcal pneumonia. Erythromycins may be given prophylactically before dental procedures to prevent bacterial endocarditis.

Adverse Effects

Erythromycins rarely can cause serious adverse effects. Nausea, vomiting, and diarrhea may occur with all forms of erythromycin.

Drug Interactions

Erythromycin inhibits the hepatic metabolism of theophylline. It may interfere with the metabolism of digoxin, corticosteroids, and cyclosporin.

Penicillins

Penicillins are natural or semisynthetic antibiotics produced by or derived from certain species of the fungus *Penicillium*. They are the most widely used antimicrobial agents; however,

---

TABLE 20-4. Most Commonly Used Macrolides

GENERIC NAME	TRADE NAME	ROUTE OF ADMINISTRATION	COMMON DOSAGE RANGE
Erythromycin base	Eryc®, E-mycin®	Oral	250 mg
Erythromycin estolate	Ilosone®	IM, IV, oral	30 mg–1 g
Erythromycin stearate	Erythrocin®	IV, oral	30 mg–1 g
Clarithromycin	Biaxin®	Oral	7.5–500 mg
Azithromycin	Zithromax®	Oral	5–2000 mg
Dirithromycin	Dynabac®	Oral	250 mg
Troleandomycin	Tao®	Oral	125–500 mg

TABLE 20-5. Common Penicillins and Routes of Administration

GENERIC NAME	TRADE NAME	ROUTE OF ADMINISTRATION	COMMON DOSAGE RANGE
Natural Penicillins			
Penicillin G	Pen®, Pfizerpen®	IM, IV	1–30 million U
Penicillin V	Beepen®, Ledercillin®	Oral	25 mg–2 g
Penicillin G procaine	Pfizerpen®	IM	200,000–24 million U
Penicillin G benzathine	Wycillin®	IM	25,000–24 million U
Penicillinase-Resistant Penicillins			
Cloxacillin	Cloxapen®	Oral	250–500 mg
Dicloxacillin	Dycill®, Dynapen®	Oral	125–500 mg
Flucloxacillin	Floxapen®	Oral, IV	PO, 250 mg qid; IV, 1–2 g for surgical prophylaxis
Methicillin	Staphcillin®	IM, IV	4–12 g daily
Nafcillin	Nafcil®, Unipen®	Oral, IM, IV	1–2 g
Oxacillin	Bactocill®, Oxacillin®	Oral, IM, IV	50 mg–1 g
Semisynthetic Penicillins			
Amoxicillin	Amoxil®, Trimox®		15–500 g
Amoxicillin/clavulanate potassium	Augmentin®	Oral	250–2000 mg
Ampicillin	Ampicil®, Omnipen®	Oral, IM, IV	300 mg–3 g
Bacampicillin	Spectrobid®	Oral	800 mg q12h
Cyclacillin	Cyclapen-W®	Oral	500 mg q8h

cephalosporin usage has increased in the last decade. Among the most important antibiotics, natural penicillins are the preferred drugs for the treatment of many infectious diseases. The major cause of resistance to penicillin is production of β-lactamases (penicillinases). Common organisms that are capable of producing penicillinase include *Staphylococcus aureus*, *E. coli*, *P. aeruginosa*, and species of *Bacillus*, *Proteus*, and *Bacteroides*. Penicillins are absorbed rapidly after parenteral administration, are distributed throughout body fluids, and penetrate the cerebrospinal fluid and the ocular fluid to a significant extent only during inflammation. Most penicillins are excreted by the kidneys, predominantly via tubular secretion. Penicillins are available as penicillin G, penicillin V, penicillin G procaine, and penicillin G benzathine. Table 20-5 shows common types of penicillins.

Mechanism of Action

Penicillins are bactericidal. They inhibit bacterial cell wall synthesis in ways similar to those of the cephalosporins. Natural penicillins are highly active against gram-positive and against some gram-negative cocci. Penicillin G is 10 times more active than penicillin V against gram-negative organisms.

Therapeutic Uses

Penicillin G is the drug of choice for all *S. pneumoniae* organisms. Penicillins G and V are highly effective against other streptococcal infections such as bacteremia, pharyngitis, otitis

media, and sinusitis. Penicillin G is also the drug of choice for many gonococcal infections, postexposure inhalational anthrax, syphilis, and gas gangrene. Penicillin G procaine is effective for syphilis and uncomplicated gonorrhea. Penicillin G benzathine is very effective for group A β-hemolytic streptococcal infections. Penicillins G and V may be indicated for prophylactic treatment to prevent streptococcal infection, rheumatic fever, and neonatal ophthalmia due to gonorrhea.

Adverse Effects

Hypersensitivity occurs in nearly 10% of patients. Reactions ranging from a simple rash to anaphylaxis can be observed from within 2 minutes and up to 3 days after administration. Anaphylaxis is a life-threatening reaction that most commonly occurs with parenteral administration. Signs and symptoms include severe hypotension, bronchoconstriction, nausea, vomiting, and abdominal pain. Before penicillin therapy begins, the patient's history should be evaluated for allergy to penicillin.

Drug Interactions

The most significant drugs that may increase or decrease the effect of penicillin include probenecid, erythromycins, tetracyclines, and chloramphenicol. Probenecid increases blood levels of natural penicillin. On the other hand, chloramphenicol, erythromycins, and tetracyclines are antagonists of the effects of penicillin.

Amoxicillin/Clavulanate Potassium

S. pneumoniae is the most common cause of acute bacterial sinusitis and community-acquired pneumonia. Amoxicillin/clavulanate potassium is the first antibiotic approved by the U.S. Food and Drug Administration for both of these infections.

Mechanism of Action   The amoxicillin component of the formulation exerts a bactericidal action against many gram-negative and gram-positive organisms. The clavulanate potassium component protects the amoxicillin from degradation by inactivating harmful β-lactamase enzymes.

Therapeutic Uses   This combination is used for the treatment of upper respiratory tract infections such as otitis media, tonsillitis, and sinusitis. It is also used to treat lower respiratory tract infections such as bronchitis and pneumonia. Urinary tract, skin, and soft tissue infections can also be treated with this combination agent.

Adverse Effects   Amoxicillin/clavulanate potassium should not be used in patients with hepatic dysfunction because of the danger of transient hepatitis and cholestatic jaundice. Serious and occasionally fatal hypersensitivity reactions have been reported in patients receiving concurrent penicillin therapy.

Drug Interactions   Concurrent use of this agent with probenecid may result in increased and prolonged blood levels of amoxicillin. This agent interacts with coumarin or indandione-derivative anticoagulants, heparin, non-steroidal anti-inflammatory agents (especially aspirin), other platelet aggregation inhibitors or thrombolytic agents, and estrogen-containing oral contraceptives.

Penicillinase-Resistant Penicillins

Resistant penicillins are used predominantly for penicillinase-producing staphylococcal infections. Most staphylococci are now resistant to benzylpenicillin because they produce a penicillinase. As their name suggests, penicillinase-resistant penicillins are resistant to the action of this enzyme and are therefore indicated in infections caused by penicillin-resistant *Staphylococcus* organisms. Oxacillin, cloxacillin, dicloxacillin, and nafcillin can be given orally. Methicillin is administered parenterally. Nafcillin is used parenterally for more serious infections. Flucloxacillin is effective in infections caused by penicillin-resistant staphylococci, is acid-stable, and, therefore, can be given by mouth as well as by injection. Penicillinase-resistant penicillins are used solely in staphylococcal infections resulting from organisms that are resistant to natural penicillins. These agents are less potent than natural penicillins against organisms susceptible to natural penicillins. Penicillinase-resistant penicillins are the preferred choice for skin and soft tissue infections caused by staphylococci. Higher doses should be used for severe infections or for

infections of the lower respiratory tract. In suspension form, these agents should be taken on an empty stomach, are stable for 14 days after mixing (but refrigeration is required), and are known for their bitter aftertaste.

Mechanism of Action   Penicillinase-resistant penicillins prevent cell wall synthesis by binding to enzymes called penicillin-binding proteins. These enzymes are essential for the synthesis of the bacterial cell wall.

Therapeutic Uses   Therapeutic uses of penicillinase-resistant penicillins include prevention and treatment of bacterial infections, including those caused by streptococcus, enterococcus, and staphylococcus strains.

Adverse Effects   The penicillinase-resistant penicillins can cause hypersensitivity reactions such as those with natural penicillins. Methicillin may cause nephrotoxicity. Oxacillin can produce hepatotoxicity. They may cause nausea, vomiting, diarrhea, or skin rash and are contraindicated in penicillin-allergic patients.

Drug Interactions   Penicillinase-resistant penicillins can inactivate aminoglycoside serum samples from patients receiving both drugs.

Semisynthetic Penicillins

The group of penicillins known as semisynthetic penicillins includes ampicillin, amoxicillin, bacampicillin, and cyclacillin. They have a wider antibacterial spectrum than narrow spectrum penicillins. The semisynthetic penicillins are known as **broad-spectrum penicillins**.

Mechanism of Action   Semisynthetic penicillins are bactericidal and inhibit bacterial cell wall synthesis.

Therapeutic Uses   Semisynthetic penicillins are used to treat gonococcal infections, upper respiratory tract infections, uncomplicated urinary tract infections, and otitis media caused by susceptible organisms. Amoxicillin is less effective than ampicillin in shigellosis. Amoxicillin is more effective against *S. aureus, Klebsiella,* and *Bacteroides fragilis* infections when administered in combination with amoxicillin/potassium clavulanate, because clavulanic acid inactivates penicillinases.

Adverse Effects   Diarrhea is most common with ampicillin. Hypersensitivity reactions may also occur with semisynthetic penicillins.

Extended-Spectrum Penicillins

This group of penicillins has the widest antibacterial spectrum. Included are the carboxypenicillins and the ureidopenicillins. See Table 20-6 for a list of extended-spectrum penicillins.

TABLE 20-6.   Extended-Spectrum Penicillins

GENERIC NAME	TRADE NAME	ROUTE OF ADMINISTRATION	COMMON DOSAGE RANGE
Carboxypenicillins			
Carbenicillin	Geocillin®	Oral	382 mg
Ticarcillin	Ticar®	IM, IV	250–400 mg/kg/day
Ticarcillin and clavulanate	Timentin®	IV	200–450 mg/kg/day
Ureidopenicillins			
Mezlocillin	Mezlin®	IM, IV	25–50 mg/kg/day
Piperacillin	Pipracil®	IM, IV	12–16 g/day

TABLE 20-7.   Classification of Sulfonamides

GENERIC NAME	TRADE NAME	ROUTE OF ADMINISTRATION	COMMON DOSAGE RANGE
Short-acting (4–8 hours)			
Sulfamethizole	Methazol®	Oral	7.5 mg–1 g
Sulfasalazine	Azulfidine®	Oral	10 mg–8 g
Sulfisoxazole	Eryzole®	Oral, vaginal	75 mg–8 g
Intermediate-acting (7–17 hours)			
Sulfadiazine	Microsulfon®	Oral	50 mg–4 g
Sulfamethoxazole	Bactrim®	Oral, IV	10–100 mg
Sulfapyridine	Dagenan®	Oral	250 mg–1 g
Long-acting (17+ hours)			
Sulfadoxine	Fansidar®	Oral	25–200 mg

Mechanism of Action   Extended-spectrum penicillins are bactericidal and inhibit bacterial cell wall synthesis.

Therapeutic Uses   They are prescribed mainly for treatment of serious infections, such as sepsis, pneumonia, peritonitis, osteomyelitis, and soft tissue infections, caused by gram-negative organisms.

Adverse Effects   As with other penicillins, hypersensitivity reactions may occur. Carbenicillin and ticarcillin may cause hypokalemia. The use of these two drugs may be a danger to patients with congestive heart failure, because of the high sodium content of carbenicillin and ticarcillin.

Drug Interactions   If given concurrently with ACE inhibitors, potassium-sparing diuretics or potassium supplements, serum potassium levels may increase. Anticoagulants increased risk of bleeding when given with high doses of parenteral carbenicillin or ticarcillin, as these drugs inhibit platelet aggregation.

Sulfonamides

Sulfonamides are the synthetic derivatives of sulfanilamide. These agents were the first drugs to prevent and cure human bacterial infection successfully. They are well-absorbed from the GI tract. Sulfonamides readily penetrate the cerebrospinal fluid. These agents are metabolized to various degrees in the liver and are eliminated by the kidneys. Sulfonamides were originally active against a wide range of gram-positive and gram-negative bacteria, but the increasing incidence of resistance in bacteria formerly susceptible to sulfonamides has decreased the clinical usefulness of the drugs. However, sulfonamides remain the drug of choice for certain infections. The major sulfonamides are generally classified as short-acting, intermediate-acting, or long-acting. Their rate of action depends on how quickly they are absorbed and eliminated. See Table 20-7 for a classification of sulfonamides.

Mechanism of Action

Sulfonamides are bacteriostatic; they suppress bacterial growth by triggering a mechanism that blocks folic acid synthesis, thereby forcing bacteria to synthesize their own folic acid.

Therapeutic Uses

Sulfonamides most often are used to treat urinary tract infections caused by E. coli, including acute and chronic cystitis, and chronic upper urinary tract infections. Prophylactic

TABLE 20-8.   Major Tetracyclines and Administration Routes

GENERIC NAME	TRADE NAME	ROUTE OF ADMINISTRATION	COMMON DOSAGE RANGE
Demeclocycline hydrochloride	Declomycin®	Oral	3 mg/lb/day–600 mg/day
Doxycycline hyclate	Vibramycin®	Oral	50 mg/day
Minocycline hydrochloride	Minocin®	Oral, IV	4 mg/kg/day–200 mg/day
Oxytetracycline	Terramycin®	Oral, IM	15 mg/kg/day–300 mg/day
Tetracycline hydrochloride	Achromycin®	Oral	250 mg/day

sulfonamide therapy has been used successfully to prevent streptococcal infections and rheumatic fever recurrences.

Adverse Effects

Sulfonamides may cause blood dyscrasias such as hemolytic anemia, aplastic anemia, thrombocytopenia, and agranulocytosis. Hypersensitivity reactions may occur with sulfonamide therapy. Hematuria and crystalluria are two of the major adverse effects of sulfonamide agents, and they should be used with caution in patients with renal impairment. The patient should be advised to take in adequate fluid to prevent or minimize these risks. Life-threatening hepatitis caused by drugs is a rare adverse effect. Patients who take sulfonamides have increased susceptibility to adverse effects from sun exposure.

Drug Interactions

Sulfonamides may increase the effects of phenytoin, oral anticoagulants, and sulfonylureas.

Tetracyclines

Tetracyclines are broad-spectrum agents that are effective against certain bacterial strains that are resistant to other antibiotics. The major tetracyclines are shown in Table 20-8.

Mechanism of Action

Tetracyclines are bacteriostatic. They inhibit bacterial protein synthesis.

Therapeutic Uses

Tetracyclines are active against gram-negative and gram-positive organisms, spirochetes, *Mycoplasma* and *Chlamydia* organisms, rickettsial species, and certain protozoa. They are the drugs of choice in rickettsial infections (e.g., Rocky Mountain spotted fever), chlamydial infections, amebiasis, cholera, brucellosis, and tularemia. Tetracyclines are prescribed as an alternative to penicillin for the treatment of anthrax, syphilis, gonorrhea, Lyme disease, and *H. influenzae* respiratory infections. Oral or topical tetracycline may be used as a treatment for acne. Doxycycline is highly effective in the prophylaxis of "traveler's diarrhea."

Adverse Effects

Abdominal discomfort, nausea, diarrhea, and anorexia are common adverse effects of tetracyclines. Cross-sensitivity within the tetracyclines are also common. Tetracyclines should not be used in children younger than 8 years of age unless other appropriate drugs are ineffective or are contraindicated. Use of the drugs in infants has resulted in retardation of bone growth. Because tetracyclines localize in the dentin and enamel of developing teeth, use of the drugs during tooth development may cause enamel hypoplasia and permanent yellow-gray to brown discoloration of the teeth. Tetracyclines can cause fetal toxicity when administered to pregnant women (e.g., retardation of skeletal development). Liver toxicity has occurred after IV administration of tetracyclines to pregnant women. Oxytetracycline is the least hepatotoxic. Phototoxicity may occur in patients when they are exposed to strong sunlight (ultraviolet), especially with demeclocycline. Minocycline can cause vestibular toxicity. Intravenous administration of tetracyclines is irritating and may cause phlebitis.

Drug Interactions

Certain foods (dairy products) and agents such as iron preparations, laxatives, and antacids that contain aluminum and calcium may reduce absorption of tetracyclines. Therefore, it is recommended that tetracyclines be taken on an empty stomach. Barbiturates and phenytoin can decrease the effectiveness of tetracyclines.

Fluoroquinolones

Fluoroquinolones are related to nalidixic acid and are bactericidal for growing bacteria. The most commonly used fluoroquinolones are shown in Table 20-9.

Mechanism of Action

Fluoroquinolones inhibit DNA enzymes.

TABLE 20-9. Most Commonly Used Quinolones

GENERIC NAME	TRADE NAME	ROUTE OF ADMINISTRATION	COMMON DOSAGE RANGE
Moxifloxacin	Avelox®	Oral, IV	400 mg and 400 mg/250 ml
Nalidixic acid	NegGram®	Oral	500 mg and 300 mg/5 mL
Cinoxacin	Cinobac®	Oral	250–500 mg
Ciprofloxacin	Cipro®	Oral	250–750 mg
Lomefloxacin	Maxaquin®	Oral	400 mg
Ofloxacin	Floxin®	Oral	200–400 mg
Norfloxacin	Noroxin®	Oral	400 mg
Trovafloxacin	Trovan®	Oral	100 mg
Levofloxacin	Levaquin®	Oral, IM, IV	250–500 mg

Therapeutic Uses

Ciprofloxacin and ofloxacin are available orally and intravenously. Ciprofloxacin is used for urinary tract infections, lower respiratory tract infections, and infections of bone, joints, and skin. Oral norfloxacin is prescribed for urinary tract infections, uncomplicated gonococcal infections, and prostatitis.

Adverse Effects

Fluoroquinolone agents may produce nausea, headache, dizziness, dyspepsia, insomnia, photosensitivity, and hypoglycemia. Crystalluria can occur with high doses at alkaline pH. Therefore, fluoroquinolones should be taken with water, and the patient should stay well hydrated. Fluoroquinolones should not be used in children or in women who are pregnant or nursing.

Drug Interactions

Ciprofloxacin may increase theophylline levels in blood. Antacids and iron can decrease the absorption of fluoroquinolones. They may increase prothrombin times in patients receiving warfarin.

Miscellaneous Antibacterial Agents

Some antibiotics are classified as miscellaneous antibacterial agents such as chloramphenicol, clindamycin, dapsone, and vancomycin.

Chloramphenicol

This antibiotic is highly effective against rickettsia as well as against many gram-positive and gram-negative organisms.

Mechanism of Action Chloramphenicol is primarily bacteriostatic and secondarily bactericidal against a few bacterial strains.

Therapeutic Uses Chloramphenicol is used only for specific infections that cannot be treated effectively with other antibiotics. These infections include typhoid fever, rickettsial infections in pregnant women, and meningococcal infections in cephalosporin-allergic patients. It can also be used for patients who have a history of allergies to tetracycline.

Adverse Effects Chloramphenicol can cause suppression of bone marrow (in high doses) with resulting pancytopenia. A rare, non-dose-related effect is aplastic anemia. Chloramphenicol therapy can also lead to gray baby syndrome in neonates.

Drug Interactions Chloramphenicol may inhibit the metabolism of phenytoin, dicumarol, and tolbutamide, leading to prolonged action and increased effects of these drugs. Phenobarbital can reduce the effect of chloramphenicol therapy. Acetaminophen elevates chloramphenicol levels and may cause toxicity. Penicillins can cause antibiotic antagonism.

Clindamycin

Clindamycin is used to treat skin, respiratory tract, and soft tissue infections caused by staphylococci, streptococci, and pneumococci.

Mechanism of Action Clindamycin is bacteriostatic and inhibits bacterial protein synthesis. This agent is active against most gram-positive and many anaerobic organisms.

Therapeutic Uses Clindamycin has marked toxicity. It is used only against infections for which it has been determined to be the most effective drug. Therefore, clindamycin is used for joint, bone, abdominal, and female genitourinary tract infections and topically for acne.

Adverse Effects Clindamycin may cause rash, nausea, vomiting, diarrhea, and pseudomembranous colitis. Leukopenia and thrombocytopenia may also occur.

Drug Interactions Clindamycin may potentiate the effects of neuromuscular blocking agents.

Dapsone

Dapsone is the primary agent for the treatment of all forms of leprosy.

Mechanism of Action Dapsone is bacteriostatic for *M. leprae* by blocking folic acid synthesis, thereby forcing microorganisms to synthesize their own folic acid.

Therapeutic Uses Dapsone is the drug of choice for treating leprosy. A dapsone-pyrimethamine product (Maloprim®) is valuable in the prophylaxis and treatment of malaria.

Adverse Effects Nausea, vomiting, and anorexia may develop. Dapsone may cause skin rash, peripheral neuropathy, blurred vision, hepatitis, and cholestatic jaundice.

Drug Interactions Probenecid can elevate blood levels of dapsone, which may result in toxicity.

Vancomycin

Vancomycin can destroy most gram-positive organisms.

Mechanism of Action Vancomycin is bactericidal. It inhibits bacterial cell wall synthesis.

Therapeutic Uses Vancomycin usually is reserved for serious infections, especially those caused by methicillin-resistant staphylococci. It is useful in patients who are allergic to penicillin or cephalosporins. Typical uses include osteomyelitis, endocarditis, and staphylococcal pneumonia.

Adverse Effects Vancomycin may cause nausea, chills, fever, ototoxicity, and nephrotoxicity. Vancomycin may cause "red man's syndrome" (also known as Stevens-Johnson syndrome). This condition is manifested by facial flushing and hypotension due to very rapid infusion of the drug. Infusion should occur a minimum of 60 minutes for a 1-gram dose. Local pain and phlebitis at the site of intravenous injection have been reported.

Drug Interactions Vancomycin increased neuromuscular blockade with atracurium, pancuronium, tubocurarine, and vecuronium.

ANTITUBERCULAR DRUGS

Antitubercular drugs are used to treat tuberculosis by suppressing or killing the slow-growing mycobacteria that cause this disease. Antitubercular agents are divided into two main categories: primary agents and retreatment agents. Because the causative organisms tend to develop resistance to any single drug, combination drug therapy has become standard for the treatment of tuberculosis. Agents chosen for therapy must eradicate mycobacteria. Drugs available include isoniazid, streptomycin, quinolones, ethambutol, rifampin, pyrazinamide, and rifabutin. Combination drug therapy is essential. Agents showing the lowest incidence of resistance such as isoniazid, rifampin, and streptomycin are usually used in combination with ethambutol or pyrazinamide. The initial agents used in most patients are isoniazid, rifampin, and pyrazinamide. A fourth drug (ethambutol or streptomycin) is added if resistance is suspected.

Primary Antitubercular Drugs

These include isoniazid, ethambutol, rifampin, pyrazinamide, and streptomycin. These drugs usually offer the greatest effectiveness with the least toxicity. In most patients, the combination of isoniazid, rifampin, and pyrazinamide is the most effective.

Isoniazid

This agent is the mainstay of antitubercular therapy and is used in all therapeutic regimens.

Mechanism of Action Isoniazid is bacteriostatic and bactericidal. The mechanism of action is not completely known.

Therapeutic Uses Isoniazid is the most widely prescribed antitubercular drug. It should be used in combination with another antitubercular agent to prevent drug resistance. In the majority of patients with tuberculosis, isoniazid should be administered for at least 6 months. The other agent, though, may continue to be administered for 6 months to 2 years depending on the severity of the disease. Prophylactic isoniazid may be given alone for up to 1 year in adults or children who have a positive tuberculin test result but lack active lesions.

Adverse Effects The most common adverse effects of isoniazid are fever, jaundice, peripheral neuritis, and skin rash. Hepatitis can be severe and fatal. Aplastic or hemolytic anemia and thrombocytopenia may occur.

Drug Interactions Isioniazid given with alcohol increases the risk of hepatotoxicity. Isioniazid may result in impaired phenytoin metabolism, leading to increased serum levels and toxicity. Isoniazid with ketoconazole may decrease serum levels of ketoconazole.

Ethambutol

Ethambutol is a synthetic water-based compound.

Mechanism of Action Ethambutol is bacteriostatic. The actual mechanism of action is unknown.

Therapeutic Uses Ethambutol is prescribed for the treatment of pulmonary tuberculosis in conjunction with at least one other antituberculosis drug.

Adverse Effects Ethambutol rarely may cause optic neuritis, drug fever, dizziness, and confusion.

Drug Interactions Ethambutol absorption is decreased with aluminum salts.

Rifampin

Rifampin is a complex macrocyclic agent.

Mechanism of Action Rifampin is bactericidal.

Therapeutic Uses The combination of rifampin and isoniazid is the most effective drug treatment for tuberculosis. Rifampin should not be given alone because it may lead to drug-resistant organisms. It may also be prescribed in combination with dapsone for the treatment of leprosy.

Adverse Effects Liver damage can result from rifampin therapy. Liver function test results should be routinely checked. Headache, fatigue, confusion, skin rash, nausea, and vomiting may occur. Rifampin may change the color of urine, tears, saliva, sweat, and feces to orange-red.

Drug Interactions Rifampin induces hepatic microsomal cytochrome P-450 enzymes; therefore, it may decrease the effect of many drugs such as warfarin, oral contraceptives, digitoxin, and corticosteroids. Probenecid may increase blood levels of rifampin.

Streptomycin

Streptomycin is an aminoglycoside that is given in combination with other antitubercular agents.

ANTIVIRAL DRUGS

These agents are used to treat viral infections; they act by influencing viral replication. Viruses are not able to independently provide their metabolic activity and can replicate only within living host cells. Therefore, antiviral agents tend to damage the host as well as viral cells. The majority of antiviral drugs are active against only one type of virus, either the DNA or the RNA type. DNA viruses include herpes simplex virus (HSV) 1 and 2, varicella-zoster virus (VZV), cytomegalovirus (CMV), and influenza A virus. Table 20-10 shows antiviral agents that are currently approved for treatment of DNA viruses.

Oseltamivir Phosphate

Oseltamivir phosphate is available as a capsule and as an oral suspension. It is indicated for the treatment of uncomplicated acute illness due to influenza infection in patients 1 year and older who have been symptomatic for no more than 2 days. It is also indicated for the prophylaxis of influenza in adult patients and adolescents 13 years and older.

Mechanism of Action

Oseltamivir phosphate is an ethyl ester prodrug; its mechanism of action is via inhibition of influenza virus neuraminidase with the possibility of alteration of virus particle aggregation and release.

Therapeutic Uses

This agent is effective against the symptoms of influenza, which include cough, nasal symptoms, sore throat, myalgia, chills, sweats, malaise, fatigue, and headache.

Adverse Effects

Adverse effects of oseltamivir phosphate include nausea and vomiting.

Drug Interactions

Because oseltamivir is excreted in the urine by glomerular filtration and tubular secretion via the anionic pathway, a potential exists for interaction with other agents excreted by this pathway.

Zanamivir

Zanamivir is used in the treatment of influenza. It is administered by oral inhalation only. A special plastic inhaler is

TABLE 20-10. Anti-DNA Viral Agents			
GENERIC NAME	**TRADE NAME**	**ROUTE OF ADMINISTRATION**	**COMMON DOSAGE RANGE**
Zanamivir	Relenza®	Inhalation	5 mg
Oseltamivir	Tamiflu®	Oral	75 mg
Rimantadine	Flumadine®	Oral—syrup and tablet	100 mg

used, into which is placed a powdered dose of the agent. The patient then inhales the dose from the inhaler.

Mechanism of Action

The proposed mechanism of action of zanamivir is via inhibition of influenza virus neuraminidase with the possibility of alteration of virus particle aggregation and release.

Therapeutic Uses

Zanamivir is indicated for the treatment of uncomplicated, acute illness due to influenza virus in patients 12 years and older who have been symptomatic for no more than 48 hours.

Adverse Effects

Adverse effects of zanamivir include bronchospasm and a decline in respiratory function.

Drug Interactions

No clinically significant pharmacokinetic drug interactions are known, based on data from *in vitro* studies.

HIV ANTIVIRAL AGENTS

RNA viruses include picornavirus (polio), rhabdovirus (rabies), paramyxoviruses (mumps and measles), and retrovirus

(HIV). Most patients with HIV infection are receiving combination therapy with different antiviral agents. Presently three classes of antiretroviral agents effective against HIV-1 and HIV-2 have been approved. These antiretroviral drugs include the nucleoside reverse transcriptase inhibitors (NRTIs), the non-nucleoside reverse transcriptase inhibitors (NNRTIs), and the protease inhibitors (PIs). Table 20-11 shows classifications of HIV antiviral agents.

Lamivudine

This agent is used in combination with other medications to treat HIV infection in patients with AIDS. It is not a cure and may not decrease the number of HIV-related illnesses. Lamivudine does not prevent the spread of HIV to other people. It is also used to treat hepatitis B infection. It is often used in combination with zidovudine.

Mechanism of Action

Lamivudine is in a class of medications called NRTIs, which work by interfering with viral reproduction by preventing the creation of new viral RNA. It should never be used alone because of viral resistance, which can occur very rapidly.

Therapeutic Uses

Lamuvidine is used to treat HIV infection, which can lead to AIDS and hepatitis B. It stops the spread of viruses responsible for both diseases.

TABLE 20-11. HIV Antiviral Agents

GENERIC NAME	TRADE NAME	ROUTE OF ADMINISTRATION	COMMON DOSAGE RANGE
NRTIs			
Abacavir	Ziagen®	Oral	300 mg bid
Zidovudine (azidothymidine, AZT)		Oral, IV	Oral: 100 mg q4h l; IV: 1 mg/kg q4h
Didanosine (DDI)	Videx®	Oral	125–200 mg q12h
Zalcitabine (ddC)	Hivid® (ddC)	Oral	0.750 mg q8h
Stavudine (d4T)	Zerit®	Oral	30–40 mg q12h
Lamivudine (3TC)	Epivir®	Oral	150 mg bid or tid
NNRTIs			
Delavirdine	Rescriptor DIV®	Oral	400 mg tid or 600 mg bid
Efavirenz	Sustiva®	Oral	600 mg/day
Nevirapine	Viramune®	Oral	200 mg bid
PIs			
Amprenavir	Agenerase®	Oral	1200 mg bid
Nelfinavir	Viracept®	Oral	750 mg tid or 1250 mg bid
Saquinavir	Invirase®, Fortovase®	Oral	1200 mg (Fortovase®) tid; 400 mg (Invirase®) bid
Ritonavir	Norvir®	Oral	600 mg bid
Indinavir	Crixivan®	Oral	800 mg q8h
Tenofovir	Viread®	Oral	300 mg once daily with meal

Adverse Effects

The most serious adverse effects of lamuvidine include rash, stomach pain, vomiting or upset stomach (in children), fever, muscle pain, and a numbness, tingling, or burning sensation in the fingers or toes.

Drug Interactions

Use of lamivudine with trimethoprim/sulfamethoxazole can increase the amount of lamivudine in the body. However, it is not necessary to change the dosages of either of these agents.

Ritonavir

Ritonavir is an anti-HIV drug that is a protease inhibitor. It is used to treat HIV infection when therapy is warranted.

Mechanism of Action

By interfering with the formation of essential proteins and enzymes, ritonavir blocks the maturation of HIV and causes formation of nonfunctional, immature, noninfectious virions.

Therapeutic Uses

Ritonavir is used to treat HIV infection in adults and children, in combination with other antiretroviral agents. Because it inhibits the metabolism of other protease inhibitors, it is being increasingly used for boosting and maintaining plasma concentrations of protease inhibitors.

Adverse Effects

One of the more serious effects of ritonavir is potentially fatal pancreatitis. Other serious adverse effects include body fat redistribution and accumulation, increased bleeding in patients with hemophilia types A and B, hyperglycemia, hyperlipidemia, new-onset diabetes mellitus, and exacerbation of existing diabetes mellitus.

Drug Interactions

When ritonavir is given in combination with other protease inhibitors, the dosage of the other protease inhibitors may be reduced. Drug interactions may occur when ritonavir is administered with a wide variety of other drugs, mostly because of pharmacokinetic interactions. Concomitant use of ritonavir with lovastatin or simvastatin is not recommended. Caution should also be taken when ritonavir is used with atorvastatin, cerivastatin, St. John's wort, sildenafil, astemizole, or cisapride.

Valganciclovir Hydrochloride

Valganciclovir hydrochloride has been approved by the FDA for the treatment of CMV retinitis in patients with AIDS.

Mechanism of Action

Valganciclovir is a prodrug of ganciclovir that exists as a mixture of two diastereomers. After oral administration, both are rapidly converted to ganciclovir by intestinal and hepatic esterases. Ganciclovir inhibits replication of human cytomegalovirus *in vitro* and *in vivo*.

Therapeutic Uses

Valganciclovir is an antiviral drug active against CMV retinitis.

Adverse Effects

Valganciclovir may cause fever, local and systemic infections, hypersensitivity reactions, convulsions, psychosis, hallucinations, neutropenia, anemia, thrombocytopenia, pancytopenia, bone marrow suppression, or aplastic anemia.

Drug Interactions

Antineoplastic agents such as amphotericin B, didanosine, trimethoprim/sulfamethoxazole, dapsone, pentamidine, probenecid, or zidovudine may increase bone marrow suppression and other toxic effects of valganciclovir. This agent may increase the risk of nephrotoxicity from cyclosporine. Antiretroviral agents may decrease valganciclovir levels or the risk of seizures due to imipenem-cilastatin.

Tenofovir

This agent is an antiviral drug that is approved for the treatment of HIV infection. It is able to reduce the HIV load in the blood, and when used in combination with other antiviral drugs, it can help prevent or reverse damage to the immune system and reduce the risk of AIDS-related illnesses. It is also being used experimentally for treatment of hepatitis B.

Mechanism of Action

Tenofovir is a potent inhibitor of retroviruses, including HIV-1. It may be active against nucleoside-resistant HIV strains. The active form of tenofovir persists in HIV-infected cells for prolonged periods; thus, it results in sustained inhibition of HIV replication. It reduces the viral load and CD4 counts.

Therapeutic Uses

Tenofovir is used in combination with other antiretroviral agents for the treatment of HIV.

Adverse Effects

Tenofovir may cause asthenia, anorexia, neutropenia, and increased creatine kinase, aspartate aminotransferase (AST), alanine aminotransferase (ALT), serum amylase, triglycerides, or serum glucose levels.

Drug Interactions

Tenofovir may increase didanosine toxicity. Use of this agent with acyclovir, amphotericin B, cidofovir, foscarnet, ganciclovir, probenecid, valacyclovir, or valganciclovir may increase tenofovir toxicity by decreasing its renal elimination.

ANTIVIRAL AGENTS IN THE UNITED STATES

Only a few antiviral agents have been successfully used in the United States. However, several viral diseases such as polio, mumps, measles, rabies, chicken pox, and smallpox are prevented by vaccines. The antiviral agents reviewed here are acyclovir, amantadine, famciclovir, ganciclovir, and ribavirin. Table 20-12 shows classifications of various antiviral drugs and their therapeutic uses.

Highly Active Antiretroviral Therapy

Antiviral agents are being used currently either alone or in combination for the treatment of HIV infection. Highly active antiretroviral therapy (HAART) has been shown to reduce viral load and increase CD4 lymphocytes in persons infected with HIV, delay the onset of AIDS, and prolong sur-

vival with AIDS. The incidence of and mortality from AIDS have declined substantially since 1996 due to HAART. The benefits of HAART, which involves the combination of three to four drugs effective against HIV, have been widely publicized. Two distinct categories of drugs are combined: nucleoside analogs and protease inhibitors. However, the use of HAART presents formidable challenges, including side effects and the potential for rapid development of drug resistance. Protease inhibitors do not work as well with a third category of HIV drugs, the non-nucleoside analogs, which should not be taken alone. If one of the drugs involved in the triple or quadruple therapy is not well tolerated or if a patient's HIV infection becomes resistant to it, a whole new set of drugs must be prescribed for the regimen to be effective. Presently, because of the limited number of HAART medications available in the United States, only a few different drug combinations are possible. HAART regimens can also fail because of lack of viral load response or the patient's poor adherence to treatment. Missing a single dose of HAART even twice a week can cause the development of drug-resistant HIV—a real danger because adherence to the drug regimen is difficult. Simplifying HIV antiretroviral therapy regimens has been shown to improve adherence. Studies have shown that patients can adhere better to regimens that require less frequent dosing (two or fewer times per day), and regimens that do not have food restrictions. Long-term side effects include lipodystrophy (a nearly complete lack of fat below the skin), diabetes, and coronary heart disease. Patients must be counseled to be aware of the

TABLE 20-12. Antiviral Drugs and Their Therapeutic Uses

GENERIC NAME	TRADE NAME	THERAPEUTIC USES	ADVERSE EFFECTS
Non-HIV Antivirals			
Abacavir	Ziagen®	HIV infection	Insomnia, hypotension
Acyclovir	Zovirax®	Herpes virus types 1 and 2	Confusion, seizures, acute renal failure
Amantadine	Symmetrel®	Influenza A	Nausea, vomiting, phlebitis at site, nephrotoxicity
Cidofovir	Vistide®	Cytomegalovirus, retinitis	Nausea, vomiting, dyspnea
Famciclovir	Famvir®	Genital herpes	Headache, dizziness, diarrhea, vomiting
Ganciclovir	Cytovene®	Cytomegalovirus	Disorientation, coma, edema
Rimantadine	Flumadine®	Influenza A	Drowsiness, nausea, vomiting
Ribavirin	Rebetol®	Influenza A and B, measles, mumps	Fatigue, anemia, jaundice, chest pain
Valacyclovir	Valtrex®	Genital herpes, herpes zoster	Acute renal failure, headache
			Palpitations, thrombophlebitis
HIV Antivirals			
Didanosine (DDI)	Videx®	Advanced HIV infection	Fatigue, headache, anemia
Indinavir	Crixivan®	HIV infection	Abdominal pain, anemia, headache
Nevirapine	Viramune®	HIV infection	Anorexia, nausea, vomiting
Stavudine	Zerit®	Advanced HIV infection	Myopathy, headache, insomnia
Zidovudine (azidothymidine, AZT)	Retrovir®	HIV infection with impaired immunity	Myopathy, headache, insomnia
Combination Medications			
Zidovudine-lamivudine	Combivir®	HIV infection	Nausea, vomiting, bone marrow depression

signs of disease and to avoid the fear of expressing their symptoms, so that their physicians may treat them properly and in time. This is especially true for life-threatening illnesses such as AIDS. Because of the stigma attached to AIDS and other diseases such as cancer, many patients avoid reporting their symptoms early enough. To treat these types of diseases, very often combinations of drugs must be used to achieve a potent effect. One combination antiviral agent approved for the treatment of HIV infection and AIDS is 2,3'-dideoxycytidine (ddC, also called zalcitabine), which is to be used only with the popular drug zidovudine (AZT). Its main side effect is peripheral neuropathy, which causes numbness, tingling, burning, or pain in the hands or feet.

Acyclovir

Acyclovir is a synthetic acyclic analog of guanosine with activity against various herpesviruses. Herpesviruses can infect neonates, children, and adults, causing a wide spectrum of diseases. Herpes simplex type 1 virus is responsible for systemic infections involving the liver and other organs, including the central nervous system, and localized infections may involve the skin, eyes, and mouth. Other medically important herpesviruses include CMV, varicella (chicken pox), and VZVt (shingles). Acyclovir is available in tablets ranging in strength from 200 to 800 mg.

Vidabrine is another agent that works similarly to acyclovir, but its action is on herpes virus type A.

Mechanism of Action

Acyclovir is taken up selectively by cells that are infected with herpesviruses. Its activity depends upon conversion to its triphosphate form when it becomes incorporated into viral DNA and inhibits viral replication.

Therapeutic Uses

Acyclovir is most active against HSV-1 and HSV-2. IV acyclovir is used for HSV encephalitis, neonatal HSV, and life-threatening HSV and VZV infections in immunocompromised patients. Oral acyclovir is indicated for the treatment of primary and recurrent genital herpes. Acyclovir ophthalmic ointment is effective for herpes simplex keratitis.

Adverse Effects

Acyclovir may cause nausea, vomiting, and headache. The drug can precipitate in the renal tubules with excessive dosages or when it is given by rapid infusion.

Drug Interactions

Amphotericin B may raise the plasma and renal concentrations of acyclovir. Probenecid reduces its renal excretion.

Amantadine

Amantadine is an antiviral agent effective for respiratory infections.

Mechanism of Action

The mechanism of the antiviral activity of amantadine is unknown. Its action appears to occur early in the course of viral infection.

Therapeutic Uses

Amantadine is indicated for the prophylaxis and treatment of influenza A viral infections, as well as for Parkinson's disease. Individuals who have not received vaccine prophylaxis can benefit from amantadine prophylaxis given for at least 10 days after a known exposure to influenza A. Amantadine is contraindicated during pregnancy.

Adverse Effects

Amantadine causes mild adverse effects including anxiety, insomnia, and dizziness. Urinary retention is another potential side effect. Serious adverse effects in patients treated for Parkinson's disease have included congestive heart failure, hypotension, depression, seizures, psychosis, and leukopenia.

Drug Interactions

Amantadine interacts with anticholinergic drugs to produce atropine-like effects unless the dosage of the anticholinergic drug is reduced. Amantadine prophylaxis or treatment does not interfere with the immune response to influenza vaccination given concurrently.

Famciclovir

Famciclovir is a prodrug (inactive or partially active drug that is metabolically changed in the body to an active drug) of the antiviral agent penciclovir.

Mechanism of Action

Famciclovir is rapidly phosphorylated in virus-infected cells by viral thymidine kinase (special enzyme) to penciclovir monophosphate.

Therapeutic Uses

Famciclovir is effective against HSV-1, HSV-2, and VZV. The drug is prescribed for management of acute VZV infections (shingles) and genital herpes infections.

Adverse Effects

Common adverse effects resulting from famciclovir use include fatigue, nausea, diarrhea, vomiting, constipation, and anorexia. Headache is also often reported.

Drug Interactions

Probenecid can increase the plasma concentration of penciclovir. Famciclovir may increase digoxin levels.

Ganciclovir

Ganciclovir is a synthetic purine nucleoside analog that is approved for the treatment of CMV infections.

Mechanism of Action

After conversion to ganciclovir triphosphate, ganciclovir is incorporated into viral DNA and inhibits viral DNA polymerase. By this mechanism, it can terminate viral replication.

Therapeutic Uses

Ganciclovir is prescribed for CMV infections such as pneumonia and retinitis.

Adverse Effects

Ganciclovir has black box warnings concerning an increased potential for dose-limited neutropenia, thrombocytopenia, and anemia. (Black box warnings are issued by the FDA when a serious problem concerning the use of a drug has been discovered, so that medical practitioners are aware of the problem and its resulting adverse effects.) Phlebitis and pain may occur at the site of infusion.

Drug Interactions

Probenecid may increase ganciclovir levels and possibly toxicity.

Ribavirin

Ribavirin is a synthetic nucleoside analog.

Mechanism of Action

Ribavirin has broad activity against both RNA and DNA viruses. It is effective against influenza A infections. Ribavirin reduces HIV replication in T lymphocyte cultures.

Therapeutic Uses

Ribavirin given by aerosol into an infant oxygen hood has been effective for the treatment of respiratory syncytial virus pneumonia.

Adverse Effects

Oral administration of ribavirin causes anemia.

Drug Interactions

No specific drug interactions have been identified, but clinical experience with the systemic administration of ribavirin is limited.

ANTIFUNGAL DRUGS

These agents are used to treat systemic, local fungal, and topical fungal infections. Antifungal drugs are listed in Table 20-13.

Voriconazole

Voriconzale is a triazole that is structurally related to fluconazole.

Mechanism of Action

As with all azole antifungal agents, voriconazole works principally by inhibiting the cytochrome P-450 enzymes used for an essential step in fungal ergosterol biosynthesis.

Therapeutic Uses

Voriconazole is active against *Aspergillus fumigatus* as well as *Aspergillus flavus, Aspergillus niger,* and *Aspergillus terreus.* Variable activity against *Scedosporium apiospermum* and *Fusarium* infections has been seen. It is used in the treatment of invasive aspergillosis.

Adverse Effects

Voriconazole may cause peripheral edema, fever, chills, hallucinations, tachycardia, hypotension, hypertension, vasodilation, cholestatic jaundice, increased alkaline phosphatase, AST, and ALT levels, hypokalemia, hypomagnesemia, rash, pruritus, abnormal vision, or photophobia.

Drug Interactions

Because of significant increased toxicity or decreased activity, the following drugs are contraindicated with use of voriconazole: barbiturates, carbamazepine, cisapride, ergot alkaloids, pimozide, quinidine, rifabutin, sirolimus, fosphenytoin, phenytoin, and rifampin. Protease inhibitors may increase voriconazole toxicity.

Oxiconazole

Oxiconazole is an antifungal agent used to treat skin infections such as athlete's foot, jock itch, and ringworm.

Mechanism of Action

This synthetic antifungal agent presumably works by altering the cellular membrane of fungi, resulting in increased membrane permeability, secondary metabolic effects, and growth inhibition.

Therapeutic Uses

Oxiconazole is used in the treatment of tinea pedis, tinea cruris, and tinea corporis. It is also used for cutaneous candidiasis.

TABLE 20-13. Antifungal Agents

GENERIC NAME	TRADE NAME	ROUTE OF ADMINISTRATION	COMMON DOSAGE RANGE
Amphotericin B	Fungizone®	IV	0.25 mg/kg/day
Griseofulvin	Grifulvin®, Fulvicin®	Oral	500 mg–1 g/day
Nystatin	Mycostatin®	Oral, vaginal	500,000–1,000,000U tid; vaginal 1–2 times daily for 2 weeks
Clioquinol	Torofor®, Vioform®	Topical	Apply thin layer to affected area bid for 1 week only
Terbinafine	Lamisil®	Oral	250 mg/day
Fluconazole	Diflucan®	Oral, IV	100–200 mg orally daily; 200 mg IV for 14–21 days. In some cases the dosage can be up to 400 mg four times daily
Butoconazole	Femstat 3®, Femstat 1®	Topical, vaginal	One applicator full vaginally before bedtime
Miconazole	Monistat®	Topical, vaginal	Apply cream or suppository in vagina daily at bedtime
Clotrimazole	Mycelex®, Lotrimin®	Topical, oral, vaginal	10 mg; topical: bid as needed; vaginal: 5–100 mg in applicator at bedtime
Tioconazole	Trosyd AF®	Topical, vaginal	5 mg once a day
Carboxybenzene (benzoic acid)		Oral	Various-combined ingredient
Econazole	Spectazole®	Topical	15–85 g (as needed)
Ketoconazole	Nizoral®	Oral	200–400 mg single dose daily
Tolciclate	Tolmicen®	Oral, topical	Oral 100 g; topical 30 g/30 mL
Tolnaftate	Absorbine®	Topical	2 oz, as needed
Caspofungin	Cancidas®	IV	35–70 mg daily
Itraconazole	Sporanox®	Oral	100–400 mg daily

Adverse Effects

Oxiconazole may cause transient burning and stinging, skin dryness, erythema, pruritus, and local irritation.

Drug Interactions

No clinically significant drug interactions have been established.

Econazole

Econazole is an antifungal agent that is applied to the skin to treat fungus infections.

Mechanism of Action

Econazole is a synthetic imidazole derivative with a broad spectrum of antifungal activity similar to that of miconazole. It exerts fungistatic action but may be fungicidal for certain microorganisms.

Therapeutic Uses

Econazole is active against dermatophytes, yeasts, and many other types of fungi. It combats athlete's foot, jock itch, ringworm of the body, and moniliasis. It also appears to be active against some gram-positive bacteria. Clinical improvement occurs within the first 1 to 2 weeks of therapy. Immune-suppressed people are at increased risk of acquiring fungal infections; included in this group are those who have had solid organ and bone marrow transplants, those with HIV infection, and those receiving cancer chemotherapy.

Adverse Effects

Econazole may cause burning or stinging sensations, pruritus, or erythema.

Drug Interactions

No clinically significant interactions with the use of econazole have been established.

Naftifine

Naftifine is an anti-infective, antibiotic, and antifungal drug used against tinea infections.

Mechanism of Action

Naftifine is a synthetic broad-spectrum antifungal agent that may be fungicidal depending on the organism. It interferes with the synthesis of ergosterol, the principal sterol in the fungus cell membrane.

Therapeutic Uses

Naftifine is used to treat tinea pedis, tinea cruris, and tinea corporis. It is also effective against tinea unguium (onychomycosis).

Adverse Effects

Naftifine may cause burning or stinging sensations, skin dryness, erythema, itching, or local irritation.

Drug Interactions

No clinically significant interactions with the use of naftifine have been established.

Tolnaftate

Tolnaftate stops the growth of fungi that cause skin infections, including athlete's foot, jock itch, and ringworm. It may be used for other conditions as well.

Mechanism of Action

Tolnaftate is a synthetic topical antifungal agent. Its mechanism of action is not clear, but clinical tests have shown that tolnaftate distorts hyphae and stunts mycelial growth on susceptible fungi. It is fungistatic or fungicidal to various types of *Microsporum*.

Therapeutic Uses

Tolnaftate is used to treat athlete's foot, jock itch, body ringworm, tinea capitis and tinea unguium, plantar or palmar lesions, and tinea versicolor.

Adverse Effects

Tolnaftate may cause local irritation and stinging of the skin from aerosol formulation.

Drug Interactions

No clinically significant interactions with the use of tolnaftate have been established.

Undecylenic Acid

Undecylenic acid is an antifungal compound used to treat various fungus infections, but it has generally been replaced by newer and more effective medicines.

Mechanism of Action

Compound undecylenic acid has a fungistatic action.

Theraputic Uses

Undecylenic acid is used for the topical treatment of fungal (ringworm) infections of the fingernails and toenails.

Adverse Effects

Among the more serious adverse effects are skin irritation and hypersensitivity reactions.

Drug Interactions

No drug interactions with the use of undecylenic acid have been established.

Amphotericin B

Amphotericin B is used for both systemic and topical fungal infections. Amphotericin B is being prescribed increasingly for severely immunocompromised patients in special clinical situations. It is also available as a 3% cream or lotion or as an oral suspension for topical uses. Liposomal amphotericin B is a lipid formulation of amphotericin B. This type reaches high concentrations in plasma and remains in the circulation longer.

Mechanism of Action

Amphotericin B is fungistatic and may be fungicidal. It is a broad-spectrum antifungal drug.

Therapeutic Uses

Amphotericin B is the most effective antifungal agent for the treatment of systemic fungal infections, particularly in immunocompromised patients. It is the drug of choice for pulmonary *Aspergillus, Blastomyces, Candida, Coccidioides*, and disseminated *Histoplasma* infections. Topical preparations are used to treat cutaneous and mucocutaneous candidiasis.

Adverse Effects

Amphotericin B can cause many serious side effects. Therefore, it should be administered in a hospital. The adverse effects include fever, nausea, vomiting, headache, hypotension, dyspnea, and tachypnea. Nephrotoxicity, anaphylactoid reactions, phlebitis, and liver damage may occur. Amphotericin B for parenteral use should only be mixed in dextrose 5% in water and should be protected from light. Sometimes patients may be premedicated with intravenous diphenhydramine or acetaminophen before administration.

Griseofulvin

Griseofulvin is a drug that is deposited in the skin and binds to keratin.

Mechanism of Action

Griseofulvin is fungistatic. It inhibits fungal cell activity. This agent is active against various strains of *Microsporum, Trichophyton*, and *Epidermophyton*.

Therapeutic Uses

Griseofulvin is effective in tinea infections of the nails, hair, and skin. It is available only in oral form. Griseofulvin may also be used to treat gout (a disease associated with an inborn error of uric acid metabolism that can cause painful, deformative, and destructive changes in the joints and surrounding tissues).

Adverse Effects

Griseofulvin may produce fatigue, headache, confusion, syncope, and lethargy. It also occasionally causes leukopenia and rarely serum sickness and hepatotoxicity.

Drug Interactions

This agent may increase the metabolism of warfarin. Barbiturates can reduce absorption of griseofulvin. Oral contraceptives may produce amenorrhea and alcohol consumption can cause flushing and tachycardia.

Nystatin

The chemical structure of nystatin is similar to that of amphotericin B. It is the common topical treatment for thrush, which can occur in the mouth or on the tongue, gums, or skin. It is not considered a systemic antifungal agent but rather acts locally. It is available in tablets or as a liquid suspension, as well as a cream, ointment, and topical powder. To be effective, therapy is usually continued for 2 weeks.

Mechanism of Action

Nystatin is fungicidal and fungistatic. It is effective against *Candida* species.

Therapeutic Uses

Nystatin is prescribed primarily as a topical drug for vaginal and oral *Candida* infections or for diaper rash caused by *Candida*. It is often used prophylactically on the area covered by a diaper when an oral *Candida* infection is present.

Adverse Effects

Nystatin can temporarily affect the sense of taste and, thus, decrease appetite. Other adverse effects include nausea, vomiting, diarrhea, and stomach pain. If nystatin is used to treat vaginal infections, the patient should avoid using sanitary napkins and refrain from sexual contact until the infection subsides.

Drug Interactions

No drug interactions with the use of nystatin have been established.

Clioquinol

Clioquinol is a topical antifungal available in a 3% ointment that can be used alone or in combination with hydrocortisone.

Mechanism of Action

The mechanism of action of clioquinol is unknown, but it is effective against dermatophytic fungi.

Therapeutic Uses

Clioquinol is used for tinea pedis and tinea cruris (ringworm infections).

Adverse Effects

Adverse effects may include local burning, irritation, redness, rash, and staining of hair and skin. Clioquinol may also cause slight enlargement of the thyroid gland and hair loss.

Caspofungin

Caspofungin is a polypeptide antifungal that is also a glucan synthesis inhibitor of the echinocandin cell structure.

Mechanism of Action

Caspofungin blocks the synthesis of a major fungal cell wall component called 1,3-β-glucan. It is fungicidal for *Candida* infections and is active against *Aspergillus* infections as well.

Therapeutic Uses

Caspofungin is used to treat invasive aspergillosis that is refractory to other treatment. It is also used in patients who are intolerant of other therapies.

Adverse Effects

Adverse effects associated with the use of caspofungin include rash, facial swelling, itching, and a sensation of warmth.

Drug Interactions

Caspofungin has been shown to increase tacrolimus levels. Cyclosporine has been shown to decrease caspofungin levels. Some patients who have received caspofungin have experienced increased values on liver function tests.

Itraconazole

Itraconazole is an antifungal agent indicated for the treatment of histoplasmosis, aspergillosis, and blastomycosis. Liver function should be monitored during treatment with itraconazole.

Mechanism of Action

Itraconazole works principally by the sterol biosynthesis pathway enzyme that leads from lanosterol to ergosterol.

Therapeutic Uses

Itraconazole is effective for infections of the skin, hair, and nails by dermatophytes and/or yeasts, ringworm, tinea versicolor, chronic mucocutaneous candidiasis, *Candida* vulvovaginitis, and oral/esophageal candidiasis.

Adverse Effects

Itraconazole may cause heart failure. With high doses, hypertension may occur. Other adverse effects include headache, dizziness, fatigue, euphoria, drowsiness, gynecomastia, hypokalemia, hypertriglyceridemia, impotence, rash, pruritus, and adrenal insufficiency.

Drug Interactions

Itraconazole may increase levels and toxicity of oral hypoglycemic agents including warfarin, terfenadine, and ritonavir. Combination with astemizole, cisapride, pimozide, or quinidine may cause severe cardiac events including cardiac arrest or sudden death.

Terbinafine

Because of its lack of drug interactions, terbinafine is the treatment of choice for several fungal infections.

Mechanism of Action

Terbinafine prevents synthesis of ergosterol, a building block for fungal cell membranes. It acts by inhibiting fungal cytochrome P-450, which is different from human cytochrome P-450.

Therapeutic Uses

Terbinafine is used to treat *Trichophyton rubrum* and *Trichophyton mentagrophytes*.

Adverse Effects

The adverse effects reported most often include severe cutaneous reactions from oral terbinafine, including Stevens-Johnson syndrome, toxic epidermal necrolysis, and allergic urticaria.

Drug Interactions

There are no major drug interaction concerns with terbinafine and no known interactions that are clinically significant.

Fluconazole

Fluconazole is indicated for treatment of oropharyngeal and esophageal candidiasis, systemic candidal infections, and cryptococcal pneumonia.

Mechanism of Action

Fluconazole inhibits fungal cytochrome P-450 synthesis of ergosterol, resulting in decreased cell wall integrity and leakage of essential cellular components.

Therapeutic Uses

Fluconazole has been shown to be effective against *Candida* and some molds such as the *Bipolaris* species and *Rhodotorula rubra*.

Adverse Effects

The most common adverse effects of fluconazole include elevated liver enzyme levels, gastrointestinal complaints, headache, and skin rash.

Drug Interactions

Drug interactions are possible when fluconazole is taken with cisapride, terfenadine, astemizole, phenytoin, rifabutin, rifampin, midazolam, triazolam, or tolbutamide.

Clotrimazole

Clotrimazole is an antifungal medication that is used to treat yeast (fungal) infections of the mouth and throat.

Mechanism of Action

Clotrimazole inhibits fungal cytochrome P-450 synthesis of ergosterol, which decreases cell wall integrity.

Therapeutic Uses

Clotrimazol is especially effective against oropharyngeal candidiasis. Oral administration over a long time necessitates periodic monitoring of liver function. Clotrimazole is also available over-the-counter as a vaginal cream. In topical form it is prescribed for ringworm.

Adverse Effects

Adverse effects of clotrimazole include hypersensitivity, nausea, vomiting, itching, and an unpleasant aftertaste.

Drug Interactions

Because clotrimazole is not absorbed by the body, drug interactions are not expected.

ANTIPROTOZOAL DRUGS

Protozoa are another type of microorganism. A protozoan is a usually motile unicellular protist. Protozoan groups that cause major diseases in humans include amoebae, sporozoa,

TABLE 20-14.	Protozoa That Cause Major Diseases and Preferred Site of Infection		
PROTOZOAN GROUP	**GENUS**	**PREFERRED SITE OF INFECTION**	**DISEASE**
Amoebae	*Entamoeba*	Intestine	Amebiasis
Sporozoa	*Plasmodium*	Bloodstream, liver	Malaria
	Toxoplasma	Intestine	
Flagellates	*Trypanosoma*	Blood	Toxoplasmosis
	Trichomonas	Genital tract	Trypanosomiasis
			Trichomoniasis
	Giardia	Intestine	Giardiasis

and flagellates. Table 20-14 shows the characteristics of each group.

Antiprotozoal agents are classified into two main categories: antimalarial agents, used to treat malaria infection, and amebicides and trichomonacides, prescribed to treat amebic and trichomonal infections.

Amebicides and Trichomonacides

These drugs are very important in the treatment of amebiasis, giardiasis, and trichomoniasis, which are the most common protozoal infections in the United States. The major amebicides include metronidazole, emetine, diloxanide, and paromomycin.

Mechanism of Action

These agents inhibit bacterial protein synthesis in specific (obligate) anaerobes and are amebicidal. The biochemical mechanism of action is not known.

Therapeutic Uses

1. *Metronidazole:* This is the drug of choice for amebic dysentery, giardiasis, and trichomoniasis.
2. *Emetine:* This is an agent commonly used to treat severe intestinal amebiasis, amebic abscess, and amebic hepatitis. Because of its toxicity, emetine is prescribed only when other drugs are contraindicated.
3. *Diloxanide:* This drug is used for extraintestinal amebiasis. It is also prescribed to treat asymptomatic carriers of amebic and giardiac cysts.
4. *Paromomycin:* This is prescribed for acute and chronic intestinal amebiasis.

Adverse Effects

1. *Metronidazole:* This may cause nausea, vomiting, diarrhea, metallic taste, and occasionally, neurological reactions. Metronidazole can cause cancer in mice and should not be used unnecessarily.
2. *Emetine:* This agent can cause severe systemic toxicity such as tachycardia, hypotension, congestive heart failure,

dizziness, headache, nausea, vomiting, and diarrhea. It is contraindicated in children and patients with renal impairment and cardiac disease.
3. *Diloxanide:* This rarely causes serious adverse effects. Vomiting and pruritus may occur.
4. *Paromomycin:* This agent may cause nausea, diarrhea, and cramping at high doses.

Drug Interactions

Paromomycin increased neuromuscular blockade with succinylcholine. It increased or decreased bioavailability of digoxin.

Antimalarial Agents

The most important human parasite among the sporozoa is *Plasmodium,* which causes malaria. There are four different types of *Plasmodium: Plasmodium falciparum, Plasmodium malariae, Plasmodium vivax,* and *Plasmodium ovale.* It has been estimated that more than 100 million people are infected and about 1 million people die annually of malaria in Africa alone. Antimalarial drugs are selectively active during different phases of the protozoan life cycle. Antimalarial drugs include chloroquine, primaquine, quinine, and hydroxychloroquine. Some agents are used for prevention of malaria. They include mefloquine, quinacrine, and folic acid antagonists. Mefloquine is chemically related to quinine. It is used both for prevention of malaria and treatment of acute malarial infections. Quinacrine was once the most popular drug for malaria prophylaxis, but its use has declined sharply with the development of safer and more effective agents. Folic acid antagonists such as pyrimethamine and sulfa drugs interfere with the synthesis of folic acid. They may be used alone or in combination to suppress and prevent malaria caused by susceptible strains of *Plasmodium.*

Mechanism of Action

Chloroquine and hydroxychloroquine bind to and alter the properties of plasmodium. The mechanism of action of primaquine and quinine is unknown.

Therapeutic Uses

Chloroquine is the drug of choice to suppress symptoms of malaria and treat acute malarial attacks resulting from *P. falciparum* and *P. malariae* infections. Chloroquine is the most useful antimalarial agent. Hydroxychloroquine is prescribed as an alternative to chloroquine in patients who cannot tolerate chloroquine or when chloroquine is unavailable. Primaquine is used to cure relapses of *P. vivax* and *P. ovale* malaria, to prevent malaria in exposed persons, and to prevent and treat malaria caused by chloroquine-resistant strains of *P. falciparum*. Quinine is prescribed for acute malaria caused by chloroquine-resistant strains. Quinine is always given in combination with another antimalarial agent.

Adverse Effects

1. *Chloroquine and hydroxychloroquine:* These drugs can concentrate in the liver and must be used carefully in patients with liver diseases. They may cause visual disturbances, headache, and skin rash.
2. *Primaquine:* Primaquine is contraindicated in patients with rheumatoid arthritis and lupus erythematosus. It may cause anemia, granulocytopenia, nausea, vomiting, and abdominal cramps.
3. *Quinine:* Overdose or hypersensitivity reactions may be fatal. Quinine toxicity includes visual and hearing disturbances, headache, fever, syncope, and cardiovascular collapse.

Other Antimalarial Agents

Malarone is a new combination drug for the prevention and treatment of acute malaria caused by *P. falciparum*. Malarone is a combination of atovaquone and proguanil HCl. Malarone is effective when resistance to other antimalarial drugs has developed.

SECONDARY APLASTIC ANEMIA

Secondary aplastic anemia is a failure of the blood cell-forming capacity of the bone marrow that affects all blood cell types. It is also known as acquired aplastic anemia. The condition is a result of injury to the stem cell, a cell that produces other blood cell types when it divides and differentiates. Causes of secondary aplastic anemia include chemotherapy, drug therapy to suppress the immune system, radiation therapy, toxins such as benzene or arsenic, drugs, pregnancy, and congenital disorders. Symptoms arise as a consequence of bone marrow failure and include fatigue, pallor, shortness of breath, rapid heart rate, rash, easy bruising, nose bleeds, bleeding of the gums, prolonged bleeding, and frequent or severe infections.

ANTIMICROBIAL CHEMOTHERAPY

Antimicrobial agents can also be classified by their range of activity. *Narrow-spectrum drugs* are only active against a relatively small number of organisms. *Moderate-spectrum drugs* are generally effective against gram-positive pathogens and most systemic, enteric, and urinary tract gram-negative pathogens. The β-lactam antibiotics belong in a third category, *narrow- and moderate-spectrum drugs*, because some of them are only effective against gram-positive organisms whereas others can also kill certain gram-negative bacteria. A fourth category is termed *broad-spectrum drugs*. These drugs are effective against all prokaryotes with two exceptions: *Mycobacterium* and *Pseudomonas* organisms. The fifth group includes drugs that are effective against *Mycobacterium* organisms. Although antimicrobial drug therapy can be life-saving, it also poses certain dangers to the patient. Some of the side effects and dangers of antimicrobial chemotherapy include overgrowth of pathogens, depression of intestinal symbiotes, nephrotoxicity, ototoxicity, ophthalmic toxicity, aplastic anemia, hypersensitivity, and bone damage.

SUMMARY

The invasion of pathogenic microorganisms may cause either local or systemic infection. The pathogen can be present in the blood circulation, causing bacteremia. Anti-infective drugs, generally called antibiotics, are used to treat infection. Selection of antibiotics depends on various factors such as pharmacologic properties and spectrum activity of the drugs and patient factors such as immunity, age, adverse drug reactions, and underlying diseases. Pregnancy and lactation also play a major role. There are broad classifications of anti-infective drugs that affect specific pathogens such as bacteria, viruses, fungi, protozoa, and rickettsia. Penicillins are the most widely used antimicrobial agents. However, cephalosporin usage has increased during the last decade. Specific antibiotics are used predominantly for penicillinase-resistant penicillins. The first drugs used successfully to prevent and treat human bacterial infections were sulfonamides.

CRITICAL THINKING

1. Explain the differences between viruses and bacteria.
2. Define the mode of transmission.
3. Classify microlides and their mechanisms of action.
4. Make a list of HIV antiviral drugs.
5. Describe antitubercular drugs.

REVIEW QUESTIONS

1. Amantadine is prescribed for the prophylaxis and treatment of
   A. malaria.
   B. *Candida* infections.
   C. HIV infection.
   D. influenza A.

2. Third-generation cephalosporins are potent against all of the following, except
   A. *Neisseria gonorrhoeae.*
   B. *Mycobacterium tuberculosis.*
   C. *Haemophilus influenzae.*
   D. enterobacteria.

3. Which of the antibiotics should not be used in children younger than age 10?
   A. Chloramphenicol
   B. Penicillins
   C. Isoniazid
   D. Ciprofloxacin

4. All of the following agents are in the class of macrolides except
   A. sulfonamide.
   B. erythromycin.
   C. troleandomycin.
   D. clarithromycin.

5. Penicillinase may be produced by
   A. streptococci.
   B. *Neisseria gonorrhoeae.*
   C. staphylococci.
   D. *Haemophilus influenzae.*

6. Streptomycin can be used for all of the following infectious diseases, except
   A. tuberculosis.
   B. plague.
   C. otitis.
   D. tularemia.

7. Which of the following antibiotics may cause enamel hypoplasia and permanent yellow-gray color of the teeth in young children?
   A. Isoniazids
   B. Streptomycins
   C. Rifampins
   D. Tetracyclines

8. Metronidazole is the drug of choice for
   A. trichomoniasis.
   B. tularemia
   C. tuberculosis.
   D. tapeworms.

9. Which of the following antibiotics may lead to gray baby syndrome?
   A. Tetracyclines
   B. Chloramphenicol
   C. Streptomycin
   D. Metronidazole

10. Which of the following antimicrobial agents has a chemical structure similar to that of amphotericin B?
    A. Ribavirin
    B. Streptomycin
    C. Amantadine
    D. Nystatin

11. A person who lacks resistance to an agent and is vulnerable to a disease is called a
    A. compromised host.
    B. susceptible host.
    C. virulent host.
    D. parasitic host.

12. The presence of viable bacteria in the circulatory system is called
    A. bacteremia.
    B. viremia.
    C. sepsis.
    D. localized infection.

13. The reservoir is a place where
    A. an infectious agent leaves the body.
    B. an organism invades the host.
    C. an agent can be spread to others.
    D. an agent can survive, colonize, and reproduce.

14. Two examples of diseases transmitted by airborne transmission are
    A. mumps and encephalitis.
    B. measles and anthrax.
    C. chicken pox and *Salmonella.*
    D. lupus and Lyme disease.

15. Anti-infective drugs derived from natural substances are called
    A. antivirals.
    B. Gram stains.
    C. antibiotics.
    D. antifungals.

Antineoplastic Agents

21

OUTLINE

OBJECTIVES

Upon completion of this chapter, the reader should be able to

1. Explain neoplasm and its classification.
2. Describe chemotherapy and the types of antineoplastic drugs.
3. List the classes of antimetabolites.
4. Explain the use of hormone therapy as an antineoplastic agent.
5. Describe the first group of antineoplastic agents.
6. List the classes of mitotic inhibitors (plant alkaloids).
7. Define radiation therapy.
8. Explain toxicity of antineoplastic agents.
9. List specific side effects of certain antineoplastic agents on particular organs or systems in the body.

GLOSSARY

alkylating agent An antineoplastic agent that affects cell growth.

antimetabolite A substance that prevents cancer growth by affecting DNA production.

antineoplastic agents Drugs used to treat cancers and malignant neoplasms.

benign Nonprogressive.

cardiac toxicity Adverse effects on the heart by drugs or chemical substances.

extravasation Leakage of fluid from vessels into surrounding tissues.

hormonal agents Substances consisting of a heterogeneous compound that either blocks hormone production or blocks hormone action.

malignant Spreading.

metastasis Uncontrollable growth characteristic of cancer cells.

neoplasm A tumor.

nitrosoureas Newer forms of alkylating agent that are lipid soluble.

pulmonary toxicity Adverse effects on the lungs by drugs or chemical substances.

OVERVIEW

A tumor, or **neoplasm**, arises from a single abnormal cell, which continues to divide indefinitely. The lack of growth controls, ability to invade local tissue, and ability to spread, or **metastasize**, are characteristics of cancer cells. These properties are not present in normal cells. Tumors are either **benign** (nonprogressive) or **malignant** (spreading). More than 100 different types of malignant neoplasms occur in man. In treating cancers, multiple drug therapy is used to take advantage of drugs that have different mechanisms of action. To properly treat any type of cancer, the physician must think about two factors: the type of cancer and its stage. A biopsy or a blood specimen can determine the type of cancer. The extent of cancer progression is referred to as the stage.

To understand cancer treatments, normal and malignant cell replication processes should be reviewed. This cell cycle may last for between 24 hours and many days. The phases of the cell cycle consist of a first growth phase (G_1), synthesis (S_1), a second growth phase (G_2), mitosis (M), and a resting phase (G_0) (see Figure 21-1).

ANTINEOPLASTIC AGENTS

Antineoplastic agents are used to treat cancers or malignant neoplasms. Many types of drug therapies are available for the treatment of cancer. The common types of antineoplastic drugs are shown in Table 21-1.

Antineoplastic agents are also called chemotherapeutic agents. They interrupt the development, growth, or spread of cancer cells. Antineoplastic agents are used for malignant tumors. Treatment of cancer includes chemotherapy, surgery, and radiation therapy. Chemotherapy may reduce the size of malignant tumors and destroy the cancer cells. Antineoplastic agents do not kill tumor cells directly but interfere with cell replication (see Figure 21-2). Each antineoplastic agent is effective at a specific stage in cell replication. It may inhibit DNA, RNA, and protein synthesis or cancer cells. Agents are most commonly given in combinations of two or more at a time. Many antineoplastic medications also have immunosuppressive properties that decrease the patient's ability to produce antibodies to attack infecting organisms. These medications are toxic to the body as a whole because they also destroy normal cells and decrease immunity.

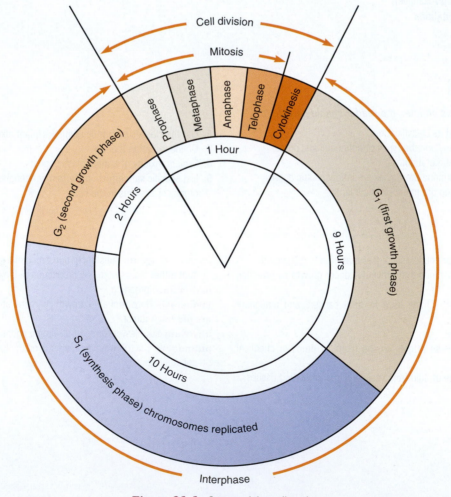

Figure 21-1. Stages of the cell cycle.

TABLE 21-1. Common Antineoplastic Agents

GENERIC NAME	TRADE NAME	ROUTE OF ADMINISTRATION	COMMON DOSAGE RANGE
Antimetabolites			
Methotrexate	Amethopterin®, Mexate®	Oral, IM, IV	2.5–30 mg/day
Mercaptopurine (6-MP)	Purinethol®	Oral	2.5 mg/kg/day
Fluorouracil (5-FU)	Efudex®, Adrucil®	IV	12 mg/kg/day for 4 days, then 6 mg/kg/qd × 4 doses
Fludarabine	Fludara®	IV	25 mg over 30 min for 5 days
Hormonal Agents			
Corticosteroids			
Dexamethasone	Provera®, Depo-Provera®	Oral, IM	PO, 0.25–4 mg bid to qid; IM, 8–16 mg q 1–3 wk
Prednisone	Deltasone®	Oral	5–60 mg/day in single or divided doses
Gonadotropin			
Danazol	Danocrine®	Oral	200–400 mg bid
Fluoxymesterone	Halotestin®	Oral	2.5–20 mg qid
Testolactone	Teslac®	Oral	250 mg qid
Estrogen			
Estramustine	Emcyt®	Oral	14 mg/kg/day
Diethylstilbestrol (DES)	Stilphostrol®	Oral, IV	50–200 mg tid
Androgen			
Testolactone	Teslac®	IM	100 mg 3 × per week
Oxymesterone	Halotestin®	Oral	10–40 mg/day
Antiestrogens			
Tamoxifen	Nolvadex®	Oral	20–40 mg/day
Raloxifene	Evista®	Oral	60 mg/day
Anastrozole	Arimidex®	Oral	1 mg/day
Antiandrogens			
Bicalutamide	Casodex®	Oral	50 mg/day
Goserelin	Zoladex®	Implant	1 implant q28ds
Flutamide	Eulexin®	Oral	250 mg tid
Progestins			
Megestrol	Megace®	Oral	40 mg/day
Antitumor Antibiotics			
Daunorubicin	Cerubidine®	IV	30–60 mg/m² BSA × 3–5 days
Doxorubicin	Adriamycin®	IV	60–75 mg/m² BSA at 21-day intervals
Bleomycin	Blenoxane®	IV, IM, SC	10–20 U/m² BSA 1–2 × per week
Plicamycin	Mithramycin®, Mithracin®	IV	25–30 mcg/kg qd for 8–10 days
Mitomycin	Mutamycin®	IV	20 mg/m2 BSA
Alkylating Agents			
Nitrogen mustards	Mustargen®	IV	0.4 mg/kg/day
Chlorambucil	Leukeran®	Oral	4–10 mg/day
Cisplatin	Platinol®	IV	20 mg–100 m²/day
Carboplatin	Paraplatin®	IV	3–8 mg/day
Busulfan	Myleran®	Oral	4–8 mg/day
Melphalan	Alkeran®	Oral	6 mg/day for 2–3 weeks
Cyclophosphamide	Cytoxan®	Oral	1–5 mg/kg
Mitotic Inhibitors (plant alkaloids)			
Vincristine	Oncovin®	IV	0.5–1.5 mg/kg/wk
Vinblastine	Velsar®, Velban®, Alkaban®	IV	0.1–0.5 mg/kg/wk
Teniposide		IV	165–250 mg/m² 2 × wk
Vinorelbine (VM-26)	Vumon®	IV	30 mg/m2 BSA/wk
Etoposide	Navelbine®	IV	Varies: patient response
Topotecan	VePesid®, Hycamtin®	IV	1.5 mg/m² over 30 min for 5 days
Paclitaxel	Taxol®	IV	135 mg/m² IV over 24 hr every 3 wk

IM, intramuscular; IV, intravenous; SC, subcutaneous; BSA, body surface area.

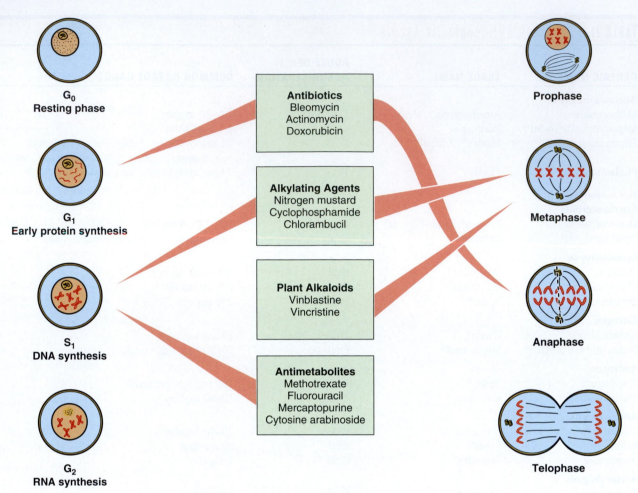

Figure 21-2. The effects of antineoplastic agents on various cell phases.

The most common types of antineoplastic agents include anti-metabolites, hormonal agents, special antibiotics, alkylating agents, and mitotic inhibitors (plant alkaloids).

Antimetabolites

Antimetabolites prevent cancer cell growth by affecting DNA production. They are only effective against cells that are actively participating in cell metabolism. The classes of antimetabolites include the following:

1. Folic acid antagonists: methotrexate
2. Purine antagonists: mercaptopurine
3. Pyrimidine antagonists: fluorouracil
4. Adenosine antagonists: fludarabine

Methotrexate

Methotrexate (MTX) is one of the most versatile antineoplastic agents because it can be used for many malignancies. MTX is the only anticancer drug for which an antidote to reduce toxicity is available. This antidote is leucovorin.

Mechanism of Action   MTX inhibits DNA, RNA, and protein synthesis.

Therapeutic Uses   This agent is used for acute lymphoblastic leukemia, meningeal leukemia, head and neck cancers, rheumatoid arthritis, psoriasis, ectopic pregnancy, and inflammatory bowel disease.

Adverse Effects   MTX commonly causes rash, hyperpigmentation, photosensitivity, hyperuricemia, decreased spermatogenesis, inflammation of the tongue, nausea, diarrhea, anorexia, and alopecia (hair loss). Serious adverse effects include severe leukopenia, bone marrow aplasia, and thrombocytopenia.

Drug Interactions   Patients should avoid alcohol, aspirin-containing products, and all nonsteroidal anti-inflammatory drugs when they are taking MTX.

Mercaptopurine

Mercaptopurine (6-MP) is one of the classes of antineoplastic, antimetabolite, and immunosuppressant drugs that probably interferes with purine nucleotide synthesis to cause cell death.

Mechanism of Action   The mechanism of action of 6-MP is most likely interference with purine nucleotide synthesis and then with RNA and DNA synthesis, leading to cell death.

Therapeutic Uses   6-MP is useful in maintenance therapy of children with acute and chronic myelocytic leukemia.

Adverse Effects   6-MP may cause anorexia, nausea, vomiting, hepatotoxicity, bone marrow depression, and hyperuricemia.

Drug Interactions   This agent may have drug interactions with antigout medications.

Fluorouracil

Fluorouracil (5-FU) is an antimetabolite and antineoplastic agent.

Mechanism of Action   5-FU inhibits DNA synthesis and cell death. It penetrates cerebrospinal fluid well. 5-FU metabolizes in the liver to inactive compounds.

Therapeutic Uses   5-FU is therapeutically useful for certain types of carcinoma, such as carcinoma of the colon, rectum, breast, stomach, and pancreas. Topical application of 5-FU is useful for treatment of premalignant keratoses, superficial basal cell carcinomas, and severe psoriasis.

Adverse Effects   5-FU causes marked myelosuppression. It can also result in gastrointestinal disturbances, alopecia (hair loss), dermatitis, and nail changes.

Drug Interactions   Allopurinol and cimetidine may increase the effects and toxicity of 5-FU.

Fludarabine

Fludarabine is an antimetabolite and antineoplastic agent.

Mechanism of Action   Fludarabine inhibits DNA synthesis and prevents cell replication.

Therapeutic Uses   Fludarabine is used for chronic lymphocytic leukemia.

Adverse Effects   Adverse effects of fludarabine use include weakness, headache, hearing loss, sleep disorders, and depression. It may also cause bone marrow toxicity, pneumonia, dyspnea, nosebleed (epistaxis), and edema.

Drug Interactions   This agent should not be used with pentostatin, because there is a risk of severe pulmonary toxicity.

Hormonal Agents

Hormonal agents are a class of heterogeneous compounds that have various effects on cells. These agents either block hormone production or block hormone action. Their action on malignant cells is highly selective. They are the least toxic of the anticancer medications. Hormones and their antagonists have various uses in the treatment of malignant diseases. Steroids are especially useful in treating acute lymphocytic leukemia. They are also used in conjunction with radiation therapy to reduce radiation edema. Sex hormones are used in carcinomas of the reproductive tract; for example estrogen is given to a patient with testicular cancer or carcinoma of the prostate. Estrogen may also be administered to postmenopausal women with breast cancer. Androgens, male hormones, are prescribed for premenopausal women with breast cancer. Major side effects include masculinization in female patients and feminization in male patients. Estrogen therapy may cause blood clots. Antiestrogens, such as tamoxifen, and antiandrogens are used to inhibit hormone production in advanced stages of cancer. Tamoxifen is prescribed for breast cancer and increases the risk of endometrial cancer; it must be used with caution.

Androgens

Androgens are chemical agents of natural and synthetic steroids responsible for the presence of primary and secondary male sex characteristics.

Mechanism of Action   Androgens stimulate receptors in androgen-responsive organs, thereby promoting growth and development of male sex organs.

Therapeutic Uses   Androgens are used for inoperable breast carcinoma, hypogonadism, and prevention of postpartum breast pain.

Adverse Effects   Androgens may cause fluid retention, nausea and vomiting, alopecia (hair loss), and acne.

Drug Interactions   Androgens have drug interactions with oral anticoagulants.

Antiandrogens

Antiandrogens are hormone antagonists used to interfere with the action of androgen in hormone therapy.

Mechanism of Action   Antiandrogens act by blocking the synthesis of endogenous testosterone.

Therapeutic Uses   Antiandrogens are used for prostate cancer.

Adverse Effects Common side effects of use of antiandrogens include diarrhea, constipation, hot flushes, bleeding, and anemia.

Drug Interactions Some antiandrogens have drug interactions with warfarin sodium.

Antiestrogens

Antiestrogens are agents that either prevent the formation of estrogen, block estrogen receptors, or produce an effect opposite to that of estrogen. Some forms of breast cancer grow faster in the presence of estrogen.

Mechanism of Action Antiestrogens work by binding to estrogen receptors, blocking estrogen from binding to these receptors. This stops estrogen from activating genes for specific growth-promoting proteins.

Therapeutic Uses Antiestrogens are commonly used to treat breast cancer.

Adverse Effects Common adverse effects resulting from the use of antiestrogens include headache, depression, bone marrow suppression, nausea, vomiting, and hot flashes.

Drug Interactions Antiestrogens such as tamoxifen may have drug interactions with estrogens. Other types of antiestrogens have none.

Corticosteroids

Corticosteroids are steroids that are secreted from the adrenal cortex.

Mechanism of Action Steroids inhibit migration of white blood cells and inhibit production of products of the arachidonic acid cascade.

Therapeutic Uses Corticosteroids are used to treat croup, respiratory failure in patients with acquired immunodeficiency syndrome (AIDS), thyroid conditions, neuropathic and cancer-related pain, alcoholic hepatitis with concomitant encephalopathy, complications of meningitis, and rheumatoid arthritis and other arthritic conditions. They also have many uses in the areas of dermatology, immunology, and oncology.

Adverse Effects Prolonged treatment with systemic steroids causes a variety of adverse effects that can be life-threatening. The most common adverse effects include insomnia, personality change, weight gain, muscle weakness, polyuria, kidney stones, diabetes mellitus, sex hormone suppression, and osteoporosis.

Drug Interactions Corticosteroids should not be used with alcohol because both of these substances can produce stomach irritation.

Estrogens

Estrogen is the primary female sex hormone. It is produced mainly in the ovaries.

Mechanism of Action Estrogen works by promoting the release of calcitonin and enhancing the availability of 1,25-dihydroxyvitamin D_3. Its effects at menopause include providing increased bone resorption and increased bone formation.

Therapeutic Uses Estrogen (estramustine) is used for prostate cancer and diethylstilbestrol (DES) may be indicated for prostate and breast cancer.

Adverse Effects Estrogens may cause fluid retention, nausea, vomiting, headache, decreased glucose tolerance, gynecomastia (enlargement of breasts) in men, and breakthrough uterine bleeding.

Drug Interactions Estrogens may have drug interactions with dairy products.

Progestins

Progestins are synthetically produced drugs that have progesterone-like properties.

Mechanism of Action Progestins inhibit secretion of pituitary gonadotropins (follicle-stimulating hormone [FSH] and luteinizing hormone [LH]) by positive feedback.

Therapeutic Uses Progestins are indicated for endometrial and breast cancer.

Adverse Effects Common adverse effects of progestin use include fluid retention, pain at the injection site, thromboembolism, nausea, and vomiting.

Drug Interactions Drug interactions with progestins are rare; no serious interactions have been established.

Gonadotropin

Gonadotropin is a hormonal substance that stimulates the function of the testes and ovaries. The gonadotropic hormones FSH and LH are produced and secreted by the anterior pituitary gland.

Mechanism of Action Gonadotropin regulates the level of estrogen in females, turning on the entire female reproductive system by stimulating pituitary gonadotropes FSH and LH.

Therapeutic Uses Gonadotropin is used therapeutically to promote fertility.

Adverse Effects Common adverse effects with use of gonadotropin include hot flashes, peripheral edema, nausea, vomiting, and headache.

Drug Interactions No drug interactions with gonadotropin have been reported.

Antitumor Antibiotics

Several antibiotics of microbial origin are very effective in the treatment of certain tumors. They are used only to treat cancer and are not used to treat infections. These antibiotics include bleomycin, doxorubicin, daunorubicin, mitomycin, and plicamycin. Their mechanism of action is to inhibit DNA and RNA synthesis (see Table 21-1).

Bleomycin

Bleomycin is an antineoplastic and antibiotic agent. Bleomycin is among the common anticancer drugs. It is a toxic drug with a low therapeutic index and is very cytotoxic. This antibiotic is widely used in combination with other chemotherapeutic drugs because it lacks significant myelosuppressive activity.

Mechanism of Action Bleomycin inhibits synthesis of DNA.

Therapeutic Uses Bleomycin is used in squamous cell carcinomas of the head, neck, penis, cervix, and vulva. It is also used for the treatment of lymphomas and testicular carcinoma.

Adverse Effects Adverse effects include ulcerations of the tongue and lips, nausea, vomiting, diarrhea, and weight loss. It may cause pneumonia and alopecia (hair loss).

Drug Interactions Bleomycin decreases the effects and toxicity of digitalis and phenytoin, but it increases the effects and toxicity of cisplatin.

Doxorubicin

Doxorubicin is the single most active agent against breast cancer.

Mechanism of Action Doxorubicin is a cytotoxic antibiotic with a wide spectrum of antitumor activity and strong immunosuppressive properties.

Therapeutic Uses Doxorubicin is used in the treatment of acute lymphoblastic and myeloblastic leukemias, soft tissue and bone cancer, carcinomas of the breast and ovary, and lymphomas. It is generally used in combination with surgery, radiation, and immunotherapy.

Adverse Effects Doxorubicin may cause serious, irreversible myocardial toxicity, hypertension, and hypotension. It also produces nausea, vomiting, diarrhea, severe myelosuppression, and hypersensitivity or anaphylactoid reactions.

Drug Interactions Doxorubicin should not be used in patients who have recently received live virus strain vaccines, such as the live oral polio vaccine, because they may then be susceptible to the virus contained in the vaccine and could contract the disease.

Dactinomycin

Dactinomycin is a potent cytotoxic antibiotic and antineoplastic agent.

Mechanism of Action Dactinomycin inhibits DNA, RNA, and protein synthesis.

Therapeutic Uses Dactinomycin is used as a single agent or in combination with other antineoplastic agents or radiation to treat carcinoma of the testes and uterus.

Adverse Effects Adverse effects with the use of dactinomycin include nausea, vomiting, abdominal pain, diarrhea, and ulceration of the tongue. Hepatitis and aplastic anemia may occur with use of dactinomycin.

Drug Interactions Dactinomycin increases the effects and toxicity of radiation therapy.

Mitomycin

Mitomycin is a potent antibiotic, antineoplastic compound. It is effective in certain tumors that are nonresponsive to surgery, radiation, or other chemotherapeutic agents.

Mechanism of Action The mechanism of action of mitomycin is not known. It may inhibit DNA and RNA synthesis.

Therapeutic Uses Mitomycin is used in combination with other chemotherapeutic agents in palliative, adjunctive treatment of cancer of the breast, stomach, and pancreas.

Adverse Effects Adverse effects with the use of mitomycin include nausea, vomiting, bone marrow toxicity, asthma, and pneumonia.

Drug Interactions Drugs that increase the effects and toxicity of mitomycin include vinca alkaloids (respiratory toxicity) and doxorubicin (cardiac toxicity).

Plicamycin

Plicamycin is a cytotoxic, antibiotic, and antineoplastic agent.

Mechanism of Action Plicamycin appears to block the hypercalcemic action of vitamin D and may inhibit the effect of parathyroid hormone on bone cells (osteoclasts). Plicamycin may interfere with synthesis of various clotting factors. Its high toxicity and low therapeutic index limits its clinical use.

Therapeutic Uses Plicamycin is used to treat hypercalcemia or hypercalcinuria associated with advanced neoplasms and to treat testicular malignancy.

Adverse Effects Drowsiness, irritability, dizziness, headache, and mental depression are common side effects of plicamycin. It can also cause nausea, vomiting, diarrhea, and intestinal hemorrhage.

Drug Interactions No serious drug interactions with the use of plicamycin have been reported.

Daunorubicin

Daunorubicin is still used in the treatment of acute myeloid leukemia. It was the first agent of the antitumor antibiotics.

Mechanism of Action Daunorubicin binds to DNA and inhibits DNA synthesis, causing cell death.

Theraputic Uses Daunorubicin is the first line treatment for advanced HIV-associated Kaposi's sarcoma.

Adverse Effects The common adverse effects of daunorubicin include depression, dizziness, fatigue, headache, palpitations, and hypertension. Daunorubicin may also cause fever, chills, cough, dyspnea, sinusitis, and red urine (not hematuria).

Drug Interactions Drug interactions have not been well studied with this agent.

Alkylating Agents

Alkylating agents were the first group of antineoplastic agents. During World War I, chemical warfare using nitrogen mustard gases was introduced. Alkylating agents came to be used for cancer therapy as a result of observations of the effects of the gases on cell growth. They are used to treat metastatic ovarian, testicular, and bladder cancers. They are also used for the palliative treatment of other cancers. The newer drugs in this category are **nitrosoureas**, lipid-soluble drugs used in treating brain tumors and testicular or ovarian cancers. The major side effects of the alkylating agents include nausea, vomiting, diarrhea, bone marrow suppression, hepatic and renal toxicity, and dermatitis. Subclassifications of alkylating agents are listed in Table 21-1.

Nitrogen Mustards

Nitrogen mustards are alkylating and antineoplastic agents.

Mechanism of Action The major cytotoxic and mutagenic effects of nitrogen mustards may result from their interactions with DNA. Mechlorethamine is the most rapidly acting and must be freshly prepared and administered into a rapidly flowing intravenous line. If extravasated, it can cause severe local tissue damage.

Therapeutic Uses The clinical uses of nitrogen mustards have been limited to the treatment of Hodgkin's disease.

Adverse Effects The dose-limiting toxicity of nitrogen mustards is bone marrow suppression. The major long-term toxicities of these drugs, as with all akylating agents, are gonadal damage and an increased risk of secondary malignancies, in particular, acute leukemia.

Drug Interactions Nitrogen mustards may interact with immunizations and alcohol. Therefore, during therapy with these agents, the patient must not receive immunizations and must avoid alcohol.

Cyclophosphamide

Cyclophosphamide, unlike the nitrogen mustards, has a wide spectrum of antitumor and immunosuppressive activity. It is an alkylating agent.

Mechanism of Action Cyclophosphamide interferes with replication of susceptible cells.

Therapeutic Uses Cyclophosphamide is used as part of combination therapy regimens to treat lymphoma, breast cancer, bladder cancer, and ovarian cancer.

Adverse Effects Among the more serious adverse reactions to cyclophosphamide are anorexia, vomiting, alopecia (hair loss), leukopenia, and potentially serious hemorrhagic cystitis. Long-term toxicity includes sterility and carcinogenesis.

Drug Interactions Cyclophosphamide has drug interaction with antigout medications.

Chlorambucil

Chlorambucil is a slow-acting nitrogen mustard. Chlorambucil is administered orally, and it is absorbed well.

Mechanism of Action Chlorambucil cross-links DNA strands, thereby interfering with DNA replication and RNA transcription.

Therapeutic Uses Chlorambucil is used primarily to treat patients with chronic lymphocytic leukemia and low-grade lymphomas.

Adverse Effects Chlorambucil is well-tolerated and usually does not cause nausea or vomiting, but there are some serious adverse effects, which include bone marrow depression, pulmonary fibrosis, interstitial pneumonia, seizures, allergic reactions, hepatic necrosis, confusion, and neuropathy.

Drug Interactions   Antigout medications and live virus vaccines may affect the toxicity of chlorambucil.

Busulfan

Busulfan is an alkylating and antineoplastic agent.

Mechanism of Action   Busulfan interacts with cellular thiol groups, causing cell death. The predominant effect of busulfan is bone marrow suppression, with little other pharmacological action.

Therapeutic Uses   Busulfan is used exclusively to treat chronic myelocytic leukemia. This agent is well absorbed orally.

Adverse Effects   Busulfan has some unusual side effects in addition to its bone marrow suppressive activity. It may cause generalized skin pigmentation, gynecomastia (enlargement of the male breasts), and pulmonary fibrosis.

Drug Interactions   Busulfan can interact with alcohol and immunizations.

Melphalan

Melphalan is an antineoplastic, alkylating agent.

Mechanism of Action   Melphalan prevents separation of strands of DNA during cell division.

Therapeutic Uses   Melphalan is well absorbed orally, and its major use has been for the treatment of multiple myeloma (a special cancer of the white blood cells that causes abnormal plasma cells to develop), usually in combination with prednisone. It has also been used to treat breast cancer and melanoma.

Adverse Effects   Nausea and vomiting are rare with melphalan, as is alopecia (hair loss). The major toxicity is similar to that of other alkylating agents (i.e., bone marrow suppression, oral ulceration, hyperuricemia, pulmonary fibrosis).

Drug Interactions   Antigout medications may increase effects and toxicity of melphalan.

Cisplatin

Cisplatin is used for various types of cancer therapy.

Mechanism of Action   Although not known for certain, there is evidence to suggest that the DNA adducts of cisplatin, which block replication and transcription, are the key mediators in the death of cancer cells.

Therapeutic Uses   Cisplatin is used to treat certain types of head and neck cancers, cervical carcinoma, lung cancer, neurological cancers, and a wide variety of other types of cancer.

Adverse Effects   Cisplatin may cause nausea, vomiting, fever, anaphylaxis, hypokalemia, hypomagnesemia, hemolysis, renal damage, sterility, teratogenesis, ototoxicity, peripheral neuropathy, Raynaud's disease, or bone marrow depression.

Drug Interactions   Use of cisplatin with other nephrotoxic or ototoxic drugs may exacerbate the adverse effects of cisplatin.

Carboplatin

Carboplatin is a chemotherapeutic agent used to treat some types of cancer.

Mechanism of Action   Although the exact mechanism of action of carboplatin is unknown, it is thought to be similar to that of bifunctional alkylating agents, meaning it most probably cross-links and interferes with DNA function.

Therapeutic Uses   Carboplatin is used to treat certain types of lung cancer, testicular cancer, head and neck cancers, Wilms' tumor, brain tumors, bladder cancer, and retinoblastoma.

Adverse Effects   The adverse effects of carboplatin include decreased white blood cell counts with increased risk of infection, decreased platelet counts with increased risk of bleeding, altered kidney function at high doses, fetal abnormalities, and infertility.

Drug Interactions   Carboplatin should not be used with hydantoins (such as phenytoin).

Mitotic Inhibitors (Plant Alkaloids)

Mitotic inhibitors are derived from plants. The primary plant alkaloids are vincristine and vinblastine. Teniposide is an analog closely related to etoposide and is active against acute leukemias in children. Topotecan is a semisynthetic plant alkaloid, used for refractory ovarian cancer, and may have activity against small-cell lung cancer. Vinblastine is toxic to the bone marrow. Vincristine is toxic to the peripheral nerves. Most plant alkaloids cause nausea and vomiting, particularly vinblastine. Examples of plant alkaloids are seen in Table 21-1.

Vinblastine

Vinblastine is a mitotic inhibitor and antineoplastic agent.

Mechanism of Action   Vinblastine disrupts cell division in metaphase by inhibition of microtubule formation.

Therapeutic Uses Vinblastine is used for the treatment of Hodgkin's disease, lymphoma, and advanced testicular carcinoma. Vinblastine is also indicated for Kaposi's sarcoma and choriocarcinoma.

Adverse Effects Peripheral neuritis, mental depression, headache, seizures, and alopecia (hair loss) are common adverse effects with the use of vinblastine. One of the most serious adverse effects is bone marrow depression.

Drug Interactions Drugs that increase the effects and toxicity of vinblastine include other antineoplastic agents (causing bone marrow suppression), mitomycin (causing bronchospasm), erythromycin, and ritonavir.

Vincristine

Vincristine is a mitotic inhibitor and antineoplastic agent.

Mechanism of Action Vincristine arrests mitotic division at the stage of metaphase. The exact mechanism of action is unknown.

Therapeutic Uses Vincristine is used for acute leukemia, Hodgkin's disease, and non-Hodgkin's lymphoma. It is also prescribed for the treatment of sarcomas.

Adverse Effects Adverse effects include headache, convulsions, foot drop, optic atrophy, and photophobia. Vincristine can also cause constipation, oral ulcerations, vomiting, and diarrhea.

Drug Interactions Vincristine may cause drug interactions with antigout medications, live virus vaccines, and doxorubicin.

Vinorelbine

Vinorelbine is an antineoplastic and mitotic inhibitor agent.

Mechanism of Action Vinorelbine affects the cell energy production required for mitosis and interferes with nucleic acid synthesis, leading to cell death.

Therapeutic Uses Vinorelbine is the first-line treatment for ambulatory patients with lung cancer.

Adverse Effects Adverse effects from the use of vinorelbine include numbness, headache, weakness, and dizziness. Nausea, vomiting, pharyngitis, diarrhea, constipation, and abdominal pain may also occur.

Drug Interactions Live virus vaccines can interact with vinorelbine.

Etoposide

Etoposide is a mitotic inhibitor and antineoplastic agent.

Mechanism of Action Etoposide inhibits cyclooxygenase, resulting in inhibition of synthesis of prostaglandins and other inflammatory mediators.

Therapeutic Uses Etoposide is used for the treatment of refractory testicular tumors as part of combination therapy.

Adverse Effects Adverse effects associated with etoposide include hypotension, fatigue, alopecia, nausea, vomiting, and liver toxicity.

Drug Interactions Drug interactions with etoposide are the same as those with other mitotic inhibitors.

Topotecan

Topotecan is an antineoplastic agent.

Mechanism of Action Topotecan inhibits the action of topoisomerase type I, an enzyme that produces reversible single-strand breaks in DNA during replication. This results in double-strand DNA breakage and cell death.

Therapeutic Uses Topotecan is used for treatment of metastatic ovarian cancer after failure of traditional chemotherapy. Topotecan is also indicated for treatment of small-cell lung cancer after failure of first-line treatment.

Adverse Effects Major adverse effects of topotecan include nausea and vomiting, diarrhea, constipation, abdominal pain, fatigue, fever, alopecia, and dyspnea.

Drug Interactions Myelosuppression is more severe when topotecan is used with cisplatin.

Paclitaxel

Paclitaxel is an antineoplastic drug that was originally isolated from the bark of the yew tree.

Mechanism of Action The drug binds to the microtubules and leads to arrest of mitosis.

Theraputic Uses Paclitaxel is used in treatment of metastatic carcinoma of the ovary after failure of first-line or subsequent therapy. It is also indicated for treatment of breast cancer after failure of other agents.

Adverse Effects The most common adverse effects of paclitaxel include nausea, vomiting, anorexia, elevated liver enzymes, bradycardia, hypotension, and peripheral sensory neuropathy.

Drug Interactions Paclitaxel increased myelosuppression with cisplatin. Drugs such as ketoconazole, verapamil, diazepam, quinidine, vincristine, and testosterone increased paclitaxel effects.

Teniposide

Teniposide is a phase-specific cytotoxic drug that prevents cells from reaching the stage of mitosis.

Mechanism of Action   Teniposide acts by inhibiting topoisomerase type II activity, relating to the number of double-stranded DNA breaks produced in cells.

Therapeutic Uses   Teniposide is used along with other anticancer agents and is indicated for induction therapy in children with refractory acute lymphoblastic leukemia.

Adverse Effects   The most severe adverse effects of teniposide include myelosuppression, leukopenia, neutropenia, thrombocytopenia, anemia, mucositis, diarrhea, nausea, and vomiting.

Drug Interactions   Caution should be used in administering teniposide with tolbutamide, sodium salicylate, and sulfamethizole.

OTHER THERAPEUTIC MODALITIES

For cancer treatment, other therapeutic modalities include surgery and radiation therapy. The purpose of surgery may be diagnosis, such as a biopsy or exploratory laparotomy for a "second look," or therapy, such as tumor debulking or removal. Surgery is often combined with chemotherapy and/or radiation.

Radiation therapy involves application of high doses of ionizing radiation to the cancerous tissue. Radiation may be combined with surgery and/or chemotherapy, depending upon the area of the body being irradiated. Adverse reactions may include stomatitis (inflammation of the oral mucosa), nausea and vomiting, diarrhea, and bone marrow suppression. See Chapter 9, "Advanced Pharmacy" (nuclear medicine).

TOXICITY

It is not possible to stop antineoplastic agents from attacking normal cells. The principles that apply to antitumor efficacy also apply to the toxicity of these agents. The bone marrow, lymphoblasts, mucous membranes, skin, and gonads are affected to a greater extent than other cells. Bone marrow depression is a major adverse effect of anti-neoplastic drugs. Skin toxicity includes alopecia (hair loss), commonly seen in patients receiving chemotherapy.

Local necrosis may result from **extravasation** of vesicant chemotherapy drugs during their administration. Cancer chemotherapy can also cause skin changes such as dryness and sensitivity to sunlight. Aspermia and amenorrhea (the absence of menstrual periods) are commonly caused by some antineoplastic agents. Immunosuppression makes the patient more vulnerable to infection. About 50% of patients with cancer die of intercurrent infections rather than from the terminal phases of the neoplastic disease. Certain antineoplastic drugs are mutagenic and carcinogenic, and the patient is subjected to the risk of future neoplasias. Hyperuricemia or renal damage may result from some antineoplastic agents. Massive destruction of certain leukemic cells may also cause an acute hypotensive crisis that is sometimes called anaphylaxis, even though it is not a true allergic response. Hypersensitivity reactions may occur with any chemotherapy agent. Life-threatening reactions, including anaphylaxis, appear to be more common with cisplatin, etoposide, paclitaxel, and teniposide. **Pulmonary toxicity** is generally irreversible, and may be fatal. **Cardiac toxicity** includes irreversible congestive heart failure. Risk factors include chest irradiation and high cumulative doses of cardiotoxic chemotherapy.

SUMMARY

A neoplasm is the result of abnormal cell division in the body. It may be benign or malignant. Only malignant tumors are capable of spreading in other organs or systems of the body. Treatment of the neoplasm depends on the progression of the tumor. Surgery, antineoplastic agents, and immunotherapy may be indicated. There are many agents used for this purpose. Many antineoplastic medications also have immunosuppressive properties that decrease the patient's ability to produce antibodies to attack infecting organisms.

Common antineoplastic agents include antimetabolites, hormonal agents, specific antibiotics, alkylating agents, and mitotic inhibitors or plant alkaloids. In some cases, surgery and radiation therapy are also necessary. Toxicity and side effects of chemotherapy and radiation therapy are the major concerns with treatment of malignant tumors.

CRITICAL THINKING

1. Define the classes of antimetabolites.
2. Explain the mechanism of action of vinblastine.
3. Name the primary plant alkaloids (mitotic inhibitors).
4. A pharmacy technician is taking chemotherapy intravenous medication to a patient's room and the IV bag begins to leak solution (approximately 30 mL) on the floor. What action should be taken?

REVIEW QUESTIONS

1. The cell cycle consists of several phases, such as G_0, G_1, S_1, G_2, and M. Which of the following explains the G_0 phase?
   A. Resting
   B. Synthesis
   C. Mitosis
   D. Growth

2. Which of the following agents is an antimetabolite?
   A. Cyclophosphamide
   B. Fluorouracil
   C. Mitomycin
   D. Nitrogen mustard

3. Which of the following is an example of an antitumor antibiotic?
   A. Vinorelbine
   B. Topotecan
   C. Bleomycin
   D. Mercaptopurine

4. Mitotic inhibitors (plant alkaloids) include
   A. mercaptopurine.
   B. testolactone.
   C. tamoxifen.
   D. vincristine.

5. Mercaptopurine may have drug interactions with which of the following agents?
   A. Amoxicillin
   B. Alcohol
   C. Antigout
   D. Estrogen

6. An adverse effect of methotrexate is
   A. bone marrow aplasia.
   B. alopecia.
   C. hypertension.
   D. hyperthyroidism.

7. Busulfan has some unusual side effects in addition to its bone marrow suppressive activity. Which of the following side effects is caused by busulfan?
   A. Peptic ulcer
   B. Testicular cancer
   C. Gynecomastia
   D. Gastrointestinal bleeding

8. Which of the following is the trade name of doxorubicin?
   A. Mutamycin®
   B. Adriamycin®
   C. Cosmegen®
   D. Blenoxane®

9. The route of administration for goserelin is
   A. oral.
   B. intramuscular.
   C. intravenous.
   D. implant.

10. Most plant alkaloids may produce
    A. nausea and vomiting.
    B. internal bleeding.
    C. hypertension.
    D. gout.

11. Which of the following antimetabolites is useful in maintenance therapy for children with acute leukemia?
    A. Fluorouracil (5-FU)
    B. Methotrexate (MTX)
    C. Mercaptopurine (6-MP)
    D. Vincristine

12. Which of the following is the best drug that may be given to a patient with testicular cancer?
    A. Tamoxifen
    B. Estrogen
    C. Progesterone
    D. Megestrol

13. The term *metastasize* means to
    A. arise.
    B. divide.
    C. spread.
    D. occur.

14. Hycamtin® is the trade name of which of the following agents?
    A. Vincristine
    B. Vinblastine
    C. Vinorelbine
    D. Topotecan

15. The single most active agent against breast cancer is
    A. dactinomycin.
    B. mitomycin.
    C. doxorubicin.
    D. bleomycin.

Allergy and Respiratory Drugs

22

OBJECTIVES

Upon completion of this chapter, the reader should be able to

1. Explain the varieties of allergic reactions.
2. Compare histamine and antihistamines.
3. Discuss the two major groups of antitussives.
4. Compare different therapies for chronic lung conditions.
5. Discuss different types of mucolytics and expectorants.
6. Explain how decongestants work and identify serious side effects.
7. Identify the most common intranasal steroid.
8. Discuss drugs used for smoking cessation.
9. Be able to list three popular asthma medications.

GLOSSARY

allergic rhinitis Inflammation of the nasal mucosa that is due to the sensitivity of the nasal tissue to an allergen.

allergy A state of hypersensitivity induced by exposure to a particular antigen.

alveolar sacs Air cells found in the lung; also known as alveoli.

alveoli Air sacs found in the lung; also known as alveolar sacs.

anaphylactic shock A severe and sometimes fatal allergic reaction.

antigen A substance that is introduced into the body and induces the formation of antibodies.

antihistamines Drugs that counteract the action of histamine.

antitussives Agents that relieve or prevent coughing.

asthma A chronic inflammatory disorder of the airways of the respiratory system.

β-adrenergic agents Drugs that work as both cardiac and respiratory agonists.

bronchodilators Agents that relax the smooth muscle of the bronchial tubes.

corticosteroids The most potent and consistently effective antiinflammatory agents that are currently available for relief of respiratory conditions.

decongestant A drug that causes vasoconstriction of nasal mucosa and reduces congestion or swelling.

dry powder inhaler (DPI) A device used to deliver medication in the form of micronized powder into the lungs.

expectorants Agents that promote the removal of mucous secretions from the lung, bronchi, and trachea, usually by coughing.

histamine A chemical substance found in all the body tissues that protects the body from factors in the environment that produce allergic and inflammatory reactions.

leukotrines Substances that contribute to the inflammation associated with asthma.

metered dose inhaler (MDI) A hand-held pressurized device used to deliver medications for inhalation.

mucolytic Destroying or dissolving the active agents that make up mucus.

xanthine derivatives A substance that is effective for relief of bronchospasm in asthma, chronic bronchitis, and emphysema.

OVERVIEW

The most important function of the respiratory system is the inspiration of oxygen and the expiration of carbon dioxide. Therefore, the respiratory tract must exchange gases and supply oxygen to the body. The effectiveness of the respiratory system affects the body's ability to function correctly and be in homeostasis. Allergic reactions occur throughout the body, but they also commonly involve individuals who are suffering from respiratory tract disorders such as rhinorrhea and allergic bronchitis.

ANATOMY REVIEW

The respiratory system consists of the nasal passages, mouth, pharynx, larynx, trachea, and lungs, as well as the accessory organs, such as the skeletal muscles of the chest wall and the diaphragm (see Figure 22-1).

The upper respiratory tract contains the nasal cavity, sinuses, mouth, and pharynx.

Bronchi and Bronchioles

The lower respiratory tract is essential for the exchange of oxygen and carbon dioxide. This system is made up of the larynx, trachea, and lungs. The lower end of the trachea separates into the right and left bronchi.

As the bronchi enter the lungs, they subdivide into bronchial tubes and small bronchioles. At the end of each bronchiole is an alveolar duct, which ends in a saclike cluster called **alveolar sacs (alveoli)** (see Figure 22-2).

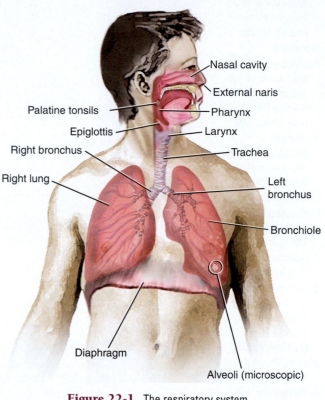

Figure labels: Nasal cavity, External naris, Palatine tonsils, Pharynx, Epiglottis, Larynx, Right bronchus, Trachea, Right lung, Left bronchus, Bronchiole, Diaphragm, Alveoli (microscopic)

Figure 22-1. The respiratory system.

ALLERGIES

An **allergy** is a state of hypersensitivity induced by exposure to a particular **antigen**, a substance that is introduced into the body and induces the formation of antibodies, resulting

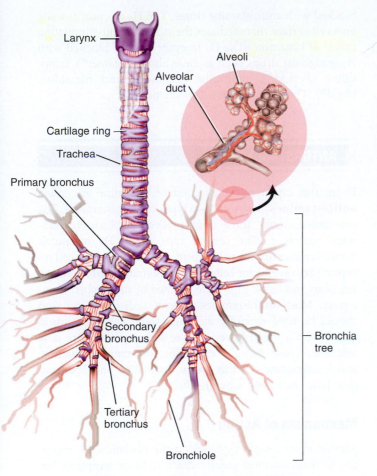

Figure 22-2. The bronchi and bronchioles.

barbiturates, iodine, anesthetics, and antibiotics (including sulfa medications).

Anaphylactic Shock

Anaphylactic shock is an allergic reaction that may be life-threatening. Its onset is sudden and severe and involves the entire body. Anaphylactic shock causes a massive release of histamine and other substances, which cause airway constriction (making breathing very difficult), abdominal cramping, vomiting, and diarrhea. Common causes of anaphylactic shock include foods, medications, insect stings, and allergies to latex. Foods that are most likely to cause this condition include nuts, fish, milk, and eggs. Individuals who have food allergies or asthma are believed to be more likely to develop anaphylactic reactions. The most common insect stings in the United States include those from bees, yellow jackets, hornets, wasps, and ants. Anaphylactic reactions often begin with tingling sensations, itching, a metallic taste sensation, hives, a sensation of warmth, symptoms of asthma, swelling of the mouth and throat, a drop in blood pressure, or a loss of consciousness. These types of reactions are usually treated with epinephrine, followed by antihistamines and steroids.

Allergic Rhinitis

Allergic rhinitis is the inflammation of the nasal mucosa that is due to the sensitivity of the nasal tissue to an allergen. It is usually associated with watery nasal discharge and itching of the nose and eyes, caused by a localized sensitivity reaction to house dust, animal dander, or an antigen, commonly pollen. The condition may be seasonal and is commonly known as "hay fever." Allergic rhinitis is caused by histamine release, whereas nonallergic rhinitis is often a symptom of the common cold.

Allergic Asthma

Asthma is defined as a chronic inflammatory disorder of the airways of the respiratory system (see Figure 22-3). It is characterized by wheezing and shortness of breath due to constriction of the bronchioles. Asthma is most commonly classified as allergic, exercise-induced, or caused by infections of the respiratory tract. Symptoms include breathlessness, cough, wheezing, and chest tightness. The airway becomes inflamed with edema and mucous plugs, and hyperactivity of the bronchial tree adds to the symptoms. During asthmatic attacks, when bronchiole constriction and increased secretions are present, bronchodilators are used for relief. Anti-inflammatory drugs, such as corticosteroids and cromolyn, may be prescribed for relief of symptoms. The majority of medications for asthma are administered by inhalation. Antiasthma medications can be divided into two categories: long-term control and quick-relief medications.

in harmful immunologic reactions on subsequent exposures. The term is usually used to refer to hypersensitivity to an environmental antigen. There are varieties of allergic reactions such as allergic rhinitis, allergic conjunctivitis, allergic asthma, and allergic dermatitis. Because this chapter focuses on respiratory disorders and drug therapy, allergic rhinitis and allergic asthma will be discussed. For the other types of allergic reactions, see other textbooks.

Allergic Reaction

An allergic reaction occurs when the immune system reacts to a foreign substance. The body attempts to get rid of the substance, whether it is an allergen from the environment or a medication. In the case of an allergic reaction to a medication, the body's response is harmful and may cause serious symptoms. Common allergic reactions include nausea, diarrhea, vomiting, headache, and lightheadedness. Other symptoms include anxiety, hives, palpitations, shortness of breath, rash, swelling, and wheezing. Items in the natural environment that most commonly cause allergies include dust, pollen, and pet dander. Medications that most commonly cause allergic reactions include anticonvulsants,

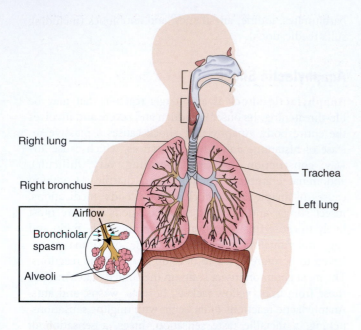

Figure 22-3. Asthma is a disease that involves bronchospasm and excessive airway secretions.

HISTAMINE

Histamine is a chemical substance found naturally in all the body tissues that protects the body from factors in the environment that produce allergic and inflammatory reactions. The greatest concentration of histamine is found in the basophils, platelets, and mast cells in skin, lungs, and the gastrointestinal tract. Histamine has several functions, including the following:

- Dilation of capillaries, which increases capillary permeability and results in hypotension
- Contraction of most smooth muscle of the bronchial tree, which may cause wheezing and difficulty breathing
- Increased stomach acid secretion
- Initiation of allergic reactions
- Acceleration of the heart rate

There are two types of histamines in our body, one that causes allergic reactions in the respiratory tract and another that works on the gastrointestinal tract (see Chapter 25). The free histamines play a role in the inflammatory process and defend exposed tissue from injury by damaging agents. Histamine causes dilation and increased permeability of capillaries. It is one of the first mediators of an inflammatory response. Antihistamine drugs inhibit this immediate, transient response. Both histamine-1 (H_1) and histamine-2 (H_2) receptors mediate the contraction of vascular smooth muscle. Histamine has also been postulated to be a neurotransmitter in the central nervous system. The H_1 receptor is a site on a cell surface that mediates the allergic response to histamine. The H_1 receptor may be

blocked with antihistamine drugs. The H_2 receptor is a site on a cell surface that mediates the stomach acid-stimulating effects of histamine. The H_2 receptor may be blocked with H_2 antagonist drugs such as cimetidine (Tagamet®), famotidine (Pepcid®), ranitidine (Zantac®), and nizatidine (Axid®). These are discussed in Chapter 25.

ANTIHISTAMINES

Drugs that counteract the action of histamine are called **antihistamines**. There are two types of antihistamines. The conventional ones, those used in allergies, block H_1 histamine receptors. The second type block H_2 receptors. Antihistamines appear to compete with histamine for cell receptor sites on effector cells. Thus, histamine-related allergic reactions and tissue injury are blocked or diminished in intensity. Most antihistamines have a sedating effect and should be used carefully, although some newer antihistamines with a much lower level of sedating effect are now available. These include acrivastine, cetirizine, loratadine, and fexofenadine. Of this group, loratadine and fexofenadine have the lowest sedating effect.

Mechanism of Action

Antihistamines work by blocking the histamine H_1 receptor, so that histamine cannot attach to these receptors, but is metabolized.

Therapeutic Uses

Antihistamines are used to relieve the symptoms resulting from the release of histamine. Antihistamines are not effective against histamines that are already attached to the receptor sites, so the antihistamine is most effective if taken before contact with the allergy-causing compounds. Therefore, these medications are more likely to be effective at the beginning of the allergy season. Allergic rhinitis is treated with antihistamines, decongestants, and nasal preparations. Antihistamines are also prescribed for relieving symptoms of allergies to insect bites and contact dermatitis.

Adverse Effects

Antihistamines are sedative agents, and one of the major side effects is sedation. Many over-the-counter (OTC) drugs contain antihistamines for sleeping aids (e.g., Nytol®). Other OTC antihistamine drugs are used to relieve nausea, vomiting, and motion sickness. Antihistamines may cause drowsiness, dizziness, headaches, and photosensitivity. They may cause the respiratory tract to dry and mucus to thicken; therefore, a person taking antihistamines should drink plenty of fluids to thin secretions and keep tissue moist. Table 22-1 shows classes of antihistamines.

TABLE 22-1.   Classification of Antihistamines

GENERIC NAME	TRADE NAME	ROUTE OF ADMINISTRATION	COMMON DOSAGE RANGE
First-generation Drugs			
Azatadine*	Optimine®	Oral	1–2 mg bid
Brompheniramine†	Dimetane®	Oral	5–40 mg 24 hr
Chlorpheniramine†	Chlor-Trimeton®	Oral	4–24 mg in 24 hr
Clemastine*,†	Tavist®	Oral	1.34–8.04 mg/day
Dexchlorpheniramine†	Polaramine®	Oral	2–6 mg/day
Dimenhydrinate*	Dramamine®	Oral	5–100 mg q4–6h PO; 50 mg IM as needed
Diphenhydramine*,†	Benadryl®	Oral	25–50 mg 4–6h
Doxylamine*	Unisom®	Oral	1 softgel hs prn
Meclizine*,†	Antivert®, Bonine®	Oral	25–100 mg daily
Phenindamine†	Nolahist®	Oral	12.5–25 mg q4–6h
Trimeprazine*	Temaril®	Oral	2.5 mg q4–6h
Triprolidine/pseudoephedrine*	Actifed®	Oral	1 tablet or 10 mL 3×/day
Second-generation Drugs			
Cetirizine*	Zyrtec®	Oral	5–10 mg daily
Fexofenadine*	Allegra®	Oral	60 mg bid or 180 mg once/day
Loratadine†	Claritin®	Oral	10 mg daily on an empty stomach
Second-generation Drugs with Decongestant			
Fexofenadine/pseudoephedrine	Allegra D®	Oral	1 tablet 2×/day
Loratadine/pseudoephedrine	Claritin D®	Oral	5–10 mg daily

IM, intramuscular; PO, oral.

*Prescription drug.

†OTC drug.

Drug Interactions

Antihistamines may interact with many drugs. Some antibiotics such as erythromycin in combination with ketoconazole or itraconazole may cause significant increases in blood concentrations of the antihistamines. Antihistamines may also interact with muscle relaxants (curare) and narcotic analgesics (morphine) that cause the release of histamine from mast cells. If patients are taking such a drug, it is not ususual for an antihistamine to be given to counteract the effects of histamine. Agents that depress the activity of the CNS such as alcohol or tranquilizers increase the occurrence of drowsiness when taken with antihistamines.

ANTITUSSIVES

Agents that relieve or prevent coughing are called **antitussives**. The initial stimulus for cough probably arises in the bronchial mucosa, where irritation results in bronchoconstriction. Antitussives are classified into two major groups: opioid and nonopioid. The cough suppression agents are classified in Table 22-2.

Mechanism of Action

The opioid cough suppressants decrease sensitivity of the central cough center to peripheral stimuli. They decrease mucosal secretions. An antitussive action occurs at doses that are lower than that required for analgesia. Examples of opiates are codeine, hydrocodone, and chlorpheniramine/hydrocodone.

Examples of nonopioid cough suppressants are dextromethorphan, benzonatate, and diphenhydramine. Dextromethorphan is generally well absorbed and is the most effective of the nonopioid cough suppressants. This agent does not suppress respiration. Dextromethorphan causes less constipation than codeine. Benzonatate chemically is similar to procaine. It reduces the activity of peripheral cough receptors and also appears to increase the threshold of the central cough center. Diphenhydramine is sedating and has anticholinergic properties.

Therapeutic Uses

Opioid cough suppressants include morphine and hydromorphone, which suppress the cough reflex, but have limited use because of unwanted side effects.

TABLE 22-2. Classification of Cough Suppressants

GENERIC NAME	TRADE NAME	ROUTE OF ADMINISTRATION	COMMON DOSAGE RANGE
Opioids			
Codeine*,†	Various with codeine	Oral, IM, IV, SC	Analgesic 15–16 mg PO, IM, IV, or SC q4–6h; Antitussive 10–12 mg PO q4–6h
Hydrocodone*	Hycodan®, Histussin®, AtussHD®	Oral	5 mg q4–6h as needed
Chlorpheniramine hydrocodone	Tussionex®	Oral	5 mL 2×/day
Nonopioids			
Dextromethorphan†	Sucrets Cough®, Benylin DM®, Robitussin DM®	Oral	10–30 mg q4–8h or 60 mg bid
Diphenhydramine†	Benadryl®, Benylin®	Oral	25–50 mg q4–8h
Benzonatate*	Tessalon®	Oral	100–200 mg tid up to 600 mg/day

IM, intramuscular; IV, intravenous; SC, subcutaneous; PO, oral.
*Prescription drug.
†OTC drug.

Codeine and hydrocodone are not as effective but are used because they elevate the cough threshold.

Nonopioid cough suppressants are used to treat or prevent motion sickness, vertigo, and reactions to blood or plasma in susceptible patients. The major nonopioid cough suppressants are found in OTC medications. Dextromethorphan is the most effective of these drugs, which are well absorbed. Diphenhydramine is the active ingredient in many OTC preparations and in some legend medications with the antitussive dosage.

Adverse Effects

Side effects of the opioid cough suppressants include constipation, nausea, and respiratory depression. Nonopioid cough suppressants do not have the gastrointestinal side effects of the codeine preparations and are nonaddicting.

Drug Interactions

Nonopioid cough suppressants such as dextromethorphan may have drug interaction with monoamine oxidase (MAO) inhibitors. Diphenhydramine is generally safe and basically has no drug interactions.

CORTICOSTEROIDS

Corticosteroids are the most potent and consistently effective anti-inflammatory agents that are currently available. There are three commonly-used devices for inhalation administration including: metered dose inhalers, dry powder

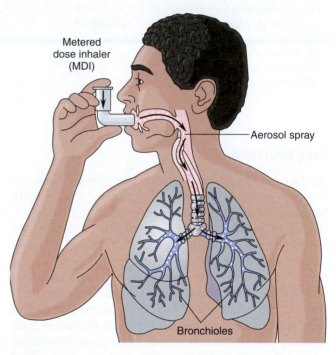

Metered dose inhaler (MDI)

Aerosol spray

Bronchioles

Figure 22-4. The metered dose inhaler aerosolizes medication for inhalation directly into the airways.

inhalers, and nebulizers. Drug administration with a **metered dose inhaler (MDI)** is often accomplished with one or two puffs from a hand-held pressurized device (see Figure 22-4).

A **dry powder inhaler (DPI)** delivers medication in the form of micronized powder into the lungs. Medications such as cromolyn and albuterol are available for use this way. DPIs are breath-activated and are easier to use than MDIs.

TABLE 22-3.   Corticosteroids for Treating Asthma

GENERIC NAME	TRADE NAME	ROUTE OF ADMINISTRATION	COMMON DOSAGE RANGE
Beclomethasone	Vanceril®, Beclovent®	MDI (inhalation)	50 mcg released at the valve delivers 42 mcg to the patient
Dextromethasone	Decadron®	MDI, powdered inhaler	3 inhalations (84 mcg each) tid-qid
Fluisolide	Nasalide®, Aerobid®	MDI	2 inhalations (500 mcg) bid: morning and evening
Fluticasone	Flovent®	MDI	100–500 mcg bid
Triamcinolone	Azmacort®	MDI	8–60 mg/day
Prednisone	Deltasone®	Oral	Initial dose: 5–60 mg/day
Prednisolone	Prelone®	Oral, IM, IV	5–60 mg/day depending on disease

Note: All of the drugs listed above are prescription drugs. IM, intramuscular; IV, intravenous.

A nebulizer uses a small machine that converts a solution into a mist. The mist droplets are inhaled either through a face mask or through a mouthpiece. Examples of inhaled corticosteroids are seen in Table 22-3.

Systematic corticosteroids are used to treat status asthmaticus, and inhaled corticosteroids are used for maintenance therapy. Inhaled corticosteroids are the most effective means of controlling asthma. Combined preparations containing a corticosteroid and a long-acting bronchodilator are considered to be useful for limiting the amount of the corticosteroid needed to control asthma.

Mechanism of Action

Corticosteroids enter target cells where they have anti-inflammatory and immunosuppressive and salt-retaining effects.

Therapeutic Uses

Inhaled corticosteroids are preferred for the long-term control of asthma and are first-line agents for treatment of patients with persistent asthma. Dosages for inhaled corticosteroids vary, depending on the specific agent and delivery device. Systemic corticosteroids are most effective for long-term asthma therapy. Long-term use of inhaled corticosteroids in children is not recommended because these agents may suppress growth and suppress production of hormones by the adrenal glands.

Adverse Effects

Adverse reactions to corticosteroid inhalation include nasal irritation and dryness, headache, nausea, epistaxis, dizziness, hoarseness, and cough.

Drug Interactions

Troleandomycin increases the therapeutic and toxic effects of corticosteroids. Corticotropin decreases the effects of anticholinesterases; profound muscular depression is possible.

BRONCHODILATORS

Bronchodilators are agents that widen the diameter of the bronchial tubes. Bronchodilators include β-adrenergic agonists, theophylline, anticholinergic drugs, and xanthine derivatives (see also Chapter 24).

Mechanism of Action

Bronchodilators relax smooth muscle of the bronchial tubes.

Therapeutic Uses

Bronchodilators are the major drugs used to treat asthma (see Table 22-4).

Adverse Effects

Adverse effects of β-adrenergic drugs such as epinephrine and isoproternol may cause restlessness, headache, dizziness, insomnia, tachycardia, palpitations, nausea, vomiting, and anorexia. The most common adverse effects of theophylline are nausea and vomiting. It also causes hypotension, headache, and flushing.

Drug Interactions

Bronchodilators increase peripheral vasoconstriction if given with ergot alkaloids. If this combination is used, monitor blood pressure carefully. Increased blood pressure response may occur if combined with tricyclic antidepressants and bretylium. Theophylline increases the effects and toxicity of cimetidine, erythromycin, troleandomycin, ciprofloxacin, and hormonal contraceptives. Theophylline decreased effects in patients who are cigarette smokers. Dosage may need to be increased 50% to 100%.

TABLE 22-4. Classification of Bronchodilators

GENERIC NAME	TRADE NAME	ROUTE OF ADMINISTRATION	COMMON DOSAGE RANGE
Epinephrine*,†	Adrenalin®	Inhalation: aerosol, nebulization	Individualized dosage Place 8–15 drops into nebulizers—opened mouth
Epinephrine*,†	Bronkaid®, Medihaler®, Primatene®	IM, SC, IV	10–150 mg/day
Ephedrine*	Vicks®, Vantronol®	Oral, IM, IV, nasal	0.25–0.5 ml or 12.5–25 mg
Isoproterenol*	Isuprel®	Oral, inhalation, IV	IV: 0.01–0.02 mg; inhalation: 1:200 solution in a dosage of 5–15 deep inhalations
Albuterol*	Proventil®	Oral, MDI	Initially 2 or 4 mg tid PO; inhalation: 90 mcg; 2 inhalations q4–6h
Salbutamol*	Ventolin®	MDI, nebulizer	2.5 mg 3–4×/day
Bitolterol*	Tornalate®	MDI	1.5–3.5 mg over 10–15 min
Isoetharine*	Bronkometer®	Nebulizer	Hand bulb nebulizers 4 inhalations
Terbutaline*	Brethaire®	MDI	Inhalation 2 separated by 60 sec q4-6h
Terbutaline sulfate*	Brethine®	Oral	0.25 mg
Metaproterenol*	Alupent®	Inhalation	2–3 inhalations q3–4h
Metaproterenol*	Metaprel®	Oral	20 mg q6–8h
Salmeterol*	Serevent®	MDI, DPI	2 inhalations bid 12 hr apart
Methylxanthines			
Theophylline/ aminophylline*	Elixophyllin®, Slo-Phyllin®, Aminophyllin®	Oral	Maintain serum levels in therapeutic range of 10–20 mcg/mL; base dosage on lean body mass
Dyphylline*	Dilor®, Lufyllin®	Oral, IM	Up to 15 mg/kg PO qid or 250–500 mg injected slowly IM (not for IV use)
Combination Bronchodilators			
Ipratropium/albuterol*	Combivent®	MDI	2 inhalations qid
Fluticasone*	Advair®	DPI	1–2 puffs bid

IM, intramuscular; IV, intravenous; PO, oral.
*Prescription drug.
†OTC drug.

ASTHMA PROPHYLACTICS

Cromolyn sodium and nedocromil are used to prevent asthma symptoms and improve airway function in patients with mild persistent asthma or exercise-induced asthma. Table 22-5 shows the most common asthma prophylactic drugs.

Mechanism of Action

Cromolyn suppresses inflammation but does not dilate the bronchial tree. It inhibits the release of histamines, so it acts as an antiallergenic. Nedocromil is also anti-inflammatory and antiallergic. Nedocromil may help reduce the dose requirements for inhaled corticosteroids.

Therapeutic Uses

Cromolyn is the drug of choice as a prophylactic for moderate allergic asthma, especially in children, because of its safety and efficacy. It is also used to reduce the symptoms of seasonal allergic attacks.

Adverse Effects

Adverse effects of cromolyn include coughing and wheezing on administration. Nedocromil has an unpleasant taste.

Drug Interactions

No clinically important drug interactions with cromolyn have been established.

LEUKOTRIENE ANTAGONISTS

Leukotrienes are a class of biologically active compounds that occur naturally in leukocytes (white blood cells) and produce allergic and inflammatory reactions similar to those of histamine. They are thought to play a role in the development of allergic and autoallergic diseases such as asthma, rheumatoid arthritis, inflammatory bowel disease, and psoriasis.

TABLE 22-5.   The Most Common Asthma Prophylactic Drugs

GENERIC NAME	TRADE NAME	ROUTE OF ADMINISTRATION	COMMON DOSAGE RANGE
Cromolyn	Aarane®, Intal®, Crolom®, Nasalcrom®	DPI, MDI, nebulizer, nasal spray	Initial: 25–300 mg/day PO; 20–330 mg/day IM; 1 spray inhaled qid; 1 spray in each nostril 3–6×/day
Nedocromil	Tilade®	MDI	2 inhalations q1d
Zafirlukast	Accolate®	Oral	20 mg bid
Zileuton	Zyflo®	Oral	600 mg qid
Montelukast	Singulair®	Oral	One 10 mg tablet/day

Note: All of the drugs listed above are prescription drugs. IM, intramuscular; PO, oral.

Mechanism of Action

Leukotriene antagonists block the bronchoconstriction, mucus production, and inflammation that occur with asthma. Zafirlukast was the first medication in this new class of anti-inflammatory agents. Zileuton is a newer drug in this class. It is rapidly absorbed via oral administration. Zileuton is used in patients older than 12 years of age. Montelukast is the latest addition to this class of drugs. Montelukast acts as a bronchodilator, respiratory stimulant, and leukotriene receptor antagonist. This medication should be given at night for maximum effectiveness.

Therapeutic Uses

Zafirlukast is prescribed as maintenance therapy for patients with chronic asthma. Montelukast is prescribed as a prophylactic drug for asthma attacks. It must not be used for acute asthma attacks.

Adverse Effects

Zafirlukast is a safe drug and has few side effects. Adverse effects of zileuton include liver toxicity and dyspepsia. The main adverse effects of montelukast are headaches and gastrointestinal symptoms.

Drug Interactions

Zafirlukast increases risk of bleeding with warfarin. It can potentially increase effects and toxicity of calcium channel-blockers and cyclosporine. Zafirlukast decreases the effectiveness of erythromycin and theophylline. Zileuton increases the effects of propranolol, theophylline, and warfarin. Montelukast decreases effects and bioavailability if taken with phenobarbital and rifampin.

◼ XANTHINE DERIVATIVES

Xanthine derivatives are chemically related to caffeine, which dilates bronchioles in the lungs. Xanthine derivatives are effective for relief of bronchospasm in several diseases.

Mechanism of Action

Xanthine derivatives relax the smooth muscles of the bronchial tree and stimulate cardiac muscle and the central nervous system. Methylxanthine is the base of xanthine derivatives, which must be converted to theophylline. Theophylline has a narrow therapeutic range and is not used as commonly today. Instead, the β_2-adrenergic agents are safer and more effective. Theophylline provides mild bronchodilation in asthmatic patients. This drug may also have important anti-inflammatory properties and enhance mucociliary clearance. Theophylline is available for oral administration in standard or sustained-release formulas with forms that last up to 24 hours. Theophylline has a small therapeutic range and β_2-agonists are safer and more effective. Therefore, the xanthines are not used as commonly today as previously.

Therapeutic Uses

These xanthine agents are used for the prevention and treatment of bronchial asthma and for the treatment of emphysema and bronchitis.

Adverse Effects

Adverse effects include tachycardia, insomnia, nervousness, headache, and nausea. Patients with hypothyroidism, acute pulmonary edema, convulsive disorders, and heart disease cannot use the xanthine derivatives. Adverse effects of theophylline at therapeutic doses include insomnia, upset stomach, aggravation of dyspepsia, and difficulties with urination in elderly men with prostatism. Dose-related toxicities are common and include nausea, vomiting, tachyarrhythmias, headache, seizures, hyperglycemia, and hypokalemia.

Drug Interactions

The xanthine drugs can produce drug interactions with caffeine, cimetidine, fluoroquinolones, antibiotics, rifampin, phenobarbital, and phenytoin.

β-ADRENERGIC AGENTS

β-Adrenergic agents work as both cardiac and respiratory agonists. These drugs or hormones act through the sympathetic nervous system. Their effects include increased heart rate, dilation of bronchial tubes in the lungs, and reduction of the force and rate of uterine contractions during labor.

Drugs with primary β_1-agonist activity act mainly on the heart, increasing heart rate and raising blood pressure. Drugs with primary β_2-agonist activity act mainly on the lungs and uterus. They are used to treat asthma and premature labor.

Mechanism of Action

The main action of β-adrenergic agents is on the smooth muscle of the bronchial tree and on the heart. A typical medication is isoproterenol, which may be taken orally or by injection. β_2-receptor drugs are the most effective medications for reducing acute bronchospasms and exercise-induced asthma. These agents provide bronchodilation by stimulating the β_2-receptors in the smooth muscle of the lung. Epinephrine and ephedrine are nonselective adrenergic agents. These agents are used to treat bronchial asthma and bronchitis and to prevent bronchospasm. Epinephrine and ephedrine have a rapid onset of action with a duration of 1 to 3 hours when used by inhalation or 1 to 4 hours when given parenterally.

Therapeutic Uses

The β_2-agonists are used to treat hypertension and a wide variety of other conditions, including asthma and bronchitis, and to prevent premature labor. Salmeterol is preferred for prophylaxis but is not effective for aborting an attack because of the slowness of its action. Salmeterol is the only agent of this class available in the United States and is indicated for long-term prevention of asthma symptoms and the prevention of exercise-induced bronchospasm. Salmeterol should not be used in place of anti-inflammatory therapy.

Adverse Effects

Adverse effects of β_2-agonists include dizziness, headache, tremor, palpitations, and sinus tachycardia. Common adverse effects of epinephrine and ephedrine include insomnia, tachycardia, nervousness, and anorexia. The cardiotoxic effects have led to the discovery and use of more specific respiratory agents that do not cause tachycardia or nervousness.

Drug Interactions

Salmeterol generally does not have interactions with other drugs. Other β_2-agonists may have drug interactions with anesthetics, digitalis, ergotamine, and MAO inhibitors.

EXPECTORANTS

Expectorants are agents that promote the removal of mucous secretions from the lungs, bronchi, and trachea, usually by coughing. These medications are available OTC and by prescription. Expectorant drugs include acetylcysteine, guaifenesin, and dornase alfa (see Table 22-6).

Mechanism of Action

Expectorants are also **mucolytic** (destroying or dissolving the active agents that make up mucous). In many cases expectorants are added to other drugs, such as antitussives, decongestants, and antihistamines, to help remove mucus. Acetylcysteine is a mucolytic agent that decreases the viscosity of mucus. It is also an antidote for acetaminophen hepatotoxicity. Guaifenesin is safer and more effective.

Therapeutic Uses

Dornase alfa is a specific expectorant for use in cystic fibrosis. Dornase alfa is able to reduce the risk of respiratory infections. The drug works within 3 to 7 days of starting treatment. It is available as a solution for inhalation by nebulizer.

Adverse Effects

The adverse effects of these expectorants are not significant.

Drug Interactions

No significant drug interactions have been reported.

DECONGESTANTS

Decongestants cause vasoconstriction of nasal mucosa and reduce congestion or swelling. These agents are available in both oral and nasal preparations. Table 22-7 shows decongestant agents.

Mechanism of Action

The majority of oral agents are adrenergic drugs that mimic the effects of the sympathetic nervous system.

Therapeutic Uses

The most common uses for decongestants are relief of nasal congestion due to infection or allergy and inflammation in the eyes. They are also used to relieve respiratory distress of bronchial asthma, chronic bronchitis, and emphysema.

TABLE 22-6.   Mucolytics and Expectorants

GENERIC NAME	TRADE NAME	ROUTE OF ADMINISTRATION	COMMON DOSAGE RANGE
Acetylcysteine†	Mucomyst®	Inhalation	1–2 mL as often as every hour
Guaifenesin*,†	Hytuss®, Robitussin®, Dura-Tuss®	Oral	100–400 mg q4h
Dornase alfa	Pulmozyme®	Inhalation	2.5 mg/day inhaled through nebulizer

*Prescription drug.
†OTC drug.

TABLE 22-7.   Decongestant Agents

GENERIC NAME	TRADE NAME	ROUTE OF ADMINISTRATION	COMMON DOSAGE RANGE
Nasal Decongestants			
Ephedrine 0.5%	Vicks®, Vatronel®	Nasal drops	Instill solution in each nostril q4h
Epinephrine 0.1%	Asthma Haler Mist®, Primatene Mist®	Oral inhalation: aerosol, nebulization	Place 8–15 drops into nebulizer
Naphazoline 0.05%	Allerest®	Nasal drops	2 drops or spray in each nostril q3–6h for no more than 3–5 days
Phenylephrine 1%	Neo-Synephrine®, Sinex®	Nasal drops	1–2 drops in each nostril q3–4h
Tetrahydrozoline 0.1%	Tyzine®	Nasal drops	2–4 drops in each nostril q3h prn
Oxymetazoline 0.05%	Afrin®, Neo-Synephrine 12 hour®	Nasal drops and spray	2–3 drops or sprays into each nostril bid for up to 3–5 days
Oral Decongestants			
Pseudophedrine	Sudafed®, Drixoral® or Sudafed-SR®	Oral; oral (sustained release)	60 mg q4–6hr; 120 mg SR q12h
Combination Decongestants			
Pseudoephedrine/ chlorpheniramine	Aller-Chlor®, Chlor-Trimeton®, Chlo-Amine®, Chlor-Pro®, Phenetron®, Sinutab Sinus Allergy®, Sudafed Plus®, Telachlor®, Teldrin®	Oral	1 tablet q4–6hr
Pseudoephedrine	Afrin®, Allerest®, Cenafed®, Contac®, Decofed®, Dorcol®, Efidac/24®, PediaCare®, Sinutab®	Oral	1 tablet q12h

Note: All of the drugs listed in this table are available OTC. SR, sustained release.

Adverse Effects

Decongestants should only be used by order of a physician for those patients with glaucoma, prostate cancer, and heart disease. Decongestants may increase blood sugar levels in patients with diabetes mellitus. Warnings on the labels of OTC preparations provide instructions for patients with hypertension, diabetes mellitus, ischemic heart disease, and hyperthyroidism. Decongestants may cause tachycardia, insomnia, nervousness, restlessness, blurred vision, and nausea or vomiting. Ephedrine is being removed from the market because of its toxicities. Phenylpropanolamine, as used in decongestants, causes a risk of hemorrhagic stroke, and the U.S. Food and Drug Administration requested removal of this drug from decongestant products starting in the year 2000. Young women are at more risk for hemorrhagic stroke from use of this drug than are other groups who have been studied.

Drug Interactions

Nasal decongestants such as ephedrine may cause severe hypertension with MAO inhibitors such as furazolidone. They may also decrease the vasopressor response with reserpine, methyldopa, and urinary acidifiers. Nasal decongestants increase the duration of action of urinary alkalinizers (sodium citrate, sodium, lactate, tromethamine, and sodium bicarbonate). They decrease antihypertensive effects of methyldopa.

DRUGS FOR SMOKING CESSATION

Cigarette smoke contains chemical compounds that affect most organs of the human body. It causes cancers of the mouth, pharynx, larynx, lungs, esophagus, pancreas, kidney, bladder, and cervix. Cigarette smoking also may cause leukemia and may increase the risk of heart disease, lung disease, or stroke. Benefits of smoking cessation include better health and a longer life. The most commonly used drugs for smoking cessation are listed in Table 22-8.

Bupropion is an antidepressant for which the dosage form for smoking cessation varies. For example, bupropion (Zyban®) is used as a tablet. Habitrol®, Nicoderm®, Nicotrol®, and Prostep® are available as transdermal patches. Nicorette® is used as a gum, and Nicotrol NS® must be used as a spray. Bupropion was the first non-nicotine drug for smoking cessation. It can be used alone or with the nicotine patch. Some nicotine inhalers may be used in combination with fluoxetine for smoking cessation. It is suspected that certain antidepressants such as fluoxetine, when added to nicotine replacement therapy, might improve abstinence rates.

Mechanism of Action

The neurochemical mechanism of the antidepressant effect of bupropion is not understood; bupropion is chemically unrelated to other antidepressant agents. It is a weak blocker of the neuronal uptake of serotonin and norepinephrine and inhibits the reuptake of dopamine to some extent.

Therapeutic Uses

Bupropion is used for treatment of depression. It also aids in treatment for smoking cessation (Zyban®).

Adverse Effects

Adverse effects of nicotine, nicotine polacrilex, and nicotine transdermal systems are headache, dizziness, lightheadedness, insomnia, irritability, tachycardia, palpitations, hypertension, nausea, salivation, vomiting, cough, hiccups, and hoarseness.

Drug Interactions

Bupropion may increase risk of adverse effects with levodopa and toxicity with MAO inhibitors. It also increases the risk of seizures with drugs that lower the seizure threshold, including alcohol.

SUMMARY

The exchange of oxygen and carbon dioxide in the lungs is one of the most important physiological tasks of the body, as this process supplies oxygen at the cell level in body tissue. Oxygen is essential to sustain life. Therefore, the respiratory tract is necessary for the inspiration of oxygen and the expiration of carbon dioxide. Respiratory system disorders such as allergic asthma and chronic obstructive pulmonary disease (COPD) are common in the United States. Antihistamines are used to relieve allergic reactions throughout the body, but they are also used commonly in patients with respiratory tract disorders to relieve rhinorrhea and allergic bronchitis. Cough-suppressing preparations are indicated for nonproductive coughs. If the cough is productive, suppression is not

TABLE 22-8. Smoking Cessation Agents

GENERIC NAME	TRADE NAME	ROUTE OF ADMINISTRATION	COMMON DOSAGE RANGE
Bupropion*	Zyban®	Oral and patch	Oral: start with 150 mg once daily ×3 days, then increase to 150 mg bid for 7–12 wk
Nicotine*,†	Nicorette®	Gum	1 piece of gum whenever urge to smoke occurs (30 days)
Nicotine*,†	Nicoderm®	Patch	Apply 1 transdermal patch q24h by the ordered schedule
Nicotine*,†	Habitrol®	Patch	Same as for Nicoderm"
Nicotine*,†	Nicotrol® NS spray	Inhaler	1 dose = 2 sprays, one per nostril; start with 1–2 doses each hour
Nicotine*,†	Prostep®	Patch	22 mg/day ×4–8 wk, then follow the ordered schedule

*Prescription drug.
†OTC drug.

warranted, and an expectorant may be used to assist in expelling the secretions.

Bronchodilators induce smooth muscle relaxation, which eases breathing. They are used to treat asthma, COPD, and chronic bronchitis. Epinephrine and β_2-agonists are indicated for acute asthma. Leukotriene agonists (new on the market), such as albuterol and cromolyn, are used for exercise-induced asthma. Glucocorticoids are administered by inhalation.

REVIEW QUESTIONS

1. Which of the following substances may cause allergic rhinitis?
   A. Epinephrine
   B. Chlorpheniramine
   C. Hydrocodone
   D. Histamine

2. Adverse reactions to corticosteroid inhalation include
   A. cough, hoarseness, and headache.
   B. cough, diarrhea, and dyspepsia.
   C. pulmonary edema, convulsive disorders, and hypothyroidism.
   D. pulmonary edema, convulsive disorders, and hyperthyroidism.

3. Which of the following drugs is an expectorant?
   A. Ephedrine
   B. Adrenalin
   C. Acetylcysteine
   D. Bupropion

4. The trade name for guaifenesin is
   A. Tussionex®.
   B. Robitussin®.
   C. Benadryl®.
   D. Tessalon®.

5. Which of the following is an example of intranasal steroids?
   A. Beclomethasone
   B. Nicotine
   C. Salmeterol
   D. Albuterol

6. Which of the following is the brand name of bupropion?
   A. Habitrol®
   B. Zyban®
   C. Nicotrol®
   D. Prostep®

7. Dextromethorphan is classified as
   A. an opioid cough suppressant.
   B. a xanthine derivative.
   C. a nonsteroid contraceptive.
   D. a nonopioid cough suppressant.

8. Another name for allergic rhinitis is
   A. contact dermatitis.
   B. hay fever.
   C. yellow fever.
   D. photosensitivity.

9. The drug of choice for chronic asthma is which of the following?
   A. Theophylline
   B. Albuterol
   C. Antihistamines
   D. Corticosteroids

10. Which of the following organs is the site of H_2 receptors?
    A. Bladder
    B. Stomach
    C. Liver
    D. Lung

11. The initial stimulus for cough probably arises from which of the following parts of the respiratory system?
    A. Bronchial mucosa
    B. Pharynx
    C. Mouth
    D. Nasal cavities

12. The trade name of fluticasone is which of the following?
    A. Combivent®
    B. Lufyllin®
    C. Advair®
    D. Serevent®

13. Which of the following devices is able to convert a solution into a mist?
    A. Mouthpiece
    B. Nebulizer
    C. Spirometer
    D. Sphygmomanometer

14. Leukotriene is part of a class of biologically active compounds that occur naturally in which of the following body cells?
    A. White blood cells
    B. Red blood cells
    C. Platelets
    D. Mast cells

15. Which of the following agents is not used as commonly today?
    A. Leukotrienes
    B. Metered dose inhalers
    C. Xanthines
    D. Mucolytics

OUTLINE

OBJECTIVES

Upon completion of this chapter, the reader should be able to

1. Explain the composition of the nervous system.
2. Describe sedative and hypnotic drugs.
3. Identify the mechanism of action of alcohol and barbiturates.
4. Describe therapeutic uses of the antipsychotic drugs.
5. Identify the mechanism of action of the antidepressants.
6. Explain therapeutic uses of the monoamine oxidase inhibitors.
7. Describe bipolar disorder and lithium therapy.
8. State five adverse effects of lithium therapy.
9. Explain therapeutic uses of levodopa.
10. Identify the mechanism of action of the narcotic analgesics.
11. Describe the four stages of anesthesia.

GLOSSARY

acetylcholine (ACh) A neurotransmitter that stimulates nerve endings.

Alzheimer's disease An illness characterized by progressive memory failure, impaired thinking, confusion, disorientation, personality changes, restlessness, speech disturbances, and inability to perform routine tasks.

anesthetics Agents that act on nervous tissue to produce a loss of sensation or unconsciousness.

anxiety A persistent and irrational fear of a specific object, activity, or situation.

aura A sensation that may precede an attack of an epileptic seizure.

convulsion Abnormal motor movements.

cross-dependence The ability of one drug to substitute for another drug in the same drug class to maintain a dependent state or prevent withdrawal.

cross-tolerance Tolerance to one drug conferring tolerance to other drugs in the same drug class.

dependence The psychological, physiological, or biochemical need to continue to take a drug.

drug abuse Nonmedical use of a drug that is deemed unacceptable by society.

endogenous depression Feelings of intense sadness, helplessness, and worthlessness that have no external cause and may be the result of genetic factors or biochemical changes in the brain.

exogenous depression Feelings of intense sadness, helplessness, and worthlessness that occur in response to a loss, disappointment, or illness.

hypnosis An increased tendency to sleep.

hypnotics Drugs that depress the central nervous system by inhibiting transmission of nerve impulses.

migraine headache A disorder characterized by unilateral throbbing or nonthrobbing pain that is often accompanied by nausea, vomiting, and sensitivity to noise and light.

neurohormones Neurotransmitters.

neuron The basic structure of a nerve consisting of dendrites, cell body, and axon.

neurosis A disease of the nerves or a mental disorder.

GLOSSARY continued

Parkinson's disease A disorder characterized by resting tremor, rigidity or resistance to passive movement, akinesia, and loss of postural reflexes.

physical dependence The necessity to continue drug use to avoid a withdrawal syndrome.

psychological dependence The overwhelming need to take a drug to maintain a sense of well-being.

psychosis A mental illness accompanied by bizarre behavior and altered personality with failure to perceive reality.

sedation A state of consciousness characterized by decreased anxiety, motor activity, and mental acuity.

sedatives Drugs that depress the central nervous system by inhibiting transmission of nerve impulses.

seizure An epileptic event.

tolerance A reduced drug effect with repeated use of a drug and a need for higher doses to produce the same effect.

OVERVIEW

Nervous system disorders include Alzheimer's disease, cerebral palsy, concussion, epilepsy, headache, and tumors. These disorders and many others often are irreversible and plague many adults throughout the aging process. A pharmacy technician should be familiar with the most common disorders of the central nervous system and the peripheral nervous system and the most effective treatments for the wide variety of disorders that are prevalent.

ANATOMY REVIEW: THE NERVOUS SYSTEM

The nervous system is composed of the brain, spinal cord, and nerves (see Figure 23-1). The nervous system is divided into two sections: the central nervous system (CNS) and the peripheral nervous system (PNS). The central nervous system is located in the dorsal cavity, the brain is enclosed in the cranium, and the spinal cord is inside the spinal cavity. The PNS is outside the CNS and connects the CNS to the remainder of the body. The nervous system controls sensory functions, integrative functions, and motor functions. Subdivision of these two systems is summarized in Figure 23-2.

The **neuron** is the basic cell of the nervous system, carrying nerve impulses from one part of the body to another. It consists of three parts: dendrites, cell body, and axons (see Figure 23-3). Dendrites are the receptors that carry information to the nerve cell body, and axons carry nerve information away from the nerve cell body. At the junction of neurons, the continuation of messages is performed by neurotransmitters such as **acetylcholine (ACh)**, which stimulates the nerve endings, and cholinesterase, which inhibits ACh. There are some other neurotransmitters, or **neurohormones**, including the catecholamines (norepinephrine, epinephrine, and dopamine), serotonin, and endorphins.

The nervous system is able to cope with different types of stressors at different times of life, which is part of normal living or mental health. Daily stressors may cause normal activities of the brain to become abnormal resulting in a mental disorder. Sensory nerves gather body information and

environmental information and carry it to the CNS. The brain puts together this information into a plan of action or movement, which is then carried out by the motor nerves. The body's muscles and glands respond to the CNS information brought to them by the motor nerves.

DRUGS THAT ACT ON THE NERVOUS SYSTEM

Many different medications are prescribed for a variety of conditions and disorders of the nervous system. These drugs are classified as sedatives and hypnotics, antipsychotics (antianxiety and antipsychosis), and antidepressants.

Sedative and Hypnotic Drugs

Sedatives and **hypnotics** are drugs that depress the CNS by inhibiting transmission of nerve impulses. Therefore, these drugs depress the action of many physiological systems that are capable of causing a wide range of desirable and undesirable effects. **Sedation** is characterized by decreased anxiety, motor activity, and mental acuity. Sedation induces calmness or sleep. **Hypnosis** is defined by an increased tendency to sleep. Insomnia is a chronic inability to sleep. It is associated with and complicates a number of medical and psychiatric disorders. It may also be caused by stress, sleep schedule, medications and ingested substances, lifestyle, and primary sleep disorders. Therefore, a number of classes of pharmacologic agents are used in the treatment of insomnia as sedatives, hypnotics, or both, including barbiturates, alcohol, and benzodiazepines. Other agents also may effectively cause sedation and sleep, such as antipsychotics, antihistamines, and antidepressants. Depression of the CNS reduces physical and mental activity; this action is often related to the use of barbiturates, alcohol, and benzodiazepines.

Barbiturates

Barbiturates are chemical derivatives of barbituric acid. Barbiturates are classified into four groups: ultra-short-acting, short-acting, intermediate-acting, and long-acting (see Table 23-1). They are also classified as either

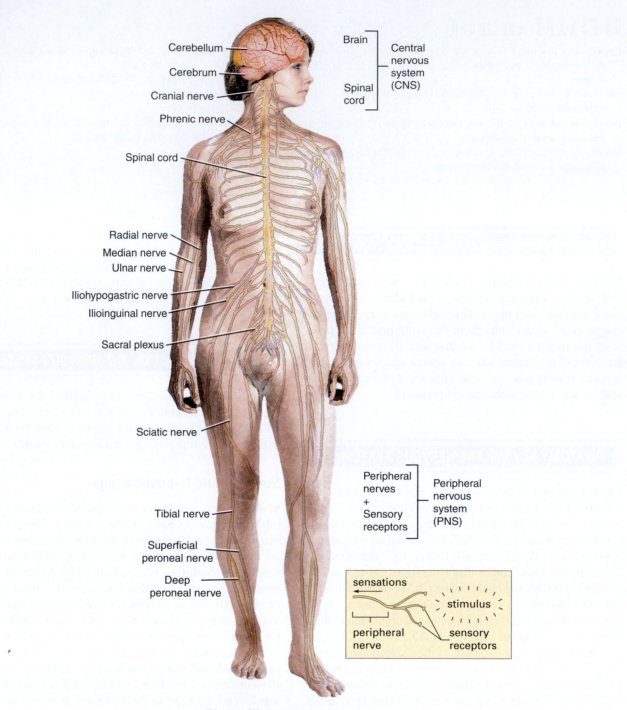

Cerebellum

Cerebrum

Cranial nerve

Phrenic nerve

Spinal cord

Radial nerve

Median nerve

Ulnar nerve

Iliohypogastric nerve

Ilioinguinal nerve

Sacral plexus

Sciatic nerve

Tibial nerve

Superficial peroneal nerve

Deep peroneal nerve

Brain

Spinal cord

Central nervous system (CNS)

Peripheral nerves + Sensory receptors

Peripheral nervous system (PNS)

sensations

stimulus

peripheral nerve

sensory receptors

Figure 23-1. The nervous system.

Schedule II or III medications. More than 2500 barbiturates have been synthesized, but only about 50 have been approved for clinical use in the United States, and fewer than a dozen are commonly used.

Mechanism of Action   All barbiturates exert a depressant effect on the CNS. The extent of their action may range from mild sedation to deep anesthesia (which will be discussed later).

Therapeutic Uses   Barbiturates are used as sedatives and hypnotics (short term for up to 2 weeks) for insomnia. Long-term treatment with certain barbiturates is prescribed in generalized tonic-clonic and cortical focal seizures. They are also indicated for emergency control of some acute convulsive episodes such as status epilepticus, eclampsia, meningitis, tetanus, and toxic reactions to local anesthetics. After prolonged use of barbiturates, withdrawal symptoms may occur.

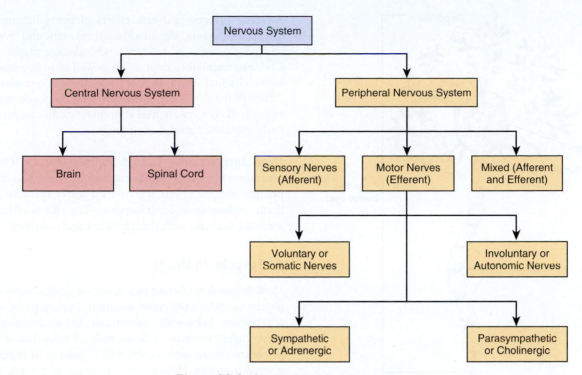

Figure 23-2. Organization of the nervous system.

Phenobarbital and mephobarbital are used for seizure disorders, congenital hyperbilirubinemia, and neonatal jaundice. Indications for intermediate-acting barbiturates are regional anesthesia, sedation, and hypnosis. Ultra-short-acting barbiturates are used for intravenous general anesthesia.

Adverse Effects   Barbiturates may cause numerous adverse effects on several different body systems. The manifestations of adverse effects include ataxia, drowsiness, dizziness, and a hangover-like effect. Some patients may have nausea and vomiting, insomnia, constipation, headache, night terrors, and faintness. Long-term use of barbiturates may cause bone pain, anorexia, muscle pain, and weight loss.

Drug Interactions   Barbiturates increase serum levels and therapeutic and toxic effects with valproic acid. They also increase CNS depression with alcohol. Barbiturates decrease the effects of the following drugs: theophyllines, oral antico-agulants, β-blockers, doxycycline, griseofulvin, corticosteroids, hormonal contraceptives, and metronidazole.

Alcohol

Alcohol is a CNS depressant that is used as an antianxiety agent and a sedative/hypnotic. Because it is a nonprescription sedative, alcohol is often a drug of abuse, permitting the body to progress through the stages of sedation from excitability to depression of the CNS to sedation, hypnosis, and possible coma.

Mechanism of Action   Alcohol depresses the CNS. The effects are dose dependent, with high doses causing depression of the medulla in the brain and the basic functions of life.

The mechanism of action of ethanol is not known. Ethanol depresses CNS activity (like other sedative and hypnotic drugs) and has antianxiety and sedative effects. It is rapidly absorbed from the stomach and small intestine and rapidly distributed in total body water. Absorption is delayed by food.

Therapeutic Uses   Alcohol (ethanol) is used primarily as an antiseptic or as a solvent for other drugs. However, it is the most seriously abused drug and will be discussed later in this chapter.

Adverse Effects   The most common concern is the non-medical chronic use of alcohol by heavy drinkers, which causes atrophy of the cerebrum (brain) and a loss of intellectual functions. In extreme doses, alcohol may produce anesthesia that could be lethal.

Drug Interactions   Drug interactions of alcohol with other medications may be additive (synergistic) or may change the effectiveness of the medications. Alcohol increases physical and psychological dependence of drugs used for sleep such as tranquilizers. The combination of alcohol and antidepressants results in rapid intoxication. Pain relievers, muscle relaxants, antiallergics, antihistamines, and metronidazole may produce nausea, vomiting, and flushing when combined with alcohol.

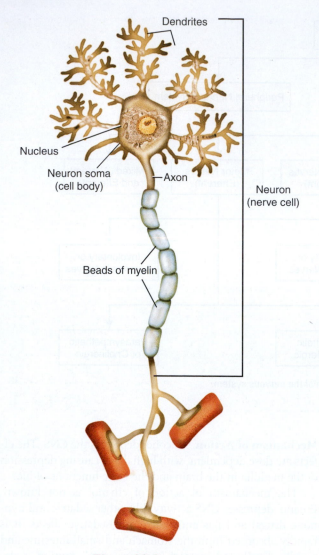

Figure 23-3. The neuron.

Dendrites

Nucleus

Neuron soma
(cell body)

Axon

Neuron
(nerve cell)

Beads of myelin

Benzodiazepines

The benzodiazepines are a widely used chemical class of drugs (see Table 23-2). The benzodiazepines are the drugs of choice to treat anxiety and are also used for hypnosis because of their great margin of safety.

Mechanism of Action   Their mechanism of action on the CNS appears to be closely related to their ability to potentiate γ-aminobutyric acid (GABA)-mediated neural inhibition. Recent research has identified specific binding sites for benzodiazepines in the CNS and has established the close relationship between the sites of action of the benzodiazepines and GABA.

Therapeutic Uses   Indications for the use of benzodiazepines include generalized anxiety disorders, panic disorders, agoraphobia (fear of open spaces), insomnia, seizures, and muscle relaxation. Table 23-3 shows some of the benzodiazepines most commonly used for sedation or as hypnotics.

Adverse Effects   Adverse effects of benzodiazepines are drowsiness, ataxia, impaired judgment, rebound insomnia, and development of tolerance. Overdosage may result in CNS and respiratory depression as well as hypotension and coma. Gradual withdrawal of these drugs is recommended. Although the use of any of the benzodiazepines during pregnancy is likely to cause fetal abnormalities, flurazepam is entirely contraindicated during pregnancy.

Drug Interactions   Benzodiazepines · increase CNS depression with alcohol and omeprazole. They also increase pharmacological effects if combined with cimetidine, disulfiram, or hormonal contraceptives. The effects of benzodiazepines decrease with theophyllines and ranitidine.

Antipsychotic Drugs

Mental disorders fall into two major categories: neurosis and psychosis. Both may cause agitation, hyperactivity, and inappropriate behaviors. Sometimes these disorders may cause violent behavior. The mentally ill individual is unable to communicate with others and is unable to function in normal activities. Medications play an important role in modern psychotherapeutic care. Antipsychotic drugs are used to reduce or alleviate symptoms and allow the mentally ill person an opportunity to participate in other psychotherapeutic treatment.

   Neurosis is a combining form meaning "a disease of the nerves" or a "mental disorder" and includes angioneurosis, psychoneurosis, and synneurosis.

   Psychosis is a mental illness accompanied by bizarre behavior and altered personality with failure to perceive reality. Psychosis involves a breakdown in personality, with thought patterns and responses to the environment unrelated to the real-life situation. The person is out of contact with reality, and communication may be impossible. The two major forms of psychosis are severe depression and schizophrenia. Various drugs may be used in treatment of mental disorders and psychosis. Antipsychotic drugs are also called *neuroleptics* (formerly called *major tranquilizers*). Neuroleptic drugs produce sedation and have a tranquilizing effect. These agents may be used for acute and chronic psychosis. The most important classes of antipsychotic medications are the phenothiazines, butyrophenones, thioxanthenes, dibenzodiazepines, and benzisoxazoles. Table 23-4 shows selected drugs used to treat psychosis.

Mechanism of Action

The mechanism of action of antipsychotic drugs is unknown, but these agents are thought to act on dopamine and serotonin (neurotransmitters in the brain).

   Chlorpromazine was the first antipsychotic agent and remains the typical phenothiazine. This agent possesses anticholinergic, antiemetic, antihistaminic, and β-adrenergic blocking effects, as well as antipsychotic actions.

TABLE 23-1.   Classification of Barbiturates

GENERIC NAME	TRADE NAME	ROUTE OF ADMINISTRATION	COMMON DOSAGE RANGE
Ultra-short-acting			
Thiopental	Pentothal®	IV	2–4 mg/kg
Methohexital	Brevital®	IV	1–30 mg/kg
Thiamylal	Surital®	IV	Used only for animals
Short-acting			
Pentobarbital	Nembutal®	Oral, IM, IV	100–150 mg/day
Secobarbital	Seconal®	Oral	8–250 mg/day
Intermediate-acting (3–4 hours)			
Amobarbital	Amytal®	Oral	50–500 mg/day
Long-acting (oral 10–16 hours)			
Phenobarbital	Bellatal®, Solfoton®	Oral, IM, SC, IV	16–300 mg/day
Mephobarbital	Mebaral®	Oral	32–100 mg/day

IM, intramuscular; IV, intravenous; SC, subcutaneous.

TABLE 23-2.   Classification of Benzodiazepines

GENERIC NAME	TRADE NAME	ROUTE OF ADMINISTRATION	COMMON DOSAGE RANGE
Short-acting			
Alprazolam	Xanax®	Oral	0.25–4 mg/day
Lorazepam	Ativan®	Oral, IM, IV	0.5–6 mg/day
Quazepam	Doral®	Oral	7.5–15 mg/day
Temazepam	Restoril®	Oral	7.5–300 mg/day
Triazolam	Halcion®	Oral	0.125–0.5 mg/day
Long-acting			
Chlordiazepoxide	Librium®	Oral	15–40 mg/day
Clonazepam	Klonopin®	Oral	0.5–20 mg/day
Chlorazepate	Tranxene®	Oral	15–60 mg/day
Prazepam	Centrax®	Oral	10–20 mg/day
Diazepam	Valium®	Oral, IM, IV	2–20 mg/day
Flurazepam	Dalmane®	Oral	15–30 mg/day
Miscellaneous Antianxiety Drugs			
Buspirone	BuSpar®	Oral	15–60 mg/day
Hydroxyzine	Atarax®	Oral, IM	2 mg/kg/day

IM, intramuscular; IV, intravenous.

Nonphenothiazines include butyrophenones, thioxanthenes, dibenzodiazepines, and benzisoxazoles. The mechanism of action for these products is often not precisely understood.

Therapeutic Uses

The antipsychotic drugs do not cure mental disorders but are used to control the symptoms related to psychosis. They are also used to relieve nausea and vomiting. Antipsychotic drugs are used to decrease the symptoms of schizophrenia and other psychotic disorders. Severe mental illnesses, such as schizophrenia, psychotic depression, mania, or psychotic brain syndrome, are commonly treated with major tranquilizers or antipsychotic drugs.

Nonphenothiazines are used mainly for schizophrenia.

Adverse Effects

The side effects of antipsychotic drugs include postural hypotension, tachycardia or bradycardia, and vertigo. Blurred vision, dry mouth, fever, constipation, and jaundice may also occur.

TABLE 23-3. Benzodiazepines Used as Hypnotic Drugs

GENERIC NAME	TRADE NAME	ROUTE OF ADMINISTRATION	COMMON DOSAGE RANGE
Diazepam	Valium®	IV, IM	2–20 mg/day
Estazolam	ProSom®	Oral	0.5–2 mg/day
Flurazepam HCl	Dalmane®	Oral	15–30 mg/day
Lorazepam	Ativan®	Oral, IM, IV, sublingual	0.5–2 mg/day
Midazolam	Versed®	IM, IV	5–40 mg/day
Quazepam	Doral®	Oral	7.5–15 mg/day
Temazepam	Restoril®	Oral	7.5–30 mg/day
Triazolam	Halcion®	Oral	7.5–30 mg/day

IM, intramuscular; IV, intravenous.

TABLE 23-4. Selected Drugs Used to Treat Psychosis

GENERIC NAME	TRADE NAME	ROUTE OF ADMINISTRATION	COMMON DOSAGE RANGE
Phenothiazines			
Chlorpromazine	Thorazine®	Oral, rectal, IM	10–200 mg/day
Fluphenazine	Prolixin®	Oral, IM	1–40 mg/day
Mesoridazine	Serentil®	Oral, IM	10–400 mg/day
Perphenazine	Trilafon®	Oral, IM	8–64 mg/day
Prochlorperazine	Compazine®	Oral	2.5–150 mg/day
Promethazine	Phenergan®	Oral, rectal, IM	6.25–50 mg/day
Thioridazine	Mellaril®	Oral	0.5–800 mg/day
Trifluoperazine	Stelazine®	Oral, IM	1–40 mg/day
Nonphenothiazines			
Butyrophenones			
Haloperidol	Haldol®	Oral, IM	0.5–100 mg/day
Thioxanthenes			
Thiothixene	Navane®	Oral, IM	2–60 mg/day
Dibenzodiazepines			
Clozapine	Clozaril®	Oral	12.5–900 mg/day
Benzisoxazoles			
Risperidone	Risperdal®	Oral	1–6 mg/day

IM, intramuscular.

When patients take antipsychotic medications over several months up to a prolonged period of time, the medications will have a tendency to cause extrapyramidal effects by blocking dopamine receptors in the brain.

Elderly patients are more prone to parkinsonian symptoms, such as tremors, muscle rigidity, and dysphagia. Children seem to be more prone to dystonic reactions, which include muscle spasms of the head with twitching, facial grimacing, torticollis, or wryneck.

Drug Interactions

Antipsychotic medications may have drug interactions with antihistamines, alcohol, analgesics, tranquilizers, narcotics, β-blockers, barbiturates, insulin, oral hypoglycemics, and epinephrine.

Antianxiety Drugs

Anxiety is defined as a persistent and irrational fear of a specific object, activity, or situation. Anxiety disorders are the most common psychiatric illnesses in the general community. The primary anxiety disorders are classified according to their duration, course, nature of precipitants, and existence.

Achievable goals of treatment are to decrease the frequency of panic attacks and to reduce their intensity. The cornerstone of drug therapy is antidepressant medications. These agents are used for the relief of anxiety and may also be used as hypnotics and sedatives to promote sleep. The difference between using the agents as anxiolytics and hypnotics is based on dosage. Higher doses have hypnotic effects and lower doses can relieve anxiety.

Mechanism of Action

Many of these medications have additive actions when combined with CNS depressants, but the mechanism of action is not known.

Therapeutic Uses

Sometimes a single medication may be prescribed both to lower anxiety and to produce sleep. Antianxiety drugs may also be used as skeletal muscle relaxants for chronic muscle pain. Occasionally, minor tranquilizers are also used as antiseizure medications to reduce the number of convulsions and as adjunctive medications in alcohol withdrawal.

A new nonbenzodiazepine, buspirone, may specifically relieve anxiety without sedation, hypnosis, or general CNS depression.

Adverse Effects

The most commonly found adverse effects of anxiolytics include drowsiness, confusion, ataxia, nausea, constipation, dry mouth, and rashes. Patients taking these medications may have sensitivity to sunlight and may require protective measures to keep from getting sunburned. Menstrual irregularities, a change in libido, and changes in liver function are less common, but may occur.

Drug Interactions

Anxiolytics (antianxiety) drugs may produce drug interactions with other CNS depressants, alcohol, cimetidine, anticoagulants, corticosteroids, digitalis, and phenytoin.

Antidepressants

Depression is one of the most common psychiatric disorders. It is characterized by feelings of intense sadness, helplessness, and worthlessness and impaired functioning. There are two types of depression: endogenous and exogenous. **Endogenous depression**, or unipolar disorder, is characterized by depression that has no external cause and may be the result of genetic factors or biochemical changes in the brain. **Exogenous depression** is often a response to a loss or disappointment, such as the death of a loved one, loss of a job, or the presence of a debilitating illness. This type of depression is often called *the blues*. After a period of adjustment, the depression resolves, and life goes on. The main antidepressant drug classes include monoamine oxidase inhibitors (MAOIs), tricyclic antidepressants (TCAs), and selective serotonin reuptake inhibitors (SSRIs). Drugs used to treat depression are shown in Table 23-5.

The therapeutic response rate with all antidepressants is similar, and the selection of the proper agent depends on the side effects that the patient experiences from the drugs.

Mechanism of Action

MAOIs reduce the activity of the enzyme monoamine oxidase. It increases CNS levels and activity of norepinephrine and serotonin. The therapeutic effect is achieved in 3 to 5 weeks.

TCAs inhibit the uptake of norepinephrine and serotonin in the CNS.

SSRIs are newer antidepressant drugs that block the reuptake and inactivation of serotonin in the brain. Unlike the TCAs, the SSRIs produce little blockage of cholinergic, adrenergic, or histamine receptors. Therefore, SSRIs produce fewer adverse effects, and they are now the most widely used antidepressant drugs. SSRIs should be administered in the morning because of the chance of nervousness and insomnia. Examples of SSRIs are fluoxetine and citalopram hydrobromide. Fluoxetine was the first SSRI drug. This medication is the most widely prescribed antidepressant in the United States because it is as effective as TCAs, with fewer side effects, and is less dangerous when taken in overdosage. Citalopram hydrobromide is one of the newer SSRI-type medications. It does not produce a sympathomimetic response or anticholinergic activity. Its only use is for depression. This medication cannot be used with MAOIs and should not be given until 2 weeks after any MAOIs are stopped.

Therapeutic Uses

MAOIs are rarely used for endogenous depression. They are generally used when TCAs are not effective. Another indication for MAOIs is narcolepsy.

TCAs are used primarily to relieve the symptoms of unipolar endogenous depression, resulting in elevation of mood, increased physical activity and mental alertness, increased appetite, increased sexual drive, and improved sleep patterns. They are effective in 70% of patients. They may also be used to treat mild exogenous depression, bipolar endogenous depression (with lithium), and nocturnal enuresis (only as a last resort and only for patients older than 6 years of age).

SSRIs are used primarily to treat major depression.

Adverse Effects

Adverse effects of MAOIs include orthostatic hypotension, drowsiness, inhibition of ejaculation, insomnia, headache, hallucinations, diarrhea, nausea, vomiting, fever, blurred vision, dry mouth, and incontinence. Overdose produces restlessness, hypotension, tachycardia, mental confusion, seizures, respiratory depression, and shock. MAOIs may cause very serious reactions if taken with certain foods or beverages. Patients must not eat foods such as chicken livers, cheese, yogurt, sour cream, bananas, raisins, and avocados and must also avoid drinking wine, because if they consume foods rich in tyramine (which is also found in wine), certain biogenic amines may be released in the body. When the breakdown of these substances is inhibited by MAOIs, the patient's blood pressure may rise rapidly to extremely high levels as these pressor substances accumulate in the body.

TABLE 23-5.   Drugs Used to Treat Depression

GENERIC NAME	TRADE NAME	ROUTE OF ADMINISTRATION	COMMON DOSAGE RANGE
Tricyclic Antidepressants			
Clomipramine	Anafranil®	Oral	25–250 mg/day
Desipramine	Norpramin®	Oral	25–300 mg/day
Nortriptyline	Aventyl®, Pamelor®	Oral	25-50 mg/day
Amitriptyline	Elavil®, Endep®	Oral	50–300 mg/day
Doxepin	Sinequan®, Adapin®	Oral	75–300 mg/day
Imipramine	Tofranil®	Oral	1–300 mg/day
Second-generation Cyclic Antidepressants			
Bupropion	Wellbutrin®, Zyban®	Oral	100–450 mg/day
Mirtazapine	Remeron®	Oral	15–45 mg/day
Nefazodone	Serzone®	Oral	100–600 mg/day
Trazodone	Desyrel®	Oral	50–600 mg/day
Venlafaxine	Effexor®	Oral	75–225 mg/day
Monoamine Oxidase Inhibitors			
Phenylzine	Nardil®	Oral	15–90 mg/day
Selective Serotonin Reuptake Inhibitors			
Fluoxetine	Prozac®	Oral	20–60 mg/day
Citalopram	Celexa®	Oral	20–40 mg/day
Fluvoxamine	Luvox®	Oral	25–300 mg/day
Paroxetine	Paxil®	Oral	10–75 mg/day
Sertraline	Zoloft®	Oral	25–200 mg/day
Medications for Bipolar Disorder			
Lithium carbonate	Eskalith®, Lithobid®	Oral	300–900 mg/day
Lithium citrate	Cibalith-S® (syrup)	Oral	300–900 mg/day
Carbamazepine	Tegretol®	Oral	100–1600 mg/day
Valproic acid	Depakene®	Oral	5–1000 mg/day
Valproate	Depakote®	Oral	5–1000 mg/day

Adverse effects of TCAs include delirium, confusion, manic reactions, sedation, weight gain, dry mouth, blurred vision, constipation, and difficulty in urination.

Adverse effects of SSRIs include sexual dysfunction, nausea, headaches, nervousness, insomnia, and anxiety.

Drug Interactions

TCAs may have drug interactions with alcohol, amphetamines, anticholinergics, antihistamines, barbiturates, phenothiazines, and antidysrhythmics. Cyclic antidepressants can have drug interactions with anticholinergics, guanethidine, and phenothiazines. SSRI drugs may be effective with and have drug interactions with alcohol, digitalis, anticholinergics, MAOIs, phenytoin, and cimetidine.

Bipolar Disorder and Lithium Therapy

Antipsychotic drugs are used primarily in the treatment of schizophrenia, organic psychoses, and the manic phase of bipolar affective disorders. These drugs appear to act by re-

ducing excessive dopamine activity through blocking of postsynaptic dopamine receptors in the brain (see Figure 23-4). In so doing, they appear to inhibit or alter the dopamine-mediated response in the brain.

Lithium is the primary drug used to treat patients in manic states. It is the drug of choice for the treatment of manic episodes such as those seen in bipolar disorder. Mania that is at some time severe enough to produce compromised functioning is necessary for diagnosis of bipolar disorder. This is a genetic disorder. The manic episode typically develops over days and may become uncontrolled and psychotic. The patient with bipolar disorder is depressed, with the depression usually being profound, but the disorder may present as a mild depressive syndrome. Attacks are usually separated by months or years, but they occasionally may cycle from one to the other over days or weeks. Bipolar disorder is a recurrent illness. A single attack is rare. The first manic episode often occurs before age 30, begins quickly, and resolves in 2 to 4 months if untreated. Suicide is the major risk during periods of depression. Drug therapy for bipolar disorder begins with lithium carbonate.

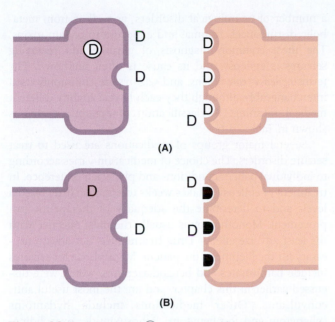

Figure 23-4. A. Dopamine Ⓓ normally combines with postsynaptic dopamine receptors in the central nervous system. B. Antipsychotic drugs ▶ appear to act by blocking postsynaptic dopamine receptors.

Mechanism of Action

The exact mechanism of action of lithium is unknown. It alters sodium transport in nerve and muscle cells. Lithium inhibits release of norepinephrine and dopamine but not serotonin from stimulated neurons.

Therapeutic Uses

Lithium is specifically used for patients with manic depressive psychosis who are in an acute manic phase. It can sometimes be useful for reducing excitement in patients suffering from schizophrenia. The therapeutic effect is seen in 2 to 3 weeks. Lithium normalizes mood in 80% of patients. It has no sedative, depressant, or euphoric actions, making it unique from all other psychiatric drugs.

Adverse Effects

Adverse effects of lithium therapy include diarrhea, tremor, anorexia, polydipsia, vomiting, polyuria, albuminuria, blurred vision, hyperglycemia, hypothyroidism, and weight gain. Overdose may produce diarrhea, vomiting, muscle weakness, drowsiness, and ataxia.

Drug Interactions

Lithium increases the risk of toxicity with thiazides diuretics because of decreased renal clearance of this agent. Drug interaction with indomethacin and some other nonsteroidal anti-inflammatory drugs (NSAIDs) (piroxicam and ibuprofen), as well as fluoxetine and methyldopa, may increase plasma lithium levels.

Alzheimer's Medication

Alzheimer's disease is a devastating illness characterized by progressive memory failure, impaired thinking, confusion, disorientation, personality changes, restlessness, speech disturbances, and the inability to perform routine tasks. Unfortunately, the disease is incurable and newly affects about one quarter million individuals per year in the United States. The current pharmacotherapy is focused on improving cognitive functioning or limiting disease progression and controlling symptoms. In Alzheimer's disease, the amount of ACh is decreased (this chemical substance is necessary for neurotransmission and for forming memories). There is no specific test for this disease; therefore, a definitive diagnosis is possible only upon autopsy. Tacrine (Cognex®) and donepezil (Aricept®) are the medications that have been approved by the Food and Drug Administration to improve memory deficits.

Mechanism of Action

Tacrine and donepezil are centrally acting reversible cholinesterase inhibitors, leading to elevated ACh levels in the brain. This action slows the neuronal degradation that occurs in Alzheimer's disease.

Therapeutic Uses

Tacrine and donepezil are used in the treatment of mild-to-moderate dementia of the Alzheimer's type.

Adverse Effects

There is significant risk of liver damage from the use of tacrine, but the benefits are worth the risk because of the devastation caused by Alzheimer's disease. Other adverse effects include nausea and vomiting, diarrhea, dyspepsia, myalgia, headache, and ataxia.

The common adverse effects of donepezil are nausea and diarrhea. Unlike tacrine, donepezil does not damage the liver.

Drug Interactions

Donepezil and tacrine increase the effects of and risk of toxicity with theophylline and cholinesterase inhibitors. They decrease the effects of anticholinergics and increase the risk of gastrointestinal bleeding with NSAIDs.

Antiepileptic Drugs

Epilepsy is a group of disorders that are characterized by hyperexcitability within the CNS. The abnormal stimuli can produce many symptoms from short periods of unconsciousness to violent convulsions. Approximately 2.5 million Americans have epilepsy, and approximately one half are seizure-free with medication. **Seizure** is a term for all epileptic events, whereas **convulsion** refers to abnormal motor movements, such as the jerking movements of grand mal attacks. Antiepileptic drugs prevent or stop a convulsive seizure. Seizures are characterized by an excessive discharge of cortical neuron activity, which can be measured by an electroencephalogram (EEG). Seizures are usually brief, with a beginning and an end. They may produce post-seizure impairment. Seizures may result acutely from any of a number of neurological disorders, as well as from metabolic disturbances, trauma, and exposure to certain toxins. The most common diagnosis of chronic and recurring seizures is epilepsy, and its cause is often unknown. The terms *epilepsy*, *convulsions*, and *seizures* are commonly used interchangeably, although they each have a slightly different medical meaning. A classification of epileptic events is shown in Table 23-6.

Several major groups of medications are used to treat seizure disorders. The choice of medication varies according to individual patient conditions and physician preference. In treatment of epilepsy, it takes weeks to establish drug plasma levels and to determine the adequacy of therapeutic improvement. Monotherapy is usually the most effective with the least adverse effects. Drug treatment is not always necessary for the lifetime of the patient. Medications for seizures include barbiturates and benzodiazepines, which were discussed earlier in this chapter, and are the most useful anticonvulsants. Other medications include hydantoins (phenytoin and fosphenytoin), ethosuximide, oxazolidinediones, and fosphenytoin (see Table 23-7).

TABLE 23-6. Classification of Epileptic Events

I. FOCAL OR PARTIAL SEIZURES	II. GENERALIZED SEIZURES
A. Simple seizures	A. Nonconvulsive
	1. Absence or petit mal seizures
B. Complex partial seizures	B. Convulsive
	1. Tonic/clonic or grand mal seizures
	2. Tonic/psychomotor seizures
	3. Status epilepticus

TABLE 23-7. Drug Treatment for Epileptic Events

GENERIC NAME	TRADE NAME	ROUTE OF ADMINISTRATION	COMMON DOSAGE RANGE
Barbiturates			
Phenobarbital	Bellatal®, Solfoton®	Oral, IM, IV, SC	30–320 mg/day
Mephobarbital	Mebaral®	Oral	16–60 mg/day
Benzodiazepines			
Diazepam	Diastat®, Diazepam®, Intensol®, Valium®	Oral, IM, IV, rectal	1–30 mg/day
Clonazepam	Klonopin®	Oral	0.25–20 mg/day
Hydantoins			
Phenytoin	Dilantin®	Oral	10 mg–1 g/day
Fosphenytoin	Cerebyx®	IM, IV	10–150 mg/day
Lamotrigine	Lamictal®	Oral	20–700 mg/day
Oxazolidinediones			
Paramethadione	Paradione®	Oral	300–2400 mg/day
Trimethadione	Tridione®	Oral	300–2400 mg/day
Succinimides			
Ethosuximide	Zarontin®	Oral	250 mg–1.5 g/day
Phensuximide	Milontin®	Oral	100–1200 mg/day
Methsuximide	Celontin®	Oral	150 mg–1.2 g/day
Miscellaneous Antiseizure Agents			
Carbamazepine	Tegretol®	Oral	100–1600 mg/day
Valproic acid	Depakene®	Oral	250–1000 mg/day
Valproate	Depakote®	Oral	250–1000 mg/day
Primidone	Mysoline®	Oral	50–500 mg/day
Gabapentin	Neurontin®	Oral	300–3600 mg/day
Tiagabine	Gabitril Filmtabs®	Oral	4–56 mg/day
Topiramate	Topamax®	Oral	25–400 mg/day

IM, intramuscular; IV, intravenous; SC, subcutaneous.

Hydantoins

The most recognizable and used drug in the hydantoin class is phenytoin. Phenytoin is a potent broad-spectrum anti-seizure medication. The newest addition to hydantoin medications is fosphenytoin, which is used parenterally for status epilepticus, and when substitution for oral antiseizure medications is necessary, such as after surgery.

Mechanism of Action   Phenytoin has antiepileptic activity without causing general CNS depression or sedation.

Therapeutic Uses   Phenytoin is used for partial and grand mal (tonic/clonic) seizures.

Adverse Effects   Adverse effects of phenytoin are related to plasma concentrations and include ataxia, mental confusion, dizziness, insomnia, gingival hyperplasia, toxic hepatitis, and pancytopenia (reduction of the blood cells).

Drug Interactions   Phenytoin increases pharmacologic effects with chloramphenicol, cimetidine, isoniazid, and sulfonamides. Complex drug interactions and effects occur when phenytoin and valproic acid are given together. Severe hypotension may occur when phenytoin is given intravenously with dopamine.

Ethosuximide

Ethosuximide is generally considered to be the safest of the succinimide drugs. It is used in the treatment of absence seizures.

Mechanism of Actions   Ethosuximide suppresses the EEG pattern associated with lapses of consciousness in absence (petit mal) seizures. Its mechanism of action is not understood, but it may act to inhibit neuronal systems.

Therapeutic Uses   Ethosuximide is used to control petit mal seizures. It may be given in combination with other anticonvulsants.

Adverse Effects   Adverse effects include ataxia, dizziness, nervousness, headache, and blurred vision. Ethosuximide can also cause pancytopenia, vaginal bleeding, muscle weakness, and abnormal liver and kidney function test results.

Drug Interactions   Ethosuximide decreases serum levels of primidone.

Antiparkinsonian Drugs

Parkinson's disease is characterized by resting tremor, rigidity or resistance to passive movement, akinesia, and loss of postural reflexes. Occasionally behavioral manifestations occur. Parkinson's disease is caused by the progressive degeneration of dopamine neurons in the brain that leads to an imbalance in the activity of dopamine and ACh in the brain (basal ganglia). Parkinsonism may also be drug induced. Because it is not possible to reverse the process, drugs are used to correct the imbalance of dopamine and ACh activity in the basal ganglia.

Table 23-8 shows some drugs for Parkinson's disease.

Mechanism of Action

Levodopa is an antiparkinsonism and anticholinergic agent. It is a metabolic precursor of dopamine, a catecholamine neurotransmitter. Unlike dopamine, levodopa readily crosses the blood-brain barrier. The precise mechanism of action is unknown.

Carbidopa is an antiparkinsonism and anticholinergic agent. When levodopa is given alone, large doses must be administered. Carbidopa prevents peripheral metabolism (decarboxylation) of levodopa and thereby makes more levodopa available for transport to the brain. Carbidopa does not cross the blood-brain barrier and, therefore, does not affect metabolism of levodopa within the brain.

Amantadine is an antiviral, anticholinergic, and antiparkinsonism agent. Its mechanism of action in parkinsonism is not understood, but it may be related to the release of dopamine and other catecholamines from neuronal storage sites.

TABLE 23-8.   Antiparkinsonism Drugs

GENERIC NAME	TRADE NAME	ROUTE OF ADMINISTRATION	COMMON DOSAGE RANGE
Levodopa	Dopar®, Larodopa®	Oral	0.5–0.8 g/day
Carbidopa	Sinemet®	Oral	10–250 mg/day
Amantadine	Symmetrel®	Oral	100–400 mg/day
Bromocriptine	Parlodel®	Oral	1.25–100 mg/day
Benztropine	Apo-Benztropine®, Cogentin®	Oral, IV	0.5–60 mg/day
Trihexyphenidyl	Trihexy®	Oral	1–15 mg/day
Ropinirole	Requip®	Oral	0.25–3 mg/day
Pramipexole	Mirapex®	Oral	0.125–1.5 mg/day
Entacapone	Comtan®	Oral	200–1600 mg/day

IV, intravenous.

Bromocriptine is an autonomic nervous system and antiparkinsonism agent. It is a semisynthetic ergot alkaloid derivative. Bromocriptine activates the dopaminergic receptors of the CNS, which may explain its action in parkinsonism.

Therapeutic Uses

Levodopa is prescribed for idiopathic Parkinson's disease and postencephalitic and arteriosclerotic parkinsonism. It is contraindicated in patients with known hypersensitivity to levodopa, narrow angle glaucoma, acute psychoses, and severe psychoneurosis.

Carbidopa is effective in the management of symptoms of Parkinson's disease and parkinsonism of secondary origin and improves life expectancy. Cabidopa used in combination with levodopa reduces the required levodopa dose to one fourth of what it would be without carbidopa.

Bromocriptine is used as an adjunct to levodopa or levodopa/carbidopa therapy to relieve symptoms of Parkinson's disease. Bromocriptine is contraindicated in patients who are hypersensitive to ergot alkaloids, or who have uncontrolled hypertension or a pituitary tumor or in women who are lactating.

Adverse Effects

Adverse effects of levodopa include increased hand tremor, grinding of teeth (bruxism), ataxia, numbness, fatigue, headache, and euphoria. Levodopa may also cause orthosta-tic hypotension, tachycardia, hypertension, nausea, vomiting, dry mouth, bitter taste, and hepatotoxicity.

Contraindications and adverse effects of carbidopa are similar to those of levodopa.

Adverse effects of bromocriptine include headache, dizziness, vertigo, fainting, sedation, nightmares, and insomnia. It may also produce blurred vision, hypertension, palpitation, arrhythmias, nausea, vomiting, and diarrhea.

Drug Interactions

Levodopa increases therapeutic effects and the possibility of a hypertensive crisis with MAOIs. Withdrawal of MAOIs is necessary at least 14 days before levodopa therapy is started. Levodopa exhibits decreased efficacy with pyridoxine (vitamin B6) and phenytoin.

Narcotic Analgesics

Opioids is the generic term for drugs with morphine-like activity that reduce pain and induce tolerance and physical dependence. They are also referred to as *narcotic analgesics*. *Opiates* is the generic term for drugs made from opium such as morphine and heroin, a powdered, dried exudate of the fruit capsule (poppy) of the plant *Papaver somniferum*. Opium alkaloids (e.g., thebaine) are used to make semisynthetic opioids.

Some opioids such as meperidine and methadone are prepared synthetically. Table 23-9 shows the most common narcotic analgesics.

TABLE 23-9. Narcotic Analgesics

GENERIC NAME	TRADE NAME	ROUTE OF ADMINISTRATION	COMMON DOSAGE RANGE
Fentanyl	Duragesic®	Transdermal patch	1 patch/3 days
Hydromorphone	Dilaudid®	Oral, SC, IM, IV, rectal	2–24 mg/day
Hydrocodone	Lortab®	Oral	5–40 mg/day
Loperamide	Imodium®	Oral	2–16 mg/day
Meperidine	Demerol®	Oral, SC, IM	50–1200 mg/day
Methadone	Dolophine®	Oral, SC, IM	20–80 mg/day
Morphine sulfate	Astramorph/PF®, Avinza®, Duramorph®, Infumorph 200®, Infumorph 500®, Kadian®, Morphine Sulfate®, MS Contin®, MS/L® (and concentrate), Oramorph SR®, Roxanol® (and SR), Morrhuate Sodium®, Scleromate®, Statex®	Oral, SC, IM, IV	2.5–180 mg/day
Camphorated opium tincture (paregoric)		Oral	5–40 mL/day
Pentazocine	Talwin®, Talacen®	Oral, SC, IM, IV	20–600 mg/day
Propoxyphene	Darvon®		65–600 mg/day
Codeine	Codeine®		10–240 mg/day
Oxycodone	OxyContin®		1.25–40 mg/day

IM, intramuscular; IV, intravenous; SC, subcutaneous.

Mechanism of Action

Narcotic analgesics are thought to change pain perception in the spinal cord, brain stem, thalamus, and limbic system. Opiate receptors in each of these areas interact with neurotransmitters of the autonomic nervous system, producing alterations in reaction to painful stimuli. The narcotic drugs relieve pain and produce sedation, euphoria, mental clouding, respiratory depression, meiosis, and constipation. They also cause depression of the cough reflex and orthostatic hypotension.

Therapeutic Uses

Narcotic analgesics are used to treat moderate-to-severe acute pain. They are prescribed for acute pain of coronary, pulmonary, hepatic, or renal vascular origin. Narcotic analgesics are also used as preoperative medications and for severe diarrhea, persistent cough (codeine), pulmonary edema, and postsurgical trauma.

Adverse Effects

Adverse reactions to narcotic analgesics include hypotension, bradycardia, anorexia, constipation, dry mouth, euphoria, vomiting, itching, syncope, and shortness of breath. Overdosage may cause respiratory depression, deep sleep, coma, meiosis, cyanosis, hypotension, oliguria, and hypothermia.

Drug Interactions

Narcotic drugs increase the likelihood of respiratory depression, hypotension, profound sedation, or coma in patients receiving barbiturate general anesthetics.

Migraine Headache Medications

Migraine headaches are characterized by unilateral throbbing or nonthrobbing pain often accompanied by nausea, vomiting, and sensitivity to noise and light. Some migraines have an **aura** (formerly known as classic migraines) and some have no aura (common migraines). The migraine without an aura is the most common type. Because migraine attacks are worst in women during menstruation and migraines seem to cease with menopause, hormones may be a component of the attacks. Some medical professionals feel that migraine headaches are vascular in origin. Ongoing migraines are treated with NSAIDs, opioid analgesics, ergot alkaloids, and sumatriptan (see Chapter 27). Drugs used for prophylaxis are β-blockers, amitriptyline, calcium channel blockers, methysergide (Sansert®), and valproic acid (see Chapter 24). Rest in a quiet, dark atmosphere is often indicated as prophylaxis early during the headache. Aspirin, acetaminophen, ibuprofen, and other aspirin-like NSAIDs can relieve mild-to-moderate migraine headaches. These drugs may be combined with metoclopramide (Reglan®) for

the enhancement of absorption of aspirin. Fiorinal is an aspirin-containing medication with an added barbiturate sedative and caffeine.

Anesthetics

Anesthesia, literally, is the unique condition of reversible unconsciousness or a loss of sensation. This condition is produced by certain chemical substances that have been called anesthetics. Anesthesia is characterized basically by four reversible actions: unconsciousness, analgesia, immobility, and amnesia. The critical factor is that there should be no significant impairment of cardiovascular or respiratory functions, especially those supplying the brain and other vital organs with adequate blood, nutrients, and gases.

Anesthetics are agents that act generally on nervous tissue. Local anesthetics act to produce a loss of sensation from a local area of the body by depressing the excitability of excitable tissues. The objective of local anesthesia is to decrease pain. A primary site of action of local anesthetics is the nerve membrane. Local anesthetics are either esters or amides that can induce neuromuscular block. They produce a transient and reversible loss of sensation (analgesia) in a circumscribed region of the body without loss of consciousness. Local anesthetics may be administered topically, by infiltration into tissues, by injection directly around nerves, and by injection into epidural or subarachnoid spaces. At therapeutic doses all local anesthetics except cocaine are vasodilators. Examples of local anesthetics are shown in Table 23-10.

General anesthetics produce a state affecting overall body function, but in anesthetic concentrations they do not produce detectable generalized effects on all nerves or all nerve cell membranes. General anesthesia produces several stages and planes. Most of the major anesthetic agents in current use are seen in Table 23-11.

Stages and Planes of Anesthesia

The use of stages and planes of anesthesia helps to describe the levels and progression of anesthesia produced by anesthetics. There are four stages of anesthesia:

Stage I—Analgesia that begins when the agent is administered and lasts until loss of consciousness.

TABLE 23-10. Examples of Local Anesthetics	
AMIDES	**ESTERS**
Lidocaine (Xylocaine®)	Procaine (Novocaine®)
Mepivacaine (Carbocaine®)	Chloroprocaine (Nesacaine®)
Prilocaine (Citanest®)	Cocaine
Bupivacaine (Marcaine®)	Tetracaine (Pontocaine®)
Etidocaine (Duranest®)	Dibucaine (Nupercaine®)
	Benzocaine (Americaine®)

TABLE 23-11. General Anesthetics Currently in Use	
ADMINISTERED BY INHALATION	**ADMINISTERED INTRAVENOUSLY**
Nitrous oxide	**Barbiturates**
Halothane (Fluothane®)	Thiopental (Pentothal®)
Enflurane (Ethrane®)	Methohexital (Brevital®)
Isoflurane (Forane®)	**Benzodiazepines**
	Diazepam (Valium®)
	Midazolam (Versed®)
	Propofol (Diprivan®)
	Ketamine (Ketalar®)

Stage I is characterized by analgesia, euphoria, perceptual distortions, and amnesia.

Stage II—Delirium begins with loss of consciousness and extends to the beginning of surgical anesthesia. There may be excitement and involuntary muscular activity. The skeletal muscle tone increases and breathing is irregular. At this stage hypertension and tachycardia may occur.

Stage III—Surgical anesthesia lasts until spontaneous respiration ceases. It is further divided into four planes based on respiration, size of the pupils, reflex characteristics, and eyeball movements.

Stage IV—Medullary depression begins with cessation of respiration and ends with circulatory collapse. The pupils are fixed and dilated. There are no lid or corneal reflexes.

The most common route of administration for general anesthesia is inhalation, although some general anesthetics are given intravenously. The major intravenous drugs are used as an aid for induction of the anesthesia or as a preoperative medication.

DRUGS OF ABUSE

Drug addiction is a chronic, relapsing disorder characterized by the compulsion to take a drug and loss of self-control in limiting drug intake. Most drugs of abuse act on the CNS to modify the user's mental state. Chronic use leads to psychological or physical dependence or both. This may result in the development of tolerance. Complications related to drug administration by the parenteral route under unsterile conditions or to the coadministration of adulterants are extremely common. These complications include the transmission of viral hepatitis, acquired immunodeficiency syndrome (AIDS), and various bacteria and fungi, as well as the development of cellulitis, thrombophlebitis, and local or systemic abscesses. The following terms are commonly used when one refers to drugs of abuse:

- **Drug abuse**: The nonmedical use of a drug that is deemed unacceptable by society.
- **Tolerance**: A reduced drug effect with repeated use of a drug and a need for higher doses to produce the same effect.
- **Cross-tolerance**: Tolerance to one drug conferring tolerance to other drugs in the same drug class.
- **Dependence**: The psychological, physiological, or biochemical need to continue to take a drug.
- **Psychological dependence**: The overwhelming need to take a drug to maintain a sense of well-being.
- **Physical dependence**: The necessity to continue drug use to avoid a withdrawal syndrome.
- **Cross-dependence**: The ability of one drug to substitute for another drug in the same drug class to maintain a dependent state or prevent withdrawal.

Drugs of abuse may affect the CNS in several different ways. Some commonly abused categories of drugs are CNS depressants, CNS stimulants, and psychodysleptics (hallucinogens).

CNS Depressants

Drugs that are able to depress the CNS are often abused. These drugs include benzodiazepines, barbiturates, and ethanol and were discussed earlier in this chapter.

Alcoholism

Tolerance to the intoxicating and euphoric effects of ethanol develops with chronic use, which is called *alcoholism*. Alcohol-related problems are common in males and peak in the 18- to 29-year-old age group, although they continue at a significant rate through middle age. Alcoholism is a maladaptive pattern of alcohol use leading to clinically significant impairment or distress, as manifested by three or more of the following occurring at any time in the same 12-month period:

1. Persistent desire or one or more unsuccessful efforts to cut down or control drinking.
2. Characteristic withdrawal syndrome for alcohol.
3. Need for a markedly increased amount of alcohol to achieve intoxication.
4. Drinking in larger amounts.
5. Important social or occupational activities given up or reduced because of drinking.

For patients who drink more than the recommended amount, the medical history should be reviewed for evidence of alcohol-related problems, including hypertension, depression, and sleep disorders. Discontinuing alcohol consumption after chronic use results in a withdrawal syndrome, indicating the development of physical dependence. Symptoms occurring over 1 to 2 days include anxiety, hyperexcitability, weakness, intestinal cramps, confusion, visual hallucinations, delirium, and convulsions. The withdrawal syndrome can be life-threatening in debilitated individuals.

CNS Stimulants

Amphetamines, cocaine, and nicotine are drugs that stimulate the CNS.

Amphetamines are called "ice," "speed," "glass," or "crystal" and have both legal and illegal uses. Legally prescribed, amphetamines are classified as Schedule II drugs and are used to treat chronic fatigue syndrome, obesity, narcolepsy, attention deficit disorder, and mental depression and to combat the side effects of narcotics in the terminally ill patient. When used illegally, they increase physical performance and psychological stimuli. Severe and life-threatening toxicity may present as hypertension, cardiac arrhythmia, ischemic stroke, convulsion, or coma.

Cocaine is a stimulant and local anesthetic with potent vasoconstrictor (contraction of blood vessel) properties. The drug produces physiological and behavioral effects when administered orally, intranasally (snorting), or intravenously or via inhalation after smoking. Cocaine abuse occurs in virtually all social and economic strata of society.

Cocaine produces a brief, dose-related stimulation, enhancement of mood, and increases in cardiac rate and blood pressure. Chronic cocaine use causes significant loss of libido and adversely affects reproductive function. Cocaine abuse by pregnant women, particularly with the smoking of "crack" (a purer form), has been associated with both an increased risk of congenital malformations in the fetus and perinatal cardiovascular and cerebrovascular disease in the mother.

Nicotine is a constituent of tobacco, along with various gases, and particulate matter. It causes CNS stimulation and sedation. Nicotine may stimulate or inhibit heart rate and blood pressure. It is able to relax skeletal muscle and increase muscle tone. Nicotine increases secretion of the gastrointestinal tract. It is rapidly metabolized in the liver and is eliminated by the kidneys. It is also excreted into breast milk.

Mechanism of Action

There is neither specific evidence that clearly establishes the mechanism whereby amphetamines produce mental and behavioral effects in children nor conclusive evidence for how these effects relate to the condition of the CNS. Their effects are mediated by release of norepinephrine from sympathetic neurons.

Cocaine blocks the initiation or conduction of the nerve impulse and causes intense vasoconstriction. Its most striking systemic effect is general CNS stimulation.

Nicotine produces complex and unpredictable pharmacological effects on the body. It stimulates the CNS and acts on the cardiovascular and other systems.

Therapeutic Uses

Amphetamine and also methamphetamine, ephedrine, and mephentermine at low oral doses are able to increase wakefulness, alertness, self-confidence, and the ability to concentrate. They also decrease appetite. Intravenous administration results in intense euphoria and a feeling of mental alertness.

Cocaine is used therapeutically for local anesthetic and vasoconstrictor activity for surgery involving mucous membranes.

Nicotine is the principal constituent of tobacco that is responsible for its addictive character. Addicted smokers regulate their nicotine intake and blood levels by adjusting the frequency and intensity of their tobacco use both to obtain the desired psychoactive effects and to avoid withdrawal. Cigarette smoke contains more than 4000 chemical compounds, including at least 43 carcinogens. Nicotine is readily absorbed in the lungs from inhaled smoke. Nicotine from smokeless tobacco products, such as chewing tobacco and snuff, is absorbed across the oral or nasal mucosa, respectively.

Cancers associated with cigarette smoking include leukemia and cancers of the mouth, pharynx, larynx, esophagus, pancreas, cervix, kidney, and bladder. Smoking also increases the risk of heart disease, lung disease, and stroke.

Adverse Effects

Adverse effects of amphetamine use usually occur after repeated intravenous administration or after overdosage and include anxiety, inability to sleep, hyperactivity, and sometimes dangerous behavior. Overdosage results in tachycardia, hypertension, hyperthermia, and tremor.

The use of cocaine is associated with atypical tolerance and withdrawal phenomena (like those for amphetamine). High-level use of this substance is characterized by episodes of repetitive self-administration that may last many hours or days, during which time the user remains continually awake, and typically continue until supplies are exhausted. Use of cocaine as "crack," by smoking, or by intravenous administration greatly increases the danger of overdosage and death. Adverse effects of cocaine use are similar to those with amphetamine, but overdosage is more often fatal because of respiratory depression, seizures, and cardiac arrest. It also may cause cerebrovascular accidents, increased occurrence of spontaneous abortions, sexual dysfunction, and toxic psychosis.

Adverse effects related to nicotine use include possible development of lung, oral cavity, bladder, and pancreatic cancer. Nicotine may cause obstructive lung disease, coronary artery disease, acceleration of atherosclerosis, and abortion. Nicotine causes strong psychological dependence. A withdrawal-like syndrome occurs within 24 hours and persists for weeks or months. The symptoms include dizziness, tremor, hypertension, irritability, anxiety, restlessness, difficulty in concentration, drowsiness, headache, increased appetite, nausea, and vomiting.

Drug Interactions

Nicotine may increase the effects of acetaminophen, β-blockers, caffeine, imipramine, labetalol, oxazepam, pentazocine, prazosin, and theophylline. It causes increased bronchodilator effects as well and may cause insulin dosages to require adjustment. Nicotine decreases the effect of isoproterenol and phenylephrine.

Psychodysleptics or Hallucinogens

People who are hallucinating have a false sensory perception that occurs in the absence of a relevant sense of reality. People may be able to identify what is in fact not a real occurrence. The classic examples of true hallucinogens are lysergic acid diethylamide (LSD) and phencyclidine (PCP).

Mechanism of Action

LSD is an extremely potent synthetic drug that, taken orally, causes altered consciousness, euphoria, and increased sensory awareness ("mind expansion").

PCP can be taken orally, intranasally, or intravenously. It also can be snorted or smoked. PCP produces euphoria, hallucinations, changed body image, and increased sense of isolation and loneliness. It impairs judgment and increases aggressiveness. Behavioral actions are thought to be related to increased activity of dopamine. The effects of PCP make it one of the most dangerous and most unpredictable of the abused substances available on the street.

Marijuana is classified as a CNS depressant that can cause euphoria, sedation, and hallucinations. No other drug produces all three of these responses, placing marijuana in a class by itself. Street names for marijuana are "pot," "grass," "weed," "Mary Jane," and "hemp." Marijuana cigarettes are known as "bowls," "stogies," "joints," or "reefers." When smoked, about 60% of marijuana is absorbed rapidly through the lungs. Tolerance occurs with marijuana and is rapidly reversed after cessation of its use. Abrupt cessation after prolonged use has been indicated in some psychological, rather than physical, dependence.

Therapeutic Uses

LSD is used only for research. No accepted medical use exists for LSD in the United States.

PCP was first studied for use as a general anesthetic for humans. Therapeutic human use was subsequently discontinued because of the high incidence of delirium. This agent is still used in veterinary practices. The use and cheapness of production of the agent by amateurs have led to wide abuse of this agent.

The active ingredient in marijuana, tetrahydrocannabinol (THC), is now being made available as a Schedule II drug for use in lessening the nausea resulting from cancer chemotherapy. It may also be used therapeutically to decrease intraocular pressure for treatment of glaucoma.

Adverse Effects

There is no physical dependence with LSD. Adverse effects include "flashback," panic reactions, misjudgment, suicide, and psychosis.

As the dosage of PCP increases, the unfavorable reactions include excitation, disorientation, anxiety, and disorganized thoughts. Bizarre behavior may occur with high doses, progressing to dysphoria, muscle rigidity, hypertensive crisis, coma, and death.

Adverse effects with chronic use of marijuana are similar to those for cigarette smoking. It impairs short-term memory and also disturbs the immune and reproductive systems.

Drug Interactions

There are no known drug interactions with LSD.

PCP use may cause drug interactions with other CNS depressants, such as alcohol and benzodiazepines, which can lead to accidental overdosage and coma.

Use of marijuana with protease inhibitors may increase THC levels, causing smaller doses of marijuana to have a greater effect. This interaction is not dangerous because overdosage of THC is impossible.

■ SUMMARY

The nervous system is composed of two divisions: the central nervous system (the brain and spinal cord) and the peripheral nervous system (nerves).

Benzodiazepines are commonly used to treat anxiety and insomnia. These agents, because of their greater effectiveness and safety, have replaced many of the sedatives of the barbiturate family that were used in the past.

The two main categories of mental illness are neurosis and psychosis, both of which produce symptoms such as hyperactivity, agitation, and inappropriate behavior. Neurosis produces fear or anxiety from either real or unknown dangers. Anxiolytics may be used to treat prolonged anxiety, but these medications may also be used as hypnotics/sedatives, as muscle relaxants, for convulsions as adjuvant medications, and with treatment for withdrawal from alcohol abuse.

Antipsychotic agents are used to suppress the symptoms of schizophrenia and other psychotic conditions. All of these drugs act on dopamine in the brain.

Alzheimer's disease is a progressive illness that causes a decline in intellectual functions. A few medications have been approved for use with this condition.

Seizures are symptoms of a discharge of disorganized electric impulses in the brain. Several drug groups are used to treat seizures. They include barbiturates, hydantoins, succinimides, benzodiazepines, and other miscellaneous medications.

With parkinsonism, the idea is to correct the imbalance of dopamine and acetylcholine found with the disease. Drugs such as anticholinergics and antihistamines are used for their central effects.

Narcotic analgesics are used to treat moderate to severe pain. If opioids or potent analgesics are used for prolonged periods, abuse, misuse, and tolerance are possible.

Anesthetics are used to interfere with conduction of nerve impulses to the CNS. General anesthesia is used in surgical procedures; anesthetic agents may be given intravenously or by inhalation. Local anesthesia is used to render a part of the body insensitive to pain. Additives, such as epinephrine, are included with local anesthetic agents to prolong their effects and to reduce bleeding by vasoconstriction.

Drug abuse is use of a drug in a way that is inconsistent with medical, social, and cultural norms of a certain population. Physical and psychological dependence occur with the chronic misuse or abuse of drugs. Dependence and tolerance lead to the need for greater doses of drugs, such as alcohol and street drugs.

CRITICAL THINKING

1. Why are substances classified as nervous system agents often abused? What can be done to prevent abuse of these agents?
2. What research is being done on new treatments and drug therapies for Alzheimer's disease, Parkinson's disease, and seizure disorders? What are the goals in research and new treatment plans?
3. Choose one of the psychiatric disorders discussed in this chapter. What are some other goals of treatment? What are three advantages and disadvantages of treatment? What risks are involved in treatment?

REVIEW QUESTIONS

1. The rigidity of the parkinsonian syndrome may be reduced by
   A. bromocriptine.
   B. amantadine.
   C. benztropine.
   D. all of the above.

2. Morphine
   A. relieves asthma attack.
   B. relieves dyspnea accompanying pulmonary edema.
   C. increases sensitivity of respiratory center to CO_2.
   D. does all of the above.

3. Orthostatic hypotension is an occasional side-effect of
   A. phenytoin.
   B. trimethadione.
   C. morphine.
   D. lithium.

4. Which of the following is useful for treatment of tonic-clonic (grand mal) seizures?
   A. Phenytoin
   B. Lithium
   C. Haloperidol
   D. Morphine

5. Buspirone (BuSpar®) is used for
   A. general central nervous system depression.
   B. sedation.
   C. hypnosis.
   D. anxiety.

6. The generic name of Librium® is
   A. clorazepate.
   B. chlordiazepoxide.
   C. diazepam.
   D. lorazepam.

7. All of the following are adverse effects of benzodiazepines, except
   A. rebound insomnia.
   B. development of tolerance.
   C. vomiting.
   D. drowsiness.

8. The primary drug used to treat patients in manic states is
   A. valproic acid.
   B. phenytoin.
   C. Valium®.
   D. lithium.

9. Which of the following is the brand name of promethazine?
   A. Phenergan®
   B. Compazine®
   C. Valium®
   D. Dilantin®

10. All of the following are amides except
    A. Xylocaine®.
    B. Duranest®.
    C. Novocaine®.
    D. Carbocaine®.

11. Which of the following is the stage of surgical anesthesia?
    A. Stage I
    B. Stage IV
    C. Stage II
    D. Stage III

12. Which of the following agents is administered by inhalation for general anesthesia?
    A. Valium®
    B. Fluothane®
    C. Ketalar®
    D. Pentothal®

Continues

13. Which of the following types of seizures is called grand mal seizure?
    A. Tonic-clonic
    B. Absence
    C. Myoclonic
    D. Atonic

14. All of the following drugs are CNS stimulants, except
    A. nicotine.
    B. cocaine.
    C. ethyl alcohol.
    D. amphetamine.

15. Which of the following drugs of abuse is now being made available as a Schedule II drug?
    A. Cocaine
    B. Marijuana
    C. LSD
    D. PCP

Cardiovascular Drugs and Diuretics

24

OBJECTIVES

Upon completion of this chapter, the reader should be able to

1. Identify the various types of antiarrhythmics and their adverse effects.
2. Discuss the action of digitalis and its side effects.
3. Describe the classification of antihypertensives.
4. Identify different types of diuretics.
5. Discuss the angiotensin-converting enzyme (ACE).
6. Differentiate between heparin and coumarin.
7. Describe vasoconstrictors and their purpose.
8. Explain the different types of coronary vasodilators.
9. Describe combination drug therapy for hyperlipidemia.

GLOSSARY

angina pectoris An episodic, reversible oxygen insufficiency.
angiotensin II receptor antagonists Drugs that block the binding of angiotensin II to the angiotensin II type 1 receptor.
angiotensin-converting enzyme inhibitors Drugs that competitively inhibit conversion of angiotensin I to angiotensin II, a potent vasoconstrictor, through the angiotensin-converting enzyme activity, with resultant lower levels of angiotensin II.
anticoagulants Agents that prevent clot formation.
antiplatelet agents Drugs used to suppress aggregation (clumping) of platelets.
arrhythmias Deviations from the normal pattern of the heartbeat.

β-adrenergic blockers Drugs used to reverse sympathetic heart action caused by exercise, stress, or physical exertion.
calcium channel blockers Drugs used to treat stable angina.
diuretics Drugs that increase sodium excretion and lower blood volume.
hyperlipidemia An increase in triglycerides.
hypertension An abnormal increase in arterial blood pressure.
ischemic heart disease A condition in which there is an insufficient supply of oxygen to the myocardium (cardiac muscle).
myocardial infarction An area of dead cardiac muscle tissue, with or without hemorrhage.
nitrates Drugs used for the treatment of angina.

GLOSSARY continued

statins A class of drugs that inhibits the activity of an enzyme that forms cholesterol in the body. Statins are named as such because all of their generic names end with "-statin" (e.g., lovastatin).

sympatholytic drugs A group of drugs that blocks or inhibits the effects of epinephrine or norepinephrine on the cells that normally react to them.

vasoconstrictors Drugs used mostly to prolong the duration of action of local anesthetics or to help control bleeding.

vasodilators Drugs used to relax or dilate vessels throughout the body.

OVERVIEW

Cardiovascular disorders are among the most common causes of death in the United States. Angina pectoris, hypertension, myocardial infarction, and hyperlipidemia are some of the most prevalent causes of death related to the cardiovascular system. There are many factors that contribute to heart disease. Some are related to age, others are related to genetics, and still others are within the individual's control. Consuming a proper diet, exercising, avoiding cigarette smoking, and getting enough rest can do a lot to keep the heart functioning for a long time. Heart disease also may be caused by other conditions or disorders such as high blood pressure, high blood cholesterol levels, obesity, and diabetes. A pharmacy technician should be familiar with the most common disorders of the cardiovascular system and the most effective agents for each of them.

ANATOMY REVIEW: THE CARDIOVASCULAR SYSTEM

The cardiovascular system consists of the heart and blood vessels. The heart is a hollow muscular organ. The blood vessels include the arteries, capillaries, and veins. The heart's pumping forces blood through the arteries, which connect to the smaller-diameter vessels. The tiniest tubes, the capillaries, are the sites of nutrient, electrolyte, gas, and waste exchange. Capillaries converge into venules, which in turn converge into veins that return blood to the heart, completing the closed system of blood circulation. The cardiovascular system brings oxygen and nutrients to all body cells and removes wastes. A functional cardiovascular system is vital for survival because, without circulation, tissues lack a supply of oxygen and nutrients and wastes accumulate. Under such conditions, the cells soon begin irreversible change,

which quickly leads to death. Figure 24-1 shows the general pattern of blood transport in the cardiovascular system.

ISCHEMIC HEART DISEASE

Ischemic heart disease is a condition in which there is an insufficient supply of oxygen to the myocardium (cardiac muscle). Ischemic heart disease decreases blood flow to the myocardium, increases oxygen demand, and decreases oxygenation of the blood. Several factors may affect functions that control myocardial oxygen demand (see Table 24-1).

Angina Pectoris

Angina pectoris is an episodic, reversible oxygen insufficiency. This condition is the most common form of ischemic heart disease. The term *angina pectoris* is applied to various forms of transient chest pain that are attributable to insufficient myocardial oxygen. Atherosclerotic lesions that produce a narrowing of the coronary arteries are the major cause of angina. However, tachycardia (increased heart rate), anemia, hyperthyroidism, and hypotension can cause an oxygen imbalance. There are three types of angina: stable (classic), unstable, and decubitus (nocturnal). The most common form is classic angina, which may be caused by exertion, emotional stress, or a heavy meal. Classic angina is relieved by rest, nitroglycerin, or both. Unstable angina is a medical emergency, and the patient must be treated in a hospital. Nocturnal angina is caused by coronary artery spasms and can be treated by calcium channel blockers and nitrates.

Treatment goals for angina include the following:

- Reducing the risk of sudden death
- Preventing myocardial infarction

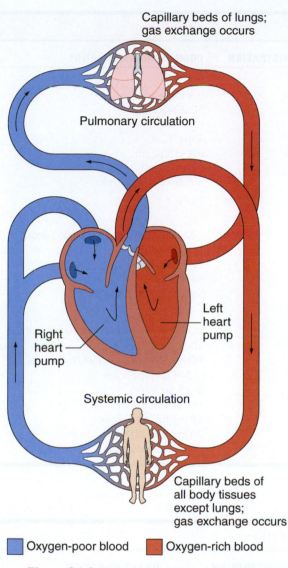

Capillary beds of lungs;
gas exchange occurs

Pulmonary circulation

Left heart pump

Right heart pump

Systemic circulation

Capillary beds of all body tissues except lungs; gas exchange occurs

■ Oxygen-poor blood ■ Oxygen-rich blood

Figure 24-1. Pulmonary and systemic circulation.

- Increasing myocardial oxygen supply
- Reducing the pain and anxiety associated with an angina attack

ANTIANGINAL DRUG THERAPY

There are three groups of medications that can help achieve the treatment goals for angina pectoris:

1. Nitrates
2. β-Adrenergic blockers
3. Calcium channel blockers

Commonly used antianginal drugs are listed in Table 24-2.

TABLE 24-1. Factors Affecting Cardiac Parameters That Control Myocardial Oxygen Demand		
FACTORS	**HEART RATE**	**BLOOD PRESSURE**
β-Blockers	Decrease	Decrease
Cold	Increase	Increase
Exercise	Increase	Increase
Nitroglycerin	Increase	Decrease
Smoking	Increase	Increase

Nitrates

Nitrates used for the treatment of angina have been available for many years and are still an important part of therapy. Table 24-3 shows nitrates commonly used in the treatment of angina.

Mechanism of Action

Nitrates primarily are effective in the venous circulation by relaxing vascular smooth muscle and reducing the work of the left ventricle. These agents are administered to dilate the blood vessels and stop attacks of angina (see Figure 24-2).

Therapeutic Uses

Nitrates are used as coronary vasodilators in the treatment of angina. The choice of nitrate preparations should be based on onset of action, duration of action, and patient compliance. Nitrate preparations are available in sublingual tablets, nitroglycerin spray bottles, topical nitroglycerin ointments, and transdermal patches. The sublingual route is the most common route of administration for nitroglycerin. This agent begins to work rapidly, and its effects last for about 1 hour. Nitroglycerin is an ideal preparation for acute anginal pain. Administration should begin as soon as the pain begins and should not be delayed until the pain is severe. If one tablet is not sufficient, one or two additional tablets should be taken at 5-minute intervals. For persistent pain, the patient should see a physician, because he or she may have signs of a myocardial infarction. The pharmacy technician should teach the patient that the sublingual tablet is to remain under the tongue until it dissolves. The shelf life of nitroglycerin is longer if it is in a dark, tightly closed container. After the container is opened, the drug is effective for approximately 6 months, and the date on which it was opened should be written on the container. Six months after the container is opened, the medication should be discarded and replaced with a new supply.

Transdermal patches contain a reservoir of nitroglycerin (Figure 24-3). The nitroglycerin is slowly released for absorption through the skin. The effects of the patches are slow in onset, and patches are not effective for an ongoing anginal attack.

Topical ointment can also be applied to the skin with an applicator and covered with plastic wrap held in place

TABLE 24-2.   Commonly Used Antianginal Drugs

GENERIC NAME	BRAND NAME	ROUTE OF ADMINISTRATION	COMMON DOSAGE RANGE
Nitrates			
Nitroglycerin	Nitrolingual®	Spray	0.4 mg/spray
	Nitrostat®	Oral	SL 0.3–0.6 mg
	Nitro-Bid®	Oral	
	Nitro-Bid", Nitrol®	Ointment	Topical 2%
	Nitro-Dur®, Nitrodisc®	Transdermal patch	0.1–0.8 mg/hr
	Nitrostat IV®, Tridil®	IV	0.5–5 mg/mL
Isosorbide dinitrate	Isordil®, Sorbitrate®	Oral	Solution: 25–200 mg
Isosorbide mononitrate	Imdur®	Oral	
β-Adrenergic Blockers			
Acebutolol	Sectral®	Oral	200–1200 mg/day in 2 divided doses
Atenolol	Tenormin®	Oral, IV	PO: 50 mg once/day; IV: 5 mg over 5 min
Metoprolol	Lopressor®, Toprol XL®	Oral, IV	PO: 100 mg/day then 100–450 mg/day
Nadolol	Corgard®	Oral	40–80 mg
Propranolol	Inderal®	Oral, IV	Various; 10–160 mg/day
Calcium-Channel Blockers			
Amlodipine	Norvasc®®	Oral	PO: 5 mg, increased over 10 mg daily
Bepridil	Vascor®	Oral	200 mg/day
Diltiazem	Cardizem®	Oral, IV	PO: 30 mg qid then 180–360 mg in 3–4 divided doses
Felodipine	Plendil®	Oral	5–15 mg daily
Nicardipine	Cardene®	Oral, IM	PO: 20–40 mg tid
Nifedipine	Adalat®, Procardia®	Oral, IV	10 mg tid initial dose
Nisoldipine	Sular®	Oral	20 mg then 20–40 mg daily
Verapamil	Calan®, Verelan®	Oral, IV	80–120 mg tid then 320–480 mg/day

IV, intravenous; PO, oral; SL, sublingual.

TABLE 24-3.   Nitrates Commonly Used in the Treatment of Angina

GENERIC NAME	TRADE NAME	ROUTE OF ADMINISTRATION	ONSET OF ACTION
Amyl nitrite	Amyl Nitrate®, Vaporole®	Inhalation	30 sec
Isosorbide dinitrate	Coronex®, Isordil®, Sorbitrate®	Oral, sublingual, chewable tablets	SL and chewable: 2–5 min; PO: 15–30 min
Nitroglycerin	Nitrogard®, Nitrol®, Nitroglyn®, Nitrolingual® spray, Transderm-Nitro®	Sublingual, transdermal, topical, oral	SL: 3 min; topical: 30–60 min; PO: slow; transdermal: 30–60 min; translingual: 2 min

SL, sublingual; PO, oral.

with adhesive tape. The sites should be rotated to prevent local irritation.

Adverse Effects

Abrupt discontinuation of long-acting nitroglycerin preparations may cause angina. Vasodilation can lead to orthostatic hypotension, tachycardia, headache, dizziness, weakness, syncope, and blushing. Nitrate-induced headache is a result of the dilation of cerebral blood vessels. Nitrates may also increase intraocular and intracranial pressure. Continuous exposure to nitrates may lead to tolerance. Large doses of nitrate drugs can produce methemoglobinemia (the presence of methemoglobin in the blood).

Drug Interactions

A combination of nitrates and sildenafil (Viagra®) can cause prolonged and potentially life-threatening hypotension. Use of sildenafil is therefore contraindicated in patients who use nitrates.

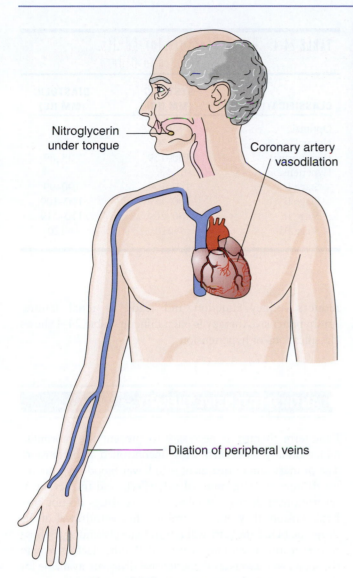

Figure 24-2. Action of nitroglycerin.

Nitroglycerin under tongue

Coronary artery vasodilation

Dilation of peripheral veins

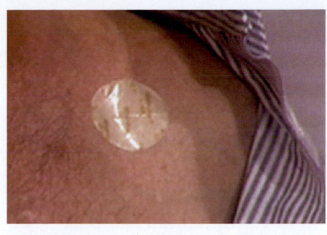

Figure 24-3. Transdermal nitroglycerin patch. (Courtesy of 3M Pharmaceuticals, St. Paul, MN.)

Adverse Effects

These agents are contraindicated for use in patients with asthma, congestive heart failure, heart block, bradycardia, or diabetes mellitus.

Drug Interactions

Generally, β-blockers may interact with cimetidine, nonsteroidal anti-inflammatory drugs (NSAIDs), epinephrine, ampicillin, antacids, calcium channel blockers, lidocaine, clonidine, prazosin, barbiturates, digoxin, anesthetics, and neuroleptics.

Calcium Channel Blockers

Calcium channel blockers are considered third-choice agents in the treatment of stable angina. For maintenance therapy of chronic stable angina, long-acting nitrates, calcium channel blocking agents, or β-blockers may be chosen; the best choice of drug will depend on the individual patient's response. Calcium channel blockers are also listed in Table 24-2.

Mechanism of Action

Calcium channel blockers are the newest type of drugs used for angina. They block the entry of calcium into smooth muscle cells and myocytes to produce arterial vasodilation and thereby reduce arterial blood pressure. They also decrease myocardial contractility, resulting in a reduction of myocardial oxygen consumption.

Therapeutic Uses

Calcium channel blockers are used for exertional angina that is not controlled by nitrates and are also used in combination with β-blockers. This combination provides the most

β-Adrenergic Blockers

β-Adrenergic blockers (β-blockers) reverse sympathetic heart action caused by exercise, stress, or physical exertion.

Mechanism of Action

β-blockers reduce oxygen demand, both at rest and during exertion.

Therapeutic Uses

The β-blockers reduce the frequency and severity of exertional angina that is not controlled by nitrates. Therefore, these agents are an important part of therapy for angina pectoris. Combined therapy with nitrates is often preferred for treatment of angina pectoris, because side effects of both agents are decreased.

effective therapy. They are considered the drug of choice for treatment of angina at rest. Diltiazem and verapamil will reduce heart rate. Nifedipine, amlodipine, and felodipine are among the most potent calcium blocking agents. β-Blockers are recommended as first-line treatment of angina pectoris, but if they are not tolerated, calcium channel blockers can be administered. Diltiazem and verapamil can also be used, but the disadvantage is that they depress contractility more than dihydropyridines do. The therapeutic goal for medication use is to reduce the frequency and intensity of anginal attacks without suppressing cardiac action too much.

Adverse Effects

Common adverse effects related to the use of calcium channel blockers include flushing, headaches, dizziness, hypotension, ankle edema, constipation, and palpitations. Combinations of nitrates, β-blockers, and calcium channel blockers are often preferred for treatment of angina pectoris, because these agents have fewer side effects. The major contraindication to combination therapy is associated with the use of β-blockers and calcium channel blockers, which may cause excessive cardiac depression.

Drug Interactions

Calcium channel blockers increase the risk of orthostatic hypotension with prazosin. Increased blood pressure may possibly occur with aspirin, bismuth subsalicylate, or magnesium salicylate. Some calcium channel blockers increase serum levels and toxicity of cyclosporine.

HYPERTENSION

Hypertension is defined as an abnormal increase in arterial blood pressure. Approximately 50 million Americans have blood pressure measurements greater than 140/90. The incidence of hypertension increases with age. In approximately 90% of patients, the cause is unknown, and more than one third of those affected have no idea that they have hypertension. Hypertension with an unknown etiology is referred to as essential or primary hypertension. Secondary hypertension may be caused by renal disease, hyperfunction of adrenal glands, and/or other disorders. Risk factors for hypertension include family history, stress, obesity, smoking, lifestyle, diabetes mellitus, and excessive blood lipids levels. Hypertension should be diagnosed in its early stages. When it is not properly treated, the risk of stroke, coronary artery disease, congestive heart failure, and renal failure increases. The risk of renal failure is increased during hypertension because the flow of the blood through the kidneys is reduced. The kidneys are very important for maintaining electrolyte balances, especially those of sodium and water. Thus, renal malfunction will increase blood pressure, which

TABLE 24-4. Blood Pressure for Adults (Aged 18 Years and Older)

CLASSIFICATION	SYSTOLIC (MM HG)	DIASTOLIC (MM HG)
Optimal	<120	<80
Normal	<130	<85
High normal	130–139	85–89
Hypertension		
Stage I	140–159	90–99
Stage II	160–179	100–109
Stage III	180–209	110–119
Stage IV	>210	>120

reduces kidney function and leads to renal failure. Antihypertensive therapy is often difficult. Table 24-4 shows classifications of hypertension.

ANTIHYPERTENSIVE THERAPY

Long-term therapy is necessary to prevent the morbidity and mortality associated with uncontrolled hypertension. The primary aim of treatment is to lower blood pressure toward "normal" with minimal side effects and to prevent or reverse organ damage. Antihypertensive drugs do not cure hypertension; they only control it. After withdrawal of the drug, the blood pressure will return to levels similar to those before treatment with medication, if all other factors remain the same. Numerous antihypertensive drugs are available for the treatment and management of all degrees of hypertension. In mild hypertension, the initial treatment regimen usually includes diet modification (restriction of salt intake), weight reduction, mild exercise programs, smoking cessation, and stress reduction. Drugs prescribed to lower blood pressure act in various ways. The drug of choice varies according to the degree of hypertension (mild, moderate, or severe). Sometimes antihypertensive drugs are combined for greater effectiveness and to reduce side effects. There are five groups of drugs that act to lower blood pressure: (1) diuretics, (2) sympatholytics, (3) angiotensin-converting enzyme inhibitors, (4) vasodilators, and (5) angiotensin II receptor antagonists. They are explained in more detail in the following sections.

Diuretics

Diuretics increase sodium excretion and lower blood volume. Diuretics are divided into four categories according to their action: thiazide, loop, potassium-sparing, and osmotic. The type of diuretic used is determined by the condition being treated. For example, carbonic anhydrase inhibitors, such as acetazolamide (Diamox®), which is recognized as a diuretic compound, are used to lower intraocular pressure.

Mechanism of Action

Thiazide agents are the most commonly used type of diuretic, increasing excretion of water, sodium, chloride, and potassium.

Loop diuretics inhibit sodium and chloride reabsorption. They are the most effective diuretics available. Potent diuretics such as furosemide (Lasix®), bumetanide (Bumex®), and ethacrynic acid (Edecrin®) are not thiazides but act in a similar way to increase excretion of water, sodium, chloride, and potassium. Their action is more rapid and effective than that of thiazides, with greater diuresis.

Potassium-sparing diuretics achieve their diuretic effects differently and are less potent than the thiazides and loop diuretics. The most pertinent feature they share with other diuretics is that they promote potassium retention.

Traditionally, substances that increase urine formation, with the excess appearing in the urine accompanied by an increased volume of water, are called osmotic diuretics.

Therapeutic Uses

Thiazides may be prescribed for the treatment of edema caused by heart failure or cirrhosis and for hypertension.

Loop diuretics are not prescribed routinely for hypertension but are used when diuresis is required. Loop diuretics are used for the treatment of edema associated with impaired renal kidney function or liver disease. They are also commonly prescribed for the treatment of congestive heart failure, pulmonary edema, and ascites caused by malignancy or cirrhosis. If thiazides are ineffective in the treatment of hypertension, loop diuretics such as furosemide or ethacrynic acid are sometimes used in combination with other antihypertensive drugs.

Potassium-sparing diuretics, which include spironolactone, triamterene, and amiloride, are sometimes administered under conditions in which potassium depletion can be dangerous. Spironolactone is a specific competitive inhibitor of aldosterone at the receptor site level. It is effective only when aldosterone is present. Triamterene and amiloride exert their effect independent of the presence or absence of aldosterone. The potassium-sparing agents are used in the management of edema associated with congestive heart failure, hepatic cirrhosis with ascites, nephritic syndrome, and idiopathic edema. Because these diuretics have little antihypertensive action of their own, they are used mainly in combination with other drugs in the management of hypertension and to correct hypokalemia often caused by other diuretic agents. Spironolactone also is used for primary hyperaldosteronism.

Mannitol has been shown to increase renal plasma flow and glomerular hydrostatic pressure. Mannitol and urea are most commonly used to reduce intracranial or intraocular pressure. Mannitol has also been used to prevent and treat acute renal failure and during certain cardiovascular surgery. Mannitol is used alone or with other diuretics to promote excretion of toxins in cases of drug poisoning.

Adverse Effects

Adverse effects of thiazides include hypokalemia, hypochloremia, muscle weakness (spasm), postural hypotension, vertigo, headache, fatigue, lethargy, and hyperglycemia. Thiazides should not be prescribed for patients with diabetes, severe renal disease, impaired liver function, and a history of gout.

Adverse effects of loop diuretics include fluid and electrolyte imbalance with dehydration, hypotension, collapse, hypokalemia, nausea, vomiting, anorexia, diarrhea, hyperglycemia, blurred vision, and hearing impairment. Loop diuretics are contraindicated in patients with liver disease, kidney impairment, and diabetes, in dehydrated patients, in pregnant and lactating women, and in children younger than 18 years of age.

Adverse effects resulting from use of potassium-sparing diuretics are hyperkalemia (which may lead to cardiac arrhythmias), dehydration, weakness, fatigue, lethargy, weight loss, nausea, vomiting, diarrhea, and hypotension. Gynecomastia and carcinoma of the breast have been reported after use of spironolactone. Potassium-sparing diuretics are contraindicated in patients with anuria, acute renal insufficiency, impaired renal function, or hyperkalemia.

The major toxic effect of osmotic diuretics is related to the amount of solute administered and its effect on the volume and distribution of body fluids. Adverse effects include fluid and electrolyte imbalance, headache, mental confusion, nausea, vomiting, tachycardia, hypertension, hypotension, allergic reactions, and severe pulmonary edema. Osmotic diuretics are contraindicated in patients with kidney failure, severe pulmonary edema, and cardiovascular disease and in pregnant and lactating women.

Drug Interactions

Significant interactions with ibuprofen diminish the effect of thiazide diuretics.

Sympatholytics (Adrenergic Blockers)

The **sympatholytic drugs** include several groups of medications: β-adrenergic blocking agents, centrally acting α-adrenergic antagonists, postganglionic adrenergic blockers, and α-adrenergic blocking agents. These drugs are listed in Table 24-5.

Mechanism of Action

β-Blockers reduce peripheral resistance and inhibit cardiac function. They also block renin secretion.

TABLE 24-5. Sympatholytic Agents

GENERIC NAME	TRADE NAME	ROUTE OF ADMINISTRATION	COMMON DOSAGE RANGE
β-Blockers			
Acebutolol	Sectral®	Oral	200–1200 mg/day in 2 divided doses
Atenolol	Tenormin®	Oral, IV	PO: 50 mg once/day; IV: 5 mg over 5 min
Betaxolol	Kerlone®	Oral	Initial 10 mg/day
Bisoprolol	Zebeta®	Oral	Initial 2.5 mg/day
Carteolol	Cartrol®	Oral	Initial 2.5 mg/day
Metoprolol	Lopressor®	Oral, IV	Initial 100 mg/day; maintenance 100–450 mg/day
Nadolol	Corgard®	Oral	40–80 mg
Penbutolol	Levatol®	Oral	Start 20 mg/day; maintenance 40–80 mg/day
Propranolol	Inderal®	Oral, IV	10–160 mg/day
Timolol	Blocadren®	Oral	10–20 mg/day
α/β-Blockers			
Labetalol	Normodyne®, Trandate®	Oral, IV	Initial 100 mg bid; maintenance 200–400 mg bid
Centrally Acting Blockers			
Clonidine	Catapres®	Oral	Initial 0.1 mg bid; maintenance 0.1–0.2 mg
Guanabenz	Wytensin®	Oral	Initial 4 mg bid; maximum 32 mg bid
Guanfacine	Tenex®	Oral	32 mg bid
Methyldopa	Aldomet®	Oral, IV	250 mg bid; maintenance 500 mg to 3 g/day, 2–4 doses
Peripherally Acting Blockers			
Doxazosin	Cardura®	Oral	Initial 1 mg/day; maintenance 2–16 mg qd
Guanadrel	Hylorel®	Oral	Start 10 mg/day; most require 20–75 mg/day
Guanethidine	Ismelin®	Oral	10 mg/day initial; average dose 25–50 mg/day
Prazosin	Minipress®	Oral	First dose limited to 1 mg hours before initial doses of 1 mg bid; maintenance 6–15 mg/day
Reserpine	Serpalan®/Serpasil®	Oral	Initial dose 0.5 mg
Terazosin	Hytrin®	Oral	Initial 1 mg hs; usual range 1–5 mg/day

IV, intravenous; PO, oral; SL, sublingual.

Centrally acting adrenergic blockers act primarily within the central nervous system on α_2-receptors to decrease sympathetic outflow to the cardiovascular system. Methyldopa decreases total peripheral resistance while having little effect on cardiac output or heart rate (except in older patients). Clonidine stimulates α_2-receptors centrally and decreases vasomotor tone and heart rate. Guanabenz and guanfacine are centrally acting α_2-adrenergic agonists that have actions similar to those of clonidine.

Peripherally acting adrenergic inhibitors are powerful antihypertensives that may interfere with the release of norepinephrine from nerve endings or may block receptors in the vascular smooth muscle. This class of antihypertensive drug is best avoided unless it is necessary to treat severe hypertension that is unresponsive to all other medications, because agents in this class are poorly tolerated by most patients. Guanethidine is one of the most potent antihypertensive drugs currently in clinical use. Guanethidine acts in peripheral neurons, where it first produces a sympathetic blockade. Guanadrel is chemically and pharmacologically similar to guanethidine.

Therapeutic Uses

β-Blockers are used for the initial treatment of hypertension. These medications can be used for angina, acute myocardial infarctions, and hypertension. Propranolol was the first β-blocking agent shown to block both β_1- and β_2-receptors. It is available both as a rapid-acting product and a long-acting product. Nadolol was the first β-blocker that could be administered as a once-daily dose. It blocks both β_1- and β_2-receptors. Timolol was the first β-blocker shown to be effective in preventing sudden death after an acute myocardial infarction.

α-/β-Blockers are drugs available for patients whose hypertension has not responded to initial antihypertensive therapy. These agents are similar to β-blockers.

Centrally acting antiadrenergic drugs have been used in the past as alternatives to initial antihypertensive therapy, but their use in mild to moderate hypertension has been reduced primarily because of the availability of other drugs. Clonidine is effective in patients with renal impairment, although they may require a reduced dose or a longer dosing interval. Clonidine is also available as a transdermal patch (Clonidine-TTS®), from which the drug is released slowly over 7 days. Guanabenz and guanfacine are recommended as adjunctive therapy with other antihypertensives for additive effects when initial therapy has failed.

Adverse Effects

β-Blockers are not totally safe in patients with bronchospastic diseases such as asthma and chronic obstructive pulmonary disease. Sudden cessation of β-blocker therapy puts the patient at risk for a withdrawal syndrome.

The adverse effects of α/β-blockers include postural hypotension, nausea, dizziness, headache, and bronchospasm.

The use of methyldopa is limited because it may produce sedation and must be administered two to four times daily. Other less common adverse effects include hemolytic anemia, hypotension and drowsiness, nausea, vomiting, sore tongue, sexual dysfunction, nasal congestion, and hepatic dysfunction. Methyldopa is contraindicated in patients with liver disease or blood dyscrasias, elderly patients, and those who are undergoing kidney dialysis. Sedation and dry mouth are common with the use of clonidine initially but usually disappear with continued therapy. Clonidine has a tendency to cause or worsen depression. Its action is apparent within 30 to 60 minutes after administration of an oral dose. The adverse effects of guanabenz and guanfacine include sedation, dry mouth, dizziness, and reduced heart rate.

Reserpine is derived from the *Rauwolfia serpentina* plant. Because of the high incidence of adverse effects, other drugs are usually chosen first. When used, reserpine is given in low doses and in conjunction with other antihypertensive agents. A history of depression is a contraindication for reserpine. It is also contraindicated in patients with peptic ulcer. Common adverse effects include drowsiness, dizziness, weakness, lethargy, memory impairment, sleep disturbances, and weight gain. Postural and exercise hypotension, fluid retention, and sexual dysfunction are common side effects when guanethidine is used. Guanadrel should be avoided in patients with congestive heart failure, angina, and stroke. Adverse effects include fainting, orthostatic hypotension, and diarrhea.

Drug Interactions

Patients taking guanethidine should avoid over-the-counter preparations that contain adrenergic substances such as cold medicines, because the combination may potentiate an acute hypertensive effect.

Angiotensin-Converting Enzyme Inhibitors

Angiotensin-converting enzyme inhibitors competitively inhibit conversion of angiotensin I to angiotensin II, a potent vasoconstrictor, through the angiotensin-converting enzyme (ACE) activity, with resultant lower levels of angiotensin II. Lower angiotensin II levels cause increased plasma renin activity and reduced aldosterone secretion.

Mechanism of Action

ACE inhibitors slow the formation of angiotensin II, which reduces vascular resistance, blood volume, and blood pressure. Renin is an enzyme that is released by the kidneys in response to reduced renal blood circulation or hyponatremia. This enzyme acts in the plasma angiotensinogen to produce angiotensin I. Then, angiotensin I is converted to angiotensin II, mostly in the lungs. Angiotensin II is a vasoconstricting agent. It causes sodium retention via release of aldosterone. In the adrenal gland, angiotensin II is converted to angiotensin III. Both angiotensin II and III stimulate the release of aldosterone. Angiotensin I is inactive in the cardiovascular system. Angiotensin II has several cardiovascular-renal actions. The most important site of the ACE is found in the lungs, but ACE also is found in the kidneys, central nervous system, and elsewhere. Figure 24-4 shows the renin-angiotensin system. Examples of ACE inhibitors are shown in Table 24-6.

Therapeutic Uses

ACE inhibitors are becoming the drugs of choice for first-line treatment of essential hypertension.

Adverse Effects

Although ACE inhibitors as a group have relatively few side effects or toxicities in most patients, these do occur, and some can be life threatening. The adverse effects of ACE

TABLE 24-6. Examples of ACE Inhibitors

GENERIC NAME	TRADE NAME	ROUTE OF ADMINISTRATION	COMMON DOSAGE RANGE
Captopril	Capoten®	Oral	Usual 25–150 mg bid-tid
Enalapril	Vasotec®	Oral, IV	PO: Initial 5 mg/day; usual 10–40 mg/day
Fosinopril	Monopril®	Oral	10–40 mg/day
Lisinopril	Prinivil®, Zestril®	Oral	Effective 5–20 mg/day
Quinapril	Accupril®	Oral	Maintenance 20–80 mg/day
Ramipril	Altace®	Oral	Initial 2.5 mg/day; usual 2.5–20 mg/day

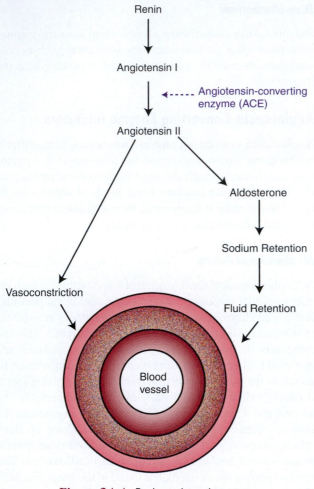

Figure 24-4. Renin-angiotensin system.

TABLE 24-7. Vasodilators

GENERIC NAME	TRADE NAME	ROUTE OF ADMINISTRATION	COMMON DOSAGE RANGE
Hydralazine	Apresoline®	Oral, IM, IV	10–15 mg/day
Minoxidil	Loniten®	Oral	Up to 100 mg/day

IM, intramuscular; IV, intravenous.

this chapter (coronary vasodilators for angina pectoris). Vasodilators are prescribed as second-line agents after initial therapy in patients taking diuretics, β-blockers, ACE inhibitors, calcium channel blockers, β-adrenergic blockers, or α/β-adrenergic blockers.

Mechanism of Action

Vasodilators block the movement of calcium into the smooth muscle of the blood vessels to cause relaxation of the smooth muscle and dilation of the resistance vessels.

Therapeutic Uses

Vasodilator agents reduce hypertension. A peripheral vasodilator is often used for the treatment of moderate to severe hypertension.

Hydralazine and minoxidil may be used for the treatment of moderate essential or early malignant hypertension and hypertensive emergencies, virtually always in conjunction with other antihypertensive drugs. However, mainly because of side effects, they are generally not used until other, safer therapy has failed. Because they increase renal blood flow, they are often used to treat toxemia of pregnancy. They are sometimes used in patients with acute congestive heart failure or after myocardial infarction (see Table 24-7).

Adverse Effects

The toxic effects of hydralazine are syndromes resembling rheumatoid arthritis or lupus erythematosus, the appearance of which necessitates withdrawal of the drug. Common adverse effects of hydralazine include headache, dizziness, tachycardia, palpitations, anxiety, nausea, vomiting, disorientation, depression, edema, impotence, and allergic reactions. Hydralazine is contraindicated in patients with systemic lupus erythematosus, renal disease, and coronary artery disease and in pregnant women (except during preeclampsia).

Drug Interactions

Hydralazine should be used with caution in patients receiving monoamine oxidase inhibitors. Profound hypotensive episodes may occur when hydralazine is used along with diazoxide injections.

inhibitors may include dizziness, angioedema, loss of taste, photosensitivity, severe hypotension, dry cough, hyperkalemia, blood dyscrasias, and renal impairment. ACE inhibitors are contraindicated in patients with renal impairment, lupus erythematosus, scleroderma, angioedema, and heart failure, in pregnant and lactating women, and in children.

Drug Interactions

ACE inhibitors increase the risk of hypersensitivity reactions with allopurinol. They decrease the antihypertensive effects of indomethacin. ACE inhibitors also increase captopril effects with probenecid. Some ACE inhibitors may increase coughing if combined with capsaicin. Fosinopril increases the risk of high potassium levels if taken with potassium-sparing diuretics. Quinapril may increase digoxin levels and decrease absorption of tetracycline.

Vasodilators

Vasodilators are used to relax or dilate vessels throughout the body. Some work on either veins or arteries; others work on both. Peripheral vasodilators were discussed earlier in

Angiotensin II Receptor Antagonists

Angiotensin II receptor antagonists block the binding of angiotensin II to the angiotensin II type 1 receptor. Angiotensin II receptor antagonists have beneficial effects on the symptoms and hemodynamics of patients with congestive heart failure.

Mechanism of Action

Angiotensin II receptor antagonist drugs work by blocking the binding of angiotensin II to the angiotensin II receptors. By blocking the receptor site, these agents inhibit the vasoconstrictor effects of angiotensin II and prevent the release of aldosterone due to angiotensin II from the adrenal glands.

Therapeutic Uses

This class of drugs has been one of the fastest growing for treatment of hypertension. Currently, six agents are available: candesartan cilexetil, eprosartan, irbesartan, losartan, telmisartan, and valsartan (see Table 24-8).

Adverse Effects

Angiotensin receptor blockers should not be used in certain populations with hypertension such as diabetics with nephropathy or congestive heart failure unless the patient cannot tolerate an ACE inhibitor.

Drug Interactions

Some of these drugs, such as losartan, decrease serum levels and effectiveness of phenobarbital. Losartan is converted to an active metabolite by cytochrome P-450, which may decrease the antihypertensive effects of losartan. Telmisartan increases serum levels and risk of toxicity of digoxin.

■ MYOCARDIAL INFARCTION

A **myocardial infarction** is an area of dead cardiac muscle tissue, with or without hemorrhage. Myocardial infarction is produced by obstruction of the coronary artery, which results in a lack of oxygen to the tissue. More than 1 million patients have a myocardial infarction every year in the United States. Despite a 50% decline in deaths due to cardiovascular causes resulting from advances in diagnosis and management of myocardial infarction over the past three decades, it is still a fatal event in one of three patients. After myocardial infarction, there are four goals that should be achieved expeditiously and simultaneously to limit myocardial necrosis and mortality:

- Relief of pain
- Confirmation of diagnosis by electrocardiogram (ECG) and measurements of serum markers
- Assessment and treatment of hemodynamic abnormalities
- Initiation of reperfusion therapy

Pain relief is best achieved with oxygen (2 L/min by nasal cannula), nitroglycerin, and morphine sulfate. The rationale for reperfusion therapy is based on the high prevalence of occlusive thrombus in early treatment. The greatest benefit is seen when this therapy is performed within the first 4 hours of the onset of pain. Antithrombotic agents should be considered for all patients with an acute myocardial infarction. Antithrombotic medications include unfractionated heparin, low molecular weight heparin, warfarin, aspirin, and antiplatelet drugs.

■ ARRHYTHMIAS

Arrhythmias are deviations from the normal pattern of the heartbeat. They may occur because of improper impulse generation, conduction, or both. Arrhythmias may result from disturbances in pacemaker function of the sinoatrial node or heart block in conduction pathways. Dysrhythmias originating at the sinoatrial node may be tachycardia, bradycardia, and even cardiac arrest. Arrhythmias may originate from different sites in the heart, causing ventricular tachycardias, atrial fibrillation, or flutter. They may also occur with digitalis toxicity or during surgery and anesthesia. When a dysrhythmia occurs, the sodium, potassium, and calcium ions that regulate the electrophysiological properties of the heart are disturbed.

TABLE 24-8. Angiotensin II Receptor Antagonists

GENERIC NAME	BRAND NAME	ROUTE OF ADMINISTRATION	COMMON DOSAGE RANGE
Candesartan cilexetil	Atacand®	Oral	8–32 mg/day
Eprosartan	Teveten®	Oral	400–800 mg/day
Irbesartan	Avapro®	Oral	150–300 mg/day
Losartan	Cozaar®	Oral	25–100 mg/day
Telmisartan	Micardis®	Oral	40–80 mg/day
Valsartan	Diovan®	Oral	80–320 mg/day

TABLE 24-9. Classification of Antiarrhythmic Drugs

CLASSES OF DRUGS	GENERIC NAME	TRADE NAME	COMMON DOSAGE RANGE
Class I			
	Quinidine	Duraquin®, Cardioquin®	2400–3600 mg/day
Subclass 1A (fast channel blockers)	Procainamide	Pronestyl®, Procan®	1000–4000 mg/day
	Disopyramide	Norpace®	400–800 mg/day
Subclass 1B	Lidocaine	Xylocaine®	50–300 mg/day
	Mexiletine	Mexitil®	50–1200 mg/day
	Tocainide	Tonocard®	400–1800 mg/day
	Phenytoin	Dilantin®	50–600 mg/day
Subclass 1C	Flecainide	Tambocor®	50–400 mg/day
Class II (β-adrenergic blockers)			
	Propranolol	Inderal®	10–640 mg/day
	Acebutolol	Sectral®	200–1200 mg/day
	Atenolol	Tenormin®	5–200 mg/day
	Esmolol	Brevibloc®	25–500 mcg/kg/min
	Nadolol	Corgard®	40–320 mg/day
	Pindolol	Visken®	10–60 mg/day
	Timolol	Blocadren®	10–60 mg/day
Class III (interfere with potassium outflow)			
	Bretylium	Bretylol®	1–30 mg/kg
	Amiodarone	Cordarone®	150–1600 mg/day
Class IV (calcium channel blockers)			
	Verapamil	Calan®, Isoptin®	5–480 mg/day
	Diltiazem	Cardizem®	120–480 mg/day
Others			
	Digoxin	Lanoxin	0.125–1.25 mg/day
	Atropine	Sal-Tropine	0.4–24 mg/day
	Magnesium	Mag-Ox 400®, Maox 420®, Uro-Mag®	400–1244 mg/day

ANTIARRHYTHMIC DRUGS

Antiarrhythmic agents do not cure dysrhythmia, but the goal of treatment is to attempt to restore normal cardiac function. These agents are classified in four distinct groups, according to their effects: class I (fast channel blockers), which are subclassified into three groups, class 1A, 1B, and 1C (see Table 24-9); class II (β-adrenergic blockers); class III (which interfere with potassium outflow); and class IV (calcium channel blockers). There are also other agents that may be used for the treatment of arrhythmias such as digoxin, atropine, and magnesium.

Mechanism of Action

Quinidine depresses the myocardium and the conduction system, resulting in slowing of the heart rate. Procainamide and disopyramide have action similar to that of quinidine.

Lidocaine is the most widely used agent for suppression and prevention of ventricular arrhythmias associated with myocardial infarction. It does not slow conduction and thus has little effect on atrial function. Lidocaine acts exclusively on the sodium channel. It is given parenterally as a bolus. Two medications that have action similar to that of lidocaine can be administered orally: mexiletine and tocainide.

Class II antiarrhythmics competitively inhibit β-adrenoreceptors and inhibit the release of norepinephrine and epinephrine. Therefore, they increase heart rate, particularly the ventricles. Major β-adrenergic blockers are listed in Table 24-10.

Class III antiarrhythmics interfere with potassium outflow during repolarization. They prolong action potential duration and effective refractory period. The prolonged period decreases the frequency of heart rate. Amiodarone decreases automaticity, prolongs atrioventricular conduction, and may even block the exchange of sodium and potassium.

Class IV antiarrhythmics selectively block slow calcium channels. Therefore, these agents can prolong nodal conduction and effective refractory period. These calcium antagonists may also decrease the ability of the heart to produce forceful

TABLE 24-10. Pharmacological Properties of β-Adrenergic Blocking Drugs

GENERIC NAME	TRADE NAME	ABSORPTION	PLASMA HALF-LIFE (hours)
Propranolol	Inderal®	Good	1–5
Nadolol	Corgard®	Incomplete	16–20
Timolol	Blocadren®	Good	4
Penbutolol	Levatol®	Complete	5
Metoprolol	Lopressor®	Good, rapid	3–4
Atenolol	Tenormin®	Incomplete	6–8
Betaxolol	Kerlone®	Good	14–22
Pindolol	Visken®	Good	3–4
Acebutolol	Sectral®	Good	3–4
Carteolol	Cartrol®	Good	6

contractions, leading to congestive heart failure. These drugs also relax smooth muscle and cause vasodilation. Verapamil works on the sinoatrial (SA) node to decrease its activity, thus decreasing the heart rate. It also decreases atrioventricular (AV) node conduction and is used for AV node dysrhythmias.

Cardiac glycosides increase the speed of myocardial contractions in both normal and failing hearts. Under normal cardiac conditions, digitalis treatment results in an increase in systemic vascular resistance and constriction of smooth muscles in veins (cardiac output may decrease). In heart failure, digitalis increases the force of myocardial contractions, slows the heart rate, and slows the conduction of electrical impulses. The increased force of contractions improves the efficiency of the heart without increasing oxygen consumption. Normal blood circulation is restored and the kidney function is increased. The most common cardiac glycosides are digoxin and digitoxin. The major active ingredients found in digitalis plants are collectively referred to as digitalis. Cardiac glycosides are able to affect beating of a congested heart more forcefully within a shorter period of time. This force increases the amount of blood pumped from the heart and improves blood circulation, thus decreasing the congestion found with heart failure.

Therapeutic Uses

Quinidine is used to treat supraventricular arrhythmias, such as atrial flutter and atrial fibrillation, and some ventricular dysrhythmias. This agent also exhibits antimalarial, antipyretic, and oxytocic actions.

Procainamide is safer to use intravenously and has fewer gastrointestinal (GI) side effects.

Disopyramide has been approved for the treatment of ventricular arrhythmias. Generally it is reserved for patients who are intolerant of quinidine or procainamide.

The dose of lidocaine must be adjusted in patients with congestive heart failure or hepatic disease. Mexiletine is used primarily for chronic treatment of ventricular arrhythmias associated with previous myocardial infarction. Tocainide is useful for the treatment of ventricular tachyarrhythmias.

Phenytoin is an antiepileptic drug that has proved to be useful in treating digitalis-induced tachyarrhythmias.

β-Adrenergic blockers are useful for treating tachyarrhythmias due to increased sympathetic activity and also are used for a variety of other arrhythmias, atrial flutter, and atrial fibrillation. These are sometimes used for digitalis toxicity. Propanolol is the most common β-blocker that is used as an antiarrhythmic.

Amiodarone is useful for severe refractory supraventricular and ventricular tachyarrhythmias. Amiodarone also possesses antianginal effects.

Calcium channel blockers are useful for angina (as discussed earlier in this chapter) and for hypertension.

Verapamil is useful for reentrant supraventricular tachycardia.

Digitalis drugs are the principal medications for the treatment of congestive heart failure and certain arrhythmias (atrial fibrillation, flutter, and paroxysmal atrial tachycardias). Digoxin is the drug prescribed most often because it can be administered orally and parenterally. It has an intermediate duration of action. The process of establishing the correct therapeutic dose of digitalis for maintaining optimal functioning of the heart without toxic effects is referred to as digitalization. The margin between effective therapy and dangerous toxicity is very narrow. Careful monitoring of the cardiac rate and rhythm with an ECG, cardiac function, side effects, and the blood digitalis level is required to determine the therapeutic maintenance dose.

Adverse Effects

Quinidine can lead to skeletal muscle weakness, especially in patients with myasthenia gravis. Rapid infusion of quinidine may cause severe hypotension and shock. It can produce ringing of the ears, dizziness, diarrhea, thrombocytopenia, and ventricular arrhythmias.

A high incidence of adverse reactions is seen with chronic use of procainamide. Procainamide may produce severe or irreversible heart failure, more than that seen with quinidine. It often causes drug-induced lupus syndrome.

Disopyramide may cause dry mouth, blurred vision, constipation, and urinary retention.

A low level of cardiotoxicity is seen with the use of lidocaine. The most common side effects are neurological, in contrast to side effects seen with quinidine and procainamide. Lidocaine has little effect on the autonomic nervous system.

The common side effects of phenytoin use are nystagmus, blurred vision, vertigo, and hyperplasia of the gums.

One adverse effect associated with the use of β-adrenergic blockers is bronchospasm. Bradycardia and myocardial depression may also occur. Atropine or isoproterenol may be used to alleviate bradycardia. The most frequent adverse cardiovascular effects with use of propranolol are hypertension and bradycardia. It may also cause mental confusion and skin rashes.

Side effects of amiodarone include GI tract disturbance, photosensitivity, gray man syndrome, corneal microdeposits, and thyroid disorders (due to iodine in drug preparations).

The side effects of verapamil are headaches, dizziness, and GI disturbances, but the most common side effect is constipation. Verapamil is contraindicated in patients with known SA or AV node problems or with congestive heart failure.

Early signs of toxicity of digitalis include anorexia, nausea, and vomiting. There are also other adverse effects such as abdominal cramping, diarrhea, fatigue, muscle weakness, headache, lethargy, vertigo, irritability, seizures, blurred vision, diplopia, bradycardia (heart rate less than 60), and electrolyte imbalance. Insomnia, mental disorders, and confusion, especially in elderly patients, are seen. Cardiac glycosides are contraindicated in patients with hypothyroidism, severe pulmonary disease, acute myocardial infarction, and impaired renal function and in pregnant and lactating women.

Vasoconstrictors

Vasoconstrictors are used mostly to prolong the duration of action of local anesthetics or to help control bleeding. Vasoconstrictors delay the absorption of local anesthetics by reducing blood flow to the area in question. They are of no value in delaying the absorption of local anesthetics from mucous membranes.

Mechanism of Action

These drugs constrict blood vessels. They predominantly affect the cardiovascular system, which causes an increase in mean arterial blood pressure. For example, they lower peripheral vascular resistance and blood pressure. The most common vasoconstrictor agents, or adrenergics, are listed in Table 24-11.

Therapeutic Uses

Several of these agents are used for maintaining blood pressure during anesthesia and for treating pronounced hypotension resulting from hemorrhage, myocardial infarction, septicemia, or drug reactions.

TABLE 24-11. Adrenergics		
GENERIC NAME	**TRADE NAME**	**INDICATIONS**
Epinephrine	Adrenalin®	Asthma, cardiac arrest, anaphylaxis
Ephedrine	Ephedrine®	Hypotension
Dopamine	Intropin®	Hypotension
Isoproterenol	Isuprel®	Asthma, ventricular arrhythmias
Metaraminol	Aramin®	Hypotension in shock
Norepinephrine	Levophed®	Severe hypotension

Adverse Effects

Adverse effects include headache, dizziness, weakness, apnea, palpitation, bradycardia, or cardiac arrhythmias.

Drug Interactions

Quinidine may cause drug interaction with β-blockers, digitalis, potassium, procainamide, and nifedipine. Administration of procainamide with pimozide, neuromuscular blockers, quinidine, alcohol, and cimetidine produces drug interactions. Disopyramide may have drug interactions with pimozide and other antiarrhythmics. Phenytoin may interact with glucocorticoids, alcohol, and antacids.

β-Adrenergic blockers interact with diuretics, NSAIDs, and xanthines.

Amiodarone can cause drug interactions with cardiac glycosides and anticoagulants.

Calcium channel blockers should be avoided with administration of β-blockers, digoxin, procainamide, quinidine, and theophylline because of their drug interactions.

HYPERLIPIDEMIA

Dietary or drug therapy of elevated plasma cholesterol levels can reduce the risk of atherosclerosis and subsequent cardiovascular disease. A patient with high serum cholesterol and increased low-density lipoprotein (LDL) levels is at risk for atherosclerotic coronary disease and myocardial infarction. Diseases associated with plasma lipids can be manifest as an elevation in the triglyceride level (**hyperlipidemia**) or as an elevation in the cholesterol level. Elevated triglyceride levels can produce life-threatening pancreatitis.

ANTIHYPERLIPIDEMIC DRUGS

Medications are not the first line of treatment for hyperlipidemia. Antihyperlipidemic drugs are used only if diet modification and exercise programs fail to lower LDL levels to normal. When medications are started, diet therapy must continue. Antihyperlipidemic drugs are the group of drugs

TABLE 24-12. Lipid-Lowering Drugs

GENERIC NAME	TRADE NAME	ROUTE OF ADMINISTRATION	COMMON DOSAGE RANGE
Bile Acid Sequestrants			
Cholestyramine	Questran®; LoCholest®, Prevalite®	Oral	4–16 g/day
Colestipol	Colestid®	Oral	2–30 g/day
Colesevelam	Welchol®	Oral	1875–4375 mg/day
Fibric Acid Derivatives			
Fenofibrate	Tricor®	Oral	54–160 mg/day
Gemfibrozil	Lopid®	Oral	1200 mg/day
Clofibrate	Atromid-S®	Oral	2 g/day
Nicotinic Acid			
Immediate release	Niacor®	Nasal spray	0.5 mg/day
Sustained release	Niaspan®, Slo-Niacin®	Transdermal patch	5–21 mg/day
Statins			
Atorvastatin	Lipito®	Oral	10–80 mg/day
Fluvastatin	Lescol®	Oral	20–80 mg/day
Lovastatin	Mevacor®	Oral	10–80 mg/day
Pravastatin	Pravachol®	Oral	10–80 mg/day
Simvastatin	Zocor®	Oral	5–80 mg/day

prescribed as adjuvant therapy to reduce elevated cholesterol levels in patients with high blood cholesterol and LDL levels. These medications are used to decrease the risk of arteriosclerosis. The major drugs for reduction of LDL cholesterol levels are bile acid sequestrants and nicotinic acid. The fibric acid derivatives and clofibrate are less effective in reducing LDL cholesterol levels. The most effective agents for reducing plasma LDL levels are the statins. Five statins are now available (see Table 24-12).

Nicotinic Acid (Niacin)

This agent can have cholesterol- and triglyceride-lowering effects at high concentrations, resulting in a decrease of LDL and very low-density lipoprotein (VLDL) levels and an increase in high-density lipoprotein (HDL) levels, but its use is limited by its side effects.

Mechanism of Action

Nicotinic acid may partially inhibit the release of free fatty acids from adipose tissue and increase lipoprotein activity, which could increase the rate of triglyceride removal from plasma. These actions reduce the concentrations of total LDL (bad cholesterol) and triglycerides, resulting in increased concentrations of HDL (good cholesterol).

Therapeutic Uses

Niacin may be prescribed as an adjunct to diet for treatment of adults with very high serum triglyceride levels who have a risk of pancreatitis and whose triglyceride concentrations do not respond adequately to dietary control.

Adverse Effects

Nicotinic acid may cause headache, anxiety, hypotension, flushing or burning feelings in the skin, dry skin, peptic ulcer, or abnormal liver function test results. Other adverse effects of this agent include hyperuricemia, glucose intolerance, nausea, vomiting, diarrhea, hyperglycemia, and elevated plasma uric acid levels.

Drug Interactions

Niacin can increase the effectiveness of antihypertensive or vasoactive drugs. It also increases the risk of bleeding with anticoagulants. Niacin decreases absorption with bile acid sequestrants and separate doses must be administered at least 4 to 6 hours apart.

Clofibrate

Clofibrate reduces hepatic synthesis of cholesterol and results in a reduction in the plasma concentrations of VLDL and triglycerides. Because more successful medications are now available, this drug is no longer the hypolipidemic drug of choice, although it is still used for patients whose condition may not respond to other medications.

Mechanism of Action

Clofibrate stimulates the liver to increase breakdown of VLDL to LDL and decreases liver synthesis of VLDL by inhibiting cholesterol formation.

Therapeutic Uses

The primary indication for clofibrate is hyperlipidemia that does not respond to diet. Clofibrate is also prescribed for patients with very high serum triglyceride concentrations with abdominal pain and pancreatitis that does not respond to diet.

Adverse Effects

The adverse effects of clofibrate include angina, arrhythmias, swelling, phlebitis, and pulmonary emboli. This agent also causes nausea, vomiting, diarrhea, flatulence, gastritis and gallstones (with long-term therapy). Clofibrate may produce impotence, dysuria, hematuria, leukopenia, and anemia.

Drug Interactions

Clofibrate may increase anticoagulant effects by lowering plasma protein binding. It increases the effect of antidiabetic drugs and exaggerates the diuretic response to furosemide. Clofibrate increases the effects of insulin. With probenecid, the therapeutic and toxic effects of clofibrate are increased. With ursodiol, there is an increased risk of gallstone formation.

Statins

Statins have become the mainstay of LDL-reducing therapy, and they are the most effective agents for reducing plasma LDL levels. The statins include atorvastatin, fluvastatin, lovastatin, pravastatin, and simvastatin. These drugs are extremely effective and well tolerated.

Mechanism of Action

Statins inhibit 3-hydroxy-3-methylglutaryl-coenzyme A, the enzyme that catalyzes the first step in the cholesterol synthesis pathway, resulting in a decrease in serum cholesterol and serum LDL levels.

Therapeutic Uses

Statins are used as adjuncts to diet in treatment of elevated total cholesterol, serum triglyceride, and LDL cholesterol levels in patients with primary hypercholesterolemia.

Adverse Effects

Statins may cause headache, flatulence, abdominal pain, cramps, constipation, nausea, and heartburn. The incidence of serious adverse effects with statins is impressively low. The most important side effects are transaminase elevation and acute myositis.

Drug Interactions

Clarithromycin, diltiazem, cyclosporine, erythromycin, nefadozone, ritonavir, and verapamil decrease statin metabolism. Clofibrate increases risk of myopathy. Gemfibrozil increases plasma lovastatin and simvastatin.

Combination Drug Therapy

Certain combinations of medications can be useful for treating markedly elevated LDL cholesterol levels. Combination therapy can maximize the reduction in LDL levels. It can also allow the limiting of dosages of individual LDL-reducing drugs, thus limiting side effects. For patients with elevations in both triglyceride and LDL levels, the addition of nicotinic acid or a fibric acid derivative to control triglyceride levels can allow the use of a bile acid sequestrant to help reduce LDL levels. The following are the most effective combinations for lowering LDL levels:

- A statin plus a bile acid sequestrant
- A statin plus nicotinic acid
- Nicotinic acid plus a bile acid sequestrant
- A statin plus a bile acid sequestrant plus nicotinic acid

The combination of a fibric acid derivative with a statin should usually be avoided because of an increased risk of myopathy.

ANTICOAGULANT DRUGS

Anticoagulants are agents that prevent formation of blood clots (thrombi). Venous thromboembolic disease occurs when vascular injury or venous stasis is present as deep venous thrombosis and/or pulmonary embolism. Risk factors for clot formation include age of patients (older than 40), obesity, immobility (bed rest for more than 4 days), pregnancy, varicose veins, high-dose estrogen therapy, trauma, surgery (especially involving the pelvis, hip, and lower limbs), malignancy, and major medical illness. Administration of thrombolytic agents reduces the tendency of blood to coagulate, thereby reducing the risk of thrombosis (clot). Anticoagulant drugs are not effective for an existing clot, but they reduce the ability of the blood to clot and prevent formation of other clots. Heparin is one of the potent anticoagulants naturally obtained from the liver and lungs of domestic animals. In humans, it is usually found in mast cells. Warfarin is a coumarin compound. It is the most widely used oral anticoagulant in the United States. Although it is primarily administered orally, an injectable preparation is available in this country. Table 24-13 shows the most commonly used anticoagulants.

Mechanism of Action

Warfarin is a vitamin K antagonist that prevents coagulation by inhibiting the formation of vitamin K-dependent clotting factors. Heparin can be given only parenterally. Injection of

TABLE 24-13. Anticoagulant Agents

GENERIC NAME	BRAND NAME	ROUTES OF ADMINISTRATION	COMMON DOSAGE RANGE
Warfarin	Coumadin®	Oral, IV	2–10 mg/day
	Dicumaro®	Oral	2–10 mg/day
Heparin	Hep-Lock®	IV, SC	1000–40,000 U/day
Lepirudin	Refludan®	IV	0.15–0.4 mg/kg
Low Molecular-weight Heparin			
Dalteparin	Fragmin®	SC	2500–10,000 IU/day
Enoxaparin	Lovenox®	SC	30–40 mg/day
Tinzaparin	Innohep®	SC	175 IU/kg/day

IV, intravenous; SC, subcutaneous.

heparin should be intravenous or subcutaneous but never intramuscular because it will cause a hematoma. The benefit of heparin administration for the patient is that it may be used as a therapeutic agent within the first 24 hours after diagnosis. Traditionally, systemic intravenous unfractionated heparin has been administered for 5 days while oral anticoagulation with warfarin is initiated. Recently, the use of three forms of low molecular-weight heparin (LMWH) has been advocated. LMWHs are fragments of standard commercial-grade heparin. These agents are approximately one third the size of heparin. Heparin is safe for use in pregnancy because it does not cross the placenta. The duration of action of heparin is short, and the onset of its effects is immediate. Oral anticoagulants are not appropriate in emergency situations because of the time between their administration and onset of action.

Therapeutic Uses

Anticoagulants are used prophylactically for deep vein thrombosis or to prevent thrombus formation in pulmonary embolus or atrial fibrillation. They are also used during heart valve replacement surgery. Warfarin is one of the most commonly used oral anticoagulants. Its levels peak a few days after initiation of treatment, and it remains in the body for 2 to 5 days after the drug is discontinued.

Adverse Effects

The adverse effects of warfarin are mainly excessive bleeding, but it may cause alopecia, GI disturbances, and dermatitis. An overdose of warfarin is treated with vitamin K.

Drug Interactions

Use of heparin with other anticoagulants may increase the anticoagulant effect to a dangerous level. They should be used with caution with salicylates (aspirin). Cholestyramine can decrease warfarin absorption, thus reducing its effects.

Colestipol and sucralfate have also been reported to interfere with warfarin absorption. Antacids appear to affect warfarin absorption but only to a minor degree.

ANTIPLATELET AGENTS

Antiplatelet agents are prescribed to suppress aggregation (clumping) of platelets. A number of drugs may be used for stopping thrombi in arteries rather than anticoagulants in veins. The most commonly used antiplatelet drug is aspirin. It has been proved effective for preventing myocardial infarctions and strokes. Other medications may be used as antiplatelet drugs, including glycoprotein antagonists, ticlopidine, and abciximab (see Table 24-14).

TABLE 24-14. Antiplatelet Agents

GENERIC NAME	TRADE NAME	ROUTE OF ADMINISTRATION	COMMON DOSAGE RANGE
Aspirin	Bayer Aspirin®, etc.	Oral, rectal	75 mg–8 g/day
Abciximab	ReoPro®	IV	0.25 mg/kg
Eptifibatide	Integrilin®	IV	0.75–2 mg/mL
Tirofiban	Aggrastat®	IV	50–250 mcg/mL
Ticlopidine	Ticlid®	Oral	250 mg/day
Clopidogrel	Plavix®	Oral	50–150 mg/day

IV, intravenous.

Mechanism of Action

Eptifibatide and tirofiban are two of the newest glycoprotein antagonists used to delay clotting by altering platelet aggregation that have received approval by the Food and Drug Administration. These agents are prescribed in conjunction with heparin and aspirin.

Therapeutic Uses

Ticlopidine prevents platelet aggregation, which reduces the risk of thrombotic stroke in patients who have experienced stroke precursors.

Abciximab is an antiplatelet drug used with heparin and aspirin to prevent coronary vessel occlusion in patients undergoing percutaneous transluminal coronary angioplasty or atherectomy.

Clopidogrel is an antiplatelet agent used in patients who have recently had a myocardial infarction or stroke.

Adverse Effects

The primary side effects associated with glycoprotein antagonists are bleeding and thrombocytopenia (a decrease in blood platelet levels).

Adverse effects of ticlopidine include neutropenia (a decrease in white blood cells), thrombocytopenia, and bleeding.

Abciximab is contraindicated in patients with allergy to this agent or those who have neutropenia, thrombocytopenia, bleeding ulcer, uncontrolled hypertension, and major trauma.

The adverse effects of clopidogrel include fatigue, arthralgic pain, headache, dizziness, hypertension, edema, and a risk of bleeding.

Drug Interactions

Aspirin has drug interactions with anticoagulants, hypoglycemic agents, uricosuric agents, spironolactone, alcohol, corticosteroids, pyrazolone derivatives, NSAIDs, urinary alkalinizers, phenobarbital, phenytoin, and propranolol. Ticlopidine potentiates the effect of aspirin and NSAIDs; it also should not be used with antacids, cimetidine, digoxin, theophylline, phenobarbital, phenytoin, or propranolol. There is no direct drug information as yet available about eptifibatide; however, its adverse effects on the body are well documented. Tirofiban, when used in combination with heparin and aspirin, has been associated with an increase in bleeding. Formal drug interaction studies with abciximab have not been conducted, although an increase in bleeding when abciximab is used concurrently with heparin, other anticoagulants, thrombolytics, and antiplatelet agents has

been documented. Use of clopidogrel with NSAIDs has caused increased GI blood loss, and it should be used with aspirin, heparin, or warfarin with caution.

SUMMARY

Diseases of the cardiovascular system are among the leading causes of death in the United States. Varieties of medications are available; some of these affect the myocardium itself, whereas others affect the blood vessels of the vascular system. Vasodilators, such as nitrates, increase the size of blood vessels to improve circulation of the blood for the management of angina pectoris. Cardiac glycosides come from digitalis and are used to increase the force of myocardial contractions in congestive heart failure. Antiarrhythmics are used to treat disorders of cardiac rhythm. These disorders may occur from coronary artery disease, electrolyte imbalances, cardiac conduction abnormalities, or even from endocrine disease (thyroid disorders). Antihypertensive drugs include diuretics (to lower blood volume), ACE inhibitors, β-blockers, and vasodilators. In some cases, calcium channel blockers must be used with care for elderly patients. Medications are used only when lifestyle changes have not adequately lowered elevated blood pressure. To reduce circulating hyperlipidemia, medications may be required. The statins reduce the amounts of enzyme necessary for cholesterol production. Nicotinic acid reduces LDL and VLDL levels. The fibric acid derivatives decrease triglyceride and VLDL levels while raising HDL levels. These medications for hyperlipidemia are long-term therapy. Anticoagulants are used to treat deep venous thrombosis by disrupting the coagulation process and the formation of fibrin.

CRITICAL THINKING

1. Choose one of the disorders discussed in this chapter. What other types of therapeutic regimens can patients participate in that could help reduce or eliminate this disorder? What type of patient education is necessary for this disorder?
2. Why is it so critical to monitor patients with cardiac conditions for adverse reactions and interactions with other medications?
3. Perform an Internet search to see if there is new research or new drugs under development and review to treat cardiac-related disorders. What did you find? What impact could these results have on the industry?

REVIEW QUESTIONS

1. Which of the following antianginal drugs are also used as antihypertensives and antiarrhythmics?
   A. Nitrates
   B. Vasoconstrictors
   C. Diuretics
   D. β-Adrenergic blockers

2. Thiazides are contraindicated in patients with all of the following conditions, except
   A. impaired liver function.
   B. edema caused by heart failure.
   C. diabetes.
   D. a history of gout.

3. Hydralazine (Apresoline®) is a/an
   A. vasodilator.
   B. vasoconstrictor.
   C. anticoagulant.
   D. antiarrhythmic.

4. Which of the following drugs is in the class of calcium channel blockers?
   A. Propranolol
   B. Isosorbide
   C. Verapamil
   D. Atenolol

5. Early signs of toxicity of digitalis include
   A. mental disorders.
   B. nausea and vomiting.
   C. tachycardia.
   D. seizures.

6. Anticoagulants are used prophylactically for all of the following conditions or disorders, except
   A. prevention of thrombus in pulmonary embolus.
   B. hypothyroidism.
   C. deep vein thrombosis.
   D. atrial fibrillation.

7. An example of the angiotensin-converting enzyme (ACE) inhibitors is
   A. captopril (Capoten®).
   B. acebutolol (Sectral®).
   C. lidocaine (Xylocaine®).
   D. procainamide (Pronestyl®).

8. Which of the following medications is not used for arrhythmia?
   A. β-Adrenergic blockers
   B. Digoxin
   C. Heparin
   D. Atropine

9. A combination of nitrates and sildenafil (Viagra®) can cause
   A. stroke.
   B. hypotension.
   C. heart murmur.
   D. hypertension.

10. Hypertension with an unknown etiology is referred to as
    A. secondary hypertension.
    B. malignant hypertension.
    C. familial hypertension.
    D. primary hypertension.

11. The trade name of clonidine is which of the following?
    A. Corgard®
    B. Catapres®
    C. Aldomet®
    D. Lopressor®

12. Which of the following agents has become the mainstay of LDL-reducing therapy?
    A. Calcium channel blockers
    B. Cardiac glycosides
    C. Angiotensin II receptor antagonists
    D. Statins

13. Which of the following is the initial treatment of hypertension?
    A. β-Blockers
    B. Antiarrhythmic drugs
    C. Antihyperlipidemic drugs
    D. Cardiac glycosides

14. Which of the following is an antagonist of warfarin?
    A. Vitamin D
    B. Vitamin A
    C. Vitamin K
    D. Niacin

15. Which of the following is the generic name of Aramine®?
    A. Dopamine
    B. Metaraminol
    C. Ephedrine
    D. Epinephrine

25

Digestive System Drugs

OBJECTIVES

Upon completion of this chapter, the reader should be able to

1. Identify the common adverse effects of major laxative, antidiarrheal, and antiemetic drugs.
2. Explain the mechanisms of action and therapeutic effects of antacids.
3. Describe H₂-receptor antagonists.
4. Explain the newest H₂-receptor antagonists.
5. Define proton pump inhibitor agents and their indications.
6. Explain treatment for the bacterium *Helicobacter pylori*.
7. Name the five major classifications of the laxatives.
8. Identify the most effective antidiarrheal agents.
9. Explain adsorbent agents and their indications.

GLOSSARY

antacid mixtures Drugs used to treat pain related to peptic ulcer disorders; provide more even sustained action than single antacids and permit lower dosage.

bulimia An eating disorder characterized by binge eating followed by purging.

bulk-forming laxatives Natural or synthetic polysaccharide derivatives that absorb water to soften the stool and increase bulk to stimulate peristalsis.

calcium carbonate A substance that causes acid rebound, which may delay ulcer-related pain relief and ulcer healing.

chemical digestion Alteration of food into different forms through chemicals and enzymes.

emollient laxatives A substance that acts as a surfactant by allowing absorption of water into the stool.

liquid antacid Drug used to treat pain related to peptic ulcer disorders; has a greater buffering capacity than tablets.

lubricant laxative A substance such as mineral oil that works by increasing water retention in the stool to soften it.

mechanical digestion The breakdown of large food particles into smaller pieces by physical means.

saline laxatives Substances that create an osmotic effect to increase water content and volume of stool.

stimulant laxatives Substances that stimulate bowel mobility and increase secretion of fluids in the bowel.

stool softeners Substances that decrease the consistency of stool by reducing surface tension.

OVERVIEW

The digestive tract is a hollow tube extending from the mouth to the anus. The purpose of the digestive system is to break down (digest) food into particles that are small and simple enough to be absorbed. The digestive system ingests food, digests it, absorbs the end-products of digestion, and eliminates waste. There are two forms of digestion: mechanical and chemical. **Mechanical digestion** is the breakdown of large food particles into smaller pieces by physical means. This process is usually achieved by chewing and by the mashing actions of the muscles in the digestive tract. **Chemical digestion** is the chemical alteration of food. For example, a protein changes chemically into amino acid. Substances such as digestive enzymes, acid, and bile accomplish chemical digestion.

The digested food is absorbed by movement across the lining of the digestive tract into the blood. Digested nutrients eventually reach every cell in the body. Elimination of waste products is the last stage of the digestive process. Some water is also eliminated in the feces.

ANATOMY REVIEW

The digestive system consists of the digestive tract (several organs) and accessory glands of digestion. It contains the digestive tube of the body through which food passes from the mouth to the esophagus, stomach, and intestines. The accessory glands secrete digestive enzymes, which break down food substances in preparation for absorption into the bloodstream.

The gastrointestinal (GI) tract digests, stores and absorbs nutrients, and eliminates wastes. Figure 25-1 is an illustration of the digestive system.

ACID PEPTIC DISEASES

In general, ulcers occur whenever there is an increase in acid secretion or a decrease in mucosal resistance. Mucosal injury in acid peptic diseases includes gastric ulcer, duodenal ulcer, and gastroesophageal reflux disease, which are mediated by gastric acid. Hydrochloric acid is secreted by the parietal cells in the body of the stomach. It is regulated by adjacent endocrines, such as gastrin, or by histamine, somatostatin, and prostaglandin E_2. Gastrin is a relatively weak stimulus of the parietal cells. It acts primarily to cause the release of histamine, which is the most potent stimulus of acid secretion, and acts as the common mediator. Histamine antagonists inhibit acid secretion that is stimulated by gastrin and acetylcholine, as well as by histamine.

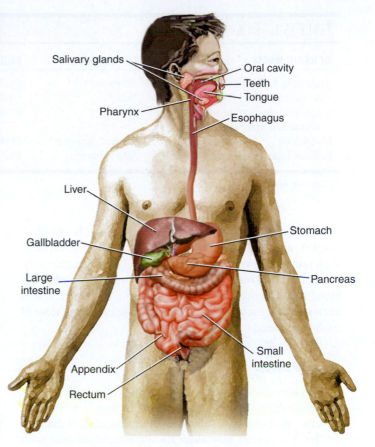

Figure 25-1. The digestive system.

Antacids

The various types of antacids differ in cation content, neutralizing capacity, duration of action, side effects, and cost. These factors must be considered when an antacid is chosen for therapeutic use. Antacids are over-the-counter (OTC) drugs. The most common antacids are shown in Table 25-1. The most widely used antacids are sodium bicarbonate, calcium carbonate, aluminum hydroxide, and magnesium hydroxide.

Mechanism of Action

Antacids neutralize hydrochloric acid and raise gastric pH, thus inhibiting pepsin (a gastric enzyme). Antacids reduce the concentration and total load of acid in the gastric contents. By increasing gastric pH, antacids also inhibit pepsin activity. In addition, they strengthen the gastric mucosal barrier.

Therapeutic Uses

These agents are used widely for the relief of heartburn and dyspepsia. The primary role of antacids in the management of acid peptic disorders is the relief of pain. Nonsystemic antacids (magnesium or aluminum substances) are preferred to systemic antacids such as sodium bicarbonate for intensive

TABLE 25-1. Common Antacids			
GENERIC NAME	**TRADE NAME**	**ROUTE OF ADMINISTRATION**	**COMMON DOSAGE RANGE**
Aluminum hydroxide	Amphojel®	Oral	500–1500 mg 3–6 ×/day
Calcium carbonate	Tums®	Oral, IV	0.5–2 g as needed
Magnesium hydroxide and aluminum hydroxide	Maalox®	Oral	5–15 mL liquid or 622–1244 mg tablets
Magaldrate	Riopan®, Iosopan®	Oral	480–1080 mg (5–10 mL)
Sodium bicarbonate (baking soda)	Alka Seltzer®	Oral, IV	300 mg–2 g/day

IV, intravenous.

ulcer therapy because the risk of alkalosis is avoided. **Liquid antacid** forms have a greater buffering capacity than tablets. However, tablets are more convenient to carry. **Antacid mixtures** such as aluminum hydroxide with magnesium hydroxide provide more even, sustained action than single-agent antacids and permit use of a lower dose of each compound.

Adverse Effects

Constipation can occur in patients using calcium carbonate- and aluminum-containing antacids. Diarrhea is a common adverse effect of magnesium-containing antacids. If diarrhea occurs, the patient may alternate the antacid mixture with aluminum hydroxide. Hypophosphatemia and osteomalacia can occur with long-term use of aluminum hydroxide, but these conditions can also occur with short-term use in severely malnourished patients, such as alcoholics. **Calcium carbonate** usually is avoided because it causes acid rebound and may delay pain relief and ulcer healing. Another potential adverse effect of this compound is hypercalcemia.

Calcium carbonate- and magnesium-containing antacids should be used cautiously in patients with severe renal disease. Sodium bicarbonate is contraindicated in patients with hypertension, congestive heart failure, severe renal disease, and edema. It should not be used for ulcer therapy. All antacids should be used cautiously in elderly patients and patients with renal impairment. Chronic administration of calcium carbonate-containing antacids should be avoided because of hypercalcemia.

Drug Interactions

Because antacids alter gastric pH and affect absorption of ingested substances, they have a high potential for drug interactions. To ensure consistent absorption and therapeutic efficacy, orally administered drugs should be given 30 to 60 minutes before antacids. These agents bind with tetracycline to inhibit its absorption, reducing its therapeutic efficacy. Antacids may destroy the coating of enteric-coated drugs, leading to premature drug dissolution in the stomach. Antacids may interfere with the absorption of many drugs, including cimetidine, ranitidine, digoxin, isoniazid, iron products, anticholinergics, and phenothiazines.

H₂-Receptor Antagonists

There are three types of histamine receptors. One of these types mediates acid secretion by gastric parietal cells and is inhibited by the H₂-receptor-blocking drugs. These drugs may be preferred to other antiulcer agents because of their convenience of use and lack of effect on GI motility. H₂-receptor antagonists are listed in Table 25-2.

Mechanism of Action

Cimetidine was the first H₂-receptor antagonist approved for clinical use. It blocks the H₂ receptor on the parietal cells of the stomach, thus decreasing gastric acid secretion.

Therapeutic Uses

H₂-receptor antagonists are used to promote healing of gastric and duodenal ulcers and for hypersecretory states such as Zollinger-Ellison syndrome. Prototypes of H₂-receptor antagonists include cimetidine, famotidine, nizatidine, and ranitidine. They are a remarkably safe group of drugs.

Cimetidines are available in OTC forms for the treatment of acute gastric ulcer, duodenal ulcer, and gastroesophageal reflux. Cimetidine is also used in the treatment of Zollinger-Ellison syndrome.

Famotidine is the most potent H₂-receptor antagonist. After a 40 mg dose, mean nocturnal gastric acid secretion is reduced by 94% for up to 10 hours. It is recommended for the short-term treatment of mucosal ulcers of the GI tract. Famotidine is absorbed incompletely. It should be used in a lower dosage and at longer dosing intervals in patients with severe renal insufficiency.

The newest H₂-receptor antagonist, nizatidine, may be used to treat and prevent recurrence of duodenal ulcers. It is also used for gastric ulcers and gastroesophageal reflux. More than 90% of an oral dose is excreted in the urine within 12 hours and 60% is excreted as unchanged drug.

TABLE 25-2. H₂-Receptor Antagonists

GENERIC NAME	BRAND NAME	ROUTE OF ADMINISTRATION	COMMON DOSAGE RANGE
Cimetidine	Tagamet®	Oral, IM, IV	PO: 300 mg qid; IM, IV: 300 mg
Famotidine	Pepcid®	Oral, IV	40 mg
Nizatidine	Axid®	Oral	150 mg bid
Ranitidine	Zantac®	Oral, IM, IV	PO: 150 mg bid; IM, IV: 50 mg q6–8h

IV, intravenous; IM, intramuscular; PO, oral.

Therefore, it should be used at a reduced dosage in patients with severe renal insufficiency.

Ranitidine is a more potent drug. It is 5 to 10 times more potent than cimetidine. Ranitidine requires less frequent dosing than cimetidine. It is an H₂-receptor antagonist indicated for the short-term treatment of duodenal ulcers and the management of hypersecretory conditions such as Zollinger-Ellison syndrome. The pharmacokinetic profile of ranitidine is similar to that of cimetidine.

Adverse Effects

The list of adverse reactions with H₂-receptor antagonists is long, but the incidence is low. Among the side effects associated with all four drugs are headache, dizziness, malaise, myalgia, nausea, diarrhea, constipation, rashes, pruritus, and impotence.

Adverse effects of cimetidine include low incidence of headache and skin rash. Cimetidine is contraindicated in patients with hypersensitivity and in pregnant and lactating women. It is not the drug of choice for elderly patients, because it may increase susceptibility to mental disturbances. It can also induce gynecomastia and impotence. Cimetidine can interact with warfarin and theophylline.

Adverse reactions from using famotidine may include headache, dizziness, constipation, and diarrhea.

Adverse reactions to nizatidine include somnolence, sweating, and urticaria. The safety and efficacy of nizatidine in children have not been established.

Adverse effects of ranitidine include headache, malaise, dizziness, constipation, nausea, abdominal pain, and rash. It should not be used during pregnancy unless needed. Ranitidine is secreted in milk; therefore, it should not be given to nursing mothers unless absolutely necessary.

Drug Interactions

Cimetidine increases the risk of decreased white blood cell counts with antimetabolites and alkylating agents. It also increases serum levels and the risk of toxicity of warfarin-type anticoagulants, phenytoin, β-adrenergic blocking agents, alcohol, quinidine, lidocaine, theophylline, chloroquine, and diazepam.

Nizatidine increases serum salicylate levels with aspirin. Ranitidine also increases effects of warfarin and toxicity of lidocaine and decreases the effectiveness of diazepam and its clearance.

Proton Pump Inhibitors

The final common pathway in gastric acid secretion is the proton pump—an H⁺/K⁺-adenosine triphosphatase. The physiological essence of this enzyme is the exchange of hydrogen ions for potassium ions. Thus, hydrogen is secreted by the parietal cell into the gastric lumen in exchange for potassium. The proton pump inhibitors should be taken before meals, because these drugs are more potent when they are taken orally and before meals. They are also absorbed more effectively in the morning.

Mechanism of Action

Proton pump inhibitors or gastric pump inhibitors inhibit H⁺ and K⁺ ions, which generate gastric acids.

Therapeutic Uses

Proton pump inhibitors are widely used in short-term therapy of duodenal and gastric ulcers. Proton pump inhibitor agents are also used in the treatment of gastroesophageal reflux disease and for long-term treatment of pathological hypersecretory conditions such as Zollinger-Ellison syndrome. Examples of proton pump inhibitors are shown in Table 25-3.

TABLE 25-3. Proton Pump Inhibitors

GENERIC NAME	TRADE NAME	ROUTE OF ADMINISTRATION	COMMON DOSAGE RANGE
Omeprazole	Prilosec®	Oral	20–40 mg/day
Lansoprazole	Prevacid®	Oral	15–30 mg/day
Rabeprazole sodium	Aciphex®	Oral	20–60 mg/day

Omeprazole is used in the treatment of acid peptic disorders. It is approved for the short-term treatment of duodenal ulcers, severe gastroesophageal reflux, and hypersecretory conditions. It is also effective in the prevention of ulcers caused by nonsteroidal anti-inflammatory drugs and their complications. The antisecretory effect of omeprazole occurs within 1 hour, with the maximum effect occurring within 2 hours.

Lansoprazole suppresses gastric acid formation in the stomach. Lansoprazole is indicated for the short-term treatment of acute duodenal ulcer, gastric ulcer, and erosive esophagitis. It is most effective if given 30 to 60 minutes before a meal. Like other proton pump inhibitors, it is very effective in the healing of acid peptic disease.

Adverse Effects

The proton pump inhibitors have many side effects, but they occur rarely. Headache, diarrhea, abdominal pain, dizziness, rash, and constipation are seen with about the same frequency as that with H_2-receptor antagonists.

Adverse reactions to omeprazole include headache, diarrhea, abdominal pain, nausea, dizziness, vomiting, and constipation. It is contraindicated for long-term use in patients with gastroesophageal reflux disease and duodenal ulcers and in lactating women.

Adverse effects of lansoprazole are fatigue, dizziness, headache, nausea, diarrhea, constipation, anorexia, or increased appetite. Contraindications include hypersensitivity to lansoprazole, lactation, pregnancy, and severe hepatic impairment.

Drug Interactions

Omeprazole increases serum levels and potentially toxicity of benzodiazepines, phenytoin, and warfarin. This agent shows decreased absorption with sucralfate (these drugs should be given at least 30 minutes apart).

Lansoprazole decreases serum levels if taken concurrently with sucralfate. It decreases serum levels of ketoconazole and theophylline.

Rabeprazole increases serum levels and potentially increases the toxicity of benzodiazepines when taken concurrently.

Treatment for *Helicobacter pylori* with Ulcer

Peptic ulcer disease has been believed to be caused by high gastric secretions. The bacterium *H. pylori* is found in 75% of duodenal ulcers. In chronic peptic ulcer, it has been found that eradication of the bacterium prevents ulcer relapse in about 95% of patients. There is also a relationship between *Helicobacter* infection and adenocarcinoma of the stomach. Treatments for patients with peptic ulcers usually are antacids, H_2-receptor antagonists, or proton pump inhibitors; other drugs are added as necessary. For eradication

of *H. pylori* and healing of duodenal and gastric ulcers in drug therapy, special antibiotics must be added. These antibiotics include amoxicillin (Amoxil®), clarithromycin (Biaxin®), tetracycline (Achromycin®), and metronidazole (Flagyl®). Bismuth products such as bismuth subsalicylate (Pepto-Bismol®) and ranitidine bismuth citrate must also be added. Bismuth compounds are highly effective when combined with proton pump inhibitors and/or antibiotics. Eradication rates with these combinations are greater than 80%. Side effects with bismuth products include neurotoxicity, dark stools and tongue, headache, diarrhea, and abdominal pain. For the treatment of *H. pylori* with ulcer, antisecretory agents (proton pump inhibitors) should be included. Therefore, combination drugs for *H. pylori* infections should be used as follows:

- Helidac® (bismuth, metronidazole, and tetracycline)
- Prevpac® (amoxicillin, clarithromycin, and lansoprazole)
- Tritec® (ranitidine bismuth)

The goals of treatment of active *H. pylori*–associated ulcers are to relieve dyspeptic symptoms, to promote ulcer healing, and to eradicate *H. pylori* infection.

DIARRHEA

Diarrhea is the manifestation of many illnesses. Its etiology includes infections (bacterial, viral, fungal, and parasitic), irritable bowel syndrome, inflammatory bowel disease (ulcerative colitis and Crohn's disease), toxins (food poisoning), drugs, and other causes. Treatment should be focused on the underlying cause.

Antidiarrheal Agents

The use of antidiarrheal agents is occasionally necessary for convenience or for conditions for which there is no primary treatment. The most commonly used antidiarrheals are anticholinergics, opioid narcotics, meperidine congeners (diphenoxylate), and loperamide. Opioid antidiarrheals are the most effective drugs for controlling diarrhea. Selected agents used to treat diarrhea are shown in Table 25-4.

Mechanism of Action

The mechanism of action for anticholinergics and opioid narcotics is discussed in Chapters 23 and 27.

Therapeutic Uses

Antidiarrheal agents are used to treat diarrhea, which is a symptom of bowel disorders and not a disorder itself. The management of diarrhea depends on finding the underlying cause, replacing water and electrolytes as needed, reducing

TABLE 25-4. Antidiarrheals

GENERIC NAME	TRADE NAME	ROUTE OF ADMINISTRATION	COMMON DOSAGE RANGE
Bismuth subsalicylate	Kaopectate;®	Oral	60–120 mL after each loose stool
	Pepto-Bismol®	Oral	15 mL every 30–60 min or 2 tablets/ 2 capsules every 30–60 min
Camphorated opium tincture (paregoric) [Schedule III]		Oral	5–10 mL after loose stool, q2h up to qid if needed
Difenoxin with atropine	Motofen®	Oral	1–8 mg/day
Diphenoxylate with atropine	Lomotil®	Oral	5–20 mg/day
Furazolidone	Furoxone®	Oral	Tablets: 25–100 mg/day; liquid 25–200 mg/day
Kaolin-pectin	Kaopectate®	Oral	60–120 mL after each loose stool
Loperamide	Imodium®	Oral	2–16 mg/day

cramping, and reducing the passage of stools. Diarrhea is usually self-limiting and resolves without further effects. Diarrhea in children may become a medical emergency in as few as 24 hours because of the loss of electrolytes.

Adverse Effects

Adverse effects of anticholinergics and opioid narcotics are discussed in Chapters 23 and 27.

Drug Interactions

Drug interactions are also discussed in Chapters 23 and 27.

GAS RETENTION

Production of excessive amounts of gas results from relief of gastric and intestinal distention. Gas retention is caused by swallowing of air, peptic ulcer, dyspepsia, irritable bowel disease, and diverticulitis (inflammation of the colon). Other factors for production of gas in the GI tract include consumption of gas-forming foods such as beans, onions, and cabbage or gas formation after gastroscopy and bowel radiography.

Antiflatulent Agents

Medications to reduce excessive gas or to prevent formation of gas in the GI tract include some antacids or carminatives (substances that stimulate the expulsion of gas from the GI tract and also increase muscle tone, thereby stimulating peristalsis) that are available as OTC drugs. Simethicone is the most common active ingredient agent used in products such as Phazyme®, Mylanta®, and Gas-X®. Simethicone disperses in the GI tract and prevents the formation of gas pockets.

Mechanism of Action

The actual mechanism of action for antiflatulents is unknown, but the predominant theory is that these agents reduce the surface tension of small air bubbles trapped in the GI tract. This allows them to coalesce into larger bubbles, which are more easily eliminated than the smaller ones.

Therapeutic Uses

Antiflatulents are used to prevent formation and retention of gas in the GI tract. Another use of antiflatulents is to relieve gas after gastroscopy and bowel radiography.

Adverse Effects

Antiflatulents are generally safe and have no side effects.

Drug Interactions

No drug interactions with the use of antiflatulents have been reported.

CONSTIPATION

Constipation is difficult or infrequent passage of stool. Normal stool frequency ranges from two to three times daily to two to three times per week. Because constipation is a symptom rather than a disease, a medical evaluation should be undertaken in patients who develop constipation.

Laxatives

Laxatives are drugs that either accelerate fecal passage or decrease fecal consistency. They work by promoting one or more of the mechanisms that cause diarrhea. Because of the wide availability and marketing of OTC laxatives, there is a potential that an appropriate diagnosis will not be sought.

Mechanism of Action

Laxatives are divided into several categories as a function of their mechanism of action: bulk-forming, saline, stimulant, emollient, and lubricant. Laxatives should not be taken if nausea, vomiting, or abdominal pain is present.

Bulk-forming laxatives are natural or synthetic polysaccharide derivatives that absorb water to soften the stool and increase bulk, which stimulates peristalsis. Bulk-forming laxatives work in both the small and large intestines. The onset of action of these agents is slow between 12 and 72 hours. All bulk-forming agents must be given with at least 8 ounces of water to minimize the possibility of constipation that is experienced by some patients. Some bulk-forming drugs may contain sugar, so diabetic patients should use sugar-free products. Bulk-forming agents should not be used if patients have an obstructing bowel lesion, intestinal strictures, or Crohn's disease, because they can make these conditions worse, which could possibly result in bowel perforation.

Saline laxatives work by creating an osmotic effect that increases the water content and volume of the stool. This increased volume results in distention of the intestinal lumen, causing increased peristalsis and bowl motility. The onset of action varies, depending on the effect and dosage form. Rectal formulations such as enemas or suppositories have an onset of action of 5 to 30 minutes, whereas oral preparations work within 3 to 6 hours.

Stimulant laxatives work in the small and large intestine to stimulate bowel motility and increase the secretion of fluids into the bowel. All stimulant laxatives can cause abdominal cramping. Also, chronic use of stimulant laxatives may cause cathartic colon, which results in poor functioning of the colon, resembling the symptoms of ulcerative colitis. Oral preparations usually have an onset of action within 6 to 10 hours. Rectal preparations usually have an onset of action within 30 to 60 minutes.

Emollient laxatives act as surfactants by allowing absorption of water into the stool, which makes the softened stool easier to pass. These agents are particularly useful for patients who must avoid straining to pass hard stools, such as those who have recently had a myocardial infarction or rectal surgery. Emollient laxatives have a slow onset of action (24 to 72 hours), which is why they are not considered the drug of choice for severe acute constipation. They are more useful for preventing constipation.

A **lubricant laxative** (e.g., mineral oil) works in the colon to increase water retention in the stool to soften it. Mineral oil has an onset of action of between 6 to 8 hours. Table 25-5 shows the most commonly used laxatives.

Stool softeners decrease the consistency of stools by reducing the surface tension. Stool softeners permit easier penetration and mixing of fats and fluids with the fecal mass. This results in a softer, more easily passed stool. Docusate acts as a detergent and stool softener. It usually takes 1 to 3 days to be effective. Stool softeners have a wide margin of safety and few potential adverse reactions. Stool softeners are combined with laxatives in medications such as Peri-Colace® and Doxidan® to soften stools while enhancing stool evacuation (see Table 25-5).

Therapeutic Uses

Laxatives are used prophylactically in patients who should avoid straining during defecation and for treatment of constipation associated with hard, dry stools.

Adverse Effects

Stool softeners have a wide margin of safety and few potential adverse reactions.

Drug Interactions

These agents may increase systemic absorption of mineral oil.

VOMITING

One of the causes of vomiting is infectious diseases that can directly irritate vomiting centers to inhibit impulses going to the stomach. Certain drugs, radiation, and chemotherapy may irritate the GI tract or stimulate the chemoreceptor trigger zone and vomiting center in the brain (medulla). After surgery, particularly abdominal surgery, nausea and vomiting are common. The main neurotransmitters that produce nausea and vomiting include dopamine, serotonin, and acetylcholine. Persistent vomiting may cause dehydration, electrolyte imbalance, metabolic alkalosis, and arrhythmias, which, in turn, may precipitate further vomiting.

Emetics

An emetic is a drug that induces vomiting. Emetics may act directly by stimulation of the medulla oblongata (such as apomorphine, morphine, and digitalis), or they may act reflexively by irritant action on the GI tract (such as copper sulfate, mustard, sodium chloride, and zinc sulfate). It should be remembered that a nasogastric tube is a safer and more efficient tool for emptying the stomach.

Mechanism of Action

Syrup of ipecac is the OTC drug used to induce vomiting. It is an emetic that is used on some occasions in the United States, but is no longer recommended for home use. This agent stimulates the chemoreceptors of the vomiting reflex,

TABLE 25-5. Laxatives and Stool Softeners

GENERIC NAME	TRADE NAME	ROUTE OF ADMINISTRATION	COMMON DOSAGE RANGE
Bulk-Forming Laxatives			
Methylcellulose	Citrucel®, Unifiber®	Oral	500–6000 mg/day
Psyllium seed	Metamucil®, Perdiem®	Oral	1 tsp in 8 oz water up to qid
Polycarbophil	Mitrolan®, Fiberall® chewable tablets	Oral	2 tablets up to qid
Fecal Softener Laxatives			
Docusate	Colace®, Dialose®, Modane®, Regutol®, Surfak®	Oral	240–960 mg/day
Saline and Osmotic Laxatives			
Magnesium citrate	Citrate of Magnesia®	Oral	1000–6000 mg/day
Magnesium hydroxide	Phillips'® Milk of Magnesia	Oral	15 mL hs
Magnesium sulfate (epsom salt)		Oral	10–30 g/day
sodium phosphate	Fleet® Enema®, Fleet® Phospho-Soda®	Rectal	133 mL/day
Glycerin		Rectal	2–4 g/day
Lactulose	Sani-Supp®	Oral	15–60 mL/day
sorbitol	Cephulac®	Oral, rectal	30–150 mL/day
Stimulant Laxatives			
Bisacodyl	Dulcolax®	Oral, rectal	PO: 10–15 mg.; rectal: 1 suppository
Cascara sagrada (bitter bark)		Oral	800–1600 mg/day
Senna	Senokot®	Oral	10–15 mL or 2 tablets hs
Castor oil	Emulsoil®, Purge®	Oral	45–60 mL/day
Oral Lubricant Laxatives			
Mineral oil	Kondremul®, Agoral®, Petrolagar®		2–15 tsp/day
Stool Softeners			
Docusate sodium	Colace®	Oral, rectal	1–4 tablets/capsules/day
Docusate calcium	Surfak®	Oral, rectal	240 mg/day
Docusate potassium	Dialose®	Oral, rectal	PO: 1–3 capsules daily; rectal: 1 suppository

and irritates the gastric mucosa to cause vomiting. Approximately 80 to 90% of people taking the medication begin vomiting within 20 to 30 minutes. The administration of ipecac should be followed by a full 8-ounce glass of water to promote vomiting. If vomiting does not occur in 30 minutes, another dose may be given. In most cases, ipecac is not absorbed because it is removed in vomitus. The effects of ipecac are stopped with activated charcoal. The misuse of ipecac has occurred in persons with eating disorders, such as **bulimia**, which may result in ipecac toxicity (muscle weakness and cardiotoxic effects).

Therapeutic Uses

Emetics are usually used for cases of poisoning or drug overdose. The nearest poison control center should be called before these medications are used. Syrup of ipecac is the OTC drug used to bring about vomiting that should be in a home emergency kit.

Adverse Effects

Emetics should not be used in patients who are unconscious or semicomatose or if coma is expected imminently. These agents should not be used in patients with severe heart disease or women in the advanced stage of pregnancy. They are contraindicated for poisoning caused by corrosive or petroleum products.

Drug Interactions

Drug interactions with emetic drugs are rare. Other medications should not be taken with syrup of ipecac, because vomiting is produced quickly, which will not allow enough time for the other medications to be absorbed.

TABLE 25-6. *Common Antiemetic Agents*

GENERIC NAME	TRADE NAME	ROUTE OF ADMINISTRATION	COMMON DOSAGE RANGE
Serotonin Antagonists			
Ondansetron	Zofran®	Oral, IV	IV: 3–0.15 mg/kg doses; PO: 8 mg tid
Granisetron	Kytril®	Oral, IV	IV: 10 mcg/kg; PO: 1 mg
Dolasetron	Anzemet®	Oral, IV	20–100 mg/day
Dopamine Antagonists			
Promethazine	Phenergan®	Oral, IM, IV	25–50 mg/day
Droperidol	Inapsine®	IM, IV	1–10 mg/day
Metoclopramide	Reglan®	Oral, IM, IV	10–30 mg/day
Antihistamine and Anticholinergics			
Diphenhydramine	Benadryl®	Oral, IM, IV	25–150 mg/day
Scopolamine patch	Transderm-Scop®, Transderm-V®	Transdermal	1 mg/3 days
Dimenhydrinate	Dramamine®	Oral, IM, IV	50–150 mg/day
Meclizine	Antivert, Antrizine®, Bonine®	Oral	25–50 mg/day
Corticosteroids			
Dexamethasone	Decadron®, Deronil®	Oral, IM, IV	PO: 0.75–9 mg/day; IM: 8–16 mg/day; IV: 0.5–9 mg/day
Sedatives			
Diazepam	Diastat®, Valium®	Oral, IM, IV, rectal	2–30 mg/day
Lorazepam	Ativan®	Oral, IM	0.5–10 mg/day

IV, intravenous; IM, intramuscular; PO; oral.

Antiemetics

Antiemetics are used to prevent or relieve nausea and vomiting that are associated with many different disorders. Table 25-6 shows the most commonly used antiemetics.

Mechanism of Action

The mechanism of action of antiemetics is largely unknown, except that they help to relax the portion of the brain controlling the muscles that cause vomiting.

Therapeutic Uses

These agents are used for treatment of drug overdose and for some types of poisoning. They are also prescribed for certain conditions that are associated with vomiting, such as motion sickness, and for postchemotherapy vomiting.

Adverse Effects

Because drowsiness is a common side effect of most of the antiemetics, patients should be cautioned not to drive or operate hazardous machinery while they are taking these drugs.

Drug Interactions

Different types of antiemetics may have differing drug interactions. For example, serotonin antagonists usually have no drug interactions whereas the effects of dopamine are altered by antiemetics, which are antagonistic.

ADSORBENTS

Adsorbent agents have the ability to adsorb gases, toxins, and bacteria. Only certain materials that possess chemical adsorptive properties are able to effectively detoxify and adsorb gases resulting from abnormal intestinal fermentation. These substances are kaolin and activated charcoal. Many of the nonsystemic antacids may operate as adsorbents and to protect internal structures. Antacids commonly are combined with kaolin or other adsorbents.

Mechanism of Action

These agents adsorb toxic substances entering the GI tract by inhibiting GI adsorption.

Therapeutic Uses

Adsorbents are used for acute treatment of many forms of poisoning, primarily as emergency antidotes. They are the emergency treatment of choice for poisoning with virtually all drugs and chemicals. Charcoal capsules also are used for the relief of flatulence and the discomfort caused by abdominal gas.

Adverse Effects

Adverse effects include vomiting (related to rapid ingestion of high doses), constipation, diarrhea, and black stools.

Drug Interactions

Adsorption with activated charcoal can inactivate the effects of syrup of ipecac and laxatives. Adsorbents decrease the effectiveness of other medications.

SUMMARY

The function of the GI tract includes digestion, storage, food absorption, and waste elimination. Varieties of drugs used include antacids, H_2-receptor antagonists, proton pump inhibitors, antidiarrheals, laxatives, antiemetics, and adsorbents. Gastric ulcer, duodenal ulcer, and gastroesophageal reflux disease are accompanied by increased secretion of hydrochloric acid for which antacids, H_2-receptor antagonists, and proton pump inhibitors should be used. Peptic ulcer, which may be caused by *Helicobacter pylori* bacteria, should be treated with the combination of special antibiotics, bismuth products, and proton pump inhibitors. Several different laxative drugs either accelerate fecal passage or decrease fecal consistency. Antiemetics are used to prevent or relieve nausea and vomiting. Adsorbents are used primarily as emergency antidotes for many forms of poisoning.

CRITICAL THINKING

1. Explain proton pump inhibitors.
2. Discuss H_2-receptor antagonists.

REVIEW QUESTIONS

1. Gastrin hormones that are released from the stomach act primarily to release
   A. histamine.
   B. pepsin.
   C. pancreatic enzymes.
   D. all of the above.

2. The generic name of Amphojel® is
   A. magaldrate.
   B. sodium bicarbonate.
   C. aluminum hydroxide.
   D. calcium carbonate.

3. Sodium bicarbonate is contraindicated in patients with
   A. congestive heart failure.
   B. severe renal disease.
   C. hypertension.
   D. all of the above.

4. Which of the following H_2-receptor antagonists was the first drug approved for clinical use?
   A. Famotidine
   B. Nizatidine
   C. Ranitidine
   D. Cimetidine

5. The generic name of Axid® is
   A. cimetidine.
   B. nizatidine.
   C. famotidine.
   D. ranitidine.

6. Which of the following laxatives is particularly useful in patients who recently had rectal surgery to avoid straining to pass hard stools?
   A. Lubricant
   B. Emollient
   C. Saline
   D. Stimulant

7. Which of the following is the generic name of Dulcolax®?
   A. Bisacodyl
   B. Docusate
   C. Senna
   D. Cascara sagrada

8. For eradication of *Helicobacter pylori* with ulcer one should combine
   A. bismuth products and proton pump inhibitors.
   B. antibiotics, bismuth, and proton pump inhibitors.
   C. proton pump inhibitors and antibiotics.
   D. antibiotics and bismuth products.

9. The generic name of Tagamet® is
   A. ranitidine.
   B. nizatidine.
   C. famotidine.
   D. cimetidine.

10. Chronic administration of calcium carbonate–containing antacids may cause
    A. hyperparathyroidism.
    B. hypercalcemia.
    C. hypertension.
    D. hyperglycemia.

Continues

11. Which of the following is the purpose of the therapeutic uses of activated charcoal?
    A. Decreased effectiveness of other medications
    B. Decreased blood sugar level
    C. Relief of vomiting and diarrhea
    D. Relief of flatulence and the discomfort of abdominal gas

12. Which of the following agents is used for treatment of vomiting after chemotherapy?
    A. Mineral oil
    B. Scopolamine patch
    C. Senna
    D. Magnesium citrate

13. The trade name of diphenoxylate with atropine is
    A. Imodium®.
    B. Furoxone®.
    C. Lomotil®.
    D. Motofen®.

14. Which of the following is an adverse effect of antiflatulents?
    A. Coma
    B. Vomiting
    C. Headache
    D. Generally none

OBJECTIVES

Upon completion of this chapter, the reader should be able to

1. Explain the location of the major endocrine glands and their hormone secretion.
2. Describe the effect of thyroxine on the body organs.
3. Define the role of calcitonin hormone in calcium metabolism.
4. Explain diabetes mellitus.
5. Name some risk factors for development of diabetes mellitus in older adults.
6. Describe different types of insulin.
7. Define gonadal hormones.
8. Explain side effects of estrogen therapy.
9. Describe indications for testosterone therapy.

GLOSSARY

acromegaly An overdevelopment of the bones of the hands, face, and feet as a result of excess growth hormone secreted as an adult.

adrenogenital syndrome A disorder resulting from excess secretion of androgens.

Conn's syndrome A disorder resulting from excess secretion of aldosterone.

Cushing's syndrome A disorder resulting from an excess of glucocorticoid hormones, which raises the blood glucose level.

depot-medroxyprogesterone (Depo-Provera®) A long-acting progestin.

dwarfism Reduction in growth of long bones as a result of too little growth hormone secretion during childhood.

ethinyl estradiol A chemical derivative of natural estrogens.

gigantism A disorder resulting from excess growth hormone secreted before puberty.

glucagon A hormone that works antagonistically with insulin and is released when blood glucose levels fall below normal.

hirsutism Excessive hair growth.

hormone A natural chemical secreted into the bloodstream from the endocrine glands to regulate and control the activity of an organ or tissues in another part of the body.

hyperactive Secretion of an excessive amount of a substance.

hypercalcemia A disorder resulting from an overactive parathyroid gland.

GLOSSARY continued

hyperpituitarism A disorder resulting from overactivity of the pituitary gland.

hypoactive Secretion of an inadequate amount of a substance.

insulin A hormone synthesized and secreted by the pancreas.

levonorgestrel A contraceptive implant; also known as the Norplant® system.

Lugol's solution A popular strong iodide solution containing 5% iodine and 10% potassium iodide and saturated solution of potassium iodide.

mestranol A chemical derivative of natural estrogens.

neurohypophysis The posterior pituitary gland.

Norplant® system A contraceptive implant; also known as levonorgestrel.

tremors Shakiness of the hands.

OVERVIEW

The endocrine system consists of specialized cell clusters, glands, hormones, and target tissues. The glands and cell clusters secrete hormones and chemical transmitters in response to stimulation from the nervous system and other sites. Together with the nervous system, the endocrine system regulates and integrates the body's metabolic activities and maintains internal homeostasis. Each target tissue has receptors for specific hormones. Hormones connect with the receptors, and the resulting hormone-receptor complex triggers the target cell's response.

ANATOMY REVIEW

The endocrine system is composed of endocrine glands, which are distributed throughout the body. Endocrine glands secrete hormones, or chemical messengers, directly into the bloodstream. The major organs of the endocrine system are the hypothalamus, the pituitary gland, the thyroid gland, the parathyroid glands, the adrenal glands, the pancreas, the testes, and the ovaries (see Figure 26-1).

Most glandular activity is controlled by the pituitary gland, which is sometimes called the *master gland*. The pituitary itself is controlled by the hypothalamus.

The body is conservative and secretes hormones only as needed. For example, **insulin** is secreted when the blood glucose level rises. Another hormone, **glucagon**, works antagonistically to insulin and is released when the blood glucose level falls below normal. Hormones are potent chemicals; thus their circulating levels must be carefully controlled. When the level of a hormone is adequate, its further release is stopped. This type of control is called a negative feedback mechanism.

Overactivity or underactivity of a gland is the malfunction that most commonly causes endocrine diseases. If a gland secretes an excessive amount of its hormone, it is **hyperactive**. When a gland fails to secrete its hormone or secretes an inadequate amount, it is **hypoactive**.

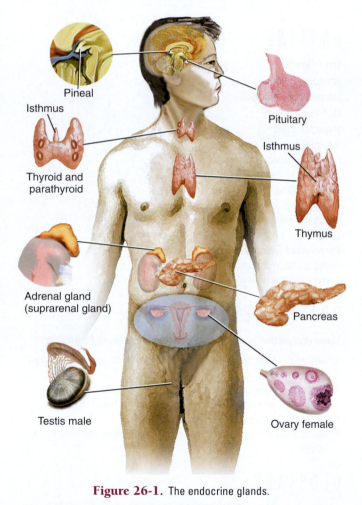

Pineal

Isthmus

Pituitary

Isthmus

Thyroid and parathyroid

Thymus

Adrenal gland (suprarenal gland)

Pancreas

Testis male

Ovary female

Figure 26-1. The endocrine glands.

HORMONAL REGULATION

The hypothalamus is the main integrative center for the endocrine and autonomic nervous systems. The hypothalamus helps control some endocrine glands by neural and hormonal pathways. Neural pathways connect the hypothalamus to the posterior pituitary gland. Neural stimulation of the posterior pituitary causes the secretion of two effector hormones: antidiuretic hormone (also known as vasopressin) and oxytocin.

The hypothalamus also exerts hormonal control at the anterior pituitary gland, by releasing and inhibiting hormones and factors, which arrive by a portal system. Hypothalamic hormones stimulate the pituitary glands to synthesize and release trophic hormones. These hormones include corticotropin (also called adrenocorticotropic hormone), thyroid-stimulating hormone, and gonadotropins, such as luteinizing hormone and follicle-stimulating hormone. Secretion of trophic hormones stimulates the adrenal cortex, thyroid gland, and gonads. Hypothalamic hormones also stimulate the pituitary gland to release or inhibit the release of effector hormones, such as growth hormone and prolactin.

HORMONES

Hormones are natural chemical substances secreted into the bloodstream from the endocrine glands that regulate and control the activity of an organ or tissues in another part of the body. The synthesis and secretion of many hormones are controlled by other hormones or changes in the concentration of essential chemicals or electrolytes in the blood. Drugs and diseases can modify hormone secretion as well as specific hormone effects at target organs. Some hormones affect nearly all the tissues of the body but the action of others is restricted to a few tissues or organs. Some hormones such as thyroxine and epinephrine are relatively simple amino acid derivatives. Several groups of hormones such as those produced by the adrenal cortex and the gonads are steroids whereas the pituitary, parathyroid, and pancreatic hormones are polypeptides or proteins. A list of major hormones and endocrine glands is provided in Table 26-1. Hormones from the various endocrine glands work together to regulate vital processes of the body and include the following:

1. Secretions in the digestive tract
2. Energy production
3. Composition and volume of extracellular fluid
4. Adaptation and immunity
5. Growth and development
6. Reproduction and lactation

Inactivation of hormones occurs enzymatically in the blood, liver, kidneys, or target tissues. Hormones are secreted primarily via the urine and, to a lesser extent, via the bile. In medicine, hormones generally are used in three ways: (1) for replacement therapy; (2) for pharmacologic effects beyond replacement; and (3) for endocrine system diagnostic testing.

TABLE 26-1. Endocrine Glands and Their Hormones

GLAND	HORMONES
Hypothalamus	Releasing and inhibiting hormones such as GnRH, GHRH, and TRH
Pituitary	
Anterior	GH
	ACTH
	TSH
	LH
	FSH
	PRL
Posterior (hormone storage site)	Oxytocin
	Vasopressin (antidiuretic hormone)
Thyroid	Thyroid hormone (T_4 and T_3)
Parathyroid	Parathyroid hormone
	Calcitonin
Thymus	Thymosin
Pancreas (islets of Langerhans)	Insulin
	Glucagon
Adrenal	
Cortex	Cortisol (a glucocorticoid)
	Aldosterone (a mineralocorticoid)
	Androgens
Medulla	Epinephrine
	Norepinephrine
Testes	Testosterone
Ovaries	Estrogen
	Progesterone

ACTH, adrenocorticotropic hormone; FSH, follicle-stimulation hormone; GH, growth hormone; GHRH, gonadotropin hormone-releasing hormone; GnRH, gonadotropin-releasing hormone; LH, luteinizing hormone; PRL, prolactin; T_3, triiodothyronine; T_4, thyroxine; TRH, thyrotropin-releasing hormone; TSH, thyroid-stimulation hormone.

HYPOTHALAMUS

The hypothalamus is a portion of the diencephalon, which is located in the deep central portion of the brain, forming the floor and part of the lateral wall of the third ventricle. It activates, controls, and integrates the peripheral autonomic nervous system, endocrine processes, and many somatic functions, such as body temperature, sleep, and appetite.

PITUITARY GLAND

The pituitary gland is a small gland situated at the base of the brain that secretes hormones directly into the bloodstream to control and regulate the other endocrine glands. It consists of two lobes, an anterior lobe (adenohypophysis) and a posterior lobe (neurohypophysis), that are under the influence of hypothalamic hormones. These hormones control the secretion of specific tropic hormones that regulate peripheral endocrine gland secretions and target tissues.

Anterior Pituitary Gland

The anterior lobe of the pituitary gland is particularly important in sustaining life. The anterior pituitary gland secretes at least six hormones: growth hormone (somatotropin, GH), adrenocorticotropic hormone (ACTH), thyroid-stimulating hormone (TSH), follicle-stimulating hormone (FSH), luteinizing hormone (LH), and prolactin (PRL). Figure 26-2

illustrates the major hormones of the pituitary gland and their principal target organs.

Hyperpituitarism

Hyperpituitarism can result from damage to the anterior lobe of the pituitary gland or from inadequate secretion of hormones. The most noticeable result of hyperpituitarism is the effect of excessive amounts of GH. This condition produces excessive growth (a "giant") if the hypersecretion of GH occurs before puberty, which is called **gigantism**. If excessive production of growth hormone occurs after puberty, it can result

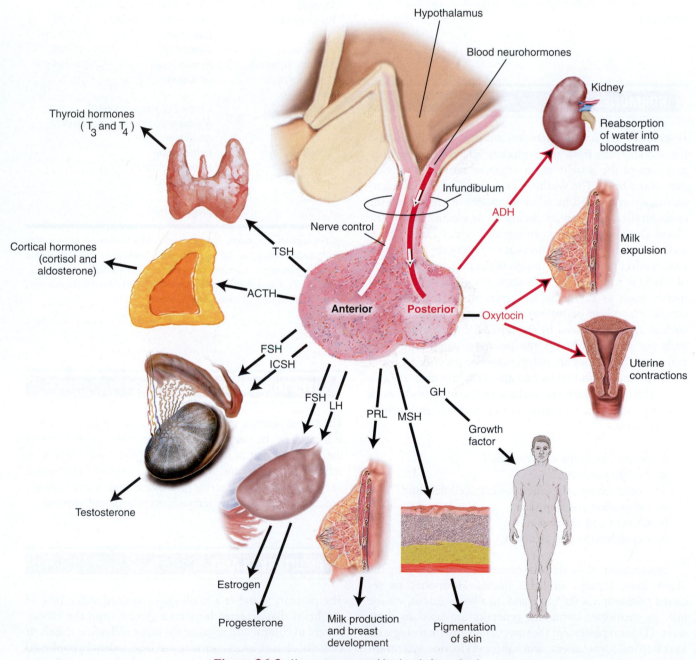

Figure 26-2. Hormones secreted by the pituitary gland.

in **acromegaly**. Treatment of these two conditions includes surgery, radiation, and medication therapy. Growth hormone insufficiency during childhood causes **dwarfism**.

Mechanism of Action.   Although still widely debated, it is believed that the mechanism of action of GH is similar to that of tryptophan, which is released by increased levels of serotonin at night.

Therapeutic Uses.   The main indication for replacement of GH is growth failure in children. Treatment is prolonged and may cause a 6-inch growth in height. Special agents used for hormone therapy of the pituitary gland are listed in Table 26-2.

Adverse Effects.   The side effects of GH therapy include headache, increased blood glucose levels, and muscle weakness.

Drug Interactions.   Depending on dosage, anabolic steroids, androgens, estrogens, and thyroid hormones may interact with GH.

Adrenocorticotropic Hormone

ACTH is another hormone from the anterior pituitary gland that stimulates the growth of the adrenal gland cortex and the secretion of corticosteroids. Under normal conditions, a diurnal rhythm occurs in ACTH secretion, with an increase beginning after the first few hours of sleep and reaching a peak at the time a person awakens. ACTH is used generally for diagnostic testing, and not for therapeutic purposes. The adverse effects include insomnia, delayed wound healing, increased susceptibility to infection, and acne (see Table 26-2).

Thyroid-Stimulating Hormone

TSH is a substance secreted by the anterior lobe of the pituitary gland that controls the release of thyroid hormone and is necessary for the growth and function of the thyroid gland. TSH stimulates the thyroid gland to increase the uptake of iodine and increase the synthesis and release of thyroid hormones. It is prescribed for hypothyroidism and diagnostic tests.

Posterior Pituitary Gland

The posterior lobe of the pituitary gland, or the **neurohypophysis**, is the release point of antidiuretic hormone (ADH, or vasopressin) and oxytocin. The neurohypophysis releases ADH when stimulated by the hypothalamus. The hormone acts on the distal and collecting tubules of the kidneys. As a result of this action, kidneys will be more permeable to water and reduce the volume of the urine. The neurohypophysis releases oxytocin under appropriate stimulation from the hypothalamus. Oxytocin produces powerful contractions of the pregnant uterus and causes milk to flow from lactating breasts. Hypofunction of the posterior pituitary gland results in diabetes insipidus.

Diabetes Insipidus

Diabetes insipidus is a disease that results from a deficiency of ADH. In the absence of ADH, water is not reabsorbed by the kidney and is excreted in the urine. Excessive water loss

---

TABLE 26-2.   Special Agents Used for Hormone Therapy of the Pituitary Gland

GENERIC NAME	TRADE NAME	ROUTE OF ADMINISTRATION	COMMON DOSAGE RANGE
Anterior Pituitary Gland			
Growth hormone			
Somatrem	Protropin®	IM, SC	0.30–0.3 mg/kg/day
Somatropin	Humatrope®	IM, SC	0.02–0.1 mg/kg/day
(DNA recombinant)	Genotropin®	IM	0.006–0.0125 mg/kg/day
Sermorelin	Geref®	SC	30 mcg/kg/day
Growth hormone inhibitor			
Octreotide	Sandostatin®	SC	50 mcg initial; 100–600 mcg/day
Adrenocortical hormones			
Corticotropin	Acthar®, ACTH-80®	IM, IV	20–80 units/day
Cosyntropin	Cortrosyn®	IM, IV (diagnostic agent)	0.25–0.75 mg/day
Posterior Pituitary Gland			
Vasopressin	Pitressin®	SC, IM, IV, intranasal	5–10 U bid or tid
Desmopressin	DDAVP®	Oral, nasal spray, IV, SC	0.1–0.4 mL/day nasally; as a single dose 0.5–1 mL/day SC or IV
Lypressin	Diapid® (is now an orphan drug; free to patients)	Nasal spray	1–2 puffs qid

IM, intramuscular; IV, intravenous; SC, subcutaneous.

can quickly lead to dehydration. Whenever possible, the underlying cause of diabetes insipidus must be corrected. ADH is used for diabetes insipidus.

THYROID GLAND

The thyroid gland is located in the anterior neck and is the largest of the endocrine glands. The thyroid gland secretes three hormones essential for proper regulation of metabolism. The thyroid gland, through its hormone, thyroxine, governs cellular oxygen consumption, and, thus, energy and heart production. The thyroid gland secretes thyroxine (T_4), triiodothyronine (T_3), and calcitonin. Iodine is essential for thyroid hormone synthesis. About 1 mg of iodine is required per week, most of which is ingested in food, water, and iodized table salt. T_3 and T_4 are controlled by THS from the anterior pituitary gland. Thyroid secretion is maintained by secretion of THS. Decreased serum levels of T_3 and T_4 stimulate release of thyrotropin-releasing hormone (TRH) from the hypothalamus, which stimulates the pituitary gland to secrete TSH. Then, TSH stimulates the thyroid gland to release thyroxine and thyroglobulin. The hormone calcitonin has a very important role in calcium metabolism. Normally, calcitonin decreases the level of blood calcium; therefore, this hormone is used to treat hypercalcemia, osteoporosis, and Paget's disease. The thyroid gland synthesizes, stores, and secretes hormones that are important to growth, development, and metabolic rate.

Hypothyroidism

Hypothyroidism is a deficiency disease that causes cretinism (mental and physical retardation) in children. It is usually due to a deficiency of iodine in the mother's diet during pregnancy. Hypothyroidism in adults results from hypothalamic pituitary or thyroid insufficiency or resistance to thyroid hormone, which is called myxedema. The disorder can progress to hyposecretion of thyroid hormone. Hypothyroidism is more common in women than in men in the United States. Hyposecretion of thyroid hormones may also be caused by lack of iodine in the diet surgical removal of the thyroid, or radiation therapy to the thyroid. It may also be due to pituitary dysfunction. Thyroid hormones are approved for supplemental or replacement needs with hypothyroidism. Thyroid hormones are usually initiated in small doses until adequate response is reached. Long-term use of thyroxine may cause osteoporosis or progressive loss of bone mass in postmenopausal women. Thyroxine is contraindicated in patients who have had a myocardial infarction. Table 26-3 shows common drugs used for disorders of the thyroid gland.

Hyperthyroidism

Hyperthyroidism is a condition of excessive amounts of thyroxine (see Figure 26-3). This condition stimulates cellular metabolism and increases respiration and body temperature. Hyperthyroidism causes nervousness and **tremors** (shakiness of the hands).

TABLE 26-3. Selected Medications Used as Drugs for the Thyroid Gland

GENERIC NAME	TRADE NAME	ROUTE OF ADMINISTRATION	COMMON DOSAGE RANGE
Natural Thyroid Replacement			
Desiccated thyroid (T_3 and T_4)	Armour Thyroid®	Oral	None; dosage is based on natural production of the hormone per patient
Synthetic Thyroid Replacement			
Levothyroxine (thyroxine, T_4)	Levothroid®, Synthroid®	Oral, IV	0.05–0.2 mg/day
Liothyronine (triiodothyronine, T_3)	Cytomel®	Oral, IV	25–75 mcg/day
Liotrix (T_3, T_4)	Cytomel®, Thyrolar®	Oral	6–120 mg/day
Thyroglobulin (T_3 and T_4)	Euthroid®, Proloid®	Oral	60–120 mg/day
Antithyroid Preparations			
Potassium iodide, iodine	Lugol's, SSKI Solution®	Oral	40–200 mcg/day
Thioamide derivatives			
Propylthiouracil	Propyl-Thyracil®	Oral	300–900 mg/day; maintenance: 100–150 mg/day
Methimazole	Tapazole®	Oral	Initial: 15–60 mg/day; maintenance: 5–15 mg/day
Calcitonin			
Calcitonin, salmon	Calcimar®	SC/IM, nasal spray	10–100 IU/day; nasal: 200 IU/day

IM, intramuscular; SC, subcutaneous.

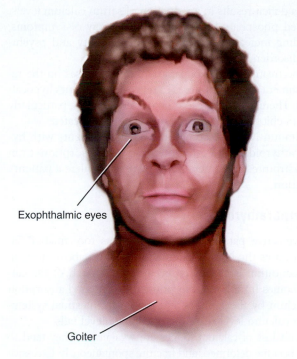

Exophthalmic eyes

Goiter

Figure 26-3. Hyperthyroidism

Graves' disease is an example of hyperthyroidism. This disease is far more common in women than in men and usually affects young women. Graves' disease can sometimes be treated with medication that inhibits the synthesis of thyroxine or by administration of radioactive iodine, which destroys the thyroid gland. Removal of the thyroid gland, however, may be necessary. If the gland is removed, hormonal supplements must be given. With partial removal of the thyroid gland, the remaining portion still secretes hormones.

Antithyroid Agents

An antithyroid drug is a chemical agent that lowers the basal metabolic rate by interfering with the formation, release, or action of thyroid hormones. A variety of compounds are known as antithyroid drugs. Iodine thyroid products (iodide ions), radioactive iodine, methimazole, and propylthiouracil are the drugs of choice for antithyroid therapy. These medications can cross the placenta and stop fetal thyroid development. They also pass through breast milk to affect the infant. Selected medications used as drugs for the thyroid gland are shown in Table 26-3.

Radioactive Iodine

Radioactive iodine is a radioactive isotope of iodine used in diagnostic radiology and radiotherapy. It is used particularly for the treatment of some thyroid conditions. Most radioactive iodine is excreted in urine, but small amounts may be found in sputum, perspiration, feces, and vomitus.

Mechanism of Action.   Destructive radiation (beta rays) is emitted by the trapped isotope, which effectively destroys thyroid cells without appreciably damaging surrounding tissue.

Therapeutic Uses.   Radioactive forms of iodides, in particular sodium iodide ^{131}I are commonly used for the diagnosis and treatment of hyperthyroidism. When administered orally or intravenously, ^{131}I is rapidly taken up and stored by the thyroid gland.

Adverse Effects.   The extent of thyroid damage can be predetermined by carefully selecting the proper dose of isotope. Low doses are used diagnostically and pose a minimal risk to thyroid tissue, although high doses can effectively destroy all thyroid function, resulting in hypothyroidism.

Drug Interactions.   Iodine interacts with selenium and possibly with vanadium.

Iodine Thyroid Products

These drugs have been shown to be useful for treatment of mild hyperthyroidism, particularly in young patients.

Mechanism of Action.   Iodine ion (Lugol's solution) inhibits the synthesis of the active thyroid hormones T_3 and T_4 and inhibits the release of these hormones into blood circulation.

Therapeutic Uses.   Iodides may be used in several different forms. The most popular are **Lugol's solution** (strong iodine solution), which contains 5% iodine and 10% potassium iodide, and saturated solution of potassium iodide (SSKI). Iodides are used as adjunctive therapy with antithyroid drugs in preparation for thyroidectomy, treatment of thyrotoxic crisis, or neonatal thyrotoxicosis.

Adverse Effects.   Lugol's solution may cause hypothyroidism, hyperthyroidism, goiter (enlargement of the thyroid), rashes, and swelling of the salivary glands.

Drug Interactions.   Lugol's solution can increase the risk of hypothyroidism if taken concurrently with lithium.

Methimazole

Methimazole is an antithyroid agent.

Mechanism of Action.   Methimazole inhibits the synthesis of thyroid hormones by coupling of iodine.

Therapeutic Uses.   Methimazole has emerged as an effective drug for controlling hyperthyroidism.

Adverse Effects.   Observation of patients using methimazole has shown that adverse effects are not common. Some patients may develop a mild skin rash and agranulocytosis has developed in a small number of patients. In very rare instances, methimazole may affect the central nervous system, causing headache, depression, drowsiness, vertigo, and neuritis.

Drug Interactions. Methimazole increases theophylline clearance and decreases effectiveness if given to hyperthyroid patients. This agent alters the effects of oral anticoagulants. It increases the therapeutic effects and toxicity of digitalis glycosides, metoprolol, and propranolol when hyperthyroid patients become euthyroid.

Propylthiouracil

Propylthiouracil (PTU) is a chemically related antithyroid drug.

Mechanism of Action. PTU inhibits the synthesis of thyroid hormones, partially inhibiting the peripheral conversion of T_4 to T_3.

Therapeutic Uses. PTU is used for treatment of hyperthyroidism.

Adverse Effects. PTU may cause neuritis, vertigo, drowsiness, depression, and headache. Other adverse effects of this agent include skin rash, skin pigmentation, loss of hair, nausea, vomiting, loss of taste, hepatitis, or nephritis.

Drug Interactions. PTU increases the risk of oral bleeding. The other side effects of PTU are similar to those of methimazole.

PARATHYROID GLAND

Four tiny glands, called the parathyroid glands, lie along the posterior surface of the thyroid gland. The parathyroid glands secrete parathyroid hormone (PTH, parathormone). The stimulus for the release of PTH is a low plasma level of calcium. PTH has three target organs: bones, digestive tract (intestines), and kidneys. The overall effect of PTH is to increase plasma calcium levels. Spontaneous atrophy or injury such as removal of the parathyroid glands is followed by a decrease in the concentration of serum calcium and an increase in the concentration of serum phosphorus. These changes can be reversed by the parenteral administration of extracts from parathyroid glands of domestic animals. The thyroid gland also produces a hormone (thyrocalcitonin) that reduces serum calcium concentrations. The biological function of calcitonin is to prevent excessive hypercalcemia from PTH activity. When plasma calcium levels are elevated, thyrocalcitonin is released in increased quantities. Thus, it tends to oppose PTH but at different cell targets.

Hypoparathyroidism

A deficiency of PTH may occur in some patients for a variety of reasons, ranging from a congenital absence of the parathyroid glands to surgery involving the thyroid gland.

Such a deficit results in a reduction of serum calcium levels, elevated phosphate levels, and a wide array of symptoms, including increased neuromuscular irritability and psychiatric disorders.

The treatment of hypoparathyroidism focuses on the replenishment of calcium stores to reverse the patient's hypocalcemia. Therefore, administration of calcium salts, particularly calcium chloride and calcium gluconate, is indicated.

Vitamin D is also commonly used in patients with hypoparathyroidism to promote calcium absorption from the gastrointestinal tract and to further stabilize a patient's condition.

Hyperparathyroidism

An overactive parathyroid gland secretes too much PTH, which raises the level of circulating calcium above normal. This condition is called **hypercalcemia**. Much of the calcium comes from bone resorption and increased absorption of calcium by the kidneys and the gastrointestinal system. As the calcium level rises, the phosphate level falls.

With loss of calcium, bones are weakened. They tend to bend, become deformed, and fracture spontaneously. Excessive amounts of calcium cause development of kidney stones because calcium forms insoluble compounds. Calcium deposited within the walls of the blood vessels makes them hard. Calcium deposits may also be found in the stomach and lungs.

Therapy for hyperparathyroidism often includes surgery. However, phosphate supplementation and/or potent diuretics, such as furosemide (Lasix®), may be administered to promote an increase in the excretion of excess calcium. Calcitonin may also be used for treating hypercalcemia.

ADRENAL GLANDS

The adrenal glands are located at the top of each kidney. They consist of two parts—the outer cortex and the inner medulla (see Figure 26-4). The adrenal cortex synthesizes three important classes of hormones: glucocorticoids (cortisol), mineralocorticoids (primarily aldosterone), and androgens. The cortex of the adrenal gland is one of the endocrine structures most vital for normal metabolic function. The medulla secretes two hormones, epinephrine and norepinephrine.

Hyperadrenalism

Overactivity of the adrenal cortex can take different forms, depending on which group of hormones is secreted in excess. **Cushing's syndrome** develops from an excess of glucocorticoids, the hormones that raise the blood glucose level. In excess, they cause hyperglycemia.

The patient with Cushing's syndrome retains salt and water, resulting in hypertension and atherosclerosis, which develops as a result of excess circulating lipids.

Conn's syndrome is another form of hyperadrenalism. In this disease, aldosterone is secreted in excess. This causes

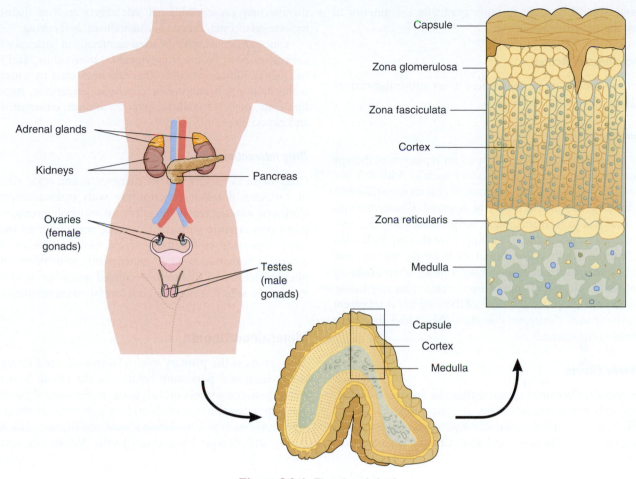

Figure 26-4. The adrenal glands.

retention of sodium and water and abnormal loss of potassium in the urine. Hypertension develops as a result of the salt imbalance and water retention. Muscles become weak to the point of paralysis.

Adrenogenital syndrome is another form of hyperadrenalism, also called adrenal virilism. In this condition, androgens (male hormones) are secreted in excess. If this excessive secretion occurs in children, it stimulates premature sexual development: The sex organs of a male child greatly enlarge, and in a girl, the clitoris enlarges, a male distribution of hair develops, and the voice deepens.

Excessive androgen secretion in a woman causes masculinization (adrenal virilism). Hair develops on the face, a condition called **hirsutism**, and the hairline recedes. The breasts diminish in size, the clitoris enlarges, and ovulation and menstruation cease.

Hypoadrenalism

Addison's disease results when the adrenal glands fail to produce corticosteroids and aldosterone. The adrenal glands may be destroyed by cancer or infection or inhibited by chronic use of steroid hormones, such as prednisone.

With aldosterone deficiency the patient is unable to retain salt and water. The kidneys are unable to concentrate urine, and eventually dehydration ensues. Severe dehydration can ultimately lead to shock. Cortisol deficiency leads to low blood glucose levels, impaired protein and carbohydrate metabolism, and generalized weakness.

Glucocorticoids

The glucocorticoids or adrenocortical steroid hormones (such as cortisone), which increase formation of glycogen from fatty acids and proteins rather than from carbohydrates (gluconeogenesis), exert an anti-inflammatory effect and influence many body functions. The glucocorticoids are controlled by release of ACTH from the pituitary gland. With stressful conditions such as trauma, major surgery, and infection, secretion of the hormone from the adrenal glands increases dramatically up to 300 mg daily (the basal production rate averages 30 mg every 24 hours). Prolonged use of glucocorticoids may suppress the pituitary gland, and the body will not produce its own hormone. If these hormones are used for extended periods of time, they cannot be stopped abruptly, and a step-down dosage should be used to taper gradually the amount of drug the patient is receiving.

Mechanism of Action

Cortisone enters target cells where it has anti-inflammatory and immunosuppressive effects.

Therapeutic Uses

The adrenal corticosteroids are used for replacement therapy in patients with adrenal insufficiency such as Addison's disease. In this condition, administration of both mineralocorticoids and glucocorticoids may be required. Glucocorticoids are also used to treat rheumatic, inflammatory, allergic, neoplastic, and other disorders as supportive therapy with other medications. These agents are of value for decreasing some cerebral edemas. Certain skin conditions are often markedly improved with use of topical or systemic glucocorticoids. Probably the most common use of these agents is treatment of arthritic and rheumatic disorders. Table 26-4 lists some adrenal corticosteroids.

Adverse Effects

Certain side effects may appear during the first week of treatment with glucocorticoids. They include euphoria, suicidal depression, psychoses, anorexia, hyperglycemia, increased susceptibility to infections, and acne. Chronic glucocorticoid therapy may cause additional side effects such as diabetes mellitus, glaucoma, cataracts, osteoporosis, and edema.

Glucocorticoids must be used cautiously in patients with congestive heart failure, hypertension, liver failure, and renal failure. Glucocorticoids are contraindicated in patients with emotional instability or psychotic tendencies, hyperlipidemia, diabetes mellitus, hypothyroidism, osteoporosis, and peptic ulcer.

Drug Interactions

Drug interactions increase the therapeutic and toxic effects of cortisone if taken concurrently with troleandomycin. Cortisone also decreases the effects of anticholinesterases if taken concurrently with corticotropin, and profound muscular depression is possible. Steroid blood levels are decreased if cortisone is taken concurrently with phenytoin, phenobarbital, and rifampin. Decreased serum levels of salicylates are seen if it is taken concurrently with cortisone.

Mineralocorticoids

Aldosterone is the primary mineralocorticoid used to regulate sodium and potassium balance in the blood. It is secreted from the adrenocortical tissue. In the normal patient, aldosterone secretion is stimulated by a decrease in circulating volume such as loss of blood, excessive diuresis, low salt intake, and increased potassium levels. Aldosterone secre-

TABLE 26-4. Steroids and Adrenal Corticosteroids

GENERIC NAME	TRADE NAME	ROUTE OF ADMINISTRATION	COMMON DOSAGE RANGE
Glucocorticosteroids			
Betamethasone	Celestone®	Oral, IM, IV, topical	PO: 0.6–7.2 mg/day; IV: up to 9 mg/day
Cortisone	Cortone®	Oral, IM	PO: 25–300 mg/day; IM: 20–330 mg/day
Dexamethasone	Decadron®	Oral, IM, IV	PO: 0.75–9 mg/day; IM: 8–16 mg/day; IV: 0.5–9 mg/day
Fluocinolone	Synalar®	Topical	15–60 g/day
Flurandrenolide ointment	Cordran®	Topical	No common range
Fluticasone	Flovent®, Vanceril®, Beclovent®	Inhaled MDI	40–250 mcg/day
Hydrocortisone	Cortisol®, Cortef®	Oral, IM, IV	PO: 4–48 mg/day; IM, IV: 10–40 mg/day
Methylprednisolone	Depo-Medrol® or Solu-Medrol®	Oral	4–80 mg/day
Paramethasone	Haldrone®	Oral	0.05–2 mg/kg/day
Prednisone	Deltasone", Colisone®, Predcor®,	Oral, topical, gingival, IM	4–60 mg/day
Triamcinolone	Azmacort®, Aristocort® Kenacort®	Oral, IM, IV	5–500 mg based on condition and response
Mineralocorticoids			
Deoxycorticosterone acetate			Not listed for humans
Fludrocortisone	Florinef®	IM, oral	0.1 mg 3 ×/wk to 0.2 mg/day

IM, intramuscular; IV, intravenous; PO, oral.

tion is suppressed by an elevation of sodium levels in the blood (e.g., by excessive dietary salt intake). The amount of aldosterone secreted by the adrenal cortex apparently is affected by the concentration of sodium in body fluids (angiotensins II and III), rather than by the stimulation of the adrenal cortex by ACTH.

Mechanism of Action

Aldosterone promotes sodium reabsorption in the kidneys to preserve extracellular fluid volume (blood). In adrenal insufficiency, an aldosterone deficit occurs, sodium reabsorption is inhibited, and potassium excretion decreases. Hyperkalemia and mild acidosis occur.

Therapeutic Uses

Mineralocorticoids are usually administered in conjunction with glucocorticosteroids for replacement therapy in adrenocortical insufficiency.

Adverse Effects

The adverse effects of mineralocorticoids are sodium and water retention, and loss of potassium (hypokalemia), which may result in edema, weakness, and hypertension. Mineralocorticoids are usually administered in conjunction with glucocorticosteroids as replacement therapy in adrenocortical insufficiency (see Table 26-4).

Drug Interaction

Mineralocorticoids interact with digitalis and diuretics such as potassium-sparing agents.

Adrenal Sex Hormones

The adrenal sex hormones are controlled by the pituitary-releasing hormones, such as FSH and LH. Androgens (male hormones) have a feedback control. Androgens are secreted in the hypothalamic-pituitary axis and circulate to the testes to produce testosterone and release it into the blood. The male produces androgens in the testes and the adrenal cortex. The female produces androgens in the ovaries and adrenal glands. Female hormones include progestin and estrogen, which will be discussed later in this chapter.

PANCREAS

The pancreas produces digestive enzymes that are deposited in the small intestine. Throughout the pancreas, there are islets of specialized cells (islets of Langerhans). The α cells produce glucagons to raise blood glucose levels and β cells

release insulin, which lowers blood glucose levels. When serum blood glucose levels decline, glucagons facilitate the breakdown of glycogen in the liver to glucose. The conversion of glycogen to glucose results in an increase in blood glucose. The release of glucagons stimulates insulin secretion, which then inhibits the release of glucagons. The most important disease involving the endocrine pancreas is diabetes mellitus, a disorder of carbohydrate metabolism that involves either insulin deficiency, insulin resistance, or both. Diabetes, if untreated or uncontrolled, leads to hyperglycemia. Severe hyperglycemia and ketoacidosis may produce diabetic coma or unconsciousness, which requires much higher doses of insulin.

Diabetes Mellitus

Diabetes mellitus is a complex disorder of carbohydrate, fat, and protein metabolism caused by lack of or inefficient use of insulin in the body. The two general classifications for diabetes mellitus are type I, or insulin-dependent diabetes mellitus (IDDM), and type II, or non–insulin-dependent diabetes mellitus (NIDDM). Type I diabetes usually occurs before age 30 and previously was called juvenile-onset diabetes. Type II diabetes was previously known as maturity-onset diabetes because its onset is usually after age 40. About 90% of the diabetic population has type II diabetes. The treatment plan for diabetes mellitus usually includes diet, exercise, and, if necessary, an oral hypoglycemic agent or insulin to help control blood glucose levels. Gestational diabetes, a form of NIDDM, occurs during pregnancy. The onset is during the second and third trimesters. Gestational diabetes affects about 4% of all pregnant women and usually resolves after delivery. It may cause low blood glucose levels, jaundice, or abnormal weight gain in the newborn. Gestational diabetes may be controlled by diet, exercise, and medications. The onset of diabetes later may also be controlled in the same manner. Note that diabetes may be a secondary effect of some drugs. These drugs include oral contraceptives, β-blockers, calcium channel blockers, glucocorticoids, diuretics, phenytoin, and niacin.

Insulin

Normally, insulin is used for treatment of type I diabetic patients whose pancreas does not produce enough insulin. Insulin needs may vary every 6 to 8 hours. Normal fasting insulin levels range from 80 to 100 mg/dL. Insulin preparations are available from three different species including cows, pigs, and humans. Human insulin now is produced by chemical conversion from porcine insulin and by *Escherichia coli*, into which the human genes for insulin have been inserted. The recombinant product has the same physiological properties as insulin from beef or pork but is much less likely to cause allergic reactions. Some patients who have type II diabetes in whom sufficient concentrations of blood glucose are not maintained with dietary regulation

TABLE 26-5. Insulin Preparations

PREPARATION	COMMON NAME	ONSET OF ACTION	DURATION OF ACTION
Short-acting Insulin			
Insulin injection	Regular	30–60 min	6–8 hr
	Regular Humulin®	15 min	6–8 hr
Prompt insulin zinc suspension	Semilente	60–90 min	12–16 hr
Crystalline zinc	Crystalline zinc	30–60 min	4–6 hr
Intermediate-acting Insulin			
Isophane insulin suspension	NPH Humulin®	60–90 min	18–24 hr
	Novolin N®	2 hr	18–24 hr
	Humulin N®	2 hr	18–24 hr
Insulin zinc suspension	Lente	60–150 min	18-24 hr
	Novolin L®	60–150 min	
Long-acting Insulin			
Protamine zinc insulin suspension	PZI	4–8 hr	36 hr
Extended insulin zinc suspension	Ultralente	4–8 hr	36 hr

and oral antidiabetic agents, also need to get insulin when they undergo surgery, have a fever, are under stress, have severe trauma, infection, serious renal or hepatic dysfunction, endocrine dysfunction, or gangrene, or are pregnant. For emergency treatment of ketoacidosis or coma, regular insulin must be administered. Insulin must be given only by injection because it is destroyed by the digestive juices. Most of the insulin used today is U-100. When an excess of insulin is present, serious or dangerous symptoms from hypoglycemia may result. Glucose administration relieves the symptoms of insulin overdosage. Glucagons may also be administered when hypoglycemia is severe after overdosage. Insulins are classified on the basis of their time of pharmacological action as short-acting, intermediate-acting, and long-acting. Most diabetic patients require a combination of short- and long-acting insulin. Table 26-5 shows varieties of insulin and their properties.

Special Consideration. Patients who will be using insulin must be instructed on the rotation method of taking their medication. Insulin is absorbed more rapidly in the arm or thigh, especially with exercise. The abdomen is used for a more consistent absorption. Glucose levels should be checked per the physician's instructions. All insulin should be checked for expiration date and clearness. Insulin should NOT be given if appears cloudy. Vials should not be shaken but rotated in between the hands to mix contents. If regular insulin is to be mixed with NPH or lente insulin, the regular insulin should be drawn into the syringe first. Unopened vials should be stored in the refrigerator, and freezing should be avoided. The vial in use can be stored at room temperature. Vials should not be put in glove compartments, suitcases, or trunks. It is imperative that the physician be called if any adverse reactions to the medications are observed.

Oral Antidiabetic Agents

Type II diabetic patients are treated with oral antidiabetic agents, diet, exercise, and, when necessary, insulin. Today, there are three types of oral antidiabetic agents: first- and second-generation sulfonylureas and a miscellaneous group that includes agents that differ from insulin in mode of action. Table 26-6 shows some examples of hypoglycemic agents and their duration of action.

The advantages of using the second-generation agents are that they have a long duration of action and fewer side effects. Of the first-generation agents, tolazamide also has advantages similar to those of second-generation drugs. Oral hypoglycemic agents are indicated for the treatment of uncomplicated type II diabetes in patients whose diabetes cannot be controlled by diet only. Side effects include nausea, vomiting, headache, blurred vision, sedation, confusion, anxiety, nightmares, and tachycardia. Oral hypoglycemic agents are contraindicated in patients who are receiving sulfonamide or thiazide-type diuretics, who are hypersensitive to the agents, and who have acidosis, severe burns, and severe diarrhea. These agents should not be used in patients with high fevers, severe infections, hyperthyroidism, or kidney function impairment.

Behavior Modification for Diabetes

Because diabetes is a lifelong disorder, education of the patient and the family is probably the most important obligation of the physician who provides initial care. This disease is markedly affected on a daily basis by fluctuations in environmental stress, exercise, diet, and the presence of infections. Therefore, the best persons to monitor and manage the disease are the patients themselves and their families. The teaching curriculum should include explanations by the

TABLE 26-6. Hypoglycemic Agents

GENERIC NAME	TRADE NAME	ROUTE OF ADMINISTRATION	COMMON DOSAGE RANGE
Sulfonylureas			
First-generation			
Acetohexamide	Dymelor®	Oral	250 mg–1.5 g/day
Chlorpropamide	Diabinese®	Oral	Initial: 250 mg/day; maintenance:100–250 mg/day
Tolazamide	Tolinase®	Oral	100–1000 mg/day
Tolbutamide	Orinase®, Mobenol®	Oral	0.25–3 g/day
Second-generation			
Glimepiride	Amaryl®	Oral	1–8 mg/day
Glipizide	Glucotrol®, Glucotrol XL®	Oral	5–30 mg/day
Glyburide	DiaBeta®, Micronase®, Glynase®	Oral	1.25–20 mg/day
Miscellaneous			
Acarbose	Precose®	Oral	25–100 mg tid
Miglitol	Glyset®	Oral	25–50 mg tid
Metformin	Glucophage®	Oral	500–2550 mg/day
Repaglinide	Prandin®	Oral	0.5–16 mg/day

physician or nurse about the nature of diabetes and its potential acute and chronic hazards. Patients should be instructed to recognize these hazards early so that they can be prevented or treated more quickly. The importance of regular testing of capillary blood specimens for glucose concentrations should be stressed and instructions on proper testing and recording of data provided. Moreover, patients should be provided with algorithms that they can use to adjust the timing and quantity of their insulin dose, food, and exercise in response to recorded blood glucose values for optimal blood glucose control. Advice on personal hygiene, including detailed instructions on foot care as well as individual instruction on diet and specific hypoglycemic therapy, should be provided. Vigorous efforts should be made to persuade patients with newly diagnosed diabetes who smoke to give up the habit, because large vessel peripheral vascular disease and debilitating retinopathy are less common in nonsmoking diabetic patients. Behavior modification to achieve adherence to an appropriate diet as well as increased physical activity to expend energy is also required. Cure can be achieved by reducing adipose stores, with consequent restoration of tissue sensitivity to insulin, but weight reduction is hard to achieve and even more difficult to maintain with our current therapies.

GONADAL HORMONES

Three main classes of steroid hormones are produced by gonadal tissues: estrogenic, progestational, and androgenic. The ovary is the primary site for synthesis and secretion of estrogen and progestin hormones in women. The menstrual cycle is regulated by the production of hypothalamic gonadotropin-releasing hormone (GnRH) that stimulates the release of FSH and LH from the anterior pituitary gland. In men and postmenopausal women, the principal source of estrogen is adipose tissue, in which the level of estrogens is regulated in part by the availability of androgenic precursors from the adrenal cortex. The most important androgenic hormone produced by the testes in men is testosterone, although the adrenal cortex also produces some androgenic hormones in both men and women. FSH and LH also regulate testosterone production by specific cells in the testes that control spermatogenesis and the development of primary and secondary sexual characteristics in men.

Ovarian Hormones

The reproductive system of the human female consists of the ovaries, fallopian tubes, uterus, and vagina. The ovaries are known as gonads. They produce ova and form endocrine secretions that initiate and maintain the secondary sex characteristics in women (see Figure 26-5).

The gonadotropins from the pituitary gland are responsible for the development and maintenance of sexual gland functions. FSH stimulates the development of the ovarian follicles up to the point of ovulation. LH promotes the growth of the interstitial cells in the follicle and the formation of the corpus luteum. Natural estrogenic hormones are produced by the ovaries and placenta. Naturally occurring estrogens include estrone, estradiol, and estriol. These substances are also synthesized by a variety of animals. They are found in the blood of both males and females. Most naturally occurring estrogens are not effective when administered orally, because they are rapidly inactivated by the liver. Chemical derivatives

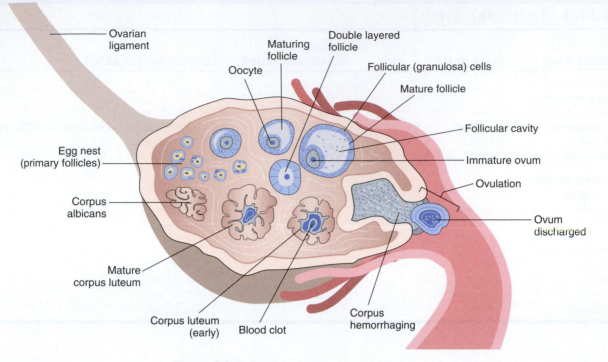

Figure 26-5. An ovary showing a developing ovum.

of the natural estrogens, such as **ethinyl estradiol** and **mestranol**, are only slowly inactivated by the liver and may be administered orally. The natural estrogens and their derivatives may be administered by the intramuscular or subcutaneous route. Estrogens can be used for a variety of conditions. They are used for the treatment of amenorrhea, dysfunctional uterine bleeding, and hirsutism, and for palliative treatment of breast cancer and prostate cancer. They are sometimes used for the relief of menopausal symptoms and also for the prevention of osteoporosis. The beneficial effects of estrogen therapy on irritability, depression, anxiety, memory, and insomnia are more unpredictable. It is not clear whether or not estrogen administration can prevent arteriosclerotic cardiovascular disease. There is a choice of compounds for estrogenic therapy. Major estrogens are listed in Table 26-7. Recently, they have been of value in maintaining healthy cardiac status of women during menopause. Estrogens are also used in primary ovarian failure, atrophic vaginitis, hypogonadism, atrophic urethritis, and prostate cancer. They should not be used in patients who have a sensitivity to any of the ingredients, are pregnant, or have breast cancer, undiagnosed abnormal uterine bleeding, thrombophlebitis, and thromboembolic disorders. The most common adverse effects are nausea, vomiting, breast swelling, fluid retention (weight gain), and thromboembolic disease.

Progesterone

Progesterone is secreted primarily by the ovarian cells in the corpus luteum at the time of ovulation during the female reproductive years. The corpus luteum secretes progesterone only during the last 2 weeks of the menstrual cycle. The greatest amount is secreted during the week after ovulation has taken place. Progesterone is responsible for the changes in the uterine endometrium during the second half of the menstrual cycle, development of the maternal placenta after implantation, and development of the mammary glands. Progesterone also causes an increase in the viscosity of cervical secretions, which impedes the movement of sperm. Progesterone in high doses suppresses the pituitary release of LH and the hypothalamic release of GnRH, thus preventing ovulation. Progesterone also decreases uterine motility. A synthetic form of progesterone produced by a chemical modification is needed because the natural type of hormone would be inactivated by the liver. These synthetic preparations are called progestins. Progesterone is used for irregular uterine bleeding and is combined with estrogen for the treatment of amenorrhea. It is also used for cases of infertility and threatened or habitual abortion. It is contraindicated in patients with thrombophlebitis, liver disease, breast cancer, reproductive organ cancer, undiagnosed vaginal bleeding, missed periods, and a hypersensitivity to the medication or any of the ingredients. Use during pregnancy and breast-feeding is not recommended. Table 26-8 shows the most commonly used progestins.

Contraceptive Agents

Combinations of estrogens and progestins may be used as oral contraceptives in women. This method is nearly 100% effective in preventing pregnancy when used as directed. Oral contraceptives are the most commonly prescribed

TABLE 26-7.   Major Estrogens

GENERIC NAME	TRADE NAME	ROUTE OF ADMINISTRATION	COMMON DOSAGE RANGE
Natural estrogens			
Estradiol	Estrace®, Gynodiol®, Alora®, Climara®	Oral, IM, vaginal	PO IM: 1–20 mg; vaginal cream: 2–4 g
Conjugated estrogens (esterified estrogens)	Premarin®	Oral, IM, vaginal	PO, 0.3 to 2.5 mg qd in cycles; IM, 25 mg; vaginal cream, 2–4 g as directed in cycles
Synthetic estrogens, ethinyl estradiol	Alesse-28®	Oral	2.5–7.5 mg/day
	Mestranol®	Oral	1–30 mg/day
	Quinestrol®	Oral	0.625-0.9 mg/day
Nonsteroidal estrogens	Chlorotrianisene®	Oral	0.2 mg/wk to 0.1 mg/day
	Dienestrol®	Oral, vaginal	12 mg/day; ½ to 2 applicators/day

IM, intramuscular; PO, oral.

TABLE 26-8.   Most Commonly-Used Progestins

GENERIC NAME	TRADE NAME	ROUTE OF ADMINISTRATION	COMMON DOSAGE RANGE
Medroxyprogesterone acetate	Provera®	Oral, IM	IM: 150–400 mg/ day q3mo; PO: 2.5–10 mg/day
Norethindrone	Ortho-Micronor®, Nor-QD®	Oral	2.5–10 mg
Norethindrone acetate	Aygestin®	Oral	2.5–10 mg
Progesterone	Gesterol®	Oral, IM	5–10 mg

IM, intramuscular; PO, oral.

contraceptive agents. Oral contraceptives contain various amounts of estrogen and progestins. The estrogen inhibits ovulation by suppressing the normal secretion of FSH. The progestin inhibits pituitary secretion of LH, causes changes in the cervical mucus that makes it unfavorable to penetration by the sperm, and alters the nature of the endometrium. The use of estrogen-progestin combinations in a cyclic fashion generally results in the inhibition of conception without prevention of menstruation. Most oral contraceptives are taken daily for 20 to 21 days, starting on the fifth day after menstrual bleeding begins. Also available are oral contraceptives with 28-day pill cycles, wherein a pill is taken every day of the cycle so that once started the pill is not stopped. In the 28 day pill cycle, an inactive pill is taken during the week of menstruation, whereas with the 20 to 21 day pill there is a week without medication, and this is when menstruation takes place. The use of oral contraceptives containing only a progestin has been advocated as a means of reducing some of the risk associated with their use. These products, which are sometimes referred to as "minipills," are generally taken continuously rather than cyclically. Because they contain no estrogen, they do not suppress ovulation. Table 26-9 shows the most commonly used contraceptive agents.

A novel form of contraception is the use of a progestin **levonorgestrel** implant, previously known as the **Norplant® system**, which has been off the market since 2002. The system consists of six small Silastic capsules. These are surgically implanted under the skin of the upper arm and may be left in place for up to 5 years. The medication is slowly released from the capsule into the bloodstream, providing constant protection from pregnancy. Like the Norplant® System, **medroxyprogesterone acetate (Depo-Provera®)** is also a long-acting progestin. It is the injectable long-acting progestin, which is approved for contraceptive use in the United States. There has been extensive worldwide experience with this method over the past three decades. The medication is given as a deep intramuscular injection of 150 mg every 3 months and has a contraceptive efficacy of 99.7%. It has been proven safe and is relatively inexpensive. Many women find this method more convenient than use of daily oral contraceptives.

Intrauterine Devices

Intrauterine devices (IUDs) are another type of contraceptive. The only IUDs currently manufactured in the United States are the Progestasert® (which secretes progesterone into the uterus) and the copper-bearing TCu380A®; the

TABLE 26-9. Most Commonly Used Contraceptive Agents

GENERIC NAME	TRADE NAME	ROUTE OF ADMINISTRATION	COMMON DOSAGE RANGE
Monophasic Agents			
Ethinyl estradiol/ norethindrone (in various strengths)	Ovcon®, Loestrin®, Nee®, Genora®, Brevicon®, Modicon®, Norinyl®, Ortho-Novum®	Oral	0.35 mg–0.75 mg/day
Ethinyl estradiol/ drospirenone	Yasmin®	Oral	3 mg/day
Ethinyl estradiol/ norelgestromin	Ortho-Evra®	Transdermal patch	20–150 mg/patch
Estinyl estradiol/ norgestrel	Lo-Ovral®, Ovral®	Oral	0.3 mg/day
Estinyl estradiol/ desogestrel	Desogen®, Ortho-Cept®, Mircette®	Oral	0.03 mg/day
Estinyl estradiol/ levonorgestrel	Alesse®, Levlen®, Nordette®	Oral	0.25–0.5 mg/day
Estinyl estradiol/ ethynodiol diacetate	Demulen®	Oral	1 mg/day
Mestranol/ norethindrone	Genora 1/50®, Norinyl®, Norethrin®, Ortho-Novum®	Oral	0.15 mg/day
Estrogen/progestin	Necon 1/35®, Ortho-Novum 1/35®, Alesse-28®	Oral	0.5–1 mg/day
Biphasic Agents			
Ethinyl estradiol/ norethindrone	Ortho-Novum 10/11®, Nelova 10/11®	Oral	0.5–1 mg/day
Triphasic Agents			
Ethinyl estradiol/ levonorgestrel	Triphasil®, Tri-Levlen®	Oral	
Ethinyl estradiol/ norgestimate	Ortho Tri-cyclin®	Oral	25 mcg/day
Ethinyl estradiol/ norethindrone	Tri/Norinyl®, Ortho-Novum 7/7/7®	Oral	0.1–0.5 mg/day
Estrophasic Agents			
Ethinyl estradiol/ norethindrone	Estrostep®	Oral	1 mg/day
Progestin Only Agents			
Norethindrone	Micronor®, Nor-QD®	Oral	0.35 mg/day
Norgestrel	Ovrette®	Oral	0.3 mg/day
Long-acting Agents			
Levonorgestrel	Norplant®	Subdermal	30–85 mcg/day
Medroxyprogesterone	Depo-Provera®	IM	150 mg/mL every 3 mo
With estradiol	Lunelle®	IM	0.5 mL/mo
Intrauterine progesterone contraceptive system	Progestasert®	IM, IUD	

IM: 5–10 mg/day for 6–8 days

mechanism of action is thought to be related to impaired fertilization due to effects on sperm motility and to abnormal development in the oviduct of ova that may have been fertilized. The TCu380A® must be replaced every 10 years for maximum efficacy. The Progestasert® must be replaced yearly, but has the advantage of causing less cramping and menstrual flow. Other methods used for prevention of pregnancy include the diaphragm and cervical cap, contraceptive foam, cream, film, sponge, jelly, and suppository, and condom.

Diaphragm and Cervical Cap

The diaphragm (with contraceptive jelly) is a safe and effective contraceptive method with features that make it acceptable to some women and not others. The advantages of this method are that it has no systemic side effects and gives significant protection against pregnancy as well as pelvic infection and cervical dysplasia. The cervical cap (with contraceptive jelly) is similar to the diaphragm, but it fits snugly over the cervix only. The cervical cap is more difficult to insert and remove than the diaphragm. The main advantage is that it can be used by women who cannot be fitted for a diaphragm. Because of a small risk of toxic shock syndrome, a cervical cap or diaphragm should not be left in the vagina for more than 12 to 18 hours nor should these devices be used during the menstrual period.

Contraceptive Foam, Cream, Film, Sponge, Jelly, and Suppository

These products are available without prescription, are easy to use, and are fairly effective. All contain the spermicides nonoxynol-9 or octoxynol-9, which also have some virucidal and bactericidal activity. The products have the advantages of being simple to use and easily available. Their disadvantage is a slightly higher failure rate than that for the diaphragm or condom.

Side Effects. The classic side effects associated with birth control drugs are nausea, weight gain, and breast tenderness, which result from the progestin. Other side effects include fluid retention, irregular vaginal bleeding, and skin discoloration. Patients with diabetes mellitus, hypertension, or hypercholesterolemia (increased blood cholesterol levels) should not take contraceptive agents. Several drugs interact with oral contraceptive agents. Some commonly prescribed drugs in this category are phenytoin, phenobarbital (and other barbiturates), primidone, carbamazepine, and rifampin. Women taking these drugs should use another means of contraception for maximum safety. Before the use of any hormonal type of contraception, the patient should have a complete history and physical examination performed. The patient should be informed of the precautions, warnings, adverse effects, and possible side effects. Patients should be made aware that smoking increases the risk of serious adverse effects on the heart and blood vessels from oral contraceptive use. The risk increases with age and heavy smoking (15 or more cigarettes per day) and is quite marked in women older than 35 years of age. Women who use oral contraceptives should not smoke. The incidence and severity of the adverse effects vary with the type of preparation. The most side effects are caused by the estrogens in combination contraceptives, but progestins also cause adverse effects. The estrogen/progestin ratio is important to the type and incidence of side effects. The most serious adverse effects of oral contraceptives include heart attack, stroke, hypertension, or other forms of thromboembolic disease. Table 26-10 summarizes the dose-related effects of oral contraceptives.

Drugs Used during Labor and Delivery

Generally, two types of medications are used during labor and delivery: uterine stimulants and uterine relaxants. Uterine stimulants cause contractions of the myometrium during labor

TABLE 26-10. Dose-Related Side Effects of Oral Contraceptives	
Estrogen Excess	**Progestin Excess**
Nausea	Increased appetite
Hypertension	Weight gain
Breast tenderness	Fatigue
Edema	Acne
Migraine headache	Hair loss
	Depression
Estrogen Deficiency	**Progestin Deficiency**
Early or midcycle bleeding	Late breakthrough bleeding
Increased spotting	Amenorrhea
Hypomenorrhea	Hypermenorrhea

and delivery. Many agents are capable of stimulating the smooth muscle of the uterus, but a few are selective, to be used for the myometrium. These agents are known as oxytocic substances. Oxytocic agents are also used to control postpartum hemorrhage, to cause uterine contraction after cesarean section, or to induce therapeutic abortion after the first trimester. There are three types of oxytocic drugs: synthetic oxytocin, ergot derivatives, and prostaglandins. Oxytocin (Pitocin®, Syntocinon®) is a hormone released from the posterior pituitary gland. Its primary effect is stimulation of the smooth muscle of the uterus and the mammary glands. When oxytocin is used to initiate or stimulate labor, it is generally administered by intravenous infusion. A nasal spray containing oxytocin (Syntocinon®) is available, but it is only indicated for inducing initial milk letdown. Ergot is a complex mixture of substances derived from a fungus. Ergot alkaloids cause powerful contractions of the uterus. This action permits them to be used to control uterine bleeding. These agents are more suitable for use postpartum or postabortion to control bleeding and maintain uterine contraction. Their use is not advised for induction of labor, because ergot agents may damage the fetus. Prostaglandins are chemically related agents that exert wide-ranging effects in the human body. The effects of these agents are comparable to those of oxytocin when they are used as oxytocic agents. The prostaglandins currently approved for use as uterine stimulants are used for induction of second-trimester abortion.

Testicular Hormone

The hypothalamus, anterior pituitary gland, and testes secrete hormones that control male reproductive functions. These hormones initiate and maintain sperm cell production and oversee the development and maintenance of male secondary sex characteristics.

The hypothalamus secretes gonadotropin-releasing hormone, which enters blood vessels leading to the anterior pituitary gland. As discussed earlier in this chapter, LH and FSH are released. Luteinizing hormone (LH) in males, also called interstitial cell-stimulating hormone (ICSH), promotes development of testicular interstitial cells, and they in turn secrete male sex hormones. FSH stimulates the supporting cells of the seminiferous tubules to respond to the effects of the male sex hormone testosterone.

Androgens are secreted mainly in the interstitial tissue of the testes in the male and secondarily in the adrenal glands of both sexes (see Figure 26-6). Androgens include testosterone and androsterone. Inadequate production of androgens in the male may be due to pituitary malfunction. Testosterone stimulates the development of the male secondary sex characteristics, initiates the production of sperm, and enhances the functional capacity of the penis and accessory sex organs. It is used for replacement therapy in androgen deficiency, for the treatment of hypogonadism and cryptorchidism, and for palliative treatment of certain metastatic breast carcinomas in women. Its use is contraindicated in patients with known hypersensitivity to any of its ingredients, in women during pregnancy and lactation, in men with cancer of the breast or suspected cancer of the prostate, and in patients with pituitary insufficiency, a history of myocardial infarction, hypercalcemia, prostatic hyperplasia, hepatic dysfunction, and nephrosis, and in infants and young children. It should be used with caution in elderly patients, in diabetic patients, in those who have hypertension, coronary artery disease, renal disease, hypercholesterolemia, and gynecomastia, and in prepubertal males. Adverse reactions in males include gynecomastia, excessive frequency and duration of penile erection, oligospermia, hirsutism, male pattern baldness, acne, increased or decreased libido, headache, anxiety, and depression. In females adverse reactions include amenorrhea, menstrual irregularities, inhibition of gonadotropin secretion, and virilization (deepening of the voice, clitoral enlargement, increased growth of facial and body hair, and male-type baldness).

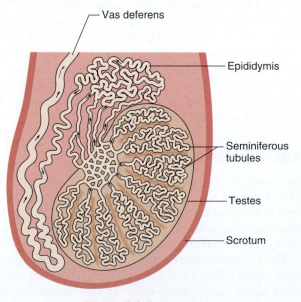

Figure 26-6. The testes.

SUMMARY

The endocrine system provides a means of chemical communication between body parts. The anterior pituitary gland controls activities of the thyroid, adrenal, and sex glands. It also stimulates growth, development, and tissue repair. The pituitary is called the *master gland* for these reasons. Pituitary activity is governed by the hypothalamus in the brain.

Hyperpituitarism causes an excess of growth hormone. This condition, if present before puberty, results in gigantism. In an adult, excessive production of growth hormone leads to acromegaly.

Severe hypopituitarism impedes growth and development in a child, causing dwarfism. Glands that depend on stimulation by the anterior pituitary are the thyroid, adrenal, and sex glands. The posterior pituitary gland releases vasopressin, also called antidiuretic hormone (ADH) and oxytocin. Insufficiency of ADH causes diabetes insipidus.

The rate of metabolism is controlled by the thyroid gland. An enlargement of this gland is called a goiter. Hyperthyroidism, which is an excess of thyroxine, accelerates heart and respiratory activity, increases metabolic rate, and raises body temperature. A congenital lack of thyroxine results in cretinism (mental and physical retardation). Myxedema is a disease of severe hypothyroidism in an adult.

Hormones of the adrenal cortex are essential to life. Aldosterone regulates salt balance and cortisol affects the metabolism of nutrients. The sex hormones estrogen and androgen are also produced by this gland. Hypoactivity of the adrenal cortex is called Addison's disease.

Hyperactivity of the adrenal cortex causes different diseases, depending on which hormones are present in excessive amounts. Cushing's syndrome results from an excess of cortisol, and Conn's syndrome results from excessive aldosterone. Precocious puberty and adrenal virilism develop from too much androgen secretion.

PTH regulates the level of circulating calcium and phosphate. Hyperactivity of the parathyroid glands causes hypercalcemia. The high level of calcium comes primarily from bone resorption that weakens the bones. Hypoparathyroidism reduces the level of calcium in the blood, which results in tetany. Hormones of the pancreas, insulin, and glucagons control the blood glucose level. Lack of insulin causes an increase in blood glucose levels, the condition called diabetes mellitus.

Hypoglycemia, an abnormally low blood glucose level, results from excess insulin. This condition can develop in diabetic patients from an overdosage of insulin.

With loss of calcium, bones are weakened. They tend to bend, become deformed, and fracture spontaneously. Excessive calcium causes formation of kidney stones because calcium forms insoluble compounds. Calcium deposited within the walls of the blood vessels makes them hard. It may also be found in the stomach and lungs.

The therapy for hyperparathyroidism often includes surgery. However, phosphate supplementation and/or potent diuretics, such as furosemide (Lasix®), may be administered to promote an increase in the excretion of excess calcium. Calcitonin may also be used to treat hypercalcemia.

CRITICAL THINKING

1. Make a list of anterior and posterior pituitary hormones.
2. Explain behavior modification for diabetes.

REVIEW QUESTIONS

1. Which of the following is secreted from the pancreas?
   A. Prolactin
   B. Growth hormone
   C. Glucagon
   D. Calcitonin

2. Another name for vasopressin is
   A. testosterone.
   B. cortisol.
   C. prolactin.
   D. antidiuretic hormone.

3. FSH and LH are released from which of the following organs?
   A. Hypothalamus
   B. Pituitary
   C. Ovaries
   D. Pancreas

4. Which of the following is a protein?
   A. Testosterone
   B. Androgen
   C. Growth hormone
   D. Cortisol

5. Which of the following hormones is released from posterior parts of the pituitary gland?
   A. Oxytocin
   B. Growth hormone
   C. Prolactin
   D. Cortisol

6. The glucocorticoid hormones are under the control of
   A. LH.
   B. TSH.
   C. ACTH.
   D. FSH.

7. Which of the following is a side effect of corticosteroids?
   A. Delayed healing with infection
   B. Hypotension
   C. Weight loss
   D. Hypertrophy of the adrenal cortex

8. Which of the following is the trade name of medroxyprogesterone?
   A. Gesterol®
   B. Provera®
   C. Norlutate®
   D. Norlutin®

9. Glucophage® is the trade name of
   A. metformin.
   B. miglitol.
   C. glimepiride.
   D. glipizide.

10. Which of the following agents is used for the diagnosis and treatment of hyperthyroidism?
    A. Thyroxine
    B. Sodium iodide
    C. Parathyroid hormone
    D. Phenytoin

11. Propylthiouracil (PTU) is chemically related to which of the following drugs?
    A. Antineoplastic
    B. Antithyroid
    C. Antiparathyroid
    D. Antidiuretic

12. Progesterone is produced in the corpus luteum, which is located in the
    A. kidneys.
    B. ovaries.
    C. uterus.
    D. testes.

13. A new type of insulin, Humulin®, is preferred because it is
    A. cheaper.
    B. taken orally.
    C. similar to human insulin.
    D. used topically.

14. Which of the following is the trade name of chlorpropamide?
    A. Diabinese®
    B. Dymelor®
    C. Tolinase®
    D. Glucotrol®

15. Insulin is used mainly in which type of diabetes?
    A. Type I
    B. NIDDM
    C. IDDM
    D. A and C

27

Muscle Relaxants and Non-Narcotic Analgesics

OBJECTIVES

Upon completion of this chapter, the reader should be able to

1. Discuss skeletal muscle relaxants.
2. Discuss neuromuscular blocking agents.
3. Name four neuromuscular blocking drugs.
4. Define centrally acting skeletal muscle relaxants.
5. Explain the major side effect of dantrolene (a direct-acting skeletal muscle relaxant).

6. Discuss nonsteroidal anti-inflammatory drugs (NSAIDs).
7. Differentiate salicylate from nonsalicylate nonsteroidal anti-inflammatory drugs.
8. Explain gold compounds.
9. Name drugs for gouty arthritis.

GLOSSARY

analgesics Pain-relieving drugs.

arthritis Disease of the joints.

bursa A closed sac with a synovial membrane lining.

corticosteroids The most potent and consistently effective anti-inflammatory agents that are currently available for relief of respiratory conditions.

derivatives Substances that are made from another substance.

haloperidol An antipsychotic drug.

nonsteroidal anti-inflammatory drugs (NSAIDs) Drugs that inhibit the synthesis of the prostaglandin responsible for causing pain and inflammation.

osteoporosis A disease characterized by a reduction in bone mass.

propoxyphene An analgesic.

spasticity A form of muscular contraction.

succinylcholine A depolarizing, noncompetitive, neuromuscular blocking agent.

tardive dyskinesia An abnormal condition characterized by involuntary repetitious movements of the muscles of the face, limbs, and trunk.

OVERVIEW

Some of the most common disorders in humans at any age are those affecting the musculoskeletal system. Medications used to treat these conditions may be classified in two broad categories: skeletal muscle relaxants and nonsteroid anti-inflammatory drugs. Drugs prescribed to treat musculoskeletal conditions such as rheumatoid arthritis, osteoarthritis, muscle spasms, gout, bursitis, and tendonitis include aspirin, nonsteroidal anti-inflammatory drugs, gold salts, and skeletal muscle relaxants.

ANATOMY REVIEW

The musculoskeletal system actually consists of two different systems that work closely together for the frame and movement of the body. The musculoskeletal system includes a collection of connective tissue, muscles, bones, and joints (see Figure 27-1).

The muscular system consists of three types of muscles: skeletal muscle, which attaches to bones and joints by connective tissue (tendons and ligaments), smooth muscle, and myocardium. Muscles require electrical impulses from motor nerves for stimulation (see Figure 27-2). When the muscles

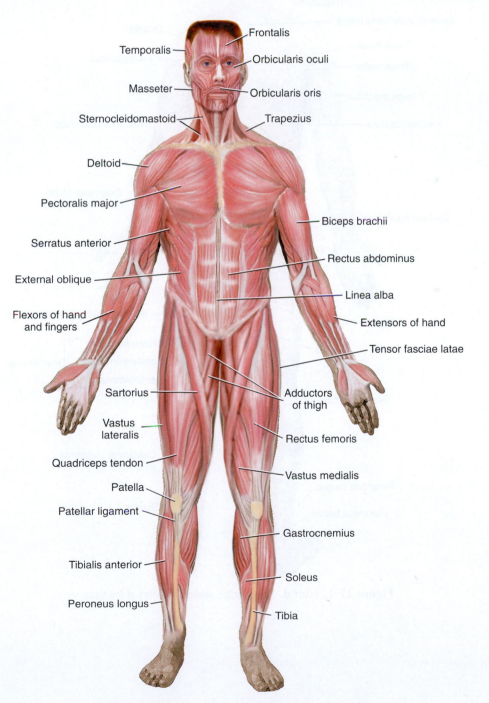

Figure 27-1. The principle skeletal muscles of the body.

Continues

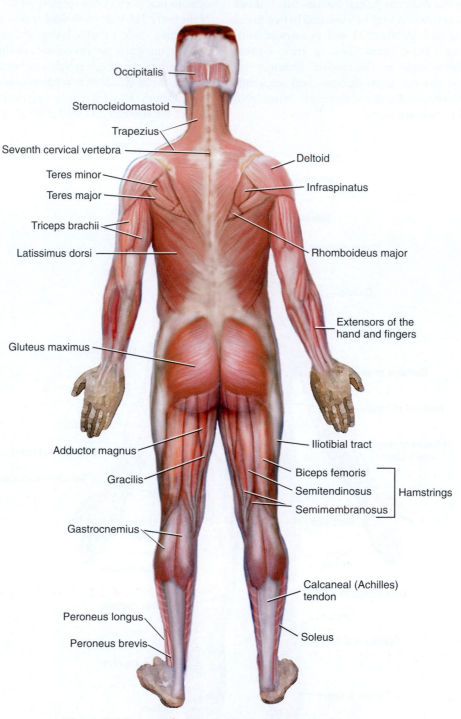

Occipitalis

Sternocleidomastoid

Trapezius

Seventh cervical vertebra

Deltoid

Teres minor

Teres major

Infraspinatus

Triceps brachii

Latissimus dorsi

Rhomboideus major

Extensors of the
hand and fingers

Gluteus maximus

Iliotibial tract

Adductor magnus

Biceps femoris

Gracilis

Semitendinosus

Hamstrings

Semimembranosus

Gastrocnemius

Calcaneal (Achilles)
tendon

Peroneus longus

Peroneus brevis

Soleus

Figure 27-1, cont'd. The principle skeletal muscles of the body.

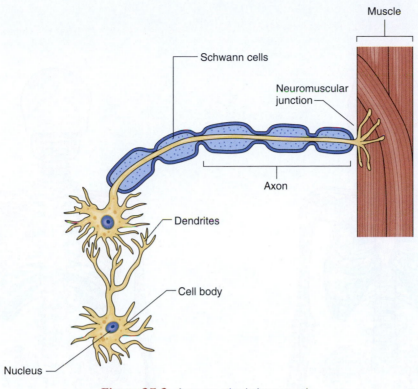

Figure 27-2. A neuron stimulating a muscle.

are excited they cause contraction and relaxation. Muscle relaxants relieve pain by relaxing muscle contractions. Skeletal muscles also have other functions. They produce movement, maintain body posture, and stabilize joints. They also produce heat and maintain body temperature.

The skeletal system consists of bones and the joints where bones meet (see Figure 27-3). The joints allow the body to be mobile and flexible. The articulation sites are covered with cartilage. The capsule or **bursa** surrounding the joints is lined with a connective membrane, called the *synovial membrane*, with fluid inside (see Figure 27-4). Diseases of joints are called **arthritis**. There are several types of arthritis. When bone mass is reduced, this condition is called **osteoporosis**.

SKELETAL MUSCLE RELAXANTS

Most muscle strains and spasms are self-limited and respond to rest, physical therapy, and short-term use of aspirin and other analgesics. However, **spasticity** (a form of muscular contraction), as the result of closed head injuries, stroke, cerebral palsy, multiple sclerosis, spinal cord injury, and other neurological conditions, requires long-term use of muscle relaxants. The skeletal muscles are voluntary muscles and are under control of the central nervous system (CNS). Skeletal muscle relaxants work by blocking somatic motor nerve impulses through depression of the right neurons

within the CNS. Transmission of an impulse from the motor nerve to each muscle cell occurs across a space known as the neuromuscular junction (see Figure 27-5). This space is sensitive to chemical changes in its immediate environment. Therefore, somatic motor nerve impulses are not able to be generated. This mechanism may also decrease the availability of calcium ions to the myofibrillar contractile system. Discontinuity of certain afferent reflex pathways by local anesthesia may also effect relaxation of limited muscle groups; local anesthetic block of efferent somatic motor outflow also is used occasionally to relieve localized skeletal muscle spasms.

Neuromuscular Blocking Agents

Neuromuscular blocking agents are chemical substances that interfere locally with the transmission or reception of impulses from motor nerves to skeletal muscles.

Mechanism of Action

Neuromuscular blocking agents prevent somatic motor nerve impulses, which affect the skeletal muscles. Some agents occupy receptor sites on the motor end plate and are able to block the action of acetylcholine. These agents are called competitive neuromuscular blocking agents. The action of other neuromuscular blocking agents resembles that of acetylcholine by depolarizing of the muscle fiber. These agents are not immediately destroyed by cholinesterase.

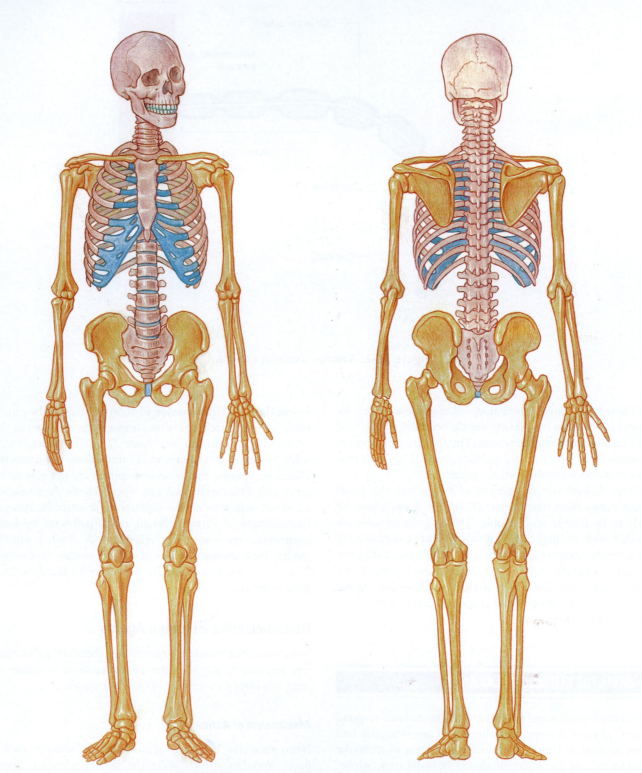

Figure 27-3. The principle bones of the body.

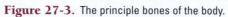

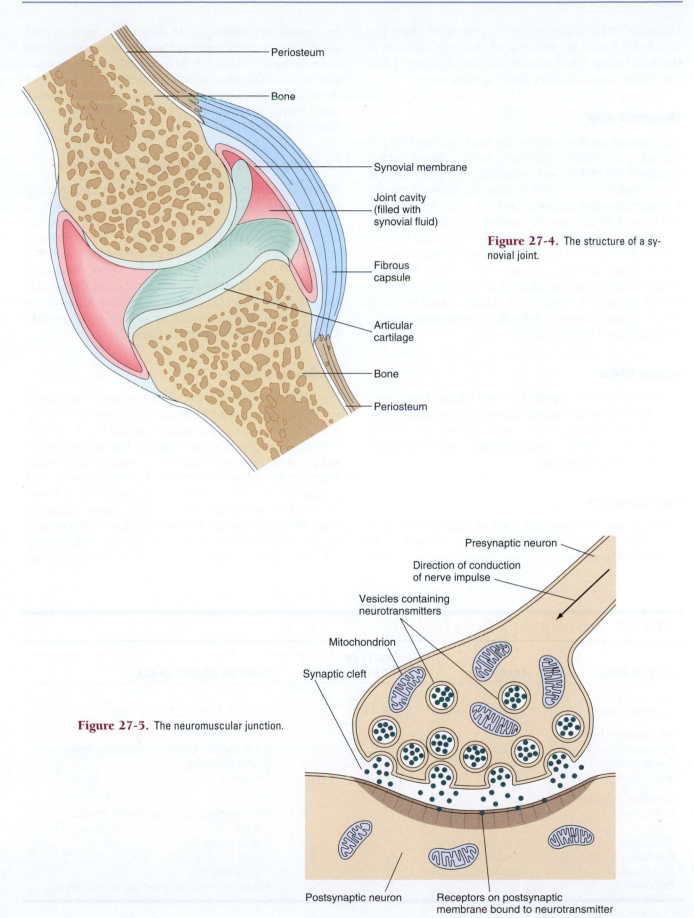

Figure 27-4. The structure of a synovial joint.

Periosteum

Bone

Synovial membrane

Joint cavity (filled with synovial fluid)

Fibrous capsule

Articular cartilage

Bone

Periosteum

Figure 27-5. The neuromuscular junction.

Presynaptic neuron

Direction of conduction of nerve impulse

Vesicles containing neurotransmitters

Mitochondrion

Synaptic cleft

Postsynaptic neuron

Receptors on postsynaptic membrane bound to neurotransmitter

Therefore, their action is more prolonged than that of acetylcholine. One example of this type of agent is **succinylcholine**, which is known as a depolarizing, or noncompetitive, neuromuscular blocking agent.

Therapeutic Uses

The principal use of neuromuscular blocking drugs is to provide adequate skeletal muscular relaxation during surgery, controlled respiration, and orthopedic manipulations. The short-acting drugs are used to relax the laryngeal muscles during endotracheal intubation and bronchoscopy. They may also be used to decrease the severity of muscle contraction during electroconvulsive treatment. Neuromuscular blocking agents have been used in the management of tetanus and for various spastic disorders, but the results usually have been disappointing. Neuromuscular blocking agents are not effective for rigidity and spasticity of muscles caused by neurological disease or trauma. Table 27-1 shows some popular neuromuscular blocking agents.

Adverse Effects

The most commonly reported adverse effects of neuromuscular blocking agents include drowsiness, increased occurrence of seizures in patients with epilepsy, dry mouth, asthenia, hypotension, muscle weakness, occasional hepatitis, and cardiac arrhythmias.

Drug Interactions

Neuromuscular blocking agents play an important role in severe adverse reactions occurring during anesthesia. Most reactions to these agents are of immunological origin, and tests for possible hypersensitivity to these drugs must be conducted before administration of anesthesia. Neuromuscular blocking agents should not be used with muscle relaxants such as succinylcholine, volatile, intravenous, or local anesthetics, other NMBAs, antibiotics, anticonvulsants, magnesium, diuretics, corticosteroids, or acetylcholine esterase inhibitors (reversal drugs).

Centrally Acting Skeletal Muscle Relaxants

Skeletal muscles are voluntarily controlled by impulses originating in the CNS. Impulses are conducted through the spinal cord in somatic neurons that eventually synapse with the muscle in a neuromuscular junction. The neurotransmitter acetylcholine (ACh) is released to combine with ACh receptors on the muscle cell membrane. When an adequate number of ACh receptors are bound, the cell then experiences sodium ion influx, causing an impulse to travel over the cell, which causes a contraction. Relaxation occurs when ACh is broken down by acetylcholinesterase.

Mechanism of Action

The exact mechanism of centrally acting muscle relaxants is unknown. They may act in the CNS at various levels to depress polysynaptic reflexes; sedative effects may be responsible for relaxation of muscle spasms. Use of the centrally acting muscle relaxants is uncertain, owing to their limited selectivity. Involuntary movement of skeletal muscles, such as that seen in palsies, chorea, or parkinsonism, is mostly the result of impairment of feedback control within the brain. When the disorder is musculoskeletal or is a result of injury or a lesion of the spinal cord, the selectivity of drugs is relatively low. However, some selectivity is achieved when

TABLE 27-1. Neuromuscular Blocking Agents

GENERIC NAME	TRADE NAME	ROUTE OF ADMINISTRATION	COMMON DOSAGE RANGE
Short Duration			
Succinylcholine	Anectine®, Quelicin®	IM, IV	IV: 0.3–1.1 mg/kg; IM: 2.5–4 mg/kg
Intermediate Duration			
Atracurium	Tracrium®	IV	0.4–0.5 mg/kg initial; then 0.08–0.1 mg/kg
Cisatracurium	Nimbex®	IV	0.15–0.20 mg/kg
Rocuronium	Zemuron®	IV	0.6 mg/kg
Extended Duration			
Doxacurium	Neuromax®	IV	0.025–0.05 mg/kg initial; then 0.005–0.01 mg/kg
Mivacurium	Mivacron®	IV	0.15–0.25 mg/kg
Pancuronium	Pavulon®	IV	0.08–0.1 mg/kg
Pipecuronium	Arduan®	IV	10–100 mcg/kg
Tubocurarine		IV	6–9 mg followed by 3–4.5 mg in 3–5 min prn

IM, intramuscular; IV, intravenous.

interneurons are involved. Most central relaxants are interneuron depressants, which will manifest variable depressant actions throughout the CNS. Many antianxiety and some sedative drugs have muscle relaxant activity. The central relaxant effects and uses of certain benzodiazepines, such as diazepam, differ from those of interneuron depressants. Table 27-2 shows some examples of centrally acting skeletal muscle relaxants. Orally, they are usually ineffective (the tolerated doses being much too low); intravenously, they have some established value in treating acute muscle spasms resulting from trauma or inflammation. Motor dysfunctions that occur with spinal cord or brain disorders are not affected very much.

Baclofen

Baclofen is a centrally acting skeletal muscle relaxant.

Mechanism of Action. The precise mechanism of baclofen is unknown.

Therapeutic Uses. Baclofen alleviates the signs and symptoms of spasticity resulting from multiple sclerosis and is used particularly for the relief of spasms and concomitant pain, spinal cord injuries, and trigeminal neuralgia (tic douloureux).

Adverse Effects. Baclofen may produce drowsiness, dizziness, weakness, confusion, insomnia, hypotension, nausea, constipation, urinary frequency, and impotence.

Drug Interactions. Baclofen increases CNS depression with alcohol and other CNS depressant agents.

Carisoprodol

Carisoprodol is a centrally acting skeletal muscle relaxant.

Mechanism of Action. The exact mechanism of action of carisoprodol is not known.

Therapeutic Uses. Carisoprodol is used to reduce discomfort associated with acute, painful musculoskeletal conditions as an adjunct to rest, physical therapy, and other measures.

Adverse Effects. The adverse effects of carisoprodol include vertigo, tremor, drowsiness, irritability, tachycardia, orthostatic hypotension, facial flushing, and nausea or vomiting.

Drug Interactions. Alcohol and other CNS depressants potentiate the CNS effects of carisoprodol.

Chlorphenesin Carbamate

This agent is a centrally acting skeletal muscle relaxant.

Mechanism of Action. The mechanism of action of chlorphenesin carbamate is unknown.

Therapeutic Uses. Chlorphenesin carbamate is a centrally active skeletal muscle relaxant. It is used to decrease skeletal muscle spasms resulting from inflammation, osteoarthritis, rheumatoid arthritis, and trauma.

Adverse Effects. This agent may cause dizziness, confusion, insomnia, headache, nausea, and pancytopenia.

Drug Interactions. Alcohol, sleep-inducing, or over-the-counter (OTC) drugs may cause dangerous drug interactions with chlorphenesin.

Chlorzoxazone

Chlorzoxazone is an autonomic, centrally acting skeletal muscle relaxant.

TABLE 27-2. Centrally Acting Skeletal Muscle Relaxants			
GENERIC NAME	**TRADE NAME**	**ROUTE OF ADMINISTRATION**	**COMMON DOSAGE RANGE**
Baclofen	Lioresal®	Oral	5 mg tid
Carisoprodol	Soma®, Rela®	Oral	350 mg tid
Chlorphenesin carbamate	Maolate®	Oral	1–4 mg qid
Chlorzoxazone	Paraflex®, Parafon Forte®	Oral	250–500 mg tid
Cyclobenzaprine hydrochloride	Flexeril®	Oral	20–40 mg bid or qid
Diazepam	Valium®, Valrelease®	Oral, IM, IV	IV, IM: 5–10 mg up to 30 mg; PO: 2–10 mg bid to qid prn
Metaxalone	Skelaxin®	Oral	800 mg tid-qid
Methocarbamol	Robaxin®	Oral, IM, IV	PO: 1.5 g qid for 2–3 days then 4–4.5 g/day tid; IM: 0.5–1 g tid; IV: 1–3 g/day
Orphenadrine citrate	Norflex®, Orfro®	Oral, IM, IV	PO: 100 mg bid; IM, IV 60 mg

IM, intramuscular; IV, intravenous; PO, oral.

Mechanism of Action. The precise mechanism of action of chlorzoxazone is unknown. It has sedative properties and acts at spinal and supraspinal levels of the CNS to depress reflex arcs involved in producing and maintaining skeletal muscle spasms.

Therapeutic Uses. Chlorzoxazone relieves discomfort associated with acute, painful musculoskeletal conditions and is used as an adjunct to rest, physical therapy, and other measures.

Adverse Effects. Chlorzoxazone may produce dizziness, light-headedness, drowsiness, anorexia, nausea, vomiting, constipation, and hepatotoxicity. It also causes urine discoloration from orange to purple-red.

Drug Interactions. Chlorzoxazone increases CNS effects with alcohol and other CNS depressants.

Cyclobenzaprine Hydrochloride

This agent is a centrally acting skeletal muscle relaxant.

Mechanism of Action. The precise mechanism of action of cyclobenzaprine hydrochloride is unknown. It does not directly relax tense skeletal muscles, but appears to act mainly at brain stem levels or in the spinal cord.

Therapeutic Uses. Cyclobenzaprine hydrochloride is used as a short-term adjunct to rest and physical therapy for relief of muscle spasm associated with acute musculoskeletal conditions. It is not effective for treatment of spasticity associated with cerebral palsy or cerebral or spinal cord diseases.

Adverse Effects. The common adverse effects of cyclobenzaprine hydrochloride are flushing and fever. It also causes drowsiness, disorientation, ataxia, psychosis, and seizures. Cyclobenzaprine hydrochloride may have cardiovascular effects and produce tachycardia and hypotension.

Drug Interactions. Cyclobenzaprine hydrochloride may interfere with the ocular antihypertensive effects of carbachol, pilocarpine, and physostigmine.

Diazepam

Diazepam is a centrally acting agent, skeletal muscle relaxant, anticonvulsant, and anxiolytic.

Mechanism of Action. Exact mechanisms of action of diazepam are not understood. It may act in the spinal cord and at supraspinal sites to produce skeletal muscle relaxation.

Therapeutic Uses. Diazepam is used adjunctively for relief of skeletal muscle spasm associated with cerebral palsy, paraplegia, and tetanus. It is also a drug of choice for status epilepticus and managing of anxiety disorders.

Adverse Effects. Diazepam may cause sedation, depression, disorientation, confusion, headache, and slurred speech. It may also produce hypotension, palpitations, edema, constipation, diarrhea, dry mouth, nausea, or vomiting. Drug dependence with withdrawal syndrome occurs when diazepam is discontinued.

Drug Interactions. Diazepam increases CNS depression with alcohol and omeprazole. Increased pharmacologic effects of diazepam occur if combined with cimetidine, disulfiram, or hormonal contraceptives. Effects of diazepam can be decreased with theophyllines and ranitidine.

Metaxalone

Metaxalone is a centrally acting drug and skeletal muscle relaxant.

Mechanism of Action. The exact mechanism of action of metaxalone is not known, but it may be due to general CNS depression.

Therapeutic Uses. Metaxalone is indicated as adjunct to rest, physical therapy, and other therapies for the relief of discomfort associated with acute, painful musculoskeletal conditions. It does not directly relax skeletal muscles and exhibits some sedative properties.

Adverse Effects. The adverse effects reported most often with metaxalone are nausea, vomiting, gastrointestinal (GI) upset, drowsiness, dizziness, headache, and nervousness.

Drug Interactions. No drug interactions with metaxalone have been reported.

Methocarbamol

Methocarbamol is classified as an autonomic nervous system agent. It is a centrally acting skeletal muscle relaxant.

Mechanism of Action. Its mechanism of action is similar to that of cyclobenzaprine, but it produces higher plasma levels more rapidly and for longer periods. It exerts skeletal muscle relaxant action by depressing multisynaptic pathways in the spinal cord and possibly by its sedative effects.

Therapeutic Uses. Methocarbamol is used as an adjunct to physical therapy and other measures in management of discomfort associated with acute musculoskeletal disorders. It is also used intravenously as an adjunct in management of neuromuscular manifestations of tetanus.

Adverse Effects. Methocarbamol may cause fever, an anaphylactic reaction, flushing, syncope, and convulsions. It also produces blurred vision, nasal congestion, drowsiness, light-headedness, headache, hypotension, and a metallic taste.

Drug Interactions. Methocarbamol may enhance CNS depression with alcohol and other CNS depressants.

Orphenadrine Citrate

Orphenadrine citrate is classified as a somatic nervous system agent. It is a centrally acting skeletal muscle relaxant.

Mechanism of Action. Orphenadrine citrate relaxes tense skeletal muscle indirectly, possibly by analgesic action or by atropine-like central action. It has some local anesthetic and antihistaminic activity, but less than that of diphenhydramine.

Therapeutic Uses. Orphenadrine citrate is used to relieve muscle spasm discomfort associated with acute musculoskeletal conditions.

Adverse Effects. Orphenadrine citrate may cause drowsiness, weakness, headache, and dizziness. It can also increase ocular tension and cause dilated pupils, blurred vision, dry mouth, nausea, vomiting, and constipation.

Drug Interactions. Orphenadrine citrate may cause increased confusion, anxiety, and tremors with **propoxyphene**. It may also worsen schizophrenic symptoms and increase the risk of **tardive dyskinesia** (an abnormal condition characterized by involuntary repetitious movements of the muscles of the face, limbs, and trunk) with **haloperidol**.

Direct Acting Skeletal Muscle Relaxants

These agents directly relax the spastic muscle. Direct acting skeletal muscle relaxants produce about a 50% decrease in contractility of skeletal muscles, but they have no effect on smooth or cardiac muscles.

Mechanism of Action

These agents do not interfere with neuromuscular transmission or the electrical excitability of muscles. They inhibit the release of calcium from the muscles. This action makes the muscle less responsive to nerve impulses. Dantrolene is one example of this group of drugs. Dantrolene sodium (Dantrium®) acts by interfering with the release of calcium from the muscles and can cause muscle weakness rather than paralysis.

Therapeutic Uses

Dantrolene is used to treat spasticity resulting from upper motor neuron lesions such as those seen with spinal cord injury, stroke, multiple sclerosis, and cerebral palsy but not spasticity resulting from musculoskeletal injury, lumbago, or rheumatoid disorders. The drug is also used to treat the neuroleptic malignant syndrome and may also be prescribed for the management of malignant hyperthermia syndrome.

Adverse Effects

The major side effect of dantrolene is muscle weakness, which may limit its therapy. Chronic use of dantrolene may result in hepatic toxicity that may be fatal. Other side effects include drowsiness, dizziness, diarrhea, seizures, and pericarditis. Dantrolene is contraindicated in patients with liver disease and respiratory muscle weakness. It may color the urine orange to red.

Drug Interactions

Interactions with dantrolene are, in most cases, minor, but caution should be used in combining this drug with warfarin, clofibrate, tolbutamide, and verapamil.

ANALGESICS, ANTIPYRETICS, AND ANTI-INFLAMMATORY DRUGS

Pain is a common problem, and one of the most common reasons for which patients see physicians. Trauma or disease patients are more likely to tolerate their pain if they know the source of the sensation and the medical course of treatment designed to manage the pain. Some pains are relieved with opioid analgesics and others with nonopioid analgesics. Pain-relieving drugs (**analgesics**) are currently available for all levels of painful stimuli. Many of these agents affect pain, fever, and inflammation depending on their properties. As a result, nonopioid analgesics, or antipyretics, and anti-inflammatory drugs are used widely for minor aches and pains, headaches, malaise, rheumatic fever, arthritis, gout, and other musculoskeletal disorders. Several drugs, such as allopurinol, colchicines, and probenecid, are pain relievers for various conditions such as gout or arthritis. These agents are not effective for other types of pain and cannot be classified as true analgesic drugs. Analgesics may be classified as opioid (narcotic) or nonopioid medications. Narcotic drugs are controlled by the Drug Enforcement Administration (DEA). They were discussed in Chapter 23. Nonopioid analgesics include salicylates and acetaminophen.

Nonsteroidal Anti-inflammatory Drugs

The inflammatory response is complex, involving the immune system. It also depends upon a variety of endogenous chemical agents. These chemical agents include prostaglandins, histamine, bradykinin, and chemotactic factors. Aspirin, other salicylates, and newer drugs with diverse structures are referred to as **nonsteroidal anti-inflammatory drugs (NSAIDs)** to distinguish them from the anti-inflammatory **corticosteroids**. The number of NSAIDs continues to increase. In addition to salicylate drugs, the NSAIDs available in the United States include indomethacin, meclofenamate, piroxicam, sulindac, and tolmetin for the treatment of arthritis and ibuprofen, fenoprofen, flurbiprofen, diclofenac, etodolac, ketorolac, and naproxen for both analgesia and arthritis. Ibuprofen and naproxen are also used for the treatment of dysmenorrhea. Currently, ibuprofen, ketoprofen, and naproxen are available OTC. NSAIDs are used to suppress the symptoms of inflammation associated with rheumatic disease. Most of these agents have analgesic and antipyretic effects. Little difference is seen between the efficacy of different NSAIDs, but some patients may respond better to one agent than to another. Anti-inflammatory effects may develop only after several weeks of treatment. Drug selection is generally dictated by the patient's ability to tolerate adverse effects.

Mechanism of Action

The mechanism of action of NSAIDs is due to irreversible inhibition of the enzyme prostaglandin H synthase, which converts arachidonic acid to prostaglandin.

Therapeutic Uses

NSAIDs are used for mild to moderate pain when opioids are not indicated. Most NSAIDs are used for inflammatory conditions such as arthritis and for dysmenorrhea and dental pain. NSAIDs are available OTC in lower doses and by prescription in larger doses. The difference between the OTC drugs and the legend medications is the strength of the drug.

Adverse Effects

The most common adverse effects of NSAIDs are primarily GI distress, gastric ulcers, and GI bleeding.

Drug Interactions

NSAIDs should not be taken with any other OTC analgesics such as acetaminophen, aspirin, or other NSAIDs. NSAIDs may result in harmful drug interactions if taken with alcohol and a wide variety of other medications.

Salicylates

Salicylates are the oldest of the nonopioid analgesics and NSAIDS. They are still often used as analgesics (Table 27-3). The salicylates include acetylsalicylic acid (aspirin), which is the most commonly used. The salicylates may be combined with caffeine to increase their action. Anacin® and Excedrin® are examples of salicylates that are combined with caffeine.

Mechanism of Action

Major actions appear to be associated primarily with inhibiting the formation of prostaglandins involved in the production of inflammation, pain, and fever.

Therapeutic Uses

Salicylates are also prescribed as NSAIDs for rheumatoid osteoarthritis and often for other inflammatory disorders. Aspirin is absorbed rapidly from the duodenum and stomach. It is used as an antipyretic and analgesic agent in a variety of conditions. Aspirin is indicated for the relief of pain from simple headache, minor muscular aches, and fever. When drug therapy is indicated for the reduction of a fever, it is one of the most effective and safest drugs. Aspirin may be useful in the prevention of coronary thrombosis by prolonging bleeding time.

Adverse Effects

The common side effects of high doses of aspirin (in 70% of patients) include nausea, vomiting, diarrhea or constipation, dyspepsia, epigastric pain, bleeding, and ulceration in the stomach. Intolerance is relatively common with aspirin and includes rash, bronchospasm, rhinitis, edema, or an anaphylactic reaction with shock, which may be life-threatening. Use of aspirin and other salicylates to control fever during viral infections in children and adolescents (influenza, common cold, and chicken pox) is associated with an increased incidence of Reye syndrome. This illness is characterized by vomiting, hepatic disturbances, and encephalopathy. Salicylates account for many accidental poisonings that may result from unordered use of large doses of these agents by the public. To avoid accidental poisoning of children, aspirin and other salicylate drugs should be kept out of their reach. The use of salicylates in children who have fever or are dehydrated must be done cautiously, because they are particularly prone to intoxication from relatively small doses

TABLE 27-3. Anti-Inflammatory and Analgesic Agent Salicylates

GENERIC NAME	TRADE NAME	ROUTE OF ADMINISTRATION	COMMON DOSAGE RANGE
Aspirin	Bayer Aspirin®, Ecotrin®, Bufferin®	Oral	350–650 mg qid (maximum 4 g/day)
Choline salicylate	Arthropan®	Oral	435–870 mg q4h
Choline magnesium salicylate	Trilisate®	Oral	1.5–2.5 g/day tid (maximum 4.5 g/day)
Magnesium salicylate	Magan®, Mobidin®	Oral	650 mg tid-qid
Salsalate	Disalcid®, Salsitab®	Oral	325–3000 mg/day tid-qid (maximum 4 g/day)

of the drugs. An allergic sensitivity to salicylates may cause a serious problem. Patients who have asthma, nasal polyps, or allergies must be very careful when they take these drugs.

Drug Interactions

Salicylates increase risk of GI ulceration with alcohol and corticosteroids. They also increase risk of toxicity with carbonic anhydrase inhibitors and valproic acid. Ammonium chloride and other acidifying agents decrease renal elimination and increase risk of salicylate toxicity. Anticoagulants increase risk of bleeding.

Cyclooxygenase-2 Inhibitors

NSAIDs inhibit both cyclooxygenase (COX)-1 and COX-2 (two enzymes that have been found to have an essential role in the inflammation process) in varying ratios. Both are present in the synovial fluid of patients with arthritis. COX-2 is more specific for prostaglandin synthesis in response to an inflammatory event. It is thought to be primarily responsible for the desired anti-inflammatory, analgesic, and antipyretic effects, whereas COX-1 has a more extensive role in the body including protection of the GI lining. As of May 2000, the U.S. Food and Drug Administration (FDA) has approved the COX-2 inhibitors celecoxib (Celebrex®) and rofecoxib (Vioxx®). However, celecoxib is not currently FDA-approved for rheumatoid arthritis, and rofecoxib is off the market because of its severe side effects. *Note:* Prostaglandins are **derivatives** of prostanoic acid. In the body, prostaglandins are principally synthesized from arachidonic acid (lipids) by the enzyme COX. Its role appears to be the daily synthesis of prostaglandins that contribute to normal homeostasis.

Mechanism of Action

These agents inhibit prostaglandin synthesis by inhibiting COX-2, but they do not inhibit COX-1.

Therapeutic Uses

COX-2 inhibitors are indicated for the treatment of osteoarthritis, rheumatoid arthritis, primary dysmenorrhea, and acute pain.

Adverse Effects

The common adverse effects of COX-2 inhibitors include fatigue, flu-like symptoms, lower extremity swelling, and back pain. Dizziness, headache, hypertension, edema, heartburn, and nausea are also seen with the use of COX-2 inhibitors.

Drug Interactions

Rofecoxib when taken with aspirin may increase the risk of GI bleeding and increase the toxicity of lithium and methotrexate.

Nonsalicylate Nonsteroidal Anti-Inflammatory Drugs

This group of NSAIDs include derivatives from propionic, acetic, and anthranilic acids, and oxicam. There is no clinical evidence to prove that any one of these drugs is consistently more effective than another, but research shows that a patient who does not respond to one NSAID may respond to another. Examples of nonsalicylate NSAIDs include ibuprofen, indomethacin, mefenamic acid, sulindac, naproxen, phenylbutazone, and piroxicam. They are absorbed rapidly after oral administration and are extensively bound in the plasma and excreted by the kidneys. Many patients tolerate effective doses of the NSAIDs better than high-dose aspirin therapy.

Mechanism of Action

Like other NSAIDs, the mechanism of action of ibuprofen probably relates to its inhibition of prostaglandin synthesis. The drug is absorbed rapidly in the digestive system. It is metabolized rapidly and eliminated from the kidneys.

Indomethacin can be absorbed rapidly after oral administration; 97% of the drug binds with plasma protein. Indomethacin is excreted unchanged in the urine.

The mechanism of action of meclofenamate is unclear.

Meloxicam is unlike ibuprofen; it inhibits prostaglandin synthesis by inhibiting COX-2. It is an NSAID agent that exhibits anti-inflammatory, analgesic, and antipyretic actions.

The exact mechanism of action of diclofenac has not been fully elucidated. It may be a potent inhibitor of cyclooxygenase, which decreases the synthesis of prostaglandins. It is an NSAID drug with analgesic and antipyretic activity.

Diflunisal is a long-acting NSAID, unlike aspirin, with which, inhibition of platelet function and effect on bleeding time are dose-related and reversible, lasting only about 24 hours after the drug is discontinued.

The exact mechanism of action of etodolac is unknown.

Fenoprofen exhibits the anti-inflammatory, analgesic, and antipyretic properties of an NSAID. The indication and adverse effects are the same as those for other NSAIDs.

Nabumetone blocks prostaglandin synthesis and is used as an anti-inflammatory, analgesic, and antipyretic agent.

Naproxen has anti-inflammatory, analgesic, and antipyretic activities. It is sold OTC. Its analgesic effects are comparable with those of aspirin or indomethacin with usual doses. It is absorbed very well from the GI tract after oral administration. More than 99% is bound to serum albumin. Almost 95% of the drug is excreted from the kidneys.

Piroxicam is an NSAID. Its exact mechanism of action is unclear.

Sulindac is an acetic acid derivative and is structurally and pharmacologically related to indomethacin. Its exact mechanism of anti-inflammatory action is not known, but is thought to result from inhibition of prostaglandin synthesis.

Tolmetin is related to indomethacin. The exact mode of anti-inflammatory action is not known.

Therapeutic Uses

Ibuprofen is effective as an analgesic and antipyretic. It is prescribed for primary dysmenorrhea, osteoarthritis, and chronic rheumatoid arthritis.

Indomethacin is a nonsteroidal drug with anti-inflammatory, antipyretic, and analgesic properties. It is not recommended as a simple analgesic or antipyretic because of the potential for severe side effects. Indomethacin is used for the treatment of rheumatoid arthritis, osteoarthritis, bursitis, tendonitis, gouty arthritis, and patent ductus arteriosus in premature neonates.

Ketoprofen is an NSAID, structurally related to ibuprofen. Its analgesic potency matches that of indomethacin and is stronger than that of aspirin. It has fewer adverse GI effects than aspirin. Ketoprofen is used in the acute or chronic treatment of rheumatoid arthritis and osteoarthritis, primary dysmenorrhea, headache, and symptomatic relief of postoperative, dental, and postpartum pain.

Meclofenamate is used for treatment of acute or chronic rheumatoid arthritis and osteoarthritis. Meclofenamate is also used in combination with gold salts or corticosteroids in treatment of rheumatoid arthritis.

Meloxicam is used for relieving the signs and symptoms of osteoarthritis.

Diclofenac is used for symptomatic treatment of rheumatoid arthritis, osteoarthritis, and ankylosing spondylitis. It is also used for acute gout and juvenile rheumatoid arthritis.

Diflunisal is used for acute and long-term relief of mild to moderate pain and symptomatic treatment of osteoarthritis and rheumatoid arthritis.

Etodolac is used for osteoarthritis and rheumatoid arthritis.

Naproxen is used for pain relief in acute and chronic rheumatoid arthritis. It is also prescribed to relieve mild postoperative and postpartum pain, primary dysmenorrhea, and headache.

Piroxicam is used in acute and chronic mild or moderate pain of osteoarthritis and rheumatoid arthritis.

Sulindac is used for the treatment of osteoarthritis, rheumatoid arthritis, ankylosing spondylitis, acute painful shoulder, and gouty arthritis.

Tolmetin is used for acute flares and management of chronic rheumatoid arthritis. It may be used alone or in combination with gold or corticosteroids.

Adverse Effects

The side effects of these agents are primarily GI distress, gastric ulcers, and GI bleeding. NSAIDs should not be taken with any other OTC analgesics (aspirin, acetaminophen, or other NSAIDs). These medications should not be used in the last 3 months of pregnancy because they could have an adverse effect on the fetus and may cause complications during delivery. The newer drugs are much more expensive than the older drugs. For example, ibuprofens are available OTC and are inexpensive when compared to Celebrex®. Table 27-4 shows nonsalicylate anti-inflammatory and analgesic agents (NSAIDs).

Ibuprofen is contraindicated in patients who are sensitive to the drug or in individuals who have nasal polyps, asthma, or angioedema. The use of ibuprofen in patients who have a history of peptic ulcer requires caution. Adverse reactions may include nausea, vomiting, epigastric pain, diarrhea or

TABLE 27-4. Nonsalicylate Anti-Inflammatory and Analgesic Agents (NSAIDs)

GENERIC NAME	TRADE NAME	ROUTE OF ADMINISTRATION	COMMON DOSAGE RANGE
Diclofenac	Voltaren®, Cataflam®	Oral	150–200 mg tid-qid
Diflunisal	Dolobid®	Oral	1000 mg followed by 500 mg tid-qid
Etodolac	Lodine®	Oral	200–400 mg tid-qid
Fenoprofen	Nalfon®	Oral	300–600 mg tid-qid`
Flurbiprofen	Ansaid®, Ocufen®	Oral	200–300 mg tid-qid
Ibuprofen	Motrin®, Rufen®, Advil®	Oral	400–800 mg tid-qid (maximum 3200 mg/day)
Indomethacin	Indocin®	Oral	25–50 mg bid-tid (maximum 200 mg/day)
Ketoprofen	Orudis®, Actron®	Oral	75 mg tid (maximum 300 mg/day)
Meclofenamate	Meclomen®, Meclofen®	Oral	200–400 mg tid-qid
Meloxicam	Mobic®	Oral	7.5–15 mg qid
Nabumetone	Relafen®	Oral	1000 mg/day single dose (maximum 2000 mg/day)
Naproxen	Naprosyn®	Oral	250–500 mg bid (maximum 1000 mg/day)
Naproxen sodium	Anaprox®, Aleve®	Oral	250–500 mg bid (maximum 1000 mg/day)
Oxaprozin	Daypro®	Oral	600–1200 mg/day (maximum 1800 mg/day)
Piroxicam	Feldene®	Oral	10–20 mg 1–2 ×/day
Sulindac	Clinoril®	Oral	150–200 mg bid (maximum 400 mg/day)
Tolmetin	Tolectin®	Oral	400 mg tid (maximum 2 g/day)

constipation, and abdominal cramps. Occasionally dizziness, headache, and nervousness are seen.

Indomethacin is contraindicated in children, pregnant women, and nursing mothers. Indomethacin must not be given to patients who are allergic to aspirin or who have GI problems. Side effects include GI ulcerations, hemorrhage, GI bleeding, nausea, vomiting, blurred vision, jaundice, aplastic anemia, and skin rashes. It may aggravate epilepsy and parkinsonism.

Adverse effects of ketoprofen include trouble in sleeping, nervousness, headache, dizziness, depression, drowsiness, and confusion. It also causes peptic ulcer, and GI bleeding, nausea, and vomiting.

Meclofenamate is contraindicated in patients with asthma, urticaria, and allergic rhinitis. Adverse effects are the same as those of other NSAIDs.

Contraindications of meloxicam are similar to those of meclofenamate.

Adverse effects of diclofenac include dizziness, headache, drowsiness, nausea, vomiting, peptic ulcer, fluid retention, and hypertension.

Contraindications of diflunisal include acute asthma attacks, urticaria, rhinitis precipitated by aspirin or other NSAIDS, or a hypersensitivity to this medication.

Etodolac is contraindicated in GI ulceration, gastritis, and lactation. Adverse effects are similar to those of other NSAIDs.

Nabumetone is contraindicated in patients with bronchospasm, severe rhinitis, angioedema, or nasal polyps. It cannot be used in patients with active peptic ulcer or bleeding abnormalities.

Adverse effects and contraindications of naproxen are generally the same as those with ibuprofen.

Piroxicam is contraindicated in patients with hemophilia, bronchospasm, nasal polyps, and angioedema. It cannot be used in patients with active peptic ulcers or GI bleeding.

Adverse effects of sulindac include drowsiness, dizziness, headache, palpitations, peripheral edema, blurred vision, nausea, vomiting, and constipation.

Adverse effects of tolmetin include allergic reaction, muscle cramps, numbness, tingling, ulcers of the mouth, rapid weight gain, seizures, bloody, black, or tarry stool, bloody urine or vomit, decreased hearing or ringing in the ears, jaundice, abdominal cramping, indigestion, or heartburn.

Drug Interactions

All nonsalicylate NSAIDs that were discussed above may cause drug interactions with oral anticoagulants. Heparin may prolong bleeding time. These agents may increase lithium and methotrexate toxicity.

Slow-Acting Antirheumatic Drugs

Slow-acting antirheumatic drugs may be prescribed for patients with rheumatoid arthritis that progresses to deformity, requiring more than an anti-inflammatory agent. Altering the disease course is attempted initially through the use of methotrexate, gold compounds, penicillamine, sulfasalazine, and hydroxychloroquine. Table 27-5 shows second-line agents for rheumatoid arthritis.

Mechanism of Action

Gold compounds (auranofin and gold sodium thiomalate) suppress or prevent inflammation in the acute forms of arthritis, but do not cure the disease. The exact mechanism is not known. The oral gold compound is available as auranofin, whereas the parenteral preparations are aurothioglucose and gold sodium thiomalate. Gold compounds that retard destruction of bone and joints by an unknown mechanism are long-latency drugs used in more advanced stages of some rheumatoid diseases. Gold sodium thiomalate is administered intramuscularly, and auranofin is administered orally.

Penicillamine is a chelating drug that is a metabolite of penicillin. It is also classified as an anti-inflammatory drug. The mechanism of action is unknown.

The mechanism of action of hydrochloroquine is unknown.

Therapeutic Uses

Penicillamine may be prescribed for advanced states of some rheumatoid disorders.

TABLE 27-5. Second-Line Agents for Rheumatoid Arthritis

GENERIC NAME	TRADE NAME	ROUTE OF ADMINISTRATION	COMMON DOSAGE RANGE
Auranofin	Rheumatrex®	Oral	6 mg/day bid
Gold sodium thiomalate	Myochrysine®	IM	10 mg week 1; 1.25 mg week 2; then 25–50 mg/wk
Methotrexate	Ridaura®	Oral	15–30 mg/day for 5 days, repeat each 12 wk for 3–5 courses
Hydroxychloroquine	Plaquenil®v	Oral	200–800 mg/day
Penicillamine	Depen®	Oral	250 mg qid
Sulfasalazine	Azulfidine®	Oral	1–2 g/day qid

Hydroxychloroquine is commonly used for the treatment of malaria and has immunosuppressant activity that may also be used for advanced phases of rheumatoid arthritis.

Corticosteroids are used in severe, progressive rheumatoid arthritis. Prednisone may afford some degree of control, but corticosteroids are usually recognized as the agents of last resort. Corticosteroids do not alter the course of rheumatoid arthritis. They may be occasionally used for elderly patients as alternatives to avoid the risks of second-line agents, for patients who cannot tolerate NSAIDs, and for patients with significant systemic manifestations of rheumatoid arthritis.

Adverse Effects

Common adverse effects of gold compounds include GI disturbances, dermatitis, and lesions of the mucous membranes. Less common side effects include aplastic anemia and nephritic syndrome. It is important to note that, except for diarrhea, serious toxicity occurs most commonly when parenteral therapy is used. If toxicity occurs, gold therapy should be stopped immediately.

The incidence of severe adverse reactions with the use of penicillamine is high, and reactions are similar to those with the gold compounds.

Long-term administration of corticosteroids may cause GI bleeding, poor wound healing, myopathy, cataracts, hyperglycemia, hypertension, and osteoporosis.

Drug Interactions

Gold compounds may have drug interactions with antimalarials and immunosuppressants. Penicillamine and phenylbutazone increase the risk of blood dyscrasias.

Methotrexate with alcohol, azathioprine, and sulfasalazine increases the risk of hepatotoxicity. Chloramphenicol, salicylates, NSAIDs, sulfonamides, phenylbutazone, phenytoin, tetracyclines, penicillin, and probenecid may increase methotrexate levels to cause increased toxicity. Folic acid may alter the response to methotrexate.

The combination of penicillamine with antimalarials and gold therapy may potentiate hematological and renal adverse effects. Iron may decrease penicillamine absorption.

Sulfasalazine absorption may be altered by iron and antibiotics.

DRUGS FOR GOUTY ARTHRITIS

There are two types of clinical gouty arthritis: acute and chronic. The initial attack for acute gout is abrupt, usually occurring at night or in the early morning as synovial fluid is reabsorbed. The most common site of the initial attack is the first metatarsophalangeal joint. Other sites that may be affected include the ankle, heel, knee, wrist, elbow, and fingers. There are two choices for therapy: general therapeutic drugs

and specific drugs. In acute gout, immobilization of the affected joint is essential. Anti-inflammatory drug therapy should begin immediately, and urate-lowering drugs should not be given until the acute attack is controlled. Specific drugs include colchicines, NSAIDs, and corticosteroids.

Colchicine

Colchicine is a gout suppressant.

Mechanism of Action

Colchicine is not an analgesic, and the precise mechanism of action is not known. The drug is well absorbed after oral administration. It is often combined with probenecid to improve prophylactic therapy of chronic gouty arthritis. Colchicine is eliminated by both urinary and fecal routes.

Therapeutic Uses

Colchicine is the traditional drug of choice for relieving pain and inflammation and ending the acute gout attack. It is most effective when initiated 12 to 36 hours after symptoms begin. It is also used in combination with either phenylbutazone or allopurinol in the management of acute gout.

Adverse Effects

The drug is very toxic, and it should be stopped at the first symptom of toxicity, such as nausea, vomiting, diarrhea, and abdominal pain. Side effects of oral colchicine include nausea, abdominal cramps, and diarrhea. It is contraindicated in patients with peptic ulcer. Local pain and necrosis can occur with administration of intravenous colchicine.

Drug Interactions

Colchicine may decrease intestinal absorption of vitamin B_{12}.

Allopurinol

Allopurinol is a xanthine oxidase inhibitor of uricosuric agent.

Mechanism of Action

This drug is not analgesic, but it relieves gouty pain because it blocks the formation of or enhances the excretion of uric acid.

Therapeutic Uses

Allopurinol is used in the treatment of gout, primary or secondary uric acid nephropathy, uric acid stone formation, and renal calculi.

Adverse Effects

Allopurinol is contraindicated in children, except those with hyperuricemia due to cancer. It should not be used by nursing mothers or by patients who develop a severe reaction to the drug. Side effects include rash, fever, leukopenia, arthralgias, and diarrhea.

Drug Interactions

Alcohol may inhibit renal excretion of uric acid. Ampicillin and amoxicillin increase the risk of skin rash. Allopurinol enhances the anticoagulant effects of warfarin. Toxicity from azathioprine, mercaptopurine, cyclophosphamide, and cyclosporin increases with allopurinol.

Acetaminophen

Another common nonopioid analgesic, acetaminophen is available OTC and is found in most households.

Mechanism of Action

Like aspirin, acetaminophen has analgesic and antipyretic actions. It can be used with relative safety in age groups from young children through older adults. Unlike aspirin, it does not have anti-inflammatory actions. The mechanism of action may be inhibition of prostaglandin in the peripheral nervous system, which makes the sensory neurons less likely to receive the pain signal. Acetaminophen is recommended as a substitute for children with fever of unknown etiology.

Acetaminophen does not displace other drugs from plasma proteins; it causes minimal GI irritation. Acetaminophen has little effect on platelet adhesion and aggregation. It can be substituted for aspirin to treat mild to moderate pain or fever for selected patients who

- are intolerant to aspirin
- have a history of peptic ulcer or hemophilia
- are using anticoagulants
- are at risk (viral infection) for Reye syndrome

Therapeutic Uses

Acetaminophen is used for fever reduction and temporary relief of mild to moderate pain. Acetaminophen may be used as a substitute for aspirin when the latter is not tolerated or is contraindicated.

Adverse Effects

Acute poisoning with acetaminophen may produce anorexia, nausea, vomiting, dizziness, chills, abdominal pain, diarrhea, hepatotoxicity, hypoglycemia, hepatic coma, and acute renal failure (rare). Chronic ingestion of acetaminophen may cause neutropenia, pancytopenia, leukopenia, and hepatotoxicity in alcoholics, as well as renal damage.

Drug Interactions

Cholestyramine may decrease acetaminophen absorption with chronic coadministration. Barbiturates, carbamazepine, phenytoin, and rifampin may increase the potential for chronic hepatotoxicity. Chronic, excessive ingestion of alcohol will increase risk of hepatotoxicity.

SUMMARY

Skeletal muscle relaxants and non-narcotic analgesics may be classified in two broad categories. One category is skeletal muscle relaxants, and another is nonsteroidal anti-inflammatory drugs (NSAIDs). Most muscle strains and spasms are self-limited and respond to rest, physical therapy, and aspirin. Spasticity resulting from closed head injuries, stroke, cerebral palsy, and others requires long-term use of muscle relaxants. Neuromuscular blocking agents prevent somatic motor nerve impulses that affect the skeletal muscles. Aspirin, other salicylates, and newer drugs with diverse structures are referred to as NSAIDs to distinguish them from the anti-inflammatory corticosteroids. Gold compounds can suppress or prevent inflammation in acute forms of rheumatoid arthritis. The drug of choice for acute gouty arthritis is colchicine. Acetaminophen has only analgesic and anti-pyretic actions. Unlike aspirin, it does not have anti-inflammatory effects.

CRITICAL THINKING

1. What is the purpose of using a neuromuscular agent?
2. Explain the mechanism of action of cyclooxygenase-2 inhibitors.
3. Describe the common adverse effects of gold compounds.

REVIEW QUESTIONS

1. The type of muscle that attaches to bones and joints by connective tissue is which of the following?
   A. Smooth
   B. Skeletal
   C. Myocardium
   D. Tendon

2. Diseases of joints are considered
   A. bursa.
   B. osteoporosis.
   C. arthritis.
   D. connective.

3. Skeletal muscles are voluntary muscles that are under the control of the
   A. central nervous system (CNS).
   B. peripheral nervous system.
   C. environment.
   D. calcium ions.

4. One of the principal uses of neuromuscular blocking agents is to provide adequate skeletal muscular relaxation during
   A. surgery.
   B. rest.
   C. epileptic seizures.
   D. exercise.

5. The abbreviation *ACh* stands for
   A. ache.
   B. aluminum chloride.
   C. acetylcholine.
   D. acetaminophen.

6. A centrally acting skeletal muscle relaxant commonly used to alleviate signs and symptoms of spasticity from multiple sclerosis is
   A. carisoprodol.
   B. baclofen.
   C. tic douloureux.
   D. codeine.

7. Which of the following may cause urine discoloration from orange to purple-red?
   A. Hepatotoxicity
   B. Diazepam
   C. Chlorzoxazone
   D. Hepatitis

8. A muscle relaxant that may worsen schizophrenic symptoms when mixed with propoxyphene is
   A. opium.
   B. orphenadrine.
   C. dantrolene sodium.
   D. calcium.

9. Pain-relieving drugs are also known as
   A. anaphylactics.
   B. antiemetics.
   C. analgesics.
   D. antitoxins.

10. NSAIDs are anti-inflammatory drugs that include
    A. corticosteroids.
    B. aspirin.
    C. opioids.
    D. haloperidol.

11. NSAIDs are used for mild to moderate pain when _____ are not indicated.
    A. prostaglandins
    B. opioids
    C. nonopioids
    D. antipyretics

12. Two enzymes that have been found to have an essential role in the inflammation process are called
    A. celecoxib and rofecoxib.
    B. prostaglandin and prostanoic.
    C. arachidonic acid and acetylcholine.
    D. COX-1 and COX-2.

13. Examples of nonsalicylate nonsteroidal anti-inflammatory drugs include
    A. ibuprofen and indomethacin.
    B. mefenamic acid and magnesium sulfate.
    C. naproxen and neomycin.
    D. piroxicam and lysergic acid.

14. Ibuprofen is prescribed for chronic rheumatoid arthritis, dysmenorrhea, and
    A. prostaglandin synthesis.
    B. bursitis.
    C. osteoarthritis.
    D. acute gout.

15. Slow-acting antirheumatic drugs may be prescribed for patients with rheumatoid arthritis that
    A. causes muscle cramps.
    B. causes numbness.
    C. exists along with palpitations.
    D. progresses to deformity.

28

Immunological Agents

OUTLINE

OBJECTIVES

Upon completion of this chapter, the reader should be able to

1. List and describe the nonspecific defenses of the human body.
2. Define the first and second lines of defense.
3. Describe the immune response or third line of defense.
4. Define antigen, antibody, and immunoglobulin.
5. Describe acquired immunity.
6. Describe active acquired immunity.
7. Differentiate between active and passive immunity.
8. Compare natural and artificial immunity.
9. List three ways in which vaccines are prepared.
10. Differentiate between immediate and delayed hypersensitivity.

GLOSSARY

active acquired immunity Immunity resulting from the development of antibodies within a person's body that renders the person immune; it may occur from exposure through a disease process or from immunizations.

anthrax A zoonotic disease caused by the anthrax bacillus that can infect humans in a number of ways and can be fatal.

antibodies Proteins that develop in response to the presence of antigen in the body and react with the antigen on the next exposure. Antibodies may be formed from infections, immunization, transfer from mother to child, or unknown antigen stimulation.

antigens Foreign substances that causes the production of specific antibodies.

antitoxin Antibodies that neutralize toxins.

attenuation The process of weakening pathogens.

B lymphocytes Cells of the adaptive immune system that express cell surface immunoglobulins specific for an epitope on an antigen.

contraindication A condition that increases the chance of a serious adverse reaction.

diphtheria An acute, toxin-mediated disease caused by *Corynebacterium diphtheriae*.

Haemophilus influenzae A gram-negative bacterium that commonly causes otitis media or bacterial meningitis in children.

hepatitis Inflammation of the liver caused by microorganisms, especially viruses, or drugs such as alcohol and other poisons.

hydrophobia A fear of water; a symptom caused by rabies as the disease progresses.

immunity An immunologic reaction that destroys or resists antigens.

379

G L O S S A R Y continued

immunogen An antigen.

immunoglobulins Blood products that contain disease-specific antibodies for passive immunity.

immunology The study of immune responses.

inactivated vaccines Vaccines in which the infectious components have been destroyed by chemical or physical treatments.

influenza A A virus causing moderate to severe illness, affecting all age groups.

influenza B A virus causing a mild illness; usually only affects children.

influenza C A viral infection of the upper respiratory tract.

killer cells Large, granular lymphocytes that appear to have the ability to destroy tumor cells.

live attenuated vaccines Vaccines containing living organisms or intact viruses that have undergone radiation or temperature conditioning to produce safe vaccinations which will help the patient become immune to a specific disease.

Mantoux test An intradermal screening for tuberculin hypersensitivity. A red, firm patch of skin at the injection site greater than 10 mm in diameter after 48 hours is a positive result that indicates current or prior exposure to tubercle bacilli.

measles An acute viral infectious disease.

meningitis An inflammation of the meninges (membranes) that surround and protect the brain. It is often caused by bacteria.

mumps An acute viral illness.

myocarditis Inflammation of the heart.

natural active acquired immunity Resistance to the causative pathogen in individuals who have had a specific infection because of the presence of antibodies and stimulated lymphocytes.

parotitis Inflammation of the salivary glands.

passive acquired immunity Immunity acquired from the injection or passage of antibodies from an immune person or animal to another for short-term immunity or immunity passed from mother to child.

pertussis An acute infectious disease caused by the bacterium *Bordetella pertussis;* also known as whooping cough.

plasma cells Differentiated B cells that secrete antibodies.

pneumonia An acute inflammation of the lungs, often caused by inhaled *Streptococcus pneumoniae.*

poliomyelitis Inflammation of the spinal cord that leads to paralysis.

precaution Specific warning to consider when medications are prescribed or administered.

rabies The only rhabdovirus that infects humans; it is a zoonotic disease characterized by fatal meningoencephalitis.

Reye syndrome A complication that occurs almost exclusively in children taking aspirin, primarily in association with influenza B or varicella zoster, and presents with severe vomiting and confusion, which may progress to coma, due to swelling of the brain.

rubella A mild, highly infectious viral disease common in childhood.

smallpox Acute viral disease that was essentially eradicated in 1979. It causes a disfiguring rash, headache, vomiting, and fever.

tetanus An acute, often fatal disease caused by an exotoxin produced by *Clostridium tetani.*

tine test In this test, the tuberculin antigen is injected just under the skin with a multipronged instrument. The antigen is located on the spikes (tines) that penetrate the skin. If results are positive, the skin around the injection site will be red and swollen like a mosquito bite 48 to 72 hours after the injection. It is not as accurate as the Mantoux test.

T lymphocytes Lymphocytes that exhibit cell surface receptors that recognize specific antigenic peptide-major histocompatibility complexes.

toxoid A toxin that has been treated with chemicals or heat to decrease its toxic effect but retain its antigenic powers.

tuberculosis A chronic granulomatous infection caused by *Mycobacterium tuberculosis.* It is generally transmitted by the inhalation or ingestion of infected droplets and usually affects the lungs.

vaccination The process of immunization for prevention of diseases.

OVERVIEW

Our environment contains a great variety of infectious microbes such as viruses, bacteria, fungi, protozoa, and multicellular parasites. These can cause disease, and if they multiply unchecked, they will eventually kill their host. Most infections in normal individuals are short-lived and leave little permanent damage. This is due to the immune system, which combats infectious agents.

Because microorganisms come in many different forms, a wide variety of immune responses are required to deal with each type of infection. For example, skin defenses of the body act as an effective barrier to most organisms, and very few infectious agents can penetrate intact skin. However, many agents gain access across the epithelia of the gastrointestinal or urogenital tracts. Others can infect the nasopharynx and lung. A small number, such as malaria and hepatitis B, can only infect the body if they enter it directly.

The site of the infection and the type of pathogen largely determine which immune responses will be effective. The most important distinction is between pathogens that invade the host's cells and those that do not. It is also important to stress that the primary function of the immune system is to eliminate infectious agents and to minimize the damage they cause.

ANATOMY REVIEW: THE IMMUNE SYSTEM

The immune system protects the body against pathogenic organisms and other foreign bodies. The principal components of the immune system include the bone marrow, the thymus, the lymph nodes, the spleen, and the lymphatic vessels (see Figure 28-1).

The spleen is the largest organ in the system. The immune system protects the body initially by creating local barriers and inflammation. Local barriers provide chemical and mechanical defenses through the skin, the mucous membranes, and the conjunctiva. Inflammation draws leukocytes to the site of injury, where these phagocytes engulf the invading

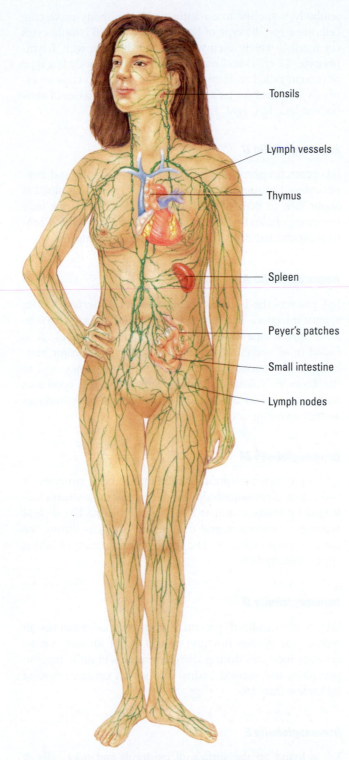

Figure 28-1. The immune system.

pathogens. Humans have three lines of defense against bacteria, viruses, fungi, and other pathogens. The first two lines of defense are nonspecific; these are ways in which the body attempts to destroy all types of substances that are foreign to it. The third line of defense, the immune response, is very specific. In the third line of defense, special proteins called **antibodies** are formed in response to particular foreign substances. These

foreign substances are called **antigens** because they cause the production of specific antibodies. If the first- and second-line defenses fail or are inadequate to protect the body, the humeral immune response and the cell-mediated response are activated.

IMMUNITY

Immunity is the condition of being immune or resistant to a particular infectious disease, usually as a result of the presence of protective antibodies that are directed against the etiological agent of that disease. The innate or native resistance to disease found in certain individuals, races, and species of animals is not a type of immunity conferred by antibodies, but rather, is a resistance resulting from natural nonspecific factors. A person who is susceptible to a disease usually has inadequate levels of protective antibodies or insufficient nonspecific defenses. In some cases, this susceptibility may simply reflect a very poor state of health or the presence of an immunodeficiency disease.

Acquired Immunity

Acquired immunity results from the active production of antibodies. If the antibodies are released within a person's body, the immunity is called **active acquired immunity**. Such protection is usually long-lasting. In **passive acquired immunity**, the person receives antibodies that were produced by another person or, in some cases, by an animal; such protection is usually only temporary. The types of acquired immunity are listed in Table 28-1.

Active Acquired Immunity

Individuals who have had a specific infection usually have some resistance to the causative pathogen because of the presence of antibodies and stimulated lymphocytes. This is called **natural active acquired immunity**. Such resistance may be permanent. Examples are immunity against poliomyelitis, whooping cough, diphtheria, mumps, and measles. Artificial active acquired immunity is another type of immunity. This results if a person receives a vaccination (the administration of a vaccine that stimulates the production of antibodies). The vaccine contains sufficient antigens of a pathogen to enable the individual to form antibodies against that pathogen. Vaccines are made from living or dead (inactivated) pathogens or from certain toxins they excrete. Vaccines made from living organisms are the most effective, but they must be prepared from harmless organisms that are antigenically closely related to the pathogens or from weakened pathogens that have been genetically changed so they are no longer pathogenic. The process of weakening pathogens is called **attenuation**, and the vaccines are referred to as attenuated vaccines. A **toxoid** vaccine is

TABLE 28-1. Acquired Immunity

ACTIVE		PASSIVE	
NATURAL	ARTIFICIAL	NATURAL	ARTIFICIAL
Clinical disease	Vaccines	Congenital (across placenta)	Antiserum
	Inactivated (killed) pathogens	Colostrum	Antitoxin Gamma globulin
	Attenuated (weakened) pathogens		
	Extracts (parts of pathogens)		
	Toxoids		

prepared from endotoxins that have been inactivated or made nontoxic by heat or chemicals. Toxoids can be injected safely to stimulate the production of antibodies that are capable of neutralizing the endotoxins of pathogens such as those that cause diphtheria and tetanus. Antibodies that neutralize toxins are called **antitoxins**.

Passive Acquired Immunity

Passive immunity is a form of acquired immunity resulting from antibodies that are transmitted naturally through the placenta to a fetus or through the colostrum to an infant or artificially by injection of antiserum (a serum containing antitoxins) for treatment or prophylaxis. Passive immunity is not permanent. It does not last as long as active immunity (see Table 28-1).

IMMUNOLOGY

Immunology is the study of immune responses. The topics of active and passive immunity to infectious agents and processes involved in antibody production were discussed earlier. Thus, under this topic, the focus is on antigens, immune responses, antibodies, hypersensitivity, and the allergic response.

Antigens

An antigen is any foreign organic substance that stimulates the production of antibodies. An antigen is also called an **immunogen**. Foreign proteins are the best antigens.

Antibodies

The terms antibody and **immunoglobulin** are used interchangeably. Antibodies are produced by lymphocytes in response to bacteria, viruses, or other antigenic substances. An antibody is specific to an antigen. The antibody-producing cells are a specific type of lymphocyte called B lymphocytes (or B cells), which often work in coordination with T lymphocytes (T cells) and macrophages. The antibody is a type of protein called an immunoglobulin (Ig). Each class of antibody is named for its action. There are five classes of antibodies: IgG, IgA, IgM, IgD, and IgE.

Immunoglobulin G

IgG protects against disease and is found in blood and lymphocytes. The normal concentration of IgG in the blood is about 70% to 80% of the total antibodies. IgG is the only immunoglobulin that crosses the placental barrier and protects against red cell antigens and white cell antigens.

Immunoglobulin A

IgA protects the mucous membranes and internal cavities against infection. The serum concentration of IgA is 15% to 20%. IgA is one of the most prevalent antibodies. It is found in all secretions of the body and is the major antibody in the mucous membranes, in the intestines, and in the bronchi, colostrum, saliva, and tears. IgA combines with a protein in the mucosa and defends body surfaces against invading microorganisms.

Immunoglobulin M

IgM is the largest immunoglobulin in molecular structure. It is the first immunoglobulin the body produces when challenged by antigens and is found in circulating blood. IgM activates complement and can destroy antigens during the initial antigen exposure. The serum concentration of IgM is approximately 10%.

Immunoglobulin D

IgD is a specialized protein found in small amounts in serum. The precise function of IgD is not known, but its quantity increases during allergic reactions to milk, insulin, penicillin, and various toxins. The serum concentration of IgD is less than 1%.

Immunoglobulin E

IgE is found on the surface of basophils and mast cells; it causes allergies, drug sensitivity, anaphylaxis, and immediate hypersensitivity. It also combats parasitic diseases. IgE is available in the serum in amounts of less than 1%. IgE is concentrated in the lungs, skin, and the cells of mucous membranes. It provides the primary defense against environmental antigens and is believed to be responsive to IgA. IgE reacts with some antigens to release certain chemical mediators (such as histamine) that cause type I hypersensitivity reactions characterized by wheal and flare. It can mediate the release of histamine in the immune response to parasites. Serum concentrations of IgE are low in the serum because the antibody is firmly fixed to the tissue surface.

IMMUNE RESPONSES

The immune system as a whole can specifically recognize many thousands of antigens. The specific cells of the immune system, the lymphocytes, undergo differentiation. Some of these cells migrate to and mature in the thymus and are referred to as thymus-derived or T lymphocytes. T lymphocytes manifest cellular immunity but also play a "helper" role in humeral immunity (an immune response that leads to the production of antibodies). Cell-mediated immunity is conferred by activated leukocytes known as **T lymphocytes**, as well as by another class of lymphocytes called **killer cells**. Most immune responses to pathogenic microorganisms include both a humeral and a cell-mediated component.

Other lymphoid stem cells influenced by fetal liver, bone marrow, or lymphoid tissue differentiate to become **B lymphocytes**. The B lymphocytes mature during immune responses and become the antibody-producing **plasma cells**. The immune response also involves three other types of immunocompetent cells: macrophages, killer cells, and natural killer cells. The macrophages (monocytes), neutrophils, and mast cells make up the inflammatory area of the immune response. The macrophage is a nonspecific, phagocytic cell. The phagocytic macrophages engulf and destroy their targets. Macrophages do not bind their targets specifically. In other words, the macrophage does not care if it is engulfing a virus or a fungal particle or a sliver of wood. In fact, it is able to phagocytize all three at once.

HYPERSENSITIVITY

Hypersensitivity is an abnormal condition characterized by an exaggerated response of the immune system to an antigen. Hypersensitivity is not manifested on first contact with the antigen, but usually appears on subsequent contact. There are four types of hypersensitivity reactions (types I, II, III, and IV), but, in practice, these types do not necessarily occur in isolation from each other. The first three are antibody-mediated; the fourth is mediated mainly by T cells and macrophages.

Type I (immediate) hypersensitivity occurs when an IgE antibody response is directed against innocuous environmental antigens such as pollen, house-dust mites, or animal dander. The resulting release of pharmacological mediators by IgE-sensitized mast cells produces an acute inflammatory reaction with symptoms such as asthma or rhinitis. Type II, or antibody-dependent cytotoxic hypersensitivity, occurs when an antibody, usually IgG, binds to either a self-antigen or a foreign antigen on cells, which leads to phagocytosis, killer cell activity, or complement-mediated lysis. Type III hypersensitivity develops when immune complexes are formed in large quantities or cannot be cleared adequately, leading to serum sickness-type reactions. Type IV or delayed type hypersensitivity (DTH) is most seriously manifested when antigens (for example, those on tubercle bacilli) are trapped in a macrophage and cannot be cleared. Other aspects of DTH reactions are seen in graft rejection and allergic contact dermatitis.

VACCINATION

A **vaccination** is the act of giving an injection or other form of antibody to protect an individual from an infectious disease. Vaccines are classified as live attenuated and inactivated. **Live attenuated vaccines** are produced from viruses or bacteria in a laboratory. Live attenuated vaccines available in the United States include live viruses and live bacteria. Examples are polio (Sabin and oral), measles/mumps/rubella (MMR), yellow fever, varicella-zoster (human herpes virus 3), and BCG (for tuberculosis). **Inactivated vaccines** can be composed of whole viruses, bacteria, or fractions of either. The more similar a vaccine is to the natural disease, the better the response to the vaccine will be. Examples are vaccines for polio (Salk), rabies, influenza, hepatitis A, typhus, pertussis, typhoid, cholera, and plague. Live attenuated vaccines are usually effective with one dose. They may cause severe reactions and may interfere with circulating antibodies. Preparations of vaccines were discussed earlier in this chapter.

An adverse reaction is an untoward effect caused by a vaccine that is extraneous to the vaccine's primary purpose of production of immunity. Adverse reactions to vaccines fall into three general categories: local, systemic, and allergic. Local reactions are generally the least severe and most frequent. Allergic reactions are the most severe and least frequent.

Recommended vaccinations and immunization schedules for both adults and children are presented in Figures 28-2 and 28-3.

Contraindications and Precautions

Generally, contraindications dictate circumstances in which vaccines will not be given. Most contraindications and precautions are temporary, and the vaccine can be given at a later time. A **contraindication** is a condition in a recipient that greatly increases the chance of a serious adverse reaction. A **precaution** is a condition in a recipient that may increase the chance of an adverse event. Permanent contraindications to vaccination include the following:

- Severe allergy to a prior dose of vaccine or to a vaccine component
- Encephalopathy after pertussis vaccine

Recommended Childhood and Adolescent Immunization Schedule — United States, 2003

Vaccine ▼ / Age ▶	Birth	1 mo	2 mos	4 mos	6 mos	12 mos	15 mos	18 mos	24 mos	4-6 yrs	11-12 yrs	13-18 yrs
Hepatitis B[1]	HepB #1	only if mother HBsAg (−)									HepB series	
		HepB #2				HepB #3						
Diphtheria, Tetanus, Pertussis[2]		DTaP	DTaP	DTaP		DTaP				DTaP	Td	
Haemophilus influenzae Type b[3]		Hib	Hib	Hib		Hib						
Inactivated Polio		IPV	IPV		IPV					IPV		
Measles, Mumps, Rubella[4]						MMR #1				MMR #2	MMR #2	
Varicella[5]						Varicella					Varicella	
Pneumococcal[6]		PCV	PCV	PCV		PCV				PCV	PPV	
Hepatitis A[7]										Hepatitis A series		
Influenza[8]						Influenza (yearly)						

Legend: range of recommended ages | catch-up vaccination | preadolescent assessment

Vaccines below this line are for selected populations

This schedule indicates the recommended ages for routine administration of currently licensed childhood vaccines, as of December 1, 2002, for children through age 18 years. Any dose not given at the recommended age should be given at any subsequent visit when indicated and feasible. ▨ Indicates age groups that warrant special effort to administer those vaccines not previously given. Additional vaccines may be licensed and recommended during the year. Licensed combination vaccines may be used whenever any components of the combination are indicated and the vaccine's other components are not contraindicated. Providers should consult the manufacturers' package inserts for detailed recommendations.

1. Hepatitis B vaccine (HepB). All infants should receive the first dose of hepatitis B vaccine soon after birth and before hospital discharge; the first dose may also be given by age 2 months if the infant's mother is HBsAg-negative. Only monovalent HepB can be used for the birth dose. Monovalent or combination vaccine containing HepB may be used to complete the series. Four doses of vaccine may be administered when a birth dose is given. The second dose should be given at least 4 weeks after the first dose, except for combination vaccines which cannot be administered before age 6 weeks. The third dose should be given at least 16 weeks after the first dose and at least 8 weeks after the second dose. The last dose in the vaccination series (third or fourth dose) should not be administered before age 6 months.

Infants born to HBsAg-positive mothers should receive HepB and 0.5 mL Hepatitis B Immune Globulin (HBIG) within 12 hours of birth at separate sites. The second dose is recommended at age 1-2 months. The last dose in the vaccination series should not be administered before age 6 months. These infants should be tested for HBsAg and anti-HBs at 9-15 months of age.

Infants born to mothers whose HBsAg status is unknown should receive the first dose of the HepB series within 12 hours of birth. Maternal blood should be drawn as soon as possible to determine the mother's HBsAg status; if the HBsAg test is positive, the infant should receive HBIG as soon as possible (no later than age 1 week). The second dose is recommended at age 1-2 months. The last dose in the vaccination series should not be administered before age 6 months.

2. Diphtheria and tetanus toxoids and acellular pertussis vaccine (DTaP). The fourth dose of DTaP may be administered as early as age 12 months, provided 6 months have elapsed since the third dose and the child is unlikely to return at age 15-18 months. **Tetanus and diphtheria toxoids (Td)** is recommended at age 11-12 years if at least 5 years have elapsed since the last dose of tetanus and diphtheria toxoid-containing vaccine. Subsequent routine Td boosters are recommended every 10 years.

3. Haemophilus influenzae type b (Hib) conjugate vaccine. Three Hib conjugate vaccines are licensed for infant use. If PRP-OMP (PedvaxHIB® or ComVax®[Merck]) is administered at ages 2 and 4 months, a dose at age 6 months is not required. DTaP/Hib combination products should not be used for primary immunization in infants at ages 2, 4 or 6 months, but can be used as boosters following any Hib vaccine.

4. Measles, mumps, and rubella vaccine (MMR). The second dose of MMR is recommended routinely at age 4-6 years but may be administered during any visit, provided at least 4 weeks have elapsed since the first dose and that both doses are administered beginning at or after age 12 months. Those who have not previously received the second dose should complete the schedule by the 11-12 year old visit.

5. Varicella vaccine. Varicella vaccine is recommended at any visit at or after age 12 months for susceptible children, i.e. those who lack a reliable history of chickenpox. Susceptible persons aged ≥13 years should receive two doses, given at least 4 weeks apart.

6. Pneumococcal vaccine. The heptavalent **pneumococcal conjugate vaccine (PCV)** is recommended for all children age 2-23 months. It is also recommended for certain children age 24-59 months. **Pneumococcal polysaccharide vaccine (PPV)** is recommended in addition to PCV for certain high-risk groups. See *MMWR* 2000;49(RR-9);1-38.

7. Hepatitis A vaccine. Hepatitis A vaccine is recommended for children and adolescents in selected states and regions, and for certain high-risk groups; consult your local public health authority. Children and adolescents in these states, regions, and high risk groups who have not been immunized against hepatitis A can begin the hepatitis A vaccination series during any visit. The two doses in the series should be administered at least 6 months apart. See *MMWR* 1999;48(RR-12);1-37.

8. Influenza vaccine. Influenza vaccine is recommended annually for children age ≥6 months with certain risk factors (including but not limited to asthma, cardiac disease, sickle cell disease, HIV, diabetes, and household members of persons in groups at high risk; see *MMWR* 2002;51(RR-3);1-31), and can be administered to all others wishing to obtain immunity. In addition, healthy children age 6-23 months are encouraged to receive influenza vaccine if feasible because children in this age group are at substantially increased risk for influenza-related hospitalizations. Children aged ≤12 years should receive vaccine in a dosage appropriate for their age (0.25 mL if age 6-35 months or 0.5 mL if aged ≥3 years). Children aged ≤8 years who are receiving influenza vaccine for the first time should receive two doses separated by at least 4 weeks.

For additional information about vaccines, including precautions and contraindications for immunization and vaccine shortages, please visit the National Immunization Program Website at www.cdc.gov/nip or call the National Immunization Information Hotline at 800-232-2522 (English) or 800-232-0233 (Spanish)

Approved by the Advisory Committee on Immunization Practices (www.cdc.gov/nip/acip), the American Academy of Pediatrics (www.aap.org), and the American Academy of Family Physicians (www.aafp.org).

Figure 28-2. Childhood immunization schedule. (Courtesy of the Centers for Disease Control and Prevention.)

Recommended Adult Immunization Schedule, United States, 2002-2003

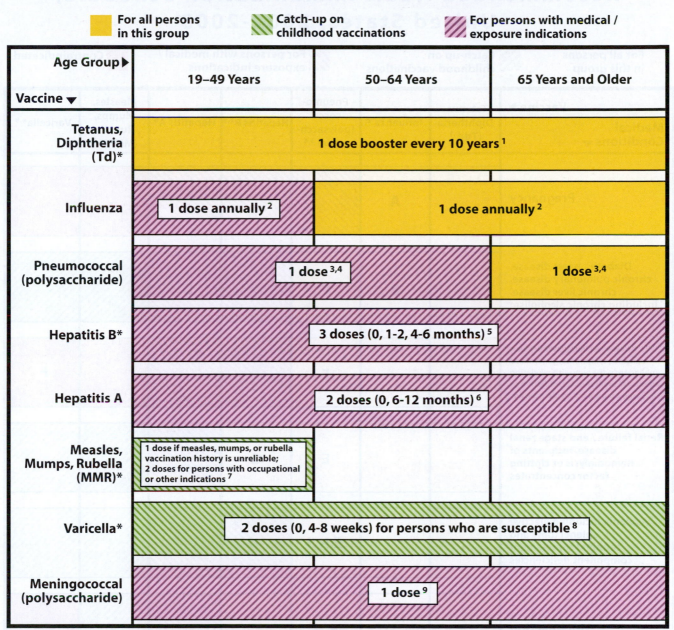

| | For all persons in this group | Catch-up on childhood vaccinations | For persons with medical / exposure indications |

Age Group ▶ Vaccine ▼	19–49 Years	50–64 Years	65 Years and Older
Tetanus, Diphtheria (Td)*	1 dose booster every 10 years [1]		
Influenza	1 dose annually [2]	1 dose annually [2]	
Pneumococcal (polysaccharide)	1 dose [3,4]		1 dose [3,4]
Hepatitis B*	3 doses (0, 1-2, 4-6 months) [5]		
Hepatitis A	2 doses (0, 6-12 months) [6]		
Measles, Mumps, Rubella (MMR)*	1 dose if measles, mumps, or rubella vaccination history is unreliable; 2 doses for persons with occupational or other indications [7]		
Varicella*	2 doses (0, 4-8 weeks) for persons who are susceptible [8]		
Meningococcal (polysaccharide)	1 dose [9]		

See Footnotes for Recommended Adult Immunization Schedule, United States, 2002-2003 on back cover.

* Covered by the Vaccine Injury Compensation Program. For information on how to file a claim call 800-228-2382. Please also visit www.hrsa.gov/osp/vicp To file a claim for vaccine injury write: U.S. Court of Federal Claims, 717 Madison Place, N.W., Washington D.C. 20005.202 219-9657.

This schedule indicates the recommended age groups for routine administration of currently licensed vaccines for persons 19 years of age and older. Licensed combination vaccines may be used whenever any components of the combination are indicated and the vaccine's other components are not contrindicated. Providers should consult the manufacturere's package inserts for detailed recommendations.

Report all clinically significant post-vaccination reactions to the Vaccine Adverse Event Reporting Sytem (VAERS). Reporting forms and instructions on filing a VAERS report are available by calling 800-822-7967 or from the VAERS website at www.vaers.org.

For additional information about the vaccines listed above and contraindications for immunization, visit the National Immunization Program Website at www.cdc.gov/nip/ or call the National Immunization Hotline at 800-232-2522 (English) or 800-232-0233 (Spanish).

Approved by the Advisory Committee on Immunization Practices (ACIP), and accepted by the American College of Obstetricians and Gynecologists (ACOG) and the American Academy of Family Physicians (AAFP)

Figure 28-3. Adult immunization schedule. (Courtesy of the Centers for Disease Control and Sprevention.)

Continues

Recommended Adult Immunization Schedule, United States, 2002-2003

▨ For all persons in this group	▨ Catch-up on childhood vaccinations	▨ For persons with medical / exposure indications	▨ Contraindicated

Medical Conditions ▼	Vaccine ▶ Tetanus-Diphtheria (Td)*,1	Influenza 2	Pneumococcal (polysaccharide) 3,4	Hepatitis B*,5	Hepatitis A6	Measles, Mumps, Rubella (MMR)*,7	Varicella*,8
Pregnancy		A					
Diabetes, heart disease, chronic pulmonary disease, chronic liver disease, including chronic alcoholism		B	C		D		
Congenital Immunodeficiency, leukemia, lymphoma, generalized malignancy, therapy with alkylating agents, antimetabolites, radiation or large amounts of corticosteroids			E				F
Renal failure / end stage renal disease, recipients of hemodialysis or clotting factor concentrates			E	G			
Asplenia including elective splenectomy and terminal complement component deficiencies			E,H,I				
HIV infection			E, J			K	

A. If pregnancy is at 2nd or 3rd trimester during influenza season.

B. Although chronic liver disease and alcholism are not indicator conditions for influenza vaccination, give 1 dose annually if the patient is ≥50 years, has other indications for influenza vaccine, or if the patient requests vaccination.

C. Asthma is an indicator condition for influenza but not for pneumococcal vaccination.

D. For all persons with chronic liver disease.

E. Revaccinate once after 5 years or more have elapsed since initial vaccination.

F. Persons with impaired humoral but not cellular immunity may be vaccinated. MMWR 1999; 48 (RR-06): 1-5.

G. Hemodialysis patients: Use special formulation of vaccine (40 ug/mL) or two 1.0 mL 20 ug doses given at one site. Vaccinate early in the course of renal disease. Assess antibody titers to hep B sufgace antigen (anti-HBs) levels annually. Administer additional doses if anti-HBs levels decline to <10 milliinternational units (mIU)/mL.

H. Also administer meningococcal vaccine.

I. Elective splenectomy: vaccinate at least 2 weeks before surgery.

J. Vaccinate as close to diagnosis as possible whe CD4 cell counts are highest.

K. Withhold MMR or other measles containing vaccines from HIV-infected persons with evidence of severe immunosuppressions. MMWR 1996; 45: 603-606, MMWR 1992; 41 (RR-17): 1-19.

Figure 28-3, cont'd. Adult immunization schedule. (Courtesy of the Centers for Disease Control and Prevention.)

Footnotes for
Recommended Adult Immunization Schedule
by Age Group and Medical Conditions, United States, 2003–2004

Tetanus and diphtheria (Td) toxoids—Adults including pregnant women with uncertain histories of a complete primary vaccination series should receive a primary series of Td. A primary series for adults is 3 doses: the first 2 doses given at least 4 weeks apart and the 3rd dose, 6-12 months after the second. Administer 1 dose if the person had received the primary series and the last vaccination was 10 years ago or longer. Consult *MMWR* 1991; 40 (RR-10): 1-21 for administering Td as prophylaxis in wound management. The ACP Task Force on Adult Immunization supports a second option for Td use in adults: a single Td booster at age 50 years for persons who have completed the full pediatric series, including the teenage/young adult booster.
Guide for Adult Immunization. 3rd ed. ACP 1994: 20.

Influenza vaccination—Medical indications: chronic disorders of the cardiovascular or pulmonary systems including asthma; chronic metabolic diseases including diabetes mellitus, renal dysfunction, hemoglobinopathies, or immunosuppression (including immunosuppression caused by medications or by human immunodeficiency virus [HIV]), requiring regular medical follow-up or hospitalization during the preceding year; women who will be in the second or third trimester of pregnancy during the influenza season. Occupational indications: health-care workers. Other indications: residents of nursing homes and other long-term care facilities; persons likely to transmit influenza to persons at high-risk (in-home care givers to persons with medical indications, household contacts and out-of-home caregivers of children birth to 23 months of age, or children with asthma or other indicator conditions for influenza vaccination, household members and care givers of elderly and adults with high-risk conditions); and anyone who wishes to be vaccinated. For healthy persons aged 5-49 years without high risk conditions, either the inactivated vaccine or the intranasally administered influenza vaccine (Flumist) may be given.
MMWR 2003; 52 (RR-8): 1-36; *MMWR* 2003; 53 (RR-13): 1-8.

Pneumococcal polysaccharide vaccination—Medical indications: chronic disorders of the pulmonary system (excluding asthma), cardiovascular diseases, diabetes mellitus, chronic liver diseases including liver disease as a result of alcohol abuse (e.g., cirrhosis), chronic renal failure or nephrotic syndrome, functional or anatomic asplenia (e.g., sickle cell disease or splenectomy), immunosuppressive conditions (e.g., congenital immunodeficiency, HIV infection, leukemia, lymphoma, multiple myeloma, Hodgkins disease, generalized malignancy, organ or bone marrow transplantation), chemotherapy with alkylating agents, anti-metabolites, or long-term systemic corticosteroids. Geographic/other indications: Alaskan Natives and certain American Indian populations. Other indications: residents of nursing homes and other long-term care facilities. *MMWR* 1997; 46 (RR-8): 1-24.
Revaccination with pneumococcal polysaccharide vaccine—One time revaccination after 5 years for persons with chronic renal failure or nephrotic syndrome, functional or anatomic asplenia (e.g., sickle cell disease or splenectomy), immunosuppressive conditions (e.g., congenital immunodeficiency, HIV infection, leukemia, lymphoma, multiple myeloma, Hodgkins disease, generalized malignancy, organ or bone marrow transplantation), chemotherapy with alkylating agents, anti-metabolites, or long-term systemic corticosteroids. For persons 65 and older, one-time revaccination if they were vaccinated 5 or more years previously and were aged less than 65 years at the time of primary vaccination. *MMWR* 1997; 46 (RR-8): 1-24.

Hepatitis B vaccination—Medical indications: hemodialysis patients, patients who receive clotting-factor concentrates. Occupational indications: health-care workers and public-safety workers who have exposure to blood in the workplace, persons in training in schools of medicine, dentistry, nursing, laboratory technology, and other allied health professions. Behavioral indications: injecting drug users, persons with more than one sex partner in the previous 6 months, persons with a recently acquired sexually-transmitted disease (STD), all clients in STD clinics, men who have sex with men. Other indications: household contacts and sex partners of persons with chronic HBV infection, clients and staff of institutions for the developmentally disabled, international travelers who will be in countries with high or intermediate prevalence of chronic HBV infection for more than 6 months, inmates of correctional facilities. *MMWR* 1991; 40 (RR-13): 1-19.
(www.cdc.gov/travel/diseases/hbv.htm)

6. **Hepatitis A vaccination**—For the combined HepA-HepB vaccine use 3 doses at 0, 1, 6 months). Medical indications: persons with clotting-factor disorders or chronic liver disease. Behavioral indications: men who have sex with men, users of injecting and noninjecting illegal drugs. Occupational indications: persons working with HAV-infected primates or with HAV in a research laboratory setting. Other indications: persons traveling to or working in countries that have high or intermediate endemicity of hepatitis A. *MMWR* 1999; 48 (RR-12): 1-37. (www.cdc.gov/travel/diseases/hav.htm)

7. **Measles, Mumps, Rubella vaccination (MMR)**—Measles component: Adults born before 1957 may be considered immune to measles. Adults born in or after 1957 should receive at least one dose of MMR unless they have a medical contraindication, documentation of at least one dose or other acceptable evidence of immunity. A second dose of MMR is recommended for adults who:
   - are recently exposed to measles or in an outbreak setting
   - were previously vaccinated with killed measles vaccine
   - were vaccinated with an unknown vaccine between 1963 and 1967
   - are students in post-secondary educational institutions
   - work in health care facilities
   - plan to travel internationally

   Mumps component: 1 dose of MMR should be adequate for protection. Rubella component: Give 1 dose of MMR to women whose rubella vaccination history is unreliable and counsel women to avoid becoming pregnant for 4 weeks after vaccination. For women of child-bearing age, regardless of birth year, routinely determine rubella immunity and counsel women regarding congenital rubella syndrome. Do not vaccinate pregnant women or those planning to become pregnant in the next 4 weeks. If pregnant and susceptible, vaccinate as early in postpartum period as possible.
   MMWR 1998; 47 (RR-8): 1-57; *MMWR* 2001; 50: 1117.

8. **Varicella vaccination**—Recommended for all persons who do not have reliable clinical history of varicella infection, or serological evidence of varicella zoster virus (VZV) infection who may be at high risk for exposure or transmission. This includes, health-care workers and family contacts of immunocompromised persons, those who live or work in environments where transmission is likely (e.g., teachers of young children, day care employees, and residents and staff members in institutional settings), persons who live or work in environments where VZV transmission can occur (e.g., college students, inmates and staff members of correctional institutions, and military personnel), adolescents and adults living in households with children, women who are not pregnant but who may become pregnant in the future, international travelers who are not immune to infection. Note: Greater than 95% of U.S. born adults are immune to VZV. Do not vaccinate pregnant women or those planning to become pregnant in the next 4 weeks. If pregnant and susceptible, vaccinate as early in postpartum period as possible. *MMWR* 1996; 45 (RR-11): 1-36; *MMWR* 1999; 48 (RR-6): 1-5.

9. **Meningococcal vaccination (quadrivalent polysaccharide vaccine for serogroups A, C, Y, and W-135)**—Consider vaccination for persons with medical indications: adults with terminal complement component deficiencies, with anatomic or functional asplenia. Other indications: travelers to countries in which disease is hyperendemic or epidemic ("meningitis belt" of sub-Saharan Africa, Mecca, Saudi Arabia for Hajj). Revaccination at 3-5 years may be indicated for persons at high risk for infection (e.g., persons residing in areas in which disease is epidemic). Counsel college freshmen, especially those who live in dormitories, regarding meningococcal disease and the vaccine so that they can make an educated decision about receiving the vaccination. *MMWR* 2000; 49 (RR-7): 1-20.
   Note: The AAFP recommends that colleges should take the lead on providing education on meningococcal infection and vaccination and offer it to those who are interested. Physicians need not initiate discussion of the meningococcal quadrivalent polysaccharide vaccine as part of routine medical car .

Figure 28-3, cont'd. Adult immunization schedule. (Courtesy of the Centers for Disease Control and Prevention.)

CURRENT VACCINES IN GENERAL USE

Several vaccines are in standard use worldwide. Table 28-2 lists vaccines in general use. Four of them—polio, measles, mumps, and rubella—are so successful that these diseases are earmarked for eradication early in the twenty-first century. If this happens, it will be an extraordinary achievement.

Diphtheria

Diphtheria is an acute, toxin-mediated disease caused by *Corynebacterium diphtheriae*. This organism is an aerobic gram-positive bacillus. Toxin production occurs only when the bacillus is itself infected by a virus (phage) carrying the genetic information for the toxin. The incubation period of diphtheria is 2 to 5 days. The disease can involve almost any mucous membrane. It is classified based on site of infection, e.g., tonsillar, pharyngeal, or cutaneous. Most complications of diphtheria, including death, are attributable to the effect of the toxin. The severity of the disease and complications are generally related to the extent of local disease. The toxin, when absorbed, affects organs and tissues distant from the site of invasion. The most common complications of diphtheria are myocarditis and neuritis.

Diphtheria Antitoxin

Diphtheria antitoxin, produced in horses, was first used in the United States in 1891. It is used only for the treatment of diphtheria. Antitoxin will not neutralize toxin that is already fixed to tissues but will neutralize circulating (unbound) toxin and will prevent progression of the disease.

Diphtheria Toxoid

Diphtheria toxoid is available combined with tetanus as pediatric DT or adult Td and with both tetanus toxoid and acellular pertussis vaccine as DtaP. Children younger than 7 years of age should receive either DtaP or pediatric DT. Persons 7 years of age or older should receive the adult formulation (adult Td), even if they have not completed a series of DtaP or pediatric DT vaccinations.

Adverse Reactions

Adverse reactions include local or severe systemic reactions. Local reactions generally result in redness and swelling with or without tenderness and are common after the administration of vaccines containing diphtheria antigen. Fever and systemic symptoms are uncommon. Severe systemic reactions are rare.

Contraindications

Persons with a history of neurological or severe allergic reactions after a previous dose should not receive additional doses of diphtheria toxoid. Pregnancy and immunosuppression are not contraindications to administration of diphtheria toxoid.

Tetanus

Tetanus is an acute, often fatal disease caused by an exotoxin produced by *Clostridium tetani*. It is characterized by generalized rigidity and convulsive spasms of the skeletal muscles. The muscle stiffness usually involves the jaw (lockjaw) and neck and then becomes generalized. *C. tetani* is an anaerobic gram-positive, spore-forming bacteria. Its spores are found in soil, dust, and animal feces. They may persist for months to years. *C. tetani* produces multiple toxins. Toxin binds in the central nervous system and leads to muscle contraction and spasm. Transmission is primarily by contaminated wounds. The wounds may be major or minor. Tetanus is not contagious from person to person. It is the only vaccine-preventable disease that is infectious but not contagious. Almost all reported cases of tetanus are in persons who either have never been vaccinated or have completed a primary series, but have not had a booster dose in the preceding 10 years. Heroin users, particularly persons who inject themselves subcutaneously, appear to be at high risk for tetanus. Quinine is used to dilute heroin and may support the growth of *C. tetani*. Neonatal tetanus is rare in the United States.

Tetanus Toxoid

Tetanus toxoid consists of a formaldehyde-treated toxin. Two types of toxoid are available: adsorbed toxoid and fluid toxoid. The adsorbed toxoid is preferred. Tetanus toxoid is available as a single antigen preparation, combined with diphtheria as pediatric DT or adult Td, and with both diphtheria toxoid and acellular pertussis vaccine as DtaP.

Adverse Reactions

Adverse reactions to vaccination may be local or systemic. Local reactions include redness, swelling, and pain at the injection site, which are common, but are usually self-limited and require no therapy. Severe systemic reactions, such as

TABLE 28-2. Vaccines Currently in General Use	
DISEASE	**VACCINE**
Tetanus	Toxoid
Diphtheria	Toxoid
Pertussis	Killed whole
Polio	Killed (Salk) or attenuated (Sabin)
Measles	Attenuated
Mumps	Attenuated
Rubella	Attenuated
Haemophilus	Polysaccharide

generalized urticaria (hives), anaphylaxis, or neurological complications, have been reported after receipt of tetanus toxoid. Severe systemic reactions are rare.

Contraindications

A severe allergic reaction (acute respiratory distress or collapse) after a previous dose of tetanus toxoid is a contraindication to further vaccination. A history of systemic allergic or neurologic reactions following a previous dose of tetanus toxoid is an absolute contraindication for further use.

Pertussis

Pertussis, or whooping cough, is an acute infectious disease caused by the bacterium *Bordetella pertussis*. This organism is a gram-negative rod, which attaches to the respiratory cilia, producing toxins that paralyze the cilia and cause inflammation of the respiratory tract. The incubation period of pertussis is commonly 7 to 10 days. Pertussis consists of three stages:

- Catarrhal stage: 1 to 2 weeks
- Paroxysmal cough stage: 1 to 6 weeks
- Convalescence: weeks to months

Complications

Young infants have the highest risk for acquiring clinical pertussis. The most common complication and the cause of most pertussis-related deaths is secondary bacterial pneumonia. Neurological complications, such as seizure and encephalopathy, may occur as a result of hypoxia from coughing or possibly from toxin.

Adverse Reactions

As with all injected vaccines, administration of DtaP may cause local reactions such as pain, redness, or swelling. Local reactions appear to be more common after the fourth or fifth dose of DtaP. Low-grade fever and drowsiness often occur. More severe adverse reactions are uncommon.

Contraindications

Contraindications to further vaccination with DtaP are a severe allergic reaction to a prior dose of vaccine or vaccine component and encephalopathy not due to another identifiable cause within 7 days of vaccination.

Poliomyelitis

Poliomyelitis is an inflammation of the spinal cord that leads to paralysis. Poliovirus enters through the mouth, and primary multiplication of the virus occurs in the pharynx, gastrointestinal tract, and local lymphatics. Replication of poliovirus in motor neurons of the spinal cord and brain stem

results in cell destruction and causes poliomyelitis. The incubation period for poliomyelitis is commonly 6 to 20 days. Up to 95% of all polio infections are unapparent or asymptomatic. Humans are the only known reservoir of poliovirus, which is transmitted most commonly by persons with unapparent infections. Person-to-person spread of poliovirus via the fecal-oral route is the most important route of transmission.

Poliovirus Vaccines

Inactivated (Salk) poliovirus vaccine (IPV) was licensed in 1955 and was used extensively from that time until the early 1960s. In 1963, oral poliovirus vaccine (OPV) was licensed and has largely replaced IPV. OPV has been the vaccine of choice in the United States and most other countries since 1963.

Adverse Reactions

Minor local reactions (pain and redness) may occur after injection of IPV. No serious adverse reactions to IPV or OPV have been documented. Allergic reactions may occur.

Contraindications

OPV should not be given to individuals or household contacts of individuals who have immune deficiency diseases, immune depression due to disease or therapy, or if there is suspected familial immune deficiency. IPV may be substituted for OPV in these circumstances. In general, neither OPV nor IPV should be given to pregnant women unless immediate protection is needed, in which case OPV is the vaccine of choice.

A serious allergic reaction to a vaccine component or after a prior dose of vaccine is a contraindication to further doses of that vaccine. Because IPV contains trace amounts of streptomycin, neomycin, and polymyxin B, there is a possibility of allergic reactions in persons sensitive to these antibiotics. Breast-feeding does not interfere with successful immunization against polio with IPV.

Measles

Measles is an acute viral infectious disease. The measles virus is rapidly inactivated by heat, light, and ether. The primary site of infection is the nasopharynx. The incubation period is 10 to 12 days. The measles rash begins on the face and upper neck and last 5 to 6 days. Measles is a human disease. There is no known animal reservoir. Transmission is primarily person-to-person via large respiratory droplets.

Complications

Approximately 30% of patients with measles have one or more complications. They are more common among children younger than 5 years of age and adults older than 20 years of age. Diarrhea, otitis media, pneumonia, and encephalitis are common complications of measles.

Measles Vaccine

The only measles virus vaccine now available in the United States is a live vaccine. It is available as a single antigen preparation, combined with rubella vaccine or combined with mumps and rubella vaccines (MMR). The vaccine contains a small amount of human albumin, neomycin, sorbitol, and gelatin. Two doses of measles vaccine as MMR, separated by at least 4 weeks, are routinely recommended for all children. The first dose of MMR should be given on or after the first birthday. Any dose of measles-containing vaccine given before 12 months of age should not be counted as part of the series.

Adverse Reactions

Adverse reactions after measles vaccine (except allergic reactions) are mild and include fever, rash, and joint symptoms. Allergic reactions after the administration of MMR or any of its component vaccines are rare. MMR is recommended for persons with asymptomatic and mildly symptomatic human immunodeficiency virus (HIV) infection. However, MMR and other measles-containing vaccines are not recommended for HIV-infected persons with evidence of severe immunosuppression.

Mumps

Mumps is an acute viral illness. Outbreaks of mumps have been reported among military personnel as recently as 1986. Mumps virus is rapidly inactivated by heat, formalin, ether, and ultraviolet light. The virus is acquired by respiratory droplets. The incubation period of mumps is 14 to 18 days. **Parotitis** (inflammation of salivary glands) is the most common manifestation of infected persons.

Complications

Aseptic meningitis is common, and adults have a higher risk for this complication than children. Testicular inflammation is the most common complication in postpubertal males.

Mumps Vaccine

Mumps vaccine is available as a single antigen preparation, combined with rubella vaccine, or combined with measles and rubella vaccine (MMR).

Adverse Reactions

Mumps vaccine is very safe. Most adverse effects are reported after MMR vaccine.

Contraindications

Persons who have experienced a severe allergic reaction after a prior dose of mumps vaccine or to a vaccine component should generally not be vaccinated with MMR.

Rubella

The term **rubella** means "little red." Rubella virus is relatively unstable and is inactivated by lipid solvents, formalin, and ultraviolet light. Rubella virus transmission is thought to occur in the nasopharynx. The incubation period of rubella is 14 days. In children, rash is usually the first manifestation, and a prodrome (an early warning symptom that may mark the beginning of a disease or illness) is rare. The rash occurs initially on the face and then progresses from head to foot. Complications are uncommon, but tend to occur more often in adults than in children.

Rubella Vaccine

Rubella vaccine is a live attenuated virus. Rubella vaccine is available as a single antigen preparation, combined with mumps and measles vaccine (MMR).

Adverse Reactions

Rubella vaccine is very safe. Most adverse events reported after MMR vaccination are attributable to the measles component. The most common complaints after rubella vaccination are fever, swelling of lymph nodes, and joint pain.

Contraindications

Persons who have experienced a severe allergic reaction after a prior dose of rubella vaccine or to a vaccine component should not be vaccinated with MMR. Women known to be pregnant or attempting to become pregnant should not receive rubella vaccine.

Haemophilus influenzae

Haemophilus influenzae is a gram-negative coccobacillus. The outermost structure of *H. influenzae* is composed of a polysaccharide, which is responsible for immunity. There are six different serotypes (a through f) of polysaccharide capsule. Type b organisms account for 95% of all strains that cause invasive disease. The organism enters the body through the nasopharynx. This disease is common in infants (at 6 to 7 months of age). *H. influenzae* type b (Hib) disease is uncommon after 5 years of age. Invasive disease caused by *H. influenzae* type b can affect many organ systems. The most common types of invasive disease are meningitis, epiglottitis, pneumonia, and arthritis. Humans are the only known reservoir.

Haemophilus influenzae *type b Conjugate Vaccine*

Since 1990, four additional conjugate Hib vaccines have been licensed for use in infants as young as 6 weeks of age. More than 95% of infants will develop protective antibody levels after a primary series of two or three doses.

Adverse Reactions

Adverse events after Hib conjugate vaccine are uncommon. Swelling, redness, and pain have been reported in 5% to 30% of recipients. Systemic reaction such as fever and irritability are infrequent.

Contraindications

Vaccination with Hib conjugate vaccine is contraindicated in persons known to have experienced anaphylaxis after a prior dose of that vaccine.

VACCINES FOR SPECIAL GROUPS ONLY

Some vaccines are targeted for selected groups of people such as travelers, nurses, and the elderly. Table 28-3 lists vaccines restricted to special groups.

In some cases, such as yellow fever or rabies, this is because of geographical restrictions, whereas in others it is because of problems in producing sufficient vaccine in time to meet the demand. For example, each influenza epidemic is caused by a different strain, requiring a new vaccine.

Hepatitis

Hepatitis is inflammation of the liver. Hepatitis may be caused by a drug or chemical toxin, but more commonly is caused by a viral infection. Many forms of viral hepatitis are highly communicable, and epidemics may be prevented by the use of vaccines.

Hepatitis A

Hepatitis A is a viral hepatitis caused by the hepatitis A virus and is characterized by slow onset of signs and symptoms. The virus may be spread through fecally contaminated food or water. Two inactivated whole virus hepatitis A vaccines are available. Both vaccines are available in pediatric and adult formulations. Neither vaccine is currently licensed for those who are younger than 2 years of age. More than 95% of adults will develop immunity. Both vaccines are highly effective in the prevention of clinical hepatitis A. Routine hepatitis A vaccination is recommended for children older than 2 years. For children and adolescents, 0.5 mL of vaccine should be administered intramuscularly into the deltoid muscle with a booster dose 6 to 12 months later. For adults, 1.0 mL of vaccine should be used.

Hepatitis A Vaccine Recommendations. Administration of hepatitis A vaccine should be strongly considered for persons 2 years of age and older who are traveling to or working in countries with a high or intermediate risk of hepatitis A virus infection. Other groups that should be offered the vaccine include men who have sex with other men, drug users, persons with occupational risk, or persons with chronic liver disease, including hepatitis C.

Adverse Reactions. The most common adverse reaction after vaccination is a local reaction at the site of injection (pain, redness, or swelling). Mild systemic complaints are fatigue, malaise, and low-grade fever. No serious adverse reactions have been reported.

Contraindications. Hepatitis A vaccine should not be administered to person with a history of a serious allergic reaction to a prior dose of hepatitis A vaccine.

Hepatitis B

Hepatitis B is a viral hepatitis caused by the hepatitis B virus (HBV). The virus is transmitted by transfusion of contaminated blood or blood products, by sexual contact with an infected person, or by the use of contaminated needles and instruments. Severe infection may cause prolonged illness, cancer, or death. Hepatitis B vaccines have

TABLE 28-3. Vaccines Restricted to Special Groups

DISEASE	VACCINE	SPECIAL GROUPS
Hepatitis B	Surface antigen	At risk (medical, nursing staff), drug addicts, male homosexuals, known contacts of carriers
Tuberculosis	BCG	United States: at-risk only
Influenza	Killed	At-risk; elderly
Rabies	Killed	At-risk postexposure (animal workers)
Hepatitis A	Killed or attenuated	Travelers
Cholera	Killed or mutant	Travelers
Meningitis	Polysaccharide	Travelers
Typhoid	Killed or mutant	Travelers
Yellow fever	Attenuated	Travelers
Pneumococcal pneumonia	Polysaccharide	Elderly

been available in the United States since 1981. From 1981 until 1991, vaccination was targeted to people in groups at high risk of HBV infection. The three major risk groups (heterosexuals with multiple partners in contact with infected persons, injection drug users, and male homosexuals) are not reached effectively by targeted programs. A plasma-derived vaccine was licensed in the United States in 1981. The vaccine was safe and effective, but was not well accepted, possibly because of unfounded fears of transmission of live HBV and other blood-borne pathogens. This vaccine was removed from the U.S. market in 1992. Recombinant hepatitis B vaccine was licensed in the United States in July 1986. Two U.S. manufacturers currently produce hepatitis B vaccine: Merck (Recombivax HB®) and SmithKline Beecham (Engerix-B®). Both vaccines are available in pediatric and adult formulations. The recommended dosage of the vaccine differs, depending on the age of the recipient, certain exposure circumstances (e.g., perinatal), and the type of vaccine.

The schedule for hepatitis B vaccine is usually three doses at 0, 1, and 6 months. Infants whose mothers are hepatitis B surface antigen-positive (carriers) should also receive hepatitis B immune globulin (HBIG) upon giving birth. Booster doses are *NOT* routinely recommended for any group. Hepatitis B vaccine indications are as follows:

- Infants at birth to 2 months of age
- Adolescents 11 to 12 years of age
- Selected adults

Prevention of Perinatal Hepatitis B Virus Infection. Infants born to women who have had acute or chronic hepatitis B have an extremely high risk of HBV transmission and chronic HBV infection. Hepatitis B vaccination and one dose of HBIG should be administered within 24 hours after birth. HBIG (0.5 mL) should be given intramuscularly, preferably within 12 hours of birth. Hepatitis B vaccine should be given intramuscularly in three doses.

Combination Hepatitis A and Hepatitis B Vaccine. In May 2001, the Food and Drug Administration approved a combination hepatitis A and hepatitis B vaccine (Twinrix®, GlaxoSmithKline). The vaccine is administered in a three-dose series at 0, 1, and 6 months. Twinrix® is approved for persons aged 18 years and older and can be used in persons in this age group with indications for both hepatitis A and B vaccines. The deltoid muscle is the recommended site for hepatitis B vaccination in adults and children, and the anterolateral thigh is recommended for infants and neonates.

Adverse Reactions. The most common adverse reaction after hepatitis B vaccine is pain at the site of injection. Low-grade fever, headache, and fatigue have also been reported.

Contraindications. A serious allergic reaction to a prior dose of hepatitis B vaccine is a contraindication to further doses of the vaccine.

Influenza

Influenza is a highly infectious viral illness. Influenza virus is a single-stranded, helically shaped RNA virus of the orthomyxovirus family. Basic antigen types A, B, and C are determined by the nuclear material. **Influenza A** causes moderate to severe illness and affects all age groups. The virus infects humans and other animals, such as pigs and birds. **Influenza B** generally causes milder disease than type A and primarily affects children. Influenza B is more stable than influenza A, with less antigenic drift and consequent immunological stability. It affects only humans. **Influenza C** is rarely reported as a cause of human illness, probably because most cases are subclinical. It has not been associated with epidemic disease. The incubation period for influenza is usually 2 days, but can vary from 1 to 5 days. The severity of influenza illness depends on the individual's prior immunological experience with antigenically related virus variants. "Classic" influenza disease is characterized by the abrupt onset of fever, myalgia, sore throat, and nonproductive cough.

The most frequent complication of influenza is pneumonia, most commonly secondary bacterial pneumonia. Primary influenza viral pneumonia is an uncommon complication with a high fatality rate. **Reye syndrome** is a complication that occurs almost exclusively in children taking aspirin, primarily in association with influenza B or varicella zoster, and presents with severe vomiting and confusion, which may progress to coma, due to swelling of the brain. Thus, aspirin should not be given to infants, children, or teenagers with influenza. Recovery is usually rapid, but some may have lingering depression and asthenia (lack of strength or energy) for several weeks. Other complications include **myocarditis** (inflammation of the heart), and worsening of chronic bronchitis and other chronic pulmonary diseases. Death is reported in 0.5 to 1 per 1000 cases. The majority of deaths occur in persons aged 65 or greater. The risk for complications and hospitalizations from influenza are higher among persons aged 65 or older, very young children, and persons of any age with certain underlying medical conditions. Influenza is spread via aerosolized or droplet transmission from the respiratory tract of infected persons. The influenza vaccines available in the United States are composed of inactivated influenza virus. Only disrupted, or split-virus, vaccines are available in the United States. Split vaccines are associated with fewer adverse events among children than previously produced whole virus vaccines. For practical purposes, immunity after inactivated influenza vaccination rarely exceeds 1 year. Influenza activity peaks in temperate areas between late December and early March.

Influenza Vaccine

This vaccine is most effective when it precedes exposure by no more than 2 to 4 months. It should be offered annually, beginning in September, for routine patient visits. Organized campaigns that are routinely accessible for high-risk persons are optimally undertaken in October and November.

Beginning in 2002, the Advisory Committee on Immunization Practices recommended that high-risk persons, health care workers, and children younger than 9 years of age being vaccinated for the first time should begin vaccinations in October. All other groups should begin vaccinations in November. The vaccination is only given intramuscularly, and the dosages are as follows:

- 6 to 35 months: one or two doses at least 1 month apart, 0.25 mL per dose
- 3 to 8 years: one or two doses at least 1 month apart, 0.50 mL per dose
- >9 years: one dose, 0.50 mL per dose

Only one dose is needed if a child received influenza vaccine during a previous influenza season.

Adverse Reactions

Local reactions are the most common adverse events after influenza vaccination. They include soreness, erythema, and induration at the site of injection. Rarely, immediate hypersensitivity, presumed to be allergic, reactions (such as hives, angioedema, allergic asthma, or systemic anaphylaxis) occur after influenza vaccination.

Contraindications

Persons with a severe allergic reaction to a previous dose of influenza vaccine or to vaccine components (such as eggs) should not receive influenza vaccine. Persons with a moderate to severe acute illness normally should not be vaccinated until their symptoms have decreased. Neither pregnancy nor breast-feeding is a contraindication to influenza vaccination.

Pneumonia

Pneumonia is an acute inflammation of the lungs, often caused by inhaled *Streptococcus pneumoniae*. The bacterium is also called *pneumococcus*. The alveoli and bronchioles of the lungs become plugged with fibrous exudates. Pneumonia may be caused by other bacteria, as well as by viruses, rickettsiae, and fungi.

Pneumococcal Vaccines

The first polysaccharide pneumococcal vaccine was licensed in the United States in 1977. Two polysaccharide vaccines are available in the United States: Pneumovax 23®, manufactured by Merck, and Pnu-Immune 23®, manufactured by Lederle. Pneumococcal vaccine is given by injection and may be administered either intramuscularly or subcutaneously. Pneumococcal polysaccharide vaccine should be administered routinely to all adults 65 years of age and older. The vaccine is also indicated for persons older than 2 years of age with normal immune systems who have chronic illnesses, including cardiovascular disease, pulmonary disease, diabetes, alcoholism, and cirrhosis.

Adverse Reactions

The most common adverse reactions after pneumococcal vaccine are local reactions.

Contraindications

A serious allergic reaction to a dose of pneumococcal vaccine is a contraindication to further doses of vaccine. Such allergic reactions are rare.

Meningitis

Meningitis is any infection or inflammation of the membranes covering the brain and spinal cord. The most common causes in adults are bacterial infection with *S. pneumoniae*, *Neisseria meningitides*, or *H. influenzae*. Nonbacterial agents such as chemical irritants, neoplasms, or viruses may cause septic meningitis. Routine vaccination with meningococcal vaccine is not recommended because of its ineffectiveness in children younger than 2 years of age. Polysaccharide meningococcal vaccine is useful for controlling serogroup C meningococcal outbreaks. Two doses should be administered 3 months apart. Adverse reactions and contraindications are the same as those for pneumococcal vaccines.

Rabies

Rabies is an acute, usually fatal viral disease of the central nervous system of animals. It is transmitted from animals to people by infected blood, tissue, or most commonly, saliva. It is also called **hydrophobia**. Local treatment of wounds infected by rabid animals may prevent the disease. The wound is cleansed with soap, water, and a disinfectant. A deep wound may be cauterized, and rabies immune globulin is injected directly into the base of the wound. For active immunization, a series of five intramuscular injections with a human diploid cell rabies vaccine are given. Studies conducted in the United States by the Centers for Disease Control and Prevention have shown that a regimen of one dose of human rabies immune globulin and five doses of vaccine over a 28-day period is effective. The schedule of rabies vaccinations is as follows:

- First dose at 0 days
- Second dose 3 days after the first
- Third dose 7 days after the first
- Fourth dose 14 days after the first
- Fifth dose 28 days after the first

Rabies vaccine should be injected IM (deltoid muscle) after exposure. Subcutaneous injection should be used for preexposure vaccination.

Tuberculosis

Tuberculosis is a chronic granulomatous infection caused by *Mycobacterium tuberculosis*. It is generally transmitted by inhalation or ingestion of infected droplets and usually affects the lungs, although infection of multiple organ systems also occurs.

BCG Vaccine

The vaccine for tuberculosis, BCG vaccine, is an active immunizing agent prepared from bacilli Calmette-Guérin.

BCG vaccine is prescribed most commonly for immunization against tuberculosis. BCG vaccination should be considered for an infant or child who has a negative tuberculin skin test. BCG vaccination is not recommended for patients infected with HIV or who are using corticosteroids concomitantly. It is not given after vaccination for smallpox, nor is it given to patients with a positive tuberculin reaction or a burn.

Tuberculin Test

A tuberculin test can determine past or present tuberculosis infection on the basis of a positive skin reaction, using one of several methods. A purified protein derivative of tubercle bacilli, called tuberculin, is introduced into the skin by scratch, puncture, or intradermal injection. If a raised, red, or hard zone forms surrounding the tuberculin test site, the person is said to be sensitive to tuberculin, and the test is read as positive. The most common tests are the Mantoux test and the **tine test**. The **Mantoux test** is performed by administration of 0.1 mL of solution into the dermis using an intradermal needle and syringe. A hardened, raised red area of 8 to 10 mm, appearing 24 to 72 hours after injection, is a positive reaction. This method is the most reliable means of testing tuberculin sensitivity.

Smallpox

Smallpox is an acute infectious disease caused by the *Variola* virus. First described in a fourth century AD Chinese text, the vaccine was developed in the late eighteenth century. The last case of smallpox in the United States was reported in Texas in 1949. In June 1966, the World Health Organization initiated an intensified global smallpox eradication program. The last indigenous case of smallpox on earth occurred in Somalia in 1977. The World Health Assembly officially certified the global eradication of smallpox in May 1980.

Humans are the only natural host. There is no chronic carrier state and no known animal reservoir. Most transmission results from face-to-face contact with infected persons. Transmission most often occurs during the first week of a rash.

Smallpox Vaccine

In 1796, Edward Jenner, a doctor in rural England, discovered that immunity to smallpox could be produced by inoculating a person with material from a cowpox lesion. Cowpox is a pox virus in the same family as *Variola*. Jenner called the material used for inoculation a vaccine. The smallpox vaccine is currently available in the United States as a live-virus preparation of infectious vaccine virus. Approximately 15 million doses of the vaccine are available now in the United States. More than 200 million additional doses of vaccine are being produced to be available in the case of an introduction of smallpox. The vaccine is administered by using a multiple-puncture technique with a special bifurcated needle, which first became available in 1965. In 1983, the smallpox vaccine was removed from the civilian market. The vaccine is currently available only from the Centers for Disease Control and Prevention under an investigational new drug protocol.

Neutralizing antibodies develop 10 days after primary vaccination and 7 days after revaccination. Antibody titers persist more than 10 years after the second dose is received and up to 30 years after three doses of vaccine are received. A high level of protection (nearly 100%) against smallpox persists for up to 5 years after the primary vaccination. Smallpox vaccine also provides protection if administered after an exposure to smallpox. The lowest disease rates are seen among persons vaccinated less than 7 days after exposure. The disease is generally less severe in persons receiving postexposure vaccinations.

Routine childhood smallpox vaccination was discontinued in the United States in 1971. Routine vaccination of health care workers was discontinued in 1976 and of military recruits in 1990. In 1980, smallpox vaccine was recommended for laboratory workers who had an occupational risk for exposure to the vaccine. The schedule for smallpox vaccine is one successful dose (i.e., a dose that results in a major reaction at the vaccination site). Under routine circumstances, the vaccine should not be administered to persons younger than 18 years of age. In an emergency (postrelease) situation, there would be no age limit for vaccination of persons exposed to a person with confirmed smallpox.

Adverse Reactions

Smallpox vaccine contains live vaccinia virus, which replicates at the site of vaccination. Adverse reactions to smallpox vaccine include the following:

- Inadvertent autoinoculation
- Eczema vaccinatum
- Generalized vaccinia
- Vaccinia necrosum
- Postvaccinal encephalitis

Contraindications

As with all vaccines, smallpox vaccine is contraindicated for persons who have experienced a serious allergic reaction to a prior dose of vaccine or to a vaccine component. Live viral vaccines are contraindicated during pregnancy. Thus, smallpox vaccine should not be administered to pregnant women for routine nonemergency indications. It is also contraindicated in

TABLE 28-4. Contraindications to and Precautions for Smallpox Vaccination

NONEMERGENCY SITUATIONS	EMERGENCY (POSTRELEASE) SITUATIONS
1. Severe allergic reaction to prior dose or vaccine component	1. Exposed persons—no contraindications
2. Immunosuppression or immunosuppressed household contact	2. Unexposed persons—same as nonemergency situations
3. Pregnancy	
4. Eczema, history of eczema, or household contact with eczema or history of eczema	
5. Other skin conditions	
6. Age younger than 18 years	

people with eczema or a past history of eczema. Smallpox vaccine should not be administered to people younger than 18 years of age. Contraindications and precautions to smallpox vaccine in nonemergency situations and emergency (postrelease) situations is seen in Table 28-4.

Anthrax

Anthrax is a zoonotic disease caused by the spore-forming bacteria *Bacillus anthracis*. A live attenuated animal vaccine was developed and tested by Louis Pasteur in 1881. A human vaccine composed of cell-free culture filtrate was developed in 1954 and improved in 1970. Anthrax was first used effectively as a bioterrorist agent in 2001. *B. anthracis* is a gram-positive aerobic bacterium. Spores may remain viable in soil for years. Humans can become infected with *B. anthracis* by skin contact, ingestion, or inhalation of spores originating from animal products of infected animals or from the environment. Spores can be inactivated by sufficient contact with paraformaldehyde vapor, 5% hypochlorite, or phenol solution or by autoclaving. The symptoms and incubation period of human anthrax are determined by the route of transmission of the organism.

Types of Anthrax

There are three clinical forms of anthrax: cutaneous (most common in natural exposure situations), gastrointestinal (rare), and inhalation. Anthrax bioterrorism attacks in the United States in 2001 totaled 22 (11 by inhalation and 11 cutaneously) in four states and Washington, DC. *B. Anthracis* was sent through the U.S. mail. Most of the patients were exposed in mail-sorting facilities or had direct contact with a contaminated envelope.

Anthrax Vaccine

Louis Pasteur successfully attenuated *B. anthracis* and produced the first live attenuated bacterial vaccine for animals in 1881. An improved cell-free vaccine was licensed for use in the United States in 1970. The duration of immunity in humans after vaccination is unknown. Primary vaccination consists of three subcutaneous injections at 0, 2, and 4 weeks, followed by doses at 6, 12, and 18 months. To maintain immunity, the manufacturer recommends an annual booster dose. The basis for the schedule of vaccinations at 0, 2, and 4 weeks and 6, 12, and 18 months, followed by the annual booster, is not well defined. Interruption of the vaccination schedule does not require restarting the entire series of anthrax vaccine injections or the addition of extra doses.

Adverse Reactions

The most common adverse reactions following anthrax vaccine are local reactions. No studies have documented occurrence of chronic diseases (e.g., cancer or infertility) after anthrax vaccination.

Contraindications

The vaccine is contraindicated in persons who had a severe allergic reaction after a previous dose or to a vaccine component. Anthrax vaccine is contraindicated in persons who have recovered from anthrax. A moderate or severe acute illness is a precaution, and vaccination should be postponed until recovery. Pregnant women should be vaccinated against anthrax only if the potential benefits of vaccination outweigh the potential risks to the fetus.

SUMMARY

Viruses, bacteria, fungi, protozoa, and multicellular parasites can cause many different diseases. The immune system combats these disease-causing microbes. Its primary function is to eliminate infectious agents and minimize the damage they cause. The principal components of the immune system include the bone marrow, thymus, lymph nodes, spleen, and lymphatic vessels. Special proteins are formed in response to particular foreign substances. These proteins are called antibodies, and active production of antibodies results in acquired immunity. Antibodies that neutralize toxins are called antitoxins. Antibodies are also known as immunoglobulins. Immunoglobulins are used in vaccinations against disease. Diseases that are commonly vaccinated against include diphtheria, tetanus, pertussis, poliomyelitis, measles, mumps, rubella, *Haemophilus influenzae* infection, hepatitis, influenza, pneumonia, meningitis, rabies, tuberculosis, smallpox, and anthrax.

CRITICAL THINKING

1. Describe how the immune system will fight off a viral infection. Will you be more or less susceptible to exposure to the virus again in the future? Why or why not?

2. Explain why the old and the young are more susceptible to infection and exposure to infectious agents.

3. Choose one of the disorders discussed in this chapter and research the origins of the disorder and the history of vaccinations related to the disorder.

REVIEW QUESTIONS

1. Which active vaccine is recommended for health care workers, but is not routinely given to infants?
   A. Measles, mumps, and rubella
   B. Influenza
   C. Diphtheria
   D. Pertussis

2. Which of the following diseases is also called hydrophobia?
   A. Smallpox
   B. Polio
   C. Anthrax
   D. Rabies

3. The first immunoglobulin produced by the body when challenged by antigens during the initial antigen exposure is
   A. IgG.
   B. IgA.
   C. IgM.
   D. IgE.

4. Which of the following is a live attenuated vaccine that is bacterial?
   A. Vaccinia
   B. Oral typhoid
   C. Oral polio
   D. Yellow fever

5. The vaccine that is allowed to be administered at birth is
   A. hepatitis B.
   B. hepatitis C.
   C. rabies.
   D. oral polio.

6. The body's first line of defense against pathogen is
   A. unbroken skin.
   B. phagocytes.
   C. antibody molecules.
   D. neutrophils.

7. Which of the following antibodies is able to cross the placenta?
   A. IgA
   B. IgM
   C. IgG
   D. IgE

8. The total number of doses of vaccine administered to an individual for anthrax is
   A. one.
   B. three.
   C. five.
   D. six.

9. Under routine circumstances, which vaccine should not be administered to children younger than 18 years of age?
   A. Influenza
   B. Smallpox
   C. BCG
   D. MMR

10. The BCG vaccine against tuberculosis is not recommended for patients infected with
    A. HIV.
    B. hepatitis B.
    C. syphilis.
    D. warts.

11. The last schedule of rabies vaccine is
    A. 1 week after the first.
    B. 2 weeks after the first.
    C. 4 weeks after the first.
    D. 6 months after the first.

12. Humeral immunity involves all of the following, except
    A. erythrocytes.
    B. antibodies.
    C. plasma cells.
    D. B cells.

13. Natural passive acquired immunity results from
    A. ingestion of colostrum.
    B. a vaccine.
    C. a gamma globulin injection.
    D. having the mumps.

14. Which of the following agents should be avoided for infants who have "classic" influenza?
    A. Penicillin
    B. Acetaminophen
    C. Aspirin
    D. Codeine preparations

15. The last vaccine in the basic schedule for anthrax administration should be administered _____ after the first vaccine.
    A. 2 months
    B. 6 months
    C. 12 months
    D. 18 months

OUTLINE

OBJECTIVES

Upon completion of this chapter, the reader should be able to

1. Understand the importance of poisons and antidotes.
2. Explain the factors of levels of toxicity.
3. Describe industrial intoxication.
4. Be familiar with poison prevention programs.
5. Describe detection of poisons.
6. Give five examples of specific poisons.
7. Explain five antidotes for specific poisons.
8. Define acute mercury poisoning.
9. Explain the most common American household poison.

GLOSSARY

aversive agent A nontoxic substance that is added to poisonous substances to cause the taste or smell of the poisonous substance to be offensive.

mutagen A substance that is capable of making changes at the cellular level.

poison Any substance that causes injury, illness, or death of a living organism.

poisoning The development of dose-related adverse effects after exposure to chemicals, drugs, or other substances foreign to the body.

salicylism Salicylate intoxication.

teratogen A substance that is capable of affecting the fetus.

toxicity The degree to which something is poisonous.

OVERVIEW

Poisoning refers to the development of dose-related adverse effects after exposure to chemicals, drugs, or other substances foreign to the body. A poisonous substance (**poison**) is defined as any substance that causes injury, illness, or death of a living organism. Poisons produce toxic effects at concentrations that alter the normal state of the organism. Approximately 70,000 different chemicals have been identified as toxic. **Toxicity** is the degree to which something is poisonous. In the United States, most exposures to poisons are acute and accidental, involve a single agent, occur in the home, result in minor or no toxicity, and involve children younger than 6 years of age. Common routes of exposure are ingestion (74%), dermal (8.2%), inhalation (6.7%), ocular (6%), and bites and stings (3.9%). Approximately 10 million people are poisoned annually, and 4000 of these poisonings are fatal. Prognosis depends on the amount of poison absorbed, the poison's toxicity, and the time interval between poisoning and treatment.

DOSE RESPONSE

For many chemicals, there is a dose at which there are no toxic effects, a dose at which the effects are reversible, and a dose at which the effects may have permanent consequences. The dose-response degree of toxicity may be affected by characteristics of the living organism consuming the poison. Some examples of these characteristics are species, weight, age, general health, and previous usage.

An example of some toxic chemicals that many members of society choose to be regularly exposed to are caffeine, tobacco, alcohol, and drugs. At doses normally consumed by the average person, the "high" effect felt by the individual response can be quite different. One person may be able to drink five cups of coffee without visible effects, whereas another person might begin to feel shaky after two cups of coffee. This is an example of how the dose and response varies from one person to the next. At some point, each of these chemicals can have a much more serious effect on the individual. At extremely high doses (much higher than the average person can consume on a regular basis), caffeine can be a **mutagen** (capable of making changes at the cellular level), a potential **teratogen** (capable of affecting the fetus), and a probable carcinogen as well. At high doses, nicotine, the active ingredient in tobacco, can be a very potent poison causing nausea, vomiting, convulsions, and even death. At high doses, alcohol can cause birth defects, brain damage, coma, and death.

When one evaluates use of drugs, the decision is made from a risk-benefit analysis because all drugs are potential poisons when used improperly or in excess dosage and can cause serious adverse effects, including death. The level of toxicity of a product depends on the dose of the product to which a person is exposed. Thus, the issue is not whether a chemical is toxic, it is the nature of the toxicity, and whether there is a less toxic alternative which, when used with the proper precautions, can have the same result.

For an average person, the use of household cleaning products is another common area of exposure to potential poisons. Many of these products definitely have a degree of toxicity, and the manufacturers have attempted to minimize the risk by providing information about safe handling procedures on the labels.

In the United States more than 1.8 million human exposures to poisons are reported each year, and approximately 70% of these exposures are managed outside of a health care facility, with the guidance of a poison center. About 60% of these poisoning victims are younger than 6 years of age; the majority of poison exposures are the result of unintentional actions. Accidental poisoning results most commonly from ingestion of toxic substances and involves children in the majority of cases.

Accidental poisoning by chemical agents causes more than 5000 deaths each year, whereas suicides by chemical agents annually number more than 6000. In addition to the victims of fatal poisoning, there is a much greater number of persons who are made seriously ill by chemical agents but recover after appropriate therapy. Unfortunately, some of these patients are left with permanent consequences of their intoxication.

In the United States, accidental poisonings occur far more often in the home than through industrial exposure and are usually acute events; industrial intoxication is more often the result of chronic exposure.

PREVENTION

The introduction of poison prevention programs has made an impact on reducing cases of accidental poisoning in the United States. One notable event was the introduction of child-resistant packaging in 1972 (see Figure 29-1). Since then, the numbers of deaths from accidental lethal poisoning with all medicines and household chemicals have been reduced, especially for children younger than 5 years of age (decrease from 216 in 1972 to 28 in 2000).

The recommended prevention guidelines for all households include the following:

1. Use child-resistant packaging properly by closing the container securely after use.
2. Keep all chemicals and medicines locked up and out of sight (see Figure 29-2).
3. Call the poison center (1-800-222-1222) immediately if poisoning is suspected.
4. When products are in use, never let young children out of your sight, even if you must take the

child or product along when answering the phone or doorbell.

5. Keep items in original containers.
6. Leave the original labels on all products, and read the label before using.
7. Do not put decorative lamps and candles that contain lamp oil where children can reach them because lamp oil is very toxic.
8. Always leave the light on when giving or taking medicine. Check the dosage every time.
9. Avoid taking medicine in front of children. Refer to medicine as "medicine" not "candy."
10. Clean out the medicine cabinet periodically, and safely dispose of unneeded medicines when the illness for which they were prescribed is over. Pour contents down the drain or toilet, and rinse the container before discarding.

Other proven poison prevention techniques include heightened parental awareness, manufacturers' modifications of product formulations, the Federal Hazardous Labeling Act, child-resistant closures, appropriate packaging and labeling, avoidance of container transfer, public education, and proper home storage of poisonous substances.

One prevention method that is causing some controversy is the introduction of aversive agents into poisons. **Aversive agents** are nontoxic substances that are added to poisonous substances to cause their taste or smell to be offensive. Most experts agree that this method of prevention should only be considered for the most toxic products. Other scientists think that aversive agents may have their maximal benefit when they are added to relatively palatable toxic substances. The controversial concerns associated with the decision to add the agents are that there are substantial data gaps. The most notable gaps that persist are long-term human safety, environmental impact, human

hypersensitivity, and teratogenicity data. The scientific community is demanding more complete information be gathered and analyzed and recommending that aversive agents be added to only a limited number of highly toxic products *before* recommending that aversive agents be added to large numbers of products.

DETECTION OF POISONS

Optimal management of the poisoned patient requires correct diagnosis. Although the toxic effects of some chemical substances are quite characteristic, most poisoning syndromes can simulate other diseases. Poisoning usually is included in the differential diagnosis of coma, convulsions, acute psychosis, acute hepatic or renal insufficiency, and bone marrow depression. Although it should be, poisoning may not be considered when the major manifestation is a mild psychiatric disturbance or neurological disorder, abdominal pain, bleeding, fever, hypotension, pulmonary congestion, or skin eruption. Furthermore, patients may be unaware of their exposure to a poison, such as with chronic

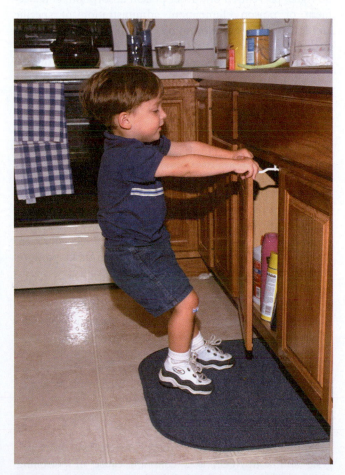

Figure 29-2. Household cabinets that contain materials that may be hazardous to children should be equipped with child safety locks.

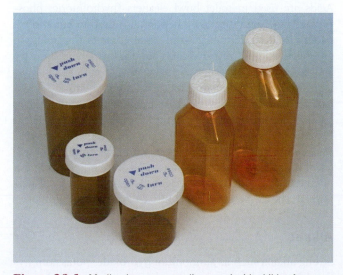

Figure 29-1. Medications are now dispensed with child safety caps to prevent accidental ingestion of medications in children.

insidious intoxications or after attempted suicide or abortion or they may be unwilling to admit it. In every instance of poisoning, identification of the toxic agent should be attempted. Specific antidotal therapy is obviously impossible without such identification.

Some poisons can produce clinical features characteristic enough to strongly suggest the diagnosis. Careful examination of the patient may reveal the unmistakable odor of cyanide; the cherry-colored flush of carboxyhemoglobin in skin and mucous membranes; or the papillary constriction, salivation, and gastrointestinal hyperactivity produced by insecticides. Chemical analysis of body fluids provides the most definite identification of the intoxicating agent. Some common poisons, such as aspirin and barbiturates, can be identified and amounts even quantitated by relatively simple laboratory procedures. Others require more complex toxicological techniques. Chemical analyses of body fluids or tissues are of particular value in the diagnosis and evaluation of chronic intoxications.

TREATMENT

Treatment goals for poisoned patients include support of vital signs, prevention of further poison absorption, enhancement of poison elimination, administration of specific antidotes, and prevention of reexposure. Specific treatment depends on the identity of the poison, the route and amount of exposure, the time of presentation relative to the time of exposure, and the severity of poisoning. Knowledge of the pharmacokinetics and pharmacodynamics of the offending agent is essential.

SPECIFIC POISONS

The most common poisons involving the general population are nonprescription drugs, household products, solvents, pesticides, and poisonous plants. The following discussions of specific poisons stress their action and the recognition or treatment of clinical poisoning. Some household products contain substances that can pose health risks if they are ingested or inhaled or if they come in contact with eyes and skin. The National Library of Medicine's Household Products Database (http://householdproducts.nlm.nih.gov) provides information in consumer-friendly language on many of these substances and their potential health effects. For more technical information users can launch a search for a product or ingredient in TOXNET from the Product Page in the database.

Acetaminophen

Acetaminophen, a popular alternative to salicylates as an analgesic and antipyretic, is a common cause of poisoning. Although the toxic and lethal doses of acetaminophen may vary from patient to patient, hepatic damage may be expected

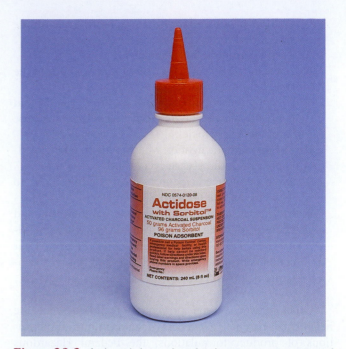

Figure 29-3. Activated charcoal can be given to treat some types of poisonings.

if an adult has taken more than 8 g as a single dose. Clinical manifestations of acetaminophen poisoning are nonspecific. In the first few hours after ingestion, lethargy, nausea, vomiting, and diaphoresis may occur. Hepatic damage, the most important manifestation of acetaminophen toxicity, becomes evident 1 to 2 days after ingestion. Treatment should begin with induction of emesis or gastric lavage followed by administration of activated charcoal (see Figure 29-3). Treatment with acetylcysteine is most effective if started within 8 to 10 hours after ingestion.

Acids

Acids are used in toilet bowl cleaners (hydrofluoric, phosphoric, and sulfuric acids). They are also used in automobile battery fluid (sulfuric acid) and stone cleaners (hydrofluoric and nitric acids). Corrosive acids are used widely in industry and laboratories. Ingestion is almost always with suicidal intent. Toxic effects are due to their direct chemical action. Ingestion of acids may produce irritation, bleeding, severe pain, and severe burns in the mouth, esophagus, and stomach. Often, profound shock develops and may be fatal. Ingested acid should be diluted immediately with large amounts of water or milk. The danger of perforation contraindicates the use of emesis or gastric lavage. Diagnostic esophagoscopy, if performed, should be done in the first 24 hours after ingestion.

Alkalis

Strong alkalis such as ammonium hydroxide, potassium hydroxide (potash), potassium carbonate, sodium hydroxide (bleach), and sodium carbonate (washing soda) are used widely in industry and in cleansers and drain cleaners. The toxic effects of alkalies are due to irritation and destruction of local tissues. Ingestion is followed by severe pain in the mouth, pharynx, chest, and abdomen. Vomiting of blood and diarrhea are common. Perforation of the esophagus or stomach may be immediate or delayed for several days. Treatment consists of immediate administration of large amounts of water or milk. Esophagoscopy should be done within the first 24 hours. Steroids are usually administered for about 3 weeks to decrease the incidence of stricture formation.

Antihistamines

There is a wide variation among patient tolerance to antihistamines and in the manifestations of poisoning. Manifestations of poisoning are central nervous system (CNS) excitement or depression. In adults, drowsiness, stupor, and coma may occur. Treatment is supportive and focused on removal of the unabsorbed drug and maintenance of vital functions. Convulsions may be controlled with phenobarbital or diazepam.

Atropine

Atropine is a widely prescribed drug. Young children are particularly susceptible to poisoning with this agent. Older persons appear to be more sensitive to the CNS effects of atropine. Manifestations usually begin within 1 hour of acute overdosage and 1 to 3 days after treatment is begun in cases of chronic poisoning. The most characteristic manifestations of atropine poisoning are dryness of mouth, thirst, dysphasia, hoarseness, dilated pupils, blurring of vision, flushing, tachycardia, hypertension, and urinary retention. Treatment includes emesis or gastric lavage followed by the administration of activated charcoal. Agitation may respond to benzodiazepine, and comatose patients may require intubation and mechanical ventilation. Cardiovascular toxicity and arrhythmias should be treated as described for antiarrhythmics (Chapter 24) and tricyclic antidepressants (Chapter 23). If symptoms are severe, physostigmine salicylate (an acetylcholinesterase inhibitor that reverses anticholinergic toxicity) should be given intravenously.

Benzene and Toluene

Benzene and toluene are solvents used in paint removers, dry-cleaning solutions, and rubber or plastic cements. Benzene is also present in most gasolines. Poisoning may result from ingestion or from the breathing of concentrated vapors. Toluene is an ingredient in some cement used by glue sniffers. Acute poisoning by these compounds causes CNS manifestations. Restlessness, excitement, euphoria, and dizziness, progressing to coma, convulsions, and respiratory failure are common. Treatment of both acute and chronic poisoning is symptomatic.

Benzodiazepines

Benzodiadepines are readily absorbed, and exhibit 85% to 99% protein binding in the plasma. They are weak acids and are lipid soluble. Benzodiazepines are eliminated mainly by hepatic metabolism. Their CNS depressant effects begin within 30 minutes of acute overdose. Coma and respiratory depression can occur with ultra-short-acting agents and when benzodiazepines are combined with other CNS depressants. Excitation may occur early in the course of poisoning. Activated charcoal absorbs benzodiazepines and is the method of choice for gastrointestinal decontamination. Respiratory support should be provided as necessary.

Bleaches

Industrial strength bleaching solutions contain 10% or more sodium hypochlorite, whereas household products (e.g., Clorox®, Purex®, and Sanichlor™) contain 3% to 6%. The solution used for chlorinating swimming pools contains 20%. Their corrosive action in the mouth, pharynx, and esophagus is similar to that of sodium hydroxide. Treatment consists of dilution of the ingested bleach with water or milk.

Carbon Monoxide

Carbon monoxide (CO) is a colorless, odorless, tasteless, and nonirritating gas that is present in the exhaust of internal combustion engines in concentrations of 3% to 7%. CO is responsible for about 3500 accidental deaths and suicides in the United States annually. The toxic effects of CO are the result of tissue hypoxia. The most characteristic sign of severe CO poisoning is the cherry color of the skin and mucous membranes. Treatment of CO poisoning requires effective ventilation in the presence of high oxygen (O_2) tensions and in the absence of CO. If necessary, ventilation should be supported artificially. Pure O_2 should be administered. Cerebral edema should be treated with diuretics and steroids.

Cyanide

The cyanide ion is an exceedingly potent and rapid-acting poison, but one for which specific and effective antidotal therapy is available. Cyanide poisoning may result from the inhalation of hydrocyanic acid or from the ingestion of soluble inorganic cyanide salts. Parts of many plants also contain substances such as amygdaline, which release cyanide upon digestion. Cyanide poisoning is a true medical emergency. However, treatment is highly effective if given rapidly. The chemical antidotes should be immediately available wherever emergency medical care is dispensed. The diagnosis may be made by the characteristic "bitter almond" odor on the breath of the victim. The objective of treatment is the production of methemoglobin by the administration of nitrite.

Supportive measures, especially artificial respiration with 100% oxygen, should be instituted as soon as possible.

Detergents and Soaps

Detergents and soaps fall into three groups: anionic, non-ionic, and cationic. The first group contains common soaps and household detergents. They may cause vomiting and diarrhea but have no serious effects, and no treatment is required. However, some laundry compounds contain phosphate water softeners whose ingestion may cause hypocalcemia. The ingestion of nonionic detergents also requires no treatment. Cationic detergents are commonly used for bactericidal purposes in hospitals and homes. These compounds are well absorbed from the gastrointestinal tract and interfere with cellular functions. The fatal oral dose is approximately 3 g. Ingestion produces nausea, vomiting, shock, coma, and convulsions and may cause death within a few hours. Treatment after ingestion of diluted preparations consists of minimizing gastrointestinal absorption by emesis and gastric lavage with ordinary soap solution, which rapidly inactivates cationic detergents. Activated charcoal should be administered.

Fluorides

Fluorides are used in insecticides. The gas fluorine is used in industry. Fluorine and fluorides are cellular poisons. Fluorides also form an insoluble precipitate with calcium and cause hypocalcemia. Ingestion of 1 to 2 g of sodium fluoride may be fatal. Inhalation of fluorine or hydrogen fluoride produces coughing and choking. After 1 or 2 days, fever, cough, cyanosis, and pulmonary edema may develop. Ingestion of fluoride salts is followed by nausea, vomiting, diarrhea, and abdominal pain. Death results from respiratory paralysis or circulatory collapse. Treatment of acute fluoride poisoning consists of immediate administration of milk, lime water, or calcium lactate solution to precipitate calcium fluoride. Gastric lavage or emesis and charcoal can be given.

Formaldehyde

Formaldehyde is a gas available as a 40% solution (formalin), which is used as a disinfectant, fumigant, or deodorant. Poisoning by formalin may be diagnosed by the characteristic odor of formaldehyde. This agent reacts chemically with cellular components and depresses cellular functions. The fatal dose of formalin is about 60 mL. Ingestion of formalin immediately causes severe abdominal pain, nausea, vomiting, and diarrhea. This may be followed by collapse, coma, severe metabolic acidosis, and anuria. Death is usually the result of circulatory failure. Because any organic material can inactivate formaldehyde, milk, bread, and soup should be administered immediately unless activated charcoal is available.

Iodine

The traditional antiseptic iodine tincture is an alcoholic solution of 2% iodine and 2% sodium iodide. Strong iodine solution (Lugol's solution) is an aqueous solution of 5% iodine and 10% potassium iodide. The fatal dose of tincture of iodine is approximately 2 g. Iodides are much less toxic, and no fatalities have been reported. The diagnosis of iodine poisoning is suggested by brown staining of the oral mucous membranes. The effects largely result from the corrosive effects of the compound on the gastrointestinal tract. Burning abdominal pain, nausea, vomiting, and bloody diarrhea may occur soon after ingestion. Fever, delirium, stupor, and anuria also have been observed. Treatment consists of the immediate administration of milk, starch, bread, or activated charcoal.

Isopropyl Alcohol and Acetone

Isopropyl alcohol is used as a sterilizing agent or as rubbing alcohol, as well as in solvents, aftershave solutions, antifreeze, and window cleaners. Acetone is found in cleaners, solvents, and nail polish removers. Both are absorbed rapidly from the stomach and the lungs and distributed in body water. Isopropyl alcohol is metabolized to acetone in the liver by the enzyme alcohol dehydrogenase. Up to 20% is excreted unchanged in urine. Acetone is excreted by the kidneys and lungs. Isopropyl alcohol and acetone are CNS depressants. Ingestion produces gastric irritation and raises the danger of vomiting with aspiration. The systemic effects of isopropyl alcohol are similar to those of ethyl alcohol, but it is twice as potent as the latter. Emesis should be induced, or gastric lavage should be performed. Activated charcoal is ineffective. Hemodialysis is effective for removing isopropyl alcohol and acetone. It should be considered in patients with high serum levels who do not respond to conservative therapy.

Lead

Lead poisoning can occur where there are old buildings, old paint, or lead pipes. Even vegetable gardens can be a source of lead. Lead poisoning in adults is rare, but unfortunately it is one of the most common and preventable childhood health problems today. It can be a problem for those who lick or eat flakes of old paint containing lead. Lead can also contaminate water flowing through old lead pipes, slowly poisoning those who drink it. Lead poisoning causes severe damage to the brain, nerves, red blood cells, and digestive system. Symptoms of acute poisoning symptoms include a metallic taste in the mouth, abdominal pain, vomiting, diarrhea, collapse, and coma. Large amounts directly affect the nervous system and cause headache, convulsions, coma, and death. Treatment usually includes the administration of medicines (called chelating agents) to help the body rid itself of lead. For mild poisoning, the chelating agent penicillamine may be used alone; for severe poisoning, it may be used in combination with edetate calcium disodium and dimercaprol. For acute poisoning, gastric lavage is performed.

Magnesium

Magnesium sulfate is used intravenously as a hypotensive agent and orally as a cathartic. The magnesium ion is a profound depressant of the CNS. Poisoning after oral or rectal administration is unlikely in the presence of normal renal function. In the presence of impaired renal function, an oral dose of 30 g may be fatal. Oral ingestion of this solution may cause gastrointestinal irritation. Systemic poisoning can cause paralysis, hypotension, hypothermia, coma, and respiratory failure. Treatment of magnesium poisoning therefore includes the intravenous administration of 10 mL of a 10% solution of calcium gluconate.

Mercury

Acute mercury poisoning usually occurs by ingestion of inorganic mercuric salts or inhalation of metallic mercury vapor. Ingestion of the mercuric salts causes a metallic taste, salivation, thirst, a burning sensation in the throat, discoloration and edema of oral mucous membranes, abdominal pain, vomiting, bloody diarrhea, and shock. Direct nephrotoxicity causes acute renal failure. Inhalation of high concentrations of metallic mercury vapor may cause acute chemical pneumonia. There is no effective specific treatment for mercury vapor pneumonitis. Ingested mercuric salts should be removed by lavage and activated charcoal should be administered. For acute ingestion of mercuric salts, dimercaprol can be given, unless the patient has severe gastroenteritis. In treating chronic poisoning, the person must be removed from exposure. Neurological toxicity is not considered to be reversible with chelation.

Methyl Alcohol

Methyl alcohol, also called wood alcohol or methanol, is the simplest of alcohols and is used as a solvent and in antifreeze and paint remover. Methyl alcohol poisoning results almost entirely from its ingestion as a substitute for ethanol or from the drinking of denatured ethyl alcohol. The toxic dose is quite variable: death has occurred after a dose of 20 mL, but 250 mL has been ingested with survival. Ingestion of as little as 15 mL of methanol has caused permanent blindness. Symptoms of methanol poisoning usually do not appear until 12 to 24 hours after ingestion, when sufficient toxic metabolites have accumulated. Manifestations include headache, dizziness, nausea, vomiting, CNS depression, and respiratory failure. Gastric aspiration is the treatment of choice in methyl alcohol intoxication for gastrointestinal decontamination. Emesis and gastric lavage are of use only within the first 2 hours after ingestion. Intravenous administration of large amounts of sodium bicarbonate combats acidosis. Intravenous ethanol therapy should be used.

Opioids

Opioids include morphine, heroin, and codeine. These drugs have widely varying potencies and durations of action. All of these agents decrease CNS and sympathetic nervous activity. Mild intoxication is characterized by euphoria, drowsiness, and constricted pupils. More severe intoxication may cause hypotension, bradycardia, hypothermia, coma, and respiratory arrest. Death is usually due to apnea or pulmonary aspiration of gastric contents. If the patient arrives for medical care shortly after ingestion, the stomach should be emptied by emesis or gastric lavage and activated charcoal should be administered. Naloxone is a specific opioid antagonist that can rapidly reverse signs of narcotic intoxication.

Organophosphate and Carbamate Insecticides

Organophosphorus compounds, such as the insecticides chlorpyrifos, phosphorothioic acid (Diazinon®), fenthion, malathion, and parathion and the chemical warfare "nerve gases" such as sarin, irreversibly inhibit acetylcholinesterase.

Organophosphates are absorbed through the skin, lungs, and gastrointestinal tract. They are distributed widely in tissues, and slowly eliminated by hepatic metabolism. The time from exposure to the onset of toxicity varies from minutes to hours, but is usually between 30 minutes and 2 hours. Organophosphates may cause nausea, vomiting, abdominal cramps, urinary and fecal incontinence, increased bronchial secretions, cough, wheezing, sweating, salivation, blurred vision, and urinary frequency. In severe poisoning, bradycardia, hypotension, and pulmonary edema may occur.

Treatment of organophosphate poisoning includes removing contaminated clothing and washing the skin with soap and water. Gastrointestinal decontamination should include use of activated charcoal. Supportive measures include oxygen administration, ventilatory assistance, and treatment of seizures.

Petroleum Distillates

Diesel oil, gasoline, kerosene, and paint thinner are all liquid petroleum distillates. Kerosene is used widely as a fuel and as a vehicle for cleaning agents, furniture polishes, insecticides, and paint thinners. Petroleum distillates are CNS depressants; they damage cells by dissolving cellular lipids. Pulmonary damage manifested by pulmonary edema or pneumonitis is a common and serious complication. Inhalation of gasoline or kerosene vapors induces a state resembling alcoholic intoxication. Headache, nausea, and a burning sensation in the chest may be present. The oral ingestion of petroleum distillates causes irritation of the mucous membranes of the upper part of the intestinal tract. In the treatment of poisoning by petroleum distillates, extreme care must be used to prevent aspiration. When large amounts have been ingested, gastric emptying is indicated. In the alert patient, emesis may be induced. Oxygen therapy should also be given.

Phenol

Phenol and related compounds (creosote, cresols, hexachlorophene, Lysol®, and tannic acid) are used as antiseptics, caustics, and preservatives. The approximate fatal oral dose ranges from 2 mL for phenol and cresols to 20 mL for tannic acid. Ingestion of these agents produces erosion of mucosa from mouth to stomach. Vomiting of blood and bloody diarrhea may occur. Hyperpnea, pulmonary edema, stupor, coma, convulsions, and shock are seen. Emesis and lavage are indicated for treatment in the absence of significant corrosive injury to the esophagus. Activated charcoal should be administered.

Phosphorus

Phosphorus occurs in two forms: a red, nonpoisonous form, and a yellow, fat-soluble, highly toxic form. The yellow form of phosphorus is used in rodent and insect poisons and in fireworks. Yellow phosphorus causes fatty degeneration and necrosis of tissues, particularly of the liver. The lethal ingested dose of yellow phosphorus is approximately 50 mg. Ingestion of yellow phosphorus may cause pain in the upper part of the gastrointestinal tract, vomiting, diarrhea, and a garlic odor to the breath. Patients may also develop hepatomegaly, jaundice, hypocalcemia, hypotension, and oliguria. Treatment includes emesis or gastric lavage and administration of activated charcoal and an osmotic cathartic.

Salicylates

Each year, 30 million pounds of aspirin are consumed in the United States, and salicylates can probably be found in most American households. Aspirin is found in many compound analgesic tablets. The ingestion of 10 to 30 g of aspirin or sodium salicylates may be fatal to adults, but survival has been reported after an oral dose of 130 g of aspirin. Salicylate intoxication may result from the cumulative effect of therapeutic administration of high doses. Toxic symptoms may begin at dosages of 3 g/day or may not appear when 10 g/day is given. Therapeutic salicylate intoxication is usually mild and is called **salicylism**. The earliest symptoms are vertigo and impairment of hearing. Further overdosage causes nausea, vomiting, sweating, diarrhea, fever, drowsiness, and headache. The CNS effects may progress to hallucinations, convulsions, coma, cardiovascular collapse, pulmonary edema, hyperthermia, and death. Treatment of salicylate poisoning consists initially of inducing emesis or of gastric lavage, after which activated charcoal and then an osmotic cathartic are administered. Respiratory depression may require artificial ventilation with oxygen. Convulsions may be treated with diazepam or phenobarbital. Peritoneal dialysis and hemodialysis are also highly effective in removing salicylates from seriously poisoned patients.

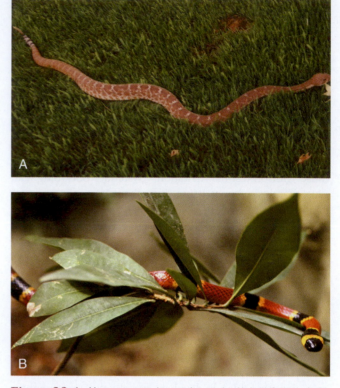

Figure 29-4. Venomous snakes native to the United States. A. Pit viper (Courtesy of Dr. Sean Bush, Loma Linda University Medical Center, Loma Linda, CA.) B. Coral snake. (Courtesy of PhotoDisk.)

Poisonous Snakebites

Each year, poisonous snakes bite about 7000 people in the United States, resulting in about 20 deaths. Such bites are most common during summer afternoons in grassy or rocky habitats. Poisonous snakebites are medical emergencies. With prompt, correct treatment, they need not be fatal. The only poisonous snakes found in the United States are pit vipers (*Crotalidae*) and coral snakes (*Elapidae*) (see Figure 29-4A and 29-4B). Most snakebites occur on the arms and legs, below the elbow or knee. Bites to the head or trunk are most dangerous, regardless of location.

Prompt and appropriate first aid can reduce venom (the poisonous matter secreted by certain creatures that is fatal or injurious to body systems and tissues) absorption and prevent severe symptoms. The victim should not be given any food, beverages, or medication orally. Remember that an incision and suction are effective only for pit viper bites and only within 1 hour of the bite. Suction is also indicated if transport time to an emergency facility would exceed 30 minutes. Mouth suction is contraindicated if the rescuer has oral ulcers, if the victim is close to a medical facility, or if antivenom can be given promptly. Never give the victim alcoholic drinks or stimulants because they speed venom absorption. Never apply ice to a snakebite because it will increase tissue damage.

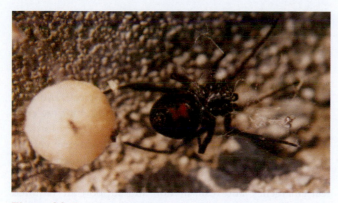

Figure 29-5. Black widow spider. (Courtesy of Dr. Sean Bush, Loma Linda University Medical Center, Loma Linda, CA.)

Insect Bites and Stings

Among the most common traumatic complaints are insect bites and stings, the more serious of which include those of ticks, brown recluse spiders, black widow spiders, scorpions, bees, wasps, and yellow jackets. In this chapter bites from black widow spiders and scorpions will be discussed.

Black Widow Spiders

Black widow spiders are common throughout the United States, particularly in warmer climates (see Figure 29-5). Females are larger than males, and the male does not bite. Mortality is less than 1% (with increased risk among the elderly, infants, and those with allergies). Treatment includes the neutralization of venom using antivenom intravenously, preceded by desensitization when skin or eye tests show sensitivity to horse serum. Calcium gluconate given intravenously is used to control muscle spasms. Muscle relaxants, adrenaline, antihistamines, oxygen, tetanus immunization, and antibiotics are also appropriate.

Scorpions

Scorpions are common throughout the United States (see Figure 29-6). There are 30 different species, but only two deadly species, which are found in the southwestern states. Most stings occur during warmer months. Antivenom (made from cat serum), calcium gluconate, and phenobarbital are appropriate. Opiates such as morphine and codeine are contraindicated because they enhance the effects of the venom.

ANTIDOTES

Specific antidotal therapy is available for only a few poisons. Some systemic antidotes are chemical and exert their therapeutic effect by reducing the concentration of the toxic substance. They may do this by combining with the poison or

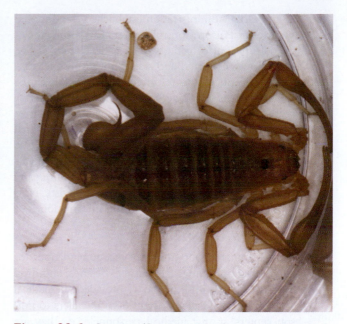

Figure 29-6. Scorpion. (Courtesy of Dr. Sean Bush, Loma Linda University Medical Center, Loma Linda, CA.)

TABLE 29-1. Poisons and Antidotes

POISON	ANTIDOTES
Acetaminophen	N-Acetylcysteine
Benzodiazepines	Flumazenil
Carbon monoxide	Oxygen
Cyanide	Amyl nitrate
Iron	Deferoxamine
Methanol	Ethanol
Opiates	Naloxone
Organophosphates	Atropine or pralidoxime

by increasing its excretion. Other systemic antidotes compete with the poison for its receptor site. Specific antidotes are listed in Table 29-1.

POISON CONTROL CENTERS

A network consisting of more than 600 poison control centers exists in the United States. Through this network, poison treatment information is available free of charge, 24 hours a day. The first poison control center was established in Chicago under the leadership of the Illinois chapter of the American Academy of Pediatrics. A few months later, the Duke University Poison Control Center was begun in North Carolina. With the appearance of these two centers, the idea of poison control centers spread across the country. In 1957, the Food and Drug Administration established the National Clearinghouse for Poison Control Centers to coordinate activities at poison control centers across the United States. The Clearinghouse collected and standardized product toxicology data, reproduced this information on large file cards, and distributed them nationwide to poison control centers.

Since 1953, poison centers have been making a positive contribution to public health in the United States. The goal of poison centers is to reduce morbidity and mortality due to poisoning. It is clear that poison centers accomplish this goal while simultaneously decreasing the cost of health care. Poison center personnel include medical toxicologists, clinical toxicologists, and specialists in poison information.

Services include the following:

1. Emergency telephone treatment recommendations for all types of poisonings, chemical exposures, and drug overdoses. This information is provided to medical and nonmedical callers. About 80% of callers to poison centers are *not* medical personnel; i.e., they are parents, grandparents, child care providers, and the poisoning victims themselves.
2. Telephone follow-up for hospitalized and nonhospitalized patients to assess progress and recommend additional treatment as necessary.
3. Research and surveillance of human poison exposures. This includes occupational and environmental exposures as well as those related to chemicals and drugs.
4. Community education in poison prevention.
5. Education in the recognition and management of poisonings for health care providers.
6. Training of future toxicologists.

SUMMARY

Poisonous substances can and do cause serious adverse consequences, including death. The most important factor in every case of poisoning is to correctly identify the toxic agent and thereby to prescribe the correct antidote. Prevention measures to avoid accidental poisoning are critical to reduce the illness and death rate, especially for children younger than 5 years of age. Poison Control centers offer valuable services for prevention and treatment of poisonous agents. Treatment of poisoning is considered a medical emergency, and resuscitation and support are required to specially prevent further absorption of poison. The management of life-threatening poisoning requires significant expertise. Consultation with a poison specialist or intensive care specialist is recommended.

CRITICAL THINKING

1. What advice would you give to new parents about how to child proof their home to prevent accidental poisoning?
2. Research an area where poisonous animal bites are a problem. What resources are available to deal with these incidences in these regions? How prevalent of a problem is it? What can people living in these areas do to prevent these emergencies?
3. Why is it difficult to detect that a poisoning has occurred? Why is it important to detect a poisoning early?

REVIEW QUESTIONS

1. Regardless of location, which of the following sites of snakebite poisonings is the most dangerous?
   A. Hand
   B. Head
   C. Knee
   D. Elbow

2. Approximately 10 million people are poisoned annually, and _____ of these are fatal poisonings.
   A. 400
   B. 4000
   C. 40,000
   D. 14,000

3. TOXNET is a
   A. prevention program.
   B. database of household products and substances.
   C. antidote for toxins.
   D. TV show.

4. Organophosphates are commonly absorbed through which of the following routes?
   A. Intravenous
   B. Skin
   C. Kidney
   D. Liver

5. Which of the following types of poisoning is a true medical emergency?
   A. Detergent or soap
   B. Lead
   C. Phenol
   D. Cyanide

6. The chelating agents that may be used for lead poisoning include
   A. penicillamine.
   B. propranolol
   C. penicillin.
   D. phenol.

Continues

7. A garlic odor of the breath is a result of ingesting
   A. salicylate.
   B. mercury.
   C. yellow phosphorus.
   D. magnesium.

8. Treatment of magnesium poisoning is
   A. formalin.
   B. calcium gluconate.
   C. active charcoal.
   D. atropin.

9. The toxic effects of carbon monoxide (CO) are the result of
   A. hypotension.
   B. anemia.
   C. hypoglycemia.
   D. tissue hypoxia.

10. The specific antidote for methanol poisoning is
    A. naloxone.
    B. ethanol.
    C. atropine.
    D. pralidoxime.

11. Accidental poisonings occur more commonly in the
    A. laboratory.
    B. pharmacy.
    C. home.
    D. workplace.

12. The cherry-colored flush of carboxyhemoglobin in skin may reveal the unmistakable poisoning of
    A. bleach.
    B. atropine.
    C. benzene.
    D. carbon monoxide.

13. Hepatic damage may be expected if an adult has taken acetaminophen in a single dose more than
    A. 2 g.
    B. 4 g.
    C. 8 g.
    D. 25 g.

14. If a poisoning occurs, one of the first measures to take is
    A. call the poison center (1-800-222-1222) immediately.
    B. tell the person to lie down.
    C. ask the person to drink some milk.
    D. call the family physician for an appointment.

15. The recommended poison prevention guidelines for all households include the following except:
    A. properly closing child-resistant containers securely after use.
    B. keeping all chemicals and medicines locked up and out of sight of the elderly.
    C. leaving the original labels on all products.
    D. avoid taking medicine in front of children.

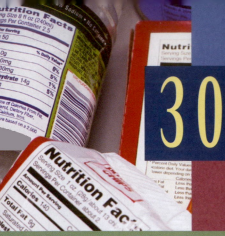

30 Nutrition

OUTLINE

Overview
Proper Nutritional Guidelines
Nutrients
  Proteins
  Carbohydrates
  Lipids (Fats)
  Vitamins
  Minerals and Electrolytes
Food Labeling
Food Additives

Malnutrition
  Marasmus
  Kwashiorkor
Weight Gain and Weight Loss
Nutritional Care
  Enteral Nutrition
  Hyperalimentation or Total Parenteral Nutrition
Pharma Food
Summary

OBJECTIVES

Upon completion of this chapter, the reader should be able to

1. Explain the classification of nutrients.
2. Describe the effects of proteins, carbohydrates, and fats in human nutrition.
3. Explain malnutrition and total parenteral nutrition therapy.
4. Classify vitamins and minerals.

5. Explain trace elements and their major effects on the body.
6. Define pharma food.
7. Explain food labeling.
8. Describe the purposes of additives in foods and supplements.
9. Explain the major complication of total parenteral nutrition therapy.

GLOSSARY

ascorbic acid A water-soluble vitamin that is essential for the formation of collagen and fibroid tissue for teeth, bones, cartilage, connective tissue, and skin. It also aids in fighting bacterial infections, bleeding gums, bruising, nosebleeds, and anemia.

biotin A water-soluble B complex vitamin that acts as a coenzyme in fatty acid production and in the oxidation of fatty acids and carbohydrates.

calciferol A fat-soluble vitamin chemically related to the steroids and essential for the normal formation of bones and teeth. It is important for the absorption of calcium and phosphorus from the gastrointestinal tract.

calcium An alkaline earth metal element. The body requires calcium ions for the transmission of nerve impulses, muscle contraction, blood coagulation, cardiac functions, and other processes.

carbohydrates Nutrients providing the main source energy in the average diet.

chloride An anion of chlorine. The most common form is sodium chloride (table salt).

cholesterol A waxy lipid found only in animal tissues. A member of a group of lipids called sterols, it is widely distributed in the body.

copper A metallic element that is a component of several important enzymes in the body and is essential to good health.

cyanocobalamin A water-soluble substance that is the common pharmaceutical form of vitamin B_{12}. It is involved in the metabolism of protein, fats, and carbohydrates. Vitamin B_{12} is also involved in normal blood formation and neural function.

electrolytes Compounds that dissociate into ions when dissolved in water.

enteral nutrition (EN) Feeding by tube directly into the patient's digestive tract.

fats Substances composed of lipids or fatty acids and occurring in various forms.

fatty acids Any of several organic acids produced by the hydrolysis of neutral fats.

fluoride A substance that prevents tooth decay and protects against osteoporosis and gum disease.

GLOSSARY continued

folacin A water-soluble vitamin essential for cell growth and the reproduction of red blood cells.

folic acid A water-soluble vitamin essential for cell growth and the reproduction of red blood cells.

food additive Any substance that becomes part of a food product.

high-density lipoproteins (HDLs) Lipoproteins that carry cholesterol from cells to the liver for eventual excretion.

hyperalimentation The administration of a nutritionally adequate hypertonic solution consisting of glucose, protein, minerals, and vitamins through an indwelling catheter into the superior vena cava.

hypervitaminosis An abnormal condition resulting from excessive intake of toxic amounts of one or more vitamins, especially over a long period.

hypovitaminosis A condition related to the deficiency of one or more vitamins.

iodine An essential micronutrient of the thyroid hormone (thyroxine).

iron A common metallic element essential for the synthesis of hemoglobin.

kwashiorkor A disease caused by extreme lack of protein.

lipids Fats.

low-density lipoproteins (LDLs) Lipoproteins that carry blood cholesterol from all cells.

magnesium A silver-white mineral element. It is the second most abundant cation of the intracellular fluids in the body and is essential for many enzyme activities.

malnutrition Ingestion of nutrients inadequate to maintain health and well-being.

marasmus Severe wasting caused by lack of protein and all nutrients or faulty absorption.

menadione A water-soluble, injectable form of the product of vitamin K_3.

minerals Inorganic substances occurring naturally in the earth's crust, having a characteristic chemical composition.

neutral fats Fats consisting of about 95% triglycerides or triacylglycerols.

niacin A part of two enzymes that regulate energy metabolism.

nutrient A chemical substance found in food that is necessary for good health.

nutrition The sum of the processes involved in the taking in of nutrients and their assimilation and use for proper body functioning and maintenance of health.

pantothenic acid A member of the vitamin B complex. It is widely distributed in plant and animal tissues and may be an important element in human nutrition.

pharma food A system of nourishing through breathing.

phospholipid A phosphorus-containing lipid.

phosphorus A nonmetallic chemical element occurring extensively in nature as a component of phosphate rock. Phosphorus is essential for the metabolism of protein, calcium, and glucose.

potassium An alkali metal element. Potassium salts are necessary to the life of all plants and animals. Potassium in the body helps to regulate neuromuscular excitability and muscle contraction.

protein The only one of six essential nutrients containing nitrogen.

pyridoxine A water-soluble vitamin that is part of the B complex. It acts as a coenzyme essential for the synthesis and breakdown of amino acids.

retinol A fat-soluble vitamin essential for skeletal growth, maintenance of normal mucosal epithelium, reproduction, and visual acuity.

riboflavin One of the heat-stable components of the B complex. It is involved as a coenzyme in the oxidative processes of carbohydrates, fats, and proteins.

sodium One of the most important elements in the body. Sodium ions are involved in acid-base balance, water balance, transmission of nerve impulses, and contraction of muscles.

thiamin A water-soluble, crystalline compound of the B complex, essential for normal metabolism and health of the cardiovascular and nervous systems.

tocopherol A fat-soluble vitamin essential for normal reproduction, muscle development, resistance of erythrocytes to hemolysis, and various other biochemical functions.

total parenteral nutrition (TPN) An intravenous feeding that supplies all the nutrients necessary for life.

triglycerides Simple fat compounds consisting of three molecules of fatty acid and glycerol. Triglycerides make up most animal and vegetable fats and are the principal lipids in the blood, where they circulate within lipoproteins.

very low-density lipoproteins (VLDLs) Lipoproteins made by the liver to transport lipids throughout the body.

vitamin A A fat-soluble vitamin essential for skeletal growth, maintenance of normal mucosal epithelium, reproduction, and visual acuity. This vitamin is also called retinol.

vitamin B complex A group of water-soluble compound vitamins.

vitamin B_1 A water-soluble, crystalline compound of the B complex, essential for normal metabolism and health of the cardiovascular and nervous systems. This vitamin is also called thiamin.

vitamin B_2 One of the heat-stable components of the B complex. It is involved as a coenzyme in the oxidative processes of carbohydrates, fats, and proteins. This vitamin is also called riboflavin.

vitamin B_3 A part of two enzymes that regulate energy metabolism. This vitamin is also called niacin.

vitamin B_6 A water-soluble vitamin that is part of the B complex. It acts as a coenzyme essential for the synthesis and breakdown of amino acids. This vitamin is also called pyridoxine.

vitamin B_7 A water-soluble, B complex vitamin that acts as a co-enzyme in fatty acid production, oxidation of fatty acids, and carbohydrates. This vitamin is also called biotin.

vitamin B_9 A water-soluble vitamin essential for cell growth and the reproduction of red blood cells. This vitamin is also called folic acid or folacin.

vitamin B_{12} A water-soluble substance that is the common pharmaceutical form of vitamin B_{12}. It is involved in the metabolism of protein, fats, and carbohydrates. Vitamin B_{12} is also involved in normal blood formation and neural function. This vitamin is also called cyanocobalamin.

vitamin C A water-soluble vitamin that is essential for the formation of collagen and fibroid tissue for teeth, bones, cartilage, connective tissue, and skin. It also aids in fighting bacterial infections, bleeding gums, bruising, nosebleeds, and anemia. This vitamin is called ascorbic acid.

vitamin D A fat-soluble vitamin chemically related to the steroids and essential for the normal formation of bones and teeth. It is important for the absorption of calcium and phosphorus from the gastrointestinal (GI) tract. This vitamin is also called calciferol.

vitamin E A fat-soluble vitamin essential for normal reproduction, muscle development, resistance of erythrocytes to hemolysis, and various other biochemical functions. This vitamin is also called tocopherol.

vitamin K A group of fat-soluble vitamins that are essential for the synthesis of prothrombin in the liver and are involved in the clotting of blood. These vitamins are also called quinones.

vitamins Organic substances necessary for life, although they do not independently provide energy.

zinc A metallic element that is an essential nutrient in the body and is used in numerous pharmaceuticals such as zinc acetate and zinc oxide.

OVERVIEW

Nutrition is the study of food and drink as related to the growth and maintenance of living organisms. **Nutrients** are chemical substances found in food that are needed for life. Life is nourished by food, and the substances in food on which life depends are the nutrients. These provide the energy and building materials for the countless substances that are essential to the growth and survival of living things. The manner in which nutrients become integral parts of the body and contribute to its function depends on the physiological and biochemical processes that govern their actions. Proteins, fats, and carbohydrates all contribute to the total energy pool, but the energy that they yield is all in the same form. Utilization and conservation of this energy to build and maintain the body require the involvement of vitamins and minerals. Pharmacy technicians are asked many questions about foods and nutrition, including specific questions about which products or supplements a client may be considering for purchase and what amount of a product to ingest.

growth and healthy life. Life expectancy is lengthening in the United States, so health promotion and disease prevention are even more important as we seek to ensure quality of life throughout our extended years.

Proper nutrition plays an important role in this matter and the U.S. Department of Agriculture (USDA) introduced the Food Guide Pyramid in 1992. This dietary guideline calls for more consumption of grains and less consumption of meat, sweets, and fats to help reach the goals of proper nutrition. The pyramid is divided into six sections. The largest sections are the foods that should be consumed in the largest quantities. The grain group, the largest section, was placed at the bottom of the pyramid, with foods high in fat and simple sugars placed at the top to emphasize the difference in importance between the two substances in the diet (see Figure 30-1).

Because of the epidemic numbers of overweight individuals in the United States, the the Food Guide Pyramid is undergoing revision by the USDA. The revised pyramid will include recommendations for physical activity levels necessary to maintain health and a proper weight. The new pyramid is scheduled to be finalized in January 2005.

PROPER NUTRITIONAL GUIDELINES

Human growth and development require both nutritional and psychosocial support. Various food patterns and habits supply the energy and nutrient requirements for normal

NUTRIENTS

Nutrients are essential for growth, reproduction, and maintenance of health. For classification purposes, nutrients are divided into six basic categories: proteins, carbohydrates,

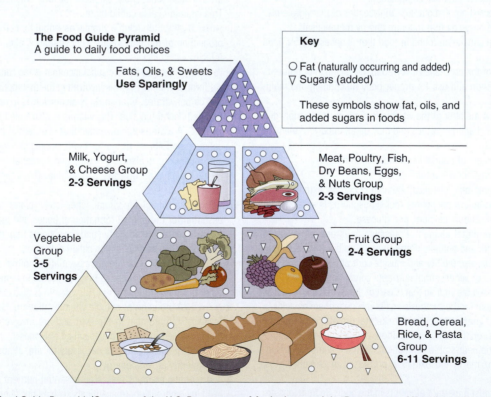

The Food Guide Pyramid
A guide to daily food choices

Fats, Oils, & Sweets
Use Sparingly

Key

○ Fat (naturally occurring and added)
▽ Sugars (added)

These symbols show fat, oils, and added sugars in foods

Milk, Yogurt, & Cheese Group
2-3 Servings

Meat, Poultry, Fish, Dry Beans, Eggs, & Nuts Group
2-3 Servings

Vegetable Group
3-5 Servings

Fruit Group
2-4 Servings

Bread, Cereal, Rice, & Pasta Group
6-11 Servings

Figure 30-1. Food Guide Pyramid. (Courtesy of the U.S. Department of Agriculture and the Department of Health and Human Services. The food guide pyramid: A guide to daily food choices. Leaflet no. 572, Washington, DC, 1992.)

lipids, vitamins, minerals, and water. The only additional substance needed for life is oxygen. Nutrient groups providing kilocalories (kcal) and thus supplying a source of energy for the body are carbohydrates, proteins, and fats. The realization that nutrients are chemicals helps the pharmacy technician to understand why they may interact with drugs, which are also composed of chemicals.

Proteins

A **protein** is a complex, organic, nitrogenous compound composed of large combinations of amino acids. Amino acids are essential components of living cells. Twenty-two amino acids have been identified as being vital for proper growth, development, and maintenance of health. The body can synthesize 13 of these, the nonessential amino acids, whereas the remaining 9 must be obtained from dietary sources and are termed essential (see Table 30-1). Protein is the major source of building material for muscles, blood, skin, hair, nails, and the internal organs. It is necessary for the formation of enzymes, antibodies, and hormones. The recommended daily requirement of protein is 0.8 g of protein for each kilogram of body weight. Protein deficiency causes abnormal growth and tissue development in children, leading to kwashiorkor, whereas in adults, it results in lack of vigor and stamina, weakness, mental depression, poor resistance to infection, impaired healing of wounds, and slow recovery from disease. Excessive intake of protein may, in some conditions, result in fluid imbalance. Amino acid solutions contain crystalline amino acids (for example, Aminosyn®); solutions are also available with electrolytes.

Carbohydrates

Carbohydrates constitute the main source of energy for all body functions, particularly brain functions, and are necessary for the metabolism of other nutrients. Most of the energy needed to move, perform work, and live is consumed in the form of carbohydrates. Carbohydrates constitute the major source of food for the people of the world. Carbohydrates are either absorbed immediately by the body or stored in the form of glycogen. Current U.S. dietary guidelines recommend that 55% to 60% of total calories should be provided by carbohydrates. Symptoms of deficiency include fatigue, depression, breakdown of essential body protein, and electrolyte imbalance. Excessive consumption of carbohydrates may be associated with tooth decay, obesity, and diabetes mellitus.

Lipids (Fats)

Lipids, or **fats**, are insoluble in water but are soluble in alcohol, chloroform, ether, and other organic solvents. Fats provide a more concentrated source of energy than carbohydrates. It is recommended that an individual's dietary fat intake should be no more than 30% of the total kilocalories ingested. However, on average, fats constitute 35% to 40% of the total calories supplied in the average American's diet. They are stored in the body and serve as an energy reserve, but fat levels are elevated in various diseases such as atherosclerosis. There are several types of lipids, such as **cholesterol**, **fatty acids**, **neutral fats**, **phospholipids**, and **triglycerides**. Table 30-2 shows the classification of lipids.

Cholesterol

Cholesterol is a waxy lipid-soluble compound found in cell membranes of all animal tissues that is also necessary for production of bile and steroid hormones. It is a member of a group of compounds called sterols. Cholesterol is a nonessential nutrient that plays a vital role in metabolic activities and facilitates the absorption and transport of fatty acids. It is found in foods of animal origin and is continuously synthesized in the body, primarily in the liver.

Fatty Acids

Fatty acids are organic acids produced by the hydrolysis of neutral fats. In a living cell, a fatty acid usually occurs in combination with another molecule, rather than in a free state.

TABLE 30-1. Amino Acids

ESSENTIAL		NONESSENTIAL	
Histidine	Phenylalanine	Alanine	Glutamine
Isoleucine	Treonine	Arginine	Glycine
Leucine	Tryptophan	Asparagine	Hydroxyproline
Lysine	Valine	Aspartic acid	Proline
Methionine		Cysteine	Serine
		Cystine	Tyrosine
		Glutamic acid	

TABLE 30-2. Classification of Lipids

CATEGORIES	EXAMPLES
Simple lipids	Fatty acids
	Neutral fats (monoglycerides, diglycerides, triglycerides)
	Waxes
	Sterol esters (cholesterol ester)
	Nonsterol ester (vitamin A ester)
Compound lipids	Phospholipids
	Glycolipids
	Lipoproteins
Sterols	Cholesterol
	Vitamin D
	Bile salts
Vitamins	Vitamin A, E, and K

Essential fatty acids are polyunsaturated molecules that cannot be produced by the body and must therefore be included in the diet. Some types are linoleic, linolenic, and arachidonic acids. Essential fatty acid deficiency is diagnosed by clinical signs of hair loss, scaly dermatitis, reduced wound healing, decreased numbers of platelets, growth retardation, and fatty liver. In this condition, the intravenous administration of a fat emulsion is essential to correct the biochemical alteration.

Neutral Fat

Most neutral fats consist of about 95% triglycerides or triacylglycerols. The remaining 5% include traces of monoglycerides, diglycerides, fatty acids, phospholipids, and sterols. Lipids important to nutrition include simple and compound lipids and the fat-soluble vitamins.

Phospholipids

Phospholipids are lipids containing fatty acids, an alcohol, and a phosphorus compound. They are widely distributed in cell membranes.

Triglycerides

Triglycerides are lipids consisting of three fatty acid chains esterified to a glycerol molecule.

Fat Intake

Cholesterol has been high on the list of dietary villains for years and has been thought to be a serious contributor to the development of heart disease. The good fats in our diet are polyunsaturated and monounsaturated fats. The bad dietary fats are cholesterol and saturated fats. The fat in our bodies is divided into two *lipoprotein* categories. The good fats, or **high-density lipoproteins (HDL)**, carry cholesterol from body tissues or the bloodstream to the liver for metabolism and excretion. The bad fats, or **low-density lipoproteins (LDLs)** and **very low-density lipoproteins (VLDLs)**, carry cholesterol to the cells. LDLs and VLDLs form atherosclerotic plaques on arterial walls that often result in heart disease, hypertension, and strokes. However, serum LDL levels can often be successfully changed through diet. Using polyunsaturated and monounsaturated fat products reduces total serum cholesterol levels. In addition, using monounsaturated fats (olive, peanut, and canola oils) reduces LDL levels. Exercise is an important tool for lowering total serum cholesterol levels, increasing LDL levels, and decreasing triglyceride levels. Another potential health risk from a high-fat diet is obesity. When too much fat is consumed in the diet, it is deposited in the body as stored adipose tissue.

Vitamins

Vitamins are organic compounds that are essential in small quantities for physiological and metabolic functioning of the body. With few exceptions, vitamins cannot be synthesized by the body and must be obtained from the diet or dietary supplements. No one food contains all the vitamins. Vitamin deficiency diseases produce specific symptoms that are usually alleviated by the administration of the appropriate vitamin. Vitamins are classified according to their fat or water solubility, their physiological effects, or their chemical structures. They are designated by alphabetic letters and chemical or other specific names. The fat-soluble vitamins are A, D, E, and K; the B complex and C vitamins are water soluble.

An abnormal condition resulting from excessive intake of toxic amounts of one or more vitamins, especially over a long period, is called **hypervitaminosis**. Serious effects may result from overdoses of fat-soluble vitamins A, D, E, or K, but adverse reactions are less likely with the water-soluble B and C vitamins, except when they are taken in megadoses. **Hypovitaminosis** may occur because of a deficiency of one or more vitamins. Examples of diseases caused by hypovitaminosis include avitaminosis, beriberi, malnutrition, scurvy, rickets, scorbutus, and moon blindness.

Fat-Soluble Vitamins

Each of the fat-soluble vitamins A, D, E, and K has a distinct and separate physiological role. For the most part, they are absorbed with other lipids, and efficient absorption requires the presence of bile and pancreatic juice. They are transported to the liver and stored in various body tissues. They are not normally excreted in the urine.

Vitamin A (retinol), one of the fat-soluble vitamins, is essential for skeletal growth, maintenance of normal mucosal epithelium, and visual acuity. Normal stores can last up to 1 year but are rapidly depleted by stress. Vitamin A has essential roles in development of vision, bone growth, maintenance of epithelial tissue, the immunological process, and normal reproduction. Deficiency leads to atrophy of epithelial tissue, resulting in keratomalacia, xerophthalmia, night blindness, and lessened resistance to infection of the mucous membranes. Plasma vitamin A concentrations are reduced in cystic fibrosis, alcohol-related cirrhosis, hepatic disease, and proteinuria. Plasma vitamin A concentrations are elevated in patients with chronic renal disease. The recommended oral intake is 2500 to 5000 IU/day. Contraindications include hypervitaminosis A, oral use in malabsorption syndrome, hypersensitivity, and intravenous use.

Vitamin D (calciferol), is another fat-soluble vitamin that is chemically related to the steroids and essential for the normal formation of bones and teeth and for the absorption of calcium and phosphorus from the GI tract. Ultraviolet rays activate a form of cholesterol in an oil of the skin and convert it to a form of the vitamin, which is then absorbed. Vitamin D is considered a hormone. Deficiency of the vitamin results in rickets in children, osteomalacia, osteoporosis, and osteodystrophy. Hypervitaminosis D produces a toxicity syndrome. Vitamin D therapy is contraindicated in hypercalcemia, malabsorption syndrome, and renal dysfunction or if an individual has evidence of vitamin D toxicity or abnormal sensitivity to the effects of vitamin D. The recommended intake is 100 to 400 IU/day. Vitamin D$_2$ is also called ergocalciferol. A fat-soluble vitamin, it is used for the prophylaxis and treatment of rickets, osteomalacia, and other hypocalcemic disorders (tetany) and hypoparathyroidism. Vitamin D$_3$ is the predominant form of vitamin D of animal origin. It is found in most fish liver oils, butter, bran, and egg yolks. It is formed in the skin exposed to sunlight or ultraviolet rays.

Vitamin E (tocopherol) is a fat-soluble vitamin that is essential for normal reproduction, muscle development, and resistance of erythrocytes to hemolysis. It is an intracellular antioxidant and acts to maintain the stability of polyunsaturated fatty acids. Deficiency results in muscle degeneration, vascular system abnormalities, megaloblastic anemia, hemolytic anemia, infertility, and liver or kidney damage. It is stored in the body for long periods so that deficiency is rare. It is considered nontoxic except in hypertensive patients and those with chronic rheumatic heart disease. The recommended oral allowance is 12 to 15 IU/day.

Vitamin K is essential for the synthesis of prothrombin in the liver. The naturally occurring forms, also called quinones, are vitamin K$_1$ (phylloquinone), which occurs in green plants, and vitamin K$_2$ (menaquinone), which is formed as the result of bacterial action in the intestinal tract. Water-soluble forms of vitamins K$_1$ and K$_2$ are also available. The fat-soluble synthetic compound, **menadione** (vitamin K$_3$), is about twice as potent biologically as the naturally occurring vitamins K$_1$ and K$_2$, on a weight basis. It is another fat-soluble vitamin. It is used for coagulation disorder and vitamin K deficiency. Such deficiency results in hypoprothrombinemia and hemorrhage. It is used to increase the clotting time in patients with obstructive jaundice and in hemorrhagic states associated with the liver diseases. It is given prophylactically to infants to prevent hemorrhagic disease of the newborn. Natural vitamin K is stored in the body and is not toxic. Excessive doses of synthetic vitamin K can cause anemia in newborns. The suggested oral intake is 0.7 to 2.0mg/day.

Water-Soluble Vitamins

Most of the water-soluble vitamins are components of essential enzyme systems. Many are involved in the reactions supporting energy metabolism. These vitamins are not normally stored in the body in appreciable amounts and are usually excreted in small quantities in the urine; thus, a daily supply is desirable to avoid depletion and interruption of normal physiological functions.

Vitamin B complex is a group of water-soluble vitamins that differ from each other structurally and in their biological effects. Heat and prolonged cooking, especially cooking with water, can destroy B vitamins.

Vitamin B$_1$ (thiamin) is a water-soluble component of the B vitamin complex that is essential for normal metabolism and health of the cardiovascular and nervous systems.

Thiamin plays a key role in the metabolic breakdown of carbohydrates. It is not stored in the body and must be supplied daily. Deficiency causes loss of appetite, irritability, sleep disturbance, dyspnea, and arrhythmia. Severe deficiency causes beriberi.

Vitamin B$_2$ (riboflavin) is one of the heat-stable components of the B vitamin complex. It is essential for certain enzyme systems in the metabolism of fats and proteins. It is sensitive to light and plays an important role in preventing some visual disorders, especially cataracts. Deficiency of riboflavin produces cheilosis, local inflammation, glossitis, photophobia, cataracts, and anemia.

Vitamin B$_3$ (niacin) contains parts of two enzymes that regulate energy metabolism. Vitamin B$_3$ is also called nicotinic acid and nicotinamide. It is essential for healthy skin, tongue, and digestive system. Severe deficiency results in pellagra, mental disturbances, various skin eruptions, and GI disturbances.

Vitamin B$_6$ (pyridoxine), is a coenzyme essential for the synthesis and breakdown of amino acids, the conversion of tryptophan to niacin, the breakdown of glycogen to glucose, and the production of antibodies. Deficiency of pyridoxine may cause anemia, anorexia, neuritis, nausea, dermatitis, and depressed immunity.

Vitamin B$_7$ (biotin) is a water-soluble vitamin that is synthesized by intestinal flora; therefore, deficiency states are rare. Biotin functions in metabolism via biotin-dependent enzymes.

Vitamin B$_9$ (folic acid) is essential for cell growth and the reproduction of red blood cells. It functions as a coenzyme with vitamins B$_{12}$ and C in the breakdown of proteins and in the formation of nucleic acid and hemoglobin. It is also essential for fetal development, particularly of the neural tube. Deficiency causes anemia and may cause spina bifida in a fetus. It is also called **folacin**.

Vitamin B$_{12}$ (cyanocobalamin) is involved in the metabolism of protein, fats, and carbohydrates. It aids in hemoglobin synthesis, is essential for normal functioning of all cells, and is important in energy metabolism. Deficiency causes pernicious anemia and neurological disorders.

Pantothenic acid is a member of the vitamin B complex. The primary role of pantothenic acid is as a constituent of coenzyme A. Thus, it is essential in many areas of cellular metabolism, including fatty acid metabolism, the synthesis of sex hormones, and the functioning of the nervous system and the adrenal glands.

Vitamin C (ascorbic acid) is essential for the formation of collagen tissue and for normal intercellular matrices in teeth, bone, cartilage, connective tissues, and skin. It protects the body against infections and helps heal wounds. Therefore, ascorbic acid has multiple functions as either a coenzyme or cofactor. Its role in enhancing absorption of iron is well recognized. Deficiency causes scurvy, lowered resistance to infections, joint tenderness, dental caries, bleeding gums, delayed wound healing, bruising, hemorrhage, and anemia.

Minerals and Electrolytes

Minerals are inorganic substances occurring naturally in the earth's crust that the body needs to help build and maintain body tissues for life functions. They are classified as major and trace elements.

Electrolytes are compounds, particularly salts, that when dissolved in water or another solvent, dissociate into ions and are able to conduct an electric current. The concentrations of electrolytes differ in blood plasma and other tissues. Sodium, potassium, and chloride are electrolytes. Minerals help keep the body's water and electrolytes in balance.

Major Minerals

The major minerals are defined as those requiring an intake of more than 100 mg/day. The six major minerals are calcium, phosphorus, chloride, sodium, potassium, and magnesium.

Calcium (Ca) is the fifth most abundant element in the human body and is present mainly in the bones. The body requires calcium ions for the transmission of nerve impulses, muscle contraction, blood coagulation, and cardiac functions. It is a component of extracellular fluid and of soft tissue cells. The normal daily requirement of calcium is 800 to 1200 mg. The following factors enhance the absorption of calcium: adequate concentrations of vitamin D, calcitonin, and parathyroid hormone; large quantities of calcium and phosphorus in the diet; and the presence of lactose. Abnormally high levels of ionized calcium in the extracellular fluid can produce muscle weakness, lethargy, and coma. Hypocalcemia can cause tetanic seizures and hypertension.

Phosphorus (P) is essential for the metabolism of protein, calcium, and glucose. It aids in building strong bones and teeth and helps in the regulation of the body's acid-base balance. Nutritional sources are dairy foods, meat, egg yolks, whole grains, and nuts. A nutritional deficiency of phosphorus can cause weight loss, anemia, and abnormal growth. Anemia, cachexia, bronchitis, and necrosis of the mandible bone characterize chronic poisoning by phosphorus.

Chloride (Cl) is involved in the maintenance of fluid and the body's acid-base balance. The most common metal chloride is sodium chloride (table salt).

Sodium (Na) is one of the most important elements in the body. Sodium ions are involved in acid-base balance, water balance, transmission of nerve impulses, and contraction of muscles. Major dietary sources of sodium are table salt (sodium chloride), catsup, mustard, cured meats and fish, cheese, and potato chips. Toxic levels may cause hypertension and renal disease. The kidney is the main regulator of sodium levels in body fluids. In high temperatures and high fever, the body loses sodium through sweat.

Potassium (K) is the major electrolyte in intracellular fluids, helping to regulate neuromuscular excitability and muscle contraction. Sources of potassium in the diet are whole grains, meat, legumes, fruit, and vegetables. Potassium is important in glycogen formation, protein synthesis, and correction of imbalances of acid-base metabolism, especially in association with the action of sodium and hydrogen ions. Potassium salts are very important as therapeutic agents but are extremely dangerous if used improperly. The kidney plays an important role in controlling the secretion and absorption of potassium by the body tissues, especially in the muscles and the liver. Increased renal excretion may be caused by diuretic therapy, large doses of anionic drugs, or renal disorders. Increased GI tract excretion of potassium may occur with the loss of GI fluid through vomiting, diarrhea, surgical drainage, or chronic use of laxatives. Potassium loss through the skin is rare, but can result from perspiration during excessive exercise in a hot environment.

Magnesium (Mg) is an important ion for the function of many enzyme systems. Magnesium is the second most abundant action of the intracellular fluids in the body. It helps to build strong bones and teeth and aids in regulating the heartbeat. It is stored in the bone and is excreted mainly by the kidneys. Renal excretion of magnesium increases during diuresis induced by ammonium chloride, glucose, and organic mercurials. Magnesium affects the central nervous, neuromuscular, and cardiovascular systems. Diarrhea, steatorrhea, chronic alcoholism, and diabetes mellitus can produce hypomagnesemia. Hypomagnesemia is often treated with administration of parenteral fluids containing magnesium sulfate or magnesium chloride. Excess magnesium (hypermagnesemia) in the body can slow the heartbeat or cause cardiac arrest. Hypermagnesemia is usually caused by renal insufficiency and is manifested by hypotension, muscle weakness, sedation, and confused mental state.

Trace Elements

Trace elements are not less important, but they occur in very small amounts in the body. Trace elements are generally defined as those having a required intake of less than 100 mg/day. Trace elements are equally essential for their specific vital tasks and include the following.

Iron (Fe) is a common metallic element essential for the synthesis of hemoglobin and myoglobin. The major role of iron is to transfer oxygen to the body tissues. Inadequate supplies of iron needed to synthesize hemoglobin, poor absorption of iron in the digestive system, or chronic bleeding can cause iron deficiency anemia. Replacement iron may be supplied by ferrous sulfate (Feosol®), preferably the oral form. Iron dextran (Imferon®) is an injectable form of iron supplement.

Iodine (I) is an essential micronutrient of the thyroid hormone (thyroxine). Almost 80% of the iodine present in the body is in the thyroid gland. Iodine deficiency can result in goiter or cretinism. Iodine is found in seafood, iodized salt, and some dairy products. Iodine is used as a contrast medium for blood vessels in computed tomography scans. Radioisotopes of iodine are used in radioisotope-scanning procedures and in palliative treatment of cancer of the thyroid.

Zinc (Zn) is essential for several enzymes, growth, glucose tolerance, wound healing, and taste acuity. It is also

TABLE 30-3.	Mineral Deficiencies
MINERAL	**SYMPTOMS AND DISEASE**
Calcium	Rickets (children), osteomalacia (adults), tetany, and osteoporosis
Iron	Iron deficiency anemia and nutritional anemia
Iodine	Goiter, cretinism (congenital myxedema in children), and acquired myxedema in adults (hypothyroidism)
Phosphorus	Weight loss, anemia, and abnormal growth
Sodium	Water intoxication, confusion, and lethargy, leading to muscle excitability, convulsions, and coma
Potassium	Impaired growth, hypertension, bone fragility, renal hypertrophy, bradycardia, and death
Magnesium	Nausea, vomiting, muscle weakness, tremors, tetany, lethargy, tachycardia, and arrhythmia
Zinc	Dwarfism, delayed growth, hypogonadism, anemia, and decreased appetite
Fluoride	Tooth decay, osteoporosis, and gum disease
Copper	Anemia and bone disease (copper deficiency is vary rare in adults)

Nutrition Facts

Serving Size ½ cup (114g)
Servings Per Container 4

Amount Per Serving

Calories 90	Calories from Fat 30

	% Daily Value
Total Fat 3g	5%
Saturated Fat 0g	0%
Cholesterol 0mg	0%
Sodium 300mg	13%
Total Carbohydrate 13g	4%
Dietary Fiber 3g	12%
Sugars 3g	
Protein 3g	

Vitamin A	80%	•	Vitamin C	60%
Calcium	4%	•	Iron	4%

* Percent Daily Values are based on a 2,000 calorie diet. Your daily values may be higher or lower depending on your calorie needs:

	Calories	2,000	2,500
Total Fat	Less than	65g	80g
Sat Fat	Less than	20g	25g
Cholesterol	Less than	300mg	300mg
Sodium	Less than	2,400mg	2,400mg
Total Carbohydrate		300g	375g
Fiber		25g	30g

Caloris per gram:
Fat 9 • Carbohydrate 4 • Protein 4

Figure 30-2. Food label. (Courtesy of the Food and Drug Administration.)

used in numerous pharmaceuticals, such as zinc acetate, zinc oxide, zinc permanganate, and zinc stearate. The best sources are protein foods. Zinc deficiency is characterized by abnormal fatigue, decreased alertness, a decrease in taste and odor sensitivity, poor appetite, retarded growth, delayed sexual maturity, prolonged healing of wounds, and susceptibility to infection and injury.

Fluoride (F) or compounds of fluoride are introduced into drinking water or applied directly to the teeth to prevent tooth decay. It also protects against osteoporosis and periodontal (gum) disease. Excessive amounts of fluoride in drinking water may result in discoloration of the teeth.

Copper (Cu) is a component of several important enzymes in the body and is essential to good health. Copper is mostly concentrated in the liver, heart, brain, and kidneys. It helps in the formation of hemoglobin and the transportation of iron to bone marrow. Copper accumulates in individuals with Wilson's disease and primary biliary cirrhosis.

Disease and symptoms associated with mineral deficiencies are listed in Table 30-3. The three minerals for which deficiencies are most common are calcium, iron, and iodine.

FOOD LABELING

Food items and supplements must be labeled in the pharmacy. By labeling these items, the technician can understand the importance of nutrition labeling regulations. Labeling of foods and supplements must be accurate and not misleading. The Nutrition Labeling and Education Act of 1990 requires that most packaged foods have a list of a specified set of nutrition

facts on the label. Setting of standards and enforcement for nutrition labeling are a responsibility of the Food and Drug Administration (FDA). All the nutrition information on the label is based on the stated serving size. Larger packages, such as cereal boxes, often include additional information not required by law. Figure 30-2 shows an example of a current food label with the minimal required facts.

FOOD ADDITIVES

Any substance that becomes part of a food product is called a **food additive**. Food additives can be added intentionally, such as when salt or cinnamon is added for flavoring, or unintentionally, such as when a pesticide used to treat crops is accidentally incorporated into the plant or when a drug given to an animal ends up in the food product supplied by the animal. One purpose of food additives is to maintain or improve nutritional value, such as the addition of vitamins and minerals to a food product. The surge in the addition of calcium to juices and other foods is a good example of this function. Another purpose of additives is to maintain freshness in the food. Antioxidants added to foods processed with fat, such as potato chips, helps to prevent the fat from becoming rancid, and preservatives help to prevent spoilage and changes in color, texture, and flavor of food. Additives also make food more appealing.

MALNUTRITION

Malnutrition is defined as a pathological state, resulting from a relative or absolute deficiency or excess of one or more essential nutrients. Malnutrition may result from an unbalanced, insufficient, or excessive diet or from impaired absorption, assimilation, or use of foods.

Marasmus

Marasmus is a chronic disease that develops over months or years as a result of a deficiency in total caloric intake. Depletion of fat stores and skeletal protein occurs to meet metabolic needs. In a hypermetabolic state (such as trauma and infection), combined with protein deprivation, this can rapidly develop into severe kwashiorkor malnutrition, characterized by hypoalbuminemia, edema, and impaired cellular immune function. In advanced stages, it is characterized by muscular wasting and absence of subcutaneous fat.

Kwashiorkor

Kwashiorkor is an acute process that can develop within weeks and is associated with protein deficiency and impaired immune function. It is due to poor protein intake with adequate to slightly inadequate caloric intake. It is characterized by hypoalbuminemia, edema, and an enlarged, fatty liver.

WEIGHT GAIN AND WEIGHT LOSS

Overweight is a state in which a person's weight exceeds a standard based on height; obesity is a condition of excessive fatness, either general or localized. It is possible to be obese at a weight within normal limits according to the standard table, just as it is possible to be overweight without being obese; however, in most people, being overweight leads to obesity. The pharmacy technician is asked many questions about weight gain and loss by clients. Technicians often are asked to help the consumer select specific food products or supplements advertised to assist with weight loss or gain, because these products are often available in the pharmacy setting. A well-balanced diet for weight loss should not require the purchase of any special product. In general, clients wanting to lose weight need professional advice if they wish to select any weight loss product or regimen. The minimum number of servings of the Food Guide Pyramid provides approximately 1200 to 1400 kcal. This amount of kilocalories would be an acceptable weight-loss regimen for most adults.

NUTRITIONAL CARE

The proper intake and assimilation of nutrients, especially for the hospitalized patient, is called nutritional care. The nutritional needs of a patient depend on the patient's condition.

Nutritional requirements may be provided by regular meals with menus selected from the ordered diet, by tube feeding, or by parenteral hyperalimentation.

Enteral Nutrition

Enteral nutrition (EN) is the delivery of nutrients through a GI tube or the ingestion of food orally. Enteral tube feeding maintains the structural and functional integrity of the GI tract. It enhances the utilization of nutrients and provides a safe and economical method of feeding. Enteral tube feedings are contraindicated in patients with the following:

- Diffused peritonitis
- Severe diarrhea
- Intractable vomiting
- Intestinal obstruction that prohibits normal bowel function

Most feeding tubes are made of silicone or polyurethane, which are durable materials and are biocompatible with formulas. The physician selects the route and type of feeding tube on the basis of the anticipated duration of feeding, the condition of the GI tract, and the potential for aspiration. The use of the GI tract to achieve total nutritional support or partial support in combination with the parenteral route should be attempted whenever possible if the patient's oral intake is adequate. Tube feedings can be administered via nasogastric, nasoduodenal, nasojejunal, esophagostomy, gastrostomy, and jejunostomy tubes (see Figure 30-3). The most common complications of EN are diarrhea and improper tube placement.

Hyperalimentation or Total Parenteral Nutrition

Hyperalimentation or **total parenteral nutrition (TPN)** is used to meet the patient's nutritional requirements when the enteral route cannot accomplish this. TPN is the treatment of choice for selected patients who are unable to tolerate and maintain adequate enteral intake. TPN is able to supply all calories, amino acids (proteins), dextrose (carbohydrates), fats, trace elements, vitamins, and other essential nutrients needed for wound healing, immunocompetence, growth, and weight gain. The basic parenteral solution may contain amino acids, carbohydrates, lipids, vitamins, and minerals. Parenteral nutrition (PN) should be undertaken within 1 to 3 days in moderately to severely malnourished patients, when the inadequacy of enteral support is anticipated for more than 5 to 7 days. There are two methods of administration for TPN. The first is the central venous route, which is used with hypertonic PN formulations such as dextrose concentrations greater than 10%. The second method is the peripheral venous route, which can be used when the dextrose concentration is 10% or less.

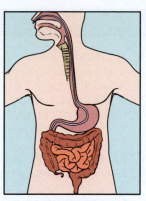

Nasogastric Route

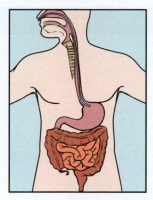

Nasoduodenal Route

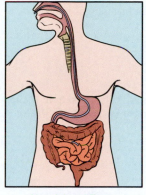

Nasojejunal Route

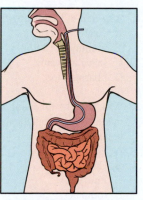

Esophagostomy Route

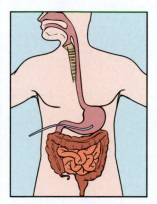

Gastrostomy Route

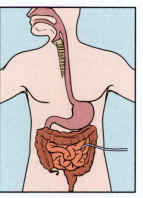

Jejunostomy Route

Figure 30-3. Enteral feeding routes.

PHARMA FOOD

Pharma food is a system of receiving nourishment through breathing. People constantly ingest microparticles that are suspended in the air, such as the dust in every home. The idea behind pharma food is to convert this act, the ingestion of polluting particles (which we are completely accustomed to and takes place in enclosed and outdoor urban areas), into a new form of nourishment.

Pharma food is composed of a type of particle that is ingested by breathing and that has beneficial effects on the organism. These particles include, in general, vitamins, amino acids, minerals, or micronutrients and constitute a volatile muesli that is released to be inhaled and reaches its destination by the mouth. For the particles to reach the stomach and avoid getting into the lungs, an element called *saliva activator* has been devised. It activates the salivary glands so that the inhaled particles adhere to saliva and are led to the stomach, where they are assimilated by the digestive system. Often, food products with pharmacological additives designed to improve health by lowering cholesterol or enhancing brain function are inhaled. Because of tough restrictions on advertising, pharma foods are not as popular as they could be, although there are continuing advances in their use. Inhaled lidocaine is now used as a treatment for asthma, which has led to a marked decline in use of steroids, the most popular type of treatment previously. Direct delivery of the lidocaine into the lungs in high concentrations results in minimal systemic exposure and toxicities, but it is nor used much anymore. A similar therapy is the use of inhaled reformulated aztreonam to treat cystic fibrosis.

SUMMARY

No single food supplies all the nutrients needed by the body. Therefore, it is important to eat various foods daily to meet all the nutrient needs of the body. Nutrients are divided into six basic categories: proteins, carbohydrates, lipids, vitamins, minerals, and water. Nutrients provide energy for the body. The main sources of energy include carbohydrates, proteins, and fat. Nutritional deficiency is known as malnutrition. Marasmus, kwashiorkor, obesity, and many disorders or conditions need special nutritional therapy. Pharmacy technicians must be familiar with basic nutrition dietary standards and pathological conditions. In pharmacy practice, there are many questions that clients may ask about foods and nutrition.

CRITICAL THINKING

1. Explain the role that nutrition plays in an individual's overall health. Why is proper nutrition so important?
2. Research some of the popular diets that are currently receiving attention in the news. What impact could these diets have on an individual's health? What advice would you provide to a customer asking questions about these diets?
3. What are the critical factors that must be accounted for in patients receiving enteral or total parenteral nutrition? What must these patients be monitored for?

REVIEW QUESTIONS

1. Which of the following nutrients is the major source of building materials for muscles, blood, skin, and hair?
    A. Vitamins
    B. Carbohydrates
    C. Proteins
    D. Oxygen

2. The nutrients necessary for the production of bile include
    A. cholesterol.
    B. vitamin D.
    C. lipoprotein.
    D. phospholipid.

3. A pathological state, resulting from a relative or absolute deficiency or excess of one or more essential nutrients, is called
    A. kwashiorkor.
    B. obesity.
    C. beriberi.
    D. marasmus.

4. The proper intake and assimilation of nutrients is known as
    A. nutrient.
    B. excretion.
    C. nutritional insufficiency.
    D. nutritional care.

5. Severe deficiency of niacin (vitamin B_3) may result in
    A. beriberi.
    B. pellagra.
    C. marasmus.
    D. pernicious anemia.

6. Which of the following nutrients helps to keep the body's water and electrolytes in balance?
    A. Lipids
    B. Carbohydrates
    C. Minerals
    D. Vitamins

7. An essential micronutrient of thyroid hormone (thyroxine) is
    A. iron.
    B. iodine.
    C. zinc.
    D. copper.

8. Calcium deficiency may cause all of the following, except
    A. rickets.
    B. osteoporosis.
    C. dwarfism.
    D. osteomalacia.

9. The Nutrition Labeling and Education Act of 1990 requires most packaged foods to list a specified set of
    A. vitamin facts on the diet.
    B. nutrition facts on the label.
    C. mineral and vitamin facts on the diet.
    D. nutritional deficiencies.

10. All of the following are the purposes of food additives, except
    A. to make food more appealing.
    B. to prevent misleading statements on the label.
    C. to maintain nutritional value.
    D. to main freshness in the food.

11. A system of nourishing through breathing is known as
    A. volatile muesli.
    B. immune activator.
    C. saliva activator.
    D. pharma food.

12. Which of the following minerals is able to help in the formation of hemoglobin and the transportation of iron to bone marrow?
    A. Fluoride (F)
    B. Copper (Cu)
    C. Zinc (Zn)
    D. Iodine (I)

13. Which of the following vitamins may protect the body against infections or help heal wounds?
    A. Vitamin C
    B. Vitamin B_{12}
    C. Vitamin K
    D. Vitamin E

14. All of the nutrition information on the label is based on which of the following?
    A. The amount of cholesterol
    B. The stated calories
    C. The stated serving size
    D. The amount of sodium

15. The purpose of food additives is
    A. to maintain nutritional value.
    B. to improve diet with low cholesterol.
    C. to improve diet with high potassium.
    D. all of the above.

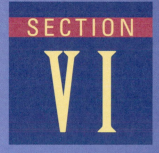

SECTION VI

Special Populations

31

Special Considerations for Pediatric and Neonatal Patients

OUTLINE

Overview
Defining the Neonatal and Pediatric Population
The Unique Characteristics of Pediatric Medication
    Administration
  Absorption
  Distribution
  Metabolism
  Excretion
Fever
Childhood Respiratory Diseases
  Apnea
  Respiratory Syncytial Virus
  Asthma
  Respiratory Distress Syndrome
  Croup
  Epiglottitis
  Pneumonia

Common Childhood Illnesses
  Otitis Media
  Diabetes Mellitus
  Seizure Disorders
Cardiovascular and Blood Disorders
  Patent Ductus Arteriosus
  Congestive Heart Failure
  Iron Deficiency Anemia
  Sickle Cell Anemia
Infectious Diseases
  Diarrhea
  Bacteremia and Septicemia
  Acute Bacterial Meningitis
  Streptococcal Infections
  Human Immunodeficiency Virus and Acquired Immunodeficiency
    Syndrome
Summary

OBJECTIVES

Upon completion of this chapter, the reader should be able to

1. Recognize common childhood respiratory diseases.
2. Identify treatment of asthma in children.
3. Describe otitis media in children.
4. Understand the factors affecting pharmacokinetics and pharmacodynamics in children.
5. Identify cardiovascular and blood disorders.

6. Define sickle cell anemia.
7. List five common examples of infectious diseases in pediatrics.
8. Explain acute bacterial meningitis.
9. Describe diabetes mellitus in pediatrics.
10. Explain international classification of seizures.

GLOSSARY

apnea The cessation of respiration for more than 20 seconds with or without cyanosis, hypotonia, or bradycardia.

asthma A chronic inflammatory disorder of the airways of the respiratory system.

bacteremia Bacteria present in the circulatory system.

congestive heart failure A disorder in which the heart cannot pump the blood returning to the right side of the heart or provide adequate circulation to meet the needs of organs and tissues in the body.

croup A viral infection that affects the larynx and the trachea.

epiglottitis An acute bacterial infection of the epiglottis (an appendage that closes the glottis while food or drink is passing through the pharynx) and the surrounding areas that causes airway obstruction.

epilepsy A disorder characterized by recurrent, unprovoked seizures, in which seizures are of primary cerebral origin, indicating underlying brain dysfunction.

insulin-dependent diabetes mellitus A disorder caused by complete lack of insulin secretion of the pancreas.

iron deficiency anemia A microcytic hypochromic anemia caused by inadequate supplies of iron needed to synthesize hemoglobin.

GLOSSARY continued

neonatal period The time from birth to approximately 28 days of age.

otitis media An inflammation of the middle ear.

patent ductus arteriosus A disorder in which the ductus remains patent when pulmonary vascular resistance falls, resulting in aortic blood being shunted into the pulmonary artery.

pediatric period The period from birth to approximately age 18.

pneumonia An acute inflammation of the lungs, often caused by inhaled Streptococcus pneumoniae.

respiratory distress syndrome (RDS) The result of the absence, deficiency, or alteration of the components of pulmonary surfactant.

respiratory syncytial virus (RSV) The major cause of bronchiolitis and pneumonia in infants younger than 1 year of age; caused by a virus and causes mild cold-like symptoms.

seizure A sudden, transient alteration in brain function as a result of abnormal neuronal activity and excessive cerebral electric discharge.

septicemia A systemic infection caused by multiplication of microorganisms in the blood circulation.

sickle cell anemia An inherited disorder characterized by the presence of abnormal hemoglobin; hemoglobin contains hemoglobin S (HbS).

OVERVIEW

Pediatric drug therapy is a special consideration in medicine. It is problematic even for practitioners with extensive experience. To put it simply, a child's age complicates drug therapy. A drug undergoes the same processes in a child as it does in an adult, but a child's body is distinctive and constantly changing, which affects how it responds to a drug. During the past few decades, drug administration, usage, and research in pediatric patients have been challenging. Children are not merely miniature adults. Therefore, knowledge about pediatric medication cannot simply be extrapolated from the adult research, literature, and clinical trials. In fact, if a label does not contain a pediatric dose, do not assume that the drug is safe for anyone younger than 12 years of age. The pharmacy technician should be sure that a drug is safe for children by asking the doctor or pharmacist. Effective and safe drug therapy in newborns, infants, and children requires an understanding of maturational changes that affect drug action, metabolism, and disposition. Pediatric drug dosage must be adjusted for the characteristics of individual drugs and for the patient's age, disease states, sex, and individual needs to prevent ineffective treatment or toxicity.

DEFINING THE NEONATAL AND PEDIATRIC POPULATION

The **neonatal period** generally covers the time from birth to approximately 28 days of age. This general category also includes premature infants of varying gestational ages. Gestational age will be a factor in dosing for various medications and may even preclude the use of some. The **pediatric period** covers a wide range of ages, from birth to approximately age 18. Accurate preparation and administration of medications to pediatric and neonatal patients requires the pharmacist or technician to have an accurate and current weight as dosages for this population are given per unit of weight. Only during a "code" situation, when the

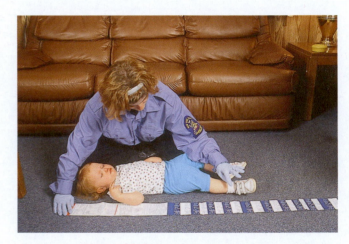

Figure 31-1. Use of the Broselow tape.

actual weight of the child is unknown, should drugs be given without knowing the accurate weight of the patient. Even in these instances, certain estimating devices are used to assure some accuracy. The Broselow tape is one such device. It is placed along the length of the child, and the corresponding color zone on the tape is used to give emergency personnel medication dosages and other pertinent information, such as catheter and endotracheal tube sizes (see Figure 31-1). Patients should be weighed daily, and this information should be sent to the pharmacy so that doses of medications can be adjusted for rapid weight gains and losses that sometimes occur with children. Pediatric liquid medicines can be given with a variety of dosing instruments: plastic medicine cups, hypodermic syringes without needles, oral syringes, oral droppers, and cylindrical dosing spoons (see Figure 31-2).

THE UNIQUE CHARACTERISTICS OF PEDIATRIC MEDICATION ADMINISTRATION

A child's body surface area, metabolism, development, and tolerance are quite different from those of an adult. For many drugs, safe and effective use in children requires additional

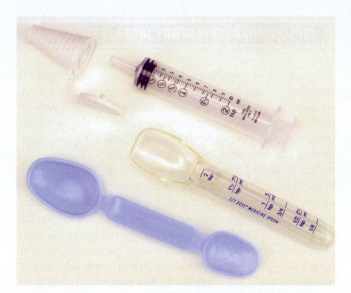

Figure 31-2. Devices for measuring medications for children.

pharmacokinetic and pharmacodynamic data. Three quarters of all medications marketed today do not have U.S. Food and Drug Administration (FDA)-approved labeling for use in neonates, infants, children, and adolescents. Only 5 of the 80 drugs most often used in newborns and infants are labeled for pediatric use. The FDA has recently made regulatory changes to facilitate labeling of drugs for pediatric use. In 1994, the FDA Center for Drug Evaluation and Research published a Pediatric Plan to encourage studies on pediatric patients during the drug development process.

To complicate matters even more, most drugs are not tested on children. In many instances, no one knows for sure if a given drug is safe or effective in children or what dosage is appropriate. Only about 30% of FDA-approved drugs have been approved for specific pediatric indications, and few approved drugs come in child-appropriate dosage forms, which means that health care professionals must formulate pediatric doses. Children younger than 2 years of age should not be given any over-the-counter drug without a doctor's approval. Certain barbiturates, for example, which make adults feel sluggish, will make a child hyperactive. Amphetamines, which stimulate adults, can calm children.

It is essential that pharmacy technicians be familiar with most common diseases and conditions of neonatal and young children, the principles of pharmacology, and the required drug therapy. The technician should also consider the four processes involved in pharmacokinetics: absorption, distribution, metabolism, and excretion.

Absorption

Absorption is the movement of a drug from its site of administration into the blood. The rate of absorption of a medication is directly related to its route of administration.

However, a child may absorb oral drugs at a different rate and to a different degree than an adult because of differences in gastrointestinal tract motility, gastric acidity, and other factors. Absorption of some drugs given intramuscularly may be erratic in newborns. Dermal and subcutaneous absorption of drugs is remarkably enhanced in newborns and young infants. For example, topically administered epinephrine may cause systemic hypertension, and dermal absorption of dyes and antibacterials may result in poisoning. Theophylline administered subcutaneously to premature newborns with apnea is well absorbed and therapeutic plasma concentrations are maintained.

Distribution

Distribution is the movement of a drug from the blood into the cells and tissues. Changes in drug distribution during growth parallel changes in body composition. The total amount of body water is greater in newborns than in adults. Therefore, to maintain equivalent drug plasma concentrations, water-soluble drugs are given in decreasing doses, per kilogram of body weight, with advancing postnatal age. This decline in total body water continues into old age.

Metabolism

Metabolism (chemical biotransformation) is the physical and chemical alteration of the drug in the body. A newborn's hepatic enzyme system can alter a drug's metabolism. Metabolism tends to be very slow in the newborn, increasing progressively during the first few months of life and exceeding adult rates by the first few years of life. Most drugs, including phenytoin, barbiturates, analgesics, and cardiac glycosides, have plasma half-lives up to three times longer in newborns than in adults.

Excretion

Excretion (elimination) is the removal of waste products of drug metabolism from the body. Renal immaturity may cause slower drug excretion and increase the risk of drug toxicity in a child. Drug elimination is still slow during adolescence and probably attains adult rates by late puberty. Whereas for some drugs, such as barbiturates and phenytoin, adult rates of elimination may be achieved 2 to 4 weeks after birth, for others, such as theophylline, adult rates may not be achieved for months. Renal elimination is the primary route for antimicrobials, which are the most commonly used drugs in newborns and young children. Effective renal blood flow affects the rate at which drugs are eliminated by the kidneys. Plasma clearance of drugs is significantly increased in early childhood after age 1; this is partly due to increased renal and hepatic elimination of drugs in young children relative to adults, especially elderly persons.

FEVER

Fever is a common reason for parents to seek medical attention for their children, and approximately 30% of visits to pediatricians are fever related. Parents believe that fever is a disease rather than a symptom. Fever is body temperature raised above its normal level by an alteration of the hypothalamic setpoint. Fever is defined as a rectal temperature greater than 100.4°F (38°C) in infants 0 to 3 months of age, and a rectal temperature of 101°F (38.3°C) in children older than 3 months.

Clinical decisions based on the presence and height of fever may be affected by the way that temperature is measured. Measuring temperature rectally appears to be the most accurate method, but it is contraindicated in struggling children and in children with anorectal anomalies. Infrared tympanometry is a rapid method for measuring temperature, but its sensitivity for detecting fever is poor.

Fever is part of the febrile response, which includes activation of numerous physiological, endocrinological, and immunological systems. Microbes, toxins, or products of microbial origin, antigen-antibody complexes, complement, and other chemical agents are pyrogens that cause fever.

This evidence indicates that fever is an important defense mechanism and that treating the fever may have detrimental effects. In varicella, for example, acetaminophen prolongs the time of crusting of skin lesions. Nevertheless, many clinicians and caregivers believe that fever is harmful. A small percentage (4%) of children between 3 months and 5 years of age will develop a seizure when they have a fever. A simple febrile seizure is not associated with central nervous system damage or future epilepsy, and in the few controlled trials conducted thus far, antipyretic therapy has not been shown to protect against recurrence of febrile seizures.

The most valid justifications for treating fever are to reassure the patient and to treat nonspecific discomfort. The Bayer Company introduced aspirin as the first commercially available antipyretic in 1899. In 1974, a significant association was noted between Reye syndrome and aspirin-containing medications in children with a viral illness.

Acetaminophen is one of the most widely used antipyretics. Like aspirin and other nonsteroidal anti-inflammatory drugs, acetaminophen blocks the conversion of arachidonic acid to prostaglandin. Current evidence still suggests that acetaminophen is the drug of choice for antipyresis in children.

Ibuprofen (Motrin®) is another option for an antipyretic. This agent has been shown to provide a greater temperature decrement in febrile children and a longer duration of antipyresis than noted with acetaminophen when the two drugs were administered in equal doses (10 mg/kg). Physical methods to reduce temperature are ineffective if shivering is not prevented, and such methods do not alter the hypothalamic setpoint.

CHILDHOOD RESPIRATORY DISEASES

The patterns of respiratory tract diseases in childhood are modified by age, sex, race, season, geography, and environmental and socioeconomic conditions. Immediately after birth, tuberculosis can be transmitted to the newborn, presenting after several weeks of life as a severe pneumonitis. Lung immaturity and other events related to the perinatal period predispose newborns to hyaline membrane disease. The incidence of respiratory tract infections also peaks during the first 2 to 3 school years. Respiratory diseases affect many children each year. Respiratory syncytial virus (RSV) and asthma are two specific problems quite often treated in the pediatric/neonatal patient population. Apnea is seen in the neonatal age group, especially in premature infants. See Chapter 22 for more information on the respiratory system.

Apnea

Apnea is the cessation of respiration for more than 20 seconds with or without cyanosis, hypotonia, or bradycardia. Apnea may be a symptom of another disorder that resolves upon treatment of the disorder. These disorders may include infection, gastroesophageal reflux, hypoglycemia, metabolic disorders, drug toxicity, hydrocephalus, or thermal instability in newborns. Immaturity of the central nervous system often accounts for apnea of the newborn, which occurs most commonly during active sleep. Obstructive apnea occurs when there is an obstruction of the airway at the level of the pharynx. About one third of infants born at less than 32 weeks' gestation have apneic episodes. More than 50% of infants weighing less than 1.5 kg require treatment for recurrent prolonged apneic episodes. Obstructive apnea is most often caused by hypertrophy of the adenoids and tonsils. Complications of apnea include hypoxia and sudden infant death syndrome.

Treatment for Apnea

The airway should be opened and cardiorespiratory resuscitation should be initiated. The treatment of central apnea that is most commonly used for premature infants includes minimizing potential causes such as temperature variances and feeding intolerance. The use of xanthine medications such as caffeine and theophylline provides central nervous system stimulation. Pulmonary function support may include the use of supplemental oxygen and continuous positive airway pressure at low pressures (see Chapter 22).

Respiratory Syncytial Virus

Respiratory syncytial virus (RSV) is the major cause of bronchiolitis and pneumonia in infants younger than 1 year of age. It is the most important respiratory tract pathogen of early childhood. It causes mild cold-like symptoms in infants and most children. However, RSV can cause a more serious respiratory disease in premature infants that sometimes requires hospitalization. The at-risk group includes infants born at less than 36 weeks' gestation or those with chronic lung disease. The respiratory disease occurs because of the immaturity of the infants' lungs and because these infants have not received sufficient antiviral substances from their mothers. Other high-risk infants include children with certain kinds of congenital heart disease, children with other chronic lung diseases such as cystic fibrosis, children who are immune-deficient, or children who are receiving immune-suppressive medication. In most parts of the United States, RSV infection occurs seasonally, generally from fall through spring (October through March). At-risk infants are now treated before discharge from the hospital to provide some immunoprophylaxis.

Treatments for Respiratory Syncytial Virus

Palivizumab (Synagis®) is used for the immunoprophylaxis against severe lower respiratory tract RSV infections. In infants with uncomplicated bronchiolitis, treatment is symptomatic. Humidified oxygen is usually indicated for hospitalized infants because most have hypoxia. Fluids should be carefully administered. Often, intravenous or tube feeding is helpful when sucking is difficult. Bronchodilators should not be routinely used. However, a course of epinephrine should be used in children with wheezing who are older than 1 year of age, and bronchodilators should be administered if found to be beneficial. The use of corticosteroids is not indicated except as a last resort in children whose condition is critical. Sedatives are rarely necessary. The antiviral drug ribavirin, delivered by small-particle aerosol and breathed along with the required concentration of oxygen for 20 to 24 hours per day for 3 to 5 days, has a beneficial effect on the course of pneumonia caused by RSV (see Chapters 22 and 24).

Asthma

Asthma is a leading cause of chronic illness in childhood and is responsible for a significant proportion of school days missed because of chronic illness. Asthma is a chronic, reversible, obstruction of the bronchial airways. The airways become over-reactive because of this inflammation and increased mucus secretion; mucosal swelling and muscle contraction then occur (see Figure 31-3). This leads to airway obstruction, chest tightness, coughing, wheezing, and, if asthma is severe, shortness of breath and low blood oxygen levels. Most children experience their first symptoms by 4 to 5 years of age. Allergies, viral respiratory infections, and airborne irritants produce the inflammation that can lead to asthma. Childhood asthma is a disease with a strong allergic component and a genetic predisposition.

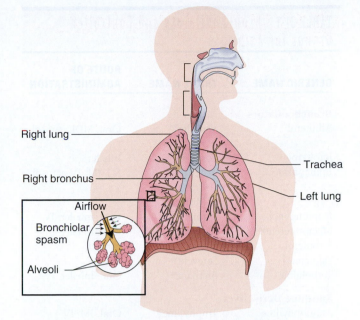

Right lung
Right bronchus
Trachea
Left lung
Airflow
Bronchiolar spasm
Alveoli

Figure 31-3. Pathophysiology of asthma.

Approximately 75% to 80% of children with asthma have allergies.

Treatment for Asthma

Treatment for asthma generally includes two types of medications: quick-relief medications (also called bronchodilators), and controller medications. Controller medications got their name because they help control inflammation to make breathing easier. These medications must be taken daily to be effective. Medications in the bronchodilators and controller groups are listed in Table 31-1.

Respiratory Distress Syndrome

Respiratory distress syndrome (RDS), or hyaline membrane disease, is the result of the absence, deficiency, or alteration of the components of pulmonary surfactant. Surfactant, a lipoprotein complex, is an ingredient of the film-like surface of each alveolus that prevents alveolar collapse. When the amount of surfactant is inadequate, alveolar collapse and hypoxia result. Pulmonary vascular constriction and decreased pulmonary perfusion then occur, leading to progressive respiratory failure. There is an inverse relationship to gestational age. The younger the infants are, the greater the incidence of RDS. However, the occurrence of RDS appears to be more dependent on lung maturity than on actual gestational age. The severity of RDS is decreased in infants whose mothers received corticosteroids 24 to 48 hours before delivery. Corticosteroids are most effective when newborns are less than 34 weeks' gestational age, and they are administered for at least 24 hours, but no longer than 7 days before delivery.

TABLE 31-1. Bronchodilators and Controller Groups for Asthma

GENERIC NAME	TRADE NAME	ROUTE OF ADMINISTRATION
Bronchodilators		
Albuterol	Ventolin®, Proventil®	Oral, MDI, aerosol
Bitolterol	Tornalate®	Inhaler
Epinephrine	Adrenalin®, Primatene Mist®	SC, IM, IV, aerosol
Isoproterenol	Isuprel®	Oral, inhaler, IV
Metaproterenol	Alupent®	Oral, inhaler
Pirbuterol	Maxair®	Inhaler
Salmeterol	Serevent®	Inhaler
Terbutaline	Brethaire®	Oral, inhaler, IV
Xanthine Derivatives		
Aminophylline	Truphylline®	Oral, IM, IV
Theophylline	Theo-Dur®	Oral
Leukotriene Inhibitors		
Montelukast	Singulair®	Oral
Zafirlukast	Accolate®	Oral
Corticosteroids		
Dexamethasone	Decadron®	Oral, inhaler
Hydrocortisone	Solu-Cortef®	Oral
Prednisolone	Pediapred®	Oral
Beclomethasone	Beclovent®	Inhaler
Budesonide	Rhinocort®	Inhaler
Fluticasone	Flovent®	Inhaler
Mast Cell Stabilizers		
Cromolyn sodium	Intal®	Inhaler, nebulizer
Nedocromil	Tilade®	Inhaler

MDI, metered dose inhaler; IM, intramuscular; IV, intravenous; SC, subcutaneous.

Treatment for Respiratory Distress Syndrome

Infants at risk for or those who have RDS as well as infants with respiratory failure due to meconium aspiration syndrome, persistent pulmonary hypertension, or pneumonia are treated with natural, animal-derived, or synthetic surfactant. Continuous positive airway pressure, via nasal prongs, is required to prevent volume loss during expiration or mechanical ventilation via endotracheal tube for severe hypoxemia and/or hypercapnia. Aerosol administration of bronchodilators is also used.

Croup

Croup, or acute laryngotracheobronchitis, is a viral infection that affects the larynx and the trachea. Subglottic edema with upper respiratory tract obstruction results, accompanied by thick secretions. Children are susceptible to airway obstruction because the diameter of the subglottic area is narrow. Croup is caused by any virus associated with upper respiratory tract infection. Spasmodic croup is a sudden attack of croup, which usually occurs during the night and can be associated with an upper respiratory tract infection, fever, or allergies. The incidence of croup is higher in the late fall and early winter. The age range of occurrence is 6 months to 6 years. The peak age of onset is 2 years of age.

Treatment for Croup

When a child with suspected croup is seen at the hospital, supplemental humidified oxygen is given as indicated by the child's appearance and result of pulse oximetry and vital signs. The child can be treated with bronchodilators, usually racemic epinephrine if humidification alone is ineffective. The use of corticosteroids is controversial. Children who receive corticosteroids need endotracheal intubation less often, and their stridor is more quickly resolved. Antibiotics are administered if secondary bacterial infection is suspected.

Epiglottitis

Epiglottitis is an acute bacterial infection of the epiglottis (an appendage that closes the glottis while food or drink is passing through the pharynx) and the surrounding areas that cause airway obstruction. The infection is caused by *Haemophilus influenzae* type B or, on rare occasions, streptococci and pneumococci. The use of *H. influenzae* type B vaccine in infants has resulted in a dramatic reduction in the incidence of epiglottitis. Onset is sudden and infection progresses rapidly, causing acute respiratory difficulty. This condition requires emergency airway stabilization and medical measures because a fatal outcome can occur. Boys between ages 2 to 7 are most often affected. The incidence of epiglottitis is highest in the winter.

Treatment for Epiglottitis

Visual examination of the throat is contraindicated until a tracheostomy is performed. The child is observed in the intensive care area until swelling of the epiglottis decreases (usually by the third day). Antibiotics are given for a total of 7 to 10 days.

Pneumonia

Pneumonia is an inflammation or infection of the pulmonary parenchyma. Pneumonia is caused by viruses, bacteria, *Mycoplasma* organisms, and aspiration of foreign substances. Pneumonia accounts for 10% to 15% of all respiratory infections, especially during the fall and winter months. Viral pneumonia occurs more often than bacterial pneumonia (about 70% to 80% of all cases). RSV, which was discussed earlier, accounts for the largest percentage of occurrences of viral pneumonia.

Treatment for Pneumonia

Medical treatment is primarily supportive and includes improving oxygenation with oxygen and respiratory treatments. Antibiotics are used to treat bacterial pneumonia based on culture and sensitivity testing. Hospitalization depends on the severity of illness, the child's age, and the suspected organism.

COMMON CHILDHOOD ILLNESSES

It is impossible to discuss all pediatric disorders and illnesses in one chapter. Therefore, some selective examples of the most common childhood illnesses will be discussed.

Otitis Media

Otitis media is an inflammation of the middle ear. Children 6 years of age and younger are at particular risk for otitis media because their Eustachian tubes are shorter and more horizontal. Otitis media is the most commonly encountered diagnosis in office visits for children younger than 15 years of age in the United States. Two types of otitis media are seen in clinical pediatric practice: acute otitis media and otitis media with effusion (fluid in the middle ear without signs and symptoms of ear infection). Otitis media occurs most often in children between 3 months and 3 years with peak incidences occurring between 5 to 24 months and 4 to 6 years. Boys have more ear infections than girls. Tympanic membrane rupture with discharge and short-term conductive hearing loss are common complications of otitis media.

Treatment for Otitis Media

The efficacy of steroid therapy, decongestants, and antihistamines for the resolution of otitis media has not been proved. Their use should not be encouraged. Surgical removal of tonsils or adenoids is not recommended for the treatment of otitis media with effusion in the absence of specific tonsil or adenoid pathological conditions. The first-line antibiotic medication most often prescribed is amoxicillin or ampicillin. The second-line medication regimen (to be used when an amoxicillin-resistant organism is suspected) includes amoxicillin with clavulanate, cefaclor, cotrimoxazole, erythromycin, or sulfisoxazole. In the penicillin-allergic child, erythromycin with a sulfonamide or trimethoprim-sulfamethoxazole may be used. Generic names, trades names, and routes of administration were discussed in Chapter 20. Myringotomy is a surgical procedure to insert pressure-equalizing tubes into the tympanic membrane. This allows ventilation of the middle ear, relieves the negative pressure, and permits drainage of fluid. The tubes usually fall out after 6 to 12 months.

Diabetes Mellitus

Insulin-dependent diabetes mellitus (IDDM), or type I (juvenile-onset) diabetes, is caused by a complete lack of insulin secretion by the pancreas. Insulin is necessary for many physiological functions of the body. Insulin deficiency results in unrestricted glucose production without appropriate use, resulting in hyperglycemia and increased production of ketones in the blood. Fifteen percent of all diabetic individuals have insulin-dependent diabetes mellitus, and 97% of all juvenile patients with newly diagnosed diabetes have insulin-dependent diabetes mellitus. Age ranges of peak incidence are 5 to 7 years and puberty. Among children 5 to 10 years of age, the disease is more commonly diagnosed in girls. Type I diabetes usually starts with polyphagia, weight loss, polydipsia, and polyuria. Symptoms caused by insulin deficiency may last from a few days to weeks before the diagnosis is made. Long-term effects of IDDM include failure to grow at a normal rate, neuropathy (the impairment of sensory and motor nerve functions), recurrent infection, renal microvascular disease, and ischemic heart disease.

Treatment for Insulin-Dependent Diabetes Mellitus

As soon as hyperglycemia or glucosuria is detected, immediate medical attention is needed because of the potential for rapid deterioration of the patient's condition. The initial therapy will depend on how early the diagnosis is made and on the state of the child. Children with initial diagnoses of IDDM are usually admitted to the hospital for stabilization of glucose levels and education but may be treated on an outpatient basis. Medical management includes the regulation of serum glucose, fluid, and electrolyte levels. Once glucose levels are stabilized, the child's insulin dose is typically dictated by a sliding scale based on the serum glucose level. Regulation of nutrition and exercise is also a key factor in managing diabetes. Age and stage of sexual development, dietary intake, and potential adherence to the treatment regimen should be taken into consideration when the individual's insulin treatment is selected. If insulin requirements and caloric intake are small (especially in the very young child), a single dose of a mixture of NPH and short-acting insulin given before breakfast, with a second dose of short-acting insulin before supper if the blood glucose values are high, is usually enough. For older children or children who are in the midst of the adolescent growth spurt a regimen of twice-daily injections of a mixture of preferably NPH and regular insulin before breakfast and before supper may be started immediately. Table 31-2 shows types and action of insulins (see also Chapter 26).

Treatment of Diabetes in the Infant

Symptomatic hyperglycemia can occur in newborn infants. These babies usually suffer from severe intrauterine malnutrition, and, therefore, are small for their gestational age. They are hypoinsulinemic, and the pancreas fails to release

TABLE 31-2. **Types and Action of Insulin**

TYPE AND ACTION	ACTION (HR)	
	PEAK	DURATION
Fast		
Regular	2–4	5–7
Semilente	2–8	8–16
Intermediate	8–12	18–24
NPH	8–12	18–28
Lente		
Slow		
Ultralente	16–18	20–36
Protamine zinc	16–20	24–36

TABLE 31-3. **International Classification of Seizures**

CLASSIFICATIONS	EXAMPLES
Partial (focal, local) seizures	Simple partial seizures
	Complex partial seizures
Generalized seizures	Absence seizures
(convulsive or	Myoclonic seizures
nonconvulsive)	Tonic-clonic seizures
	(grand mal)
	Atonic seizures
	Status epilepticus

insulin in response to any of the standard body demands. They must be treated with divided doses of exogenous insulin of up to 1 to 2 U/kg/24 hr. Insulin requirements are best established by starting a continuous intravenous insulin infusion at rates to provide at least 0.5 U/kg/24 hr. Insulin treatment is simplified by using diluted insulin so that inadvertent overdoses do not occur. In most cases, pancreas function develops sometime between the age of 6 and 12 weeks. The children do well after the newborn period and do not appear to be at increased risk of developing type I diabetes at a later age. See Chapter 26 for more information on the endocrine system, hormones, and related subjects.

Seizure Disorders

Seizure is a sudden, transient alteration in brain function as a result of abnormal neuronal activity and excessive cerebral electric discharge. The causes of seizure include perinatal factors, infectious disease (encephalitis and meningitis), febrile illness, metabolic disorders, trauma, neoplasms, toxins, circulatory disturbances, and degenerative diseases of the nervous system. **Epilepsy** is a disorder characterized by recurrent, unprovoked seizures, in which seizures are of primary cerebral origin, indicating underlying brain dysfunction. Epilepsy is not a disease in itself. Table 31-3 shows the international classification of seizures.

Treatment for Epilepsy

Antiepileptic drug therapy is the mainstay of medical management. Single-drug therapy is the most desirable, with the goal of establishing a balance between seizure control and adverse side effects. The drug of choice is based on seizure type, epileptic syndrome, and patient variables. Drug combinations may be needed to achieve seizure control. Complete control is achieved in only 50% to 75% of children with

epilepsy. The most commonly used anticonvulsants are discussed in Chapter 23.

CARDIOVASCULAR AND BLOOD DISORDERS

Medications to support cardiovascular functions in the pediatric/neonatal patient population differ little from those used with adults. Digoxin, diuretics, and, occasionally, antihypertensives are used. Their indications and dosage generally are the same for all groups. Discussion in this section will focus on a topic unique to the neonatal population, the patent ductus arteriosus, and the use of inotropic agents to support blood pressure. The pharmacy technician may need to recognize the medications used and to prepare them for proper use.

Patent Ductus Arteriosus

During fetal life most of the pulmonary arterial blood is shunted through the ductus arteriosus into the aorta. Functional closure of the ductus normally occurs soon after birth, but if the ductus remains patent when pulmonary vascular resistance falls, aortic blood is shunted into the pulmonary artery (see Figure 31-4). **Patent ductus arteriosus** (PDA) is one of the most common congenital cardiovascular anomalies associated with maternal rubella (German measles) during early pregnancy. After birth and after a series of physiological changes, the pulmonary and systemic circulations become arranged into two circuits, so that oxygenated blood returns from the lungs and is ejected from the left side of the heart to the systemic circulation. Deoxygenated blood returns from the systemic circulation and is ejected from the right side of the heart to the lungs (the pulmonary circuit). After birth, the onset of breathing causes an increase in pulmonary blood flow and pressure which, among other complex reactions, helps the ductus ar-

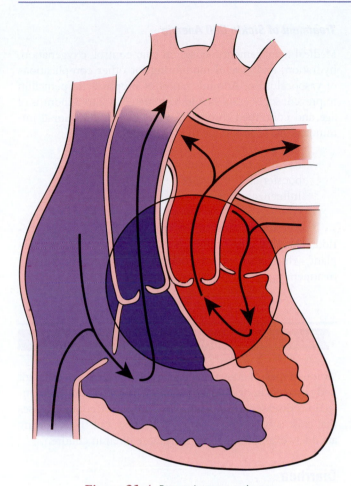

Figure 31-4. Patent ductus arteriosus.

teriosus to close. A decrease in the level of one particular chemical, prostaglandin, specifically aids in this closure. The entire phenomenon of transition is not completely understood, and the transition period of infants is a particularly important time. In uncomplicated PDA, the ductus closes spontaneously within the first weeks or months of life.

Treatment for Patent Ductus Arteriosus

When a large symptomatic PDA is present, general treatment may include fluid restriction, correction of anemia, digitalization, and diuretic therapy. Ductus arteriosus patency is mediated through prostaglandins, and the ductus arteriosus in the preterm infant with respiratory distress syndrome can be constricted and closed by administration of inhibitors of prostaglandin synthesis such as indomethacin. Early administration of indomethacin in the course of respiratory distress syndrome associated with large ductal left to right shunts is approximately 80% effective in closing the ductus. Surgical closure is a safe and effective backup technique for management when indomethacin is contraindicated or indomethacin treatment has not been successful. Administration is by intravenous infusion over at least 30 minutes to minimize adverse

effects on cerebral, renal, and gastrointestinal blood flow. Usually, three doses per course are given, with a maximum of two courses. Urine output must be closely monitored and if anuria (no urine output) or oliguria occurs, subsequent doses should be delayed.

Congestive Heart Failure

Congestive heart failure (CHF) occurs when the heart cannot pump the blood returning to the right side of the heart or provide adequate circulation to meet the needs of organs and tissues in the body. Causes of CHF include the following:

1. High output state, usually related to congenital heart diseases in which there is increased pulmonary blood flow, returning to the right side of the heart
2. Low output state, related to (1) congenital heart diseases in which there are left-side heart obstructions causing the heart to pump harder to bypass the restrictive area, such as with coarctation of the aorta or aortic valve stenosis, (2) a primary heart muscle disease, such as a cardiomyopathy, or (3) rhythm disturbances (tachycardia or bradycardia). Ninety percent of infants with congenital heart defects develop CHF within the first year of life. The majority of affected infants manifest symptoms within the first few months of life.

Treatment for Congestive Heart Failure

The initial management of CHF is accomplished by the use of pharmacological agents that act to improve the function of the heart muscle and reduce the workload on the heart. Digitalis is given to increase cardiac output by slowing conduction through the atrioventricular node to make each contraction stronger. Diuretics decrease preload volume because their actions result in decreased extracellular fluid volume. Fluids are usually restricted to two thirds of maintenance levels, and attention is given to nutrition and rest. Medical management continues with the plan for interventional cardiac catheterization or surgical intervention if indicated. See Chapter 24 for more information about the cardiovascular system and related subjects.

Iron Deficiency Anemia

Iron deficiency anemia is the most common anemia affecting children in North America. The full-term infant born of a well-nourished, nonanemic mother has sufficient iron stores until birth weight is doubled, generally at 4 to 6 months. Iron deficiency anemia is generally not evident until 9 months of age. After that period, iron must be available from the diet to meet the child's nutritional needs. If dietary iron intake is insufficient, iron deficiency anemia results.

Preterm infants, infants with significant perinatal blood loss, or infants born to a poorly nourished mother with iron deficiency may have inadequate iron stores. This infant would have a significantly higher risk for iron deficiency anemia before the age of 6 months. Iron deficiency anemia may also result from chronic blood loss. In the infant, this may be due to chronic intestinal bleeding caused by a heat-labile protein in cow's milk. Other causes of iron deficiency anemia include nutritional deficiencies such as folate (vitamin B_{12}) deficiency, sickle cell anemia, infections, and chronic inflammation.

Treatment for Iron Deficiency Anemia

Treatment efforts are focused on prevention and intervention. Prevention includes encouraging mothers to breast-feed (only until the infant is between 4 and 6 months), to eat foods that are rich in iron, and to take iron-fortified prenatal vitamins (approximately 1 mg/kg of iron supplement per day). Therapy to treat iron deficiency anemia consists of a medication regimen. Iron is administered by mouth in doses of 2 to 3 mg/kg of elemental iron. All forms of iron (ferrous sulfate, ferrous fumarate, ferrous succinate, and ferrous gluconate) are equally effective. Vitamin C must be administered simultaneously with iron (ascorbic acid increases iron absorption). Iron is best absorbed when it is taken 1 hour before a meal. Iron therapy should continue for a minimum of 6 weeks after the anemia is corrected to replenish iron stores. Injectable iron is seldom used unless small bowel malabsorption disease is present.

Sickle Cell Anemia

Sickle cell anemia is an inherited disorder. Children with sickle cell anemia have abnormal hemoglobin. Their hemoglobin contains hemoglobin S (HbS). Sickled red blood cells are crescent shaped, have decreased oxygen-carrying capacity, and are destroyed at a higher rate than that for normal red blood cells. In addition, the life span of sickled cells is diminished to 16 to 20 days compared with that for normal red blood cells. Sickle cell crises result from physiological changes that produce a decrease in the amount of oxygen available to the hemoglobin. Sickling results in clumping of red blood cells in the vessels, decreased oxygen transport, and increased destruction of red blood cells. Ischemia and tissue death result from the obstruction of vessels and decreased blood flow. The incidence of sickle cell disease among African Americans is estimated to be 1 in 375 to 650. This disease has also been occasionally reported in natives of India, Greeks, and Arabs. Sickle cell traits occur in 8% to 10% of African Americans. Most commonly, death occurs in children at 1 to 3 years of age from organ failure or thrombosis of major organs, usually the lungs and brain. With new treatments, 85% of affected individuals survive to age 20; 50% survive beyond 50 years of age.

Treatment of Sickle Cell Anemia

Medical management focuses on pain control, oxygenation, hydration, and careful monitoring for other complications of vasoocclusion. Administration of prophylactic penicillin to prevent septicemia should be initiated at 2 to 3 months of age and continued through 5 years of life. Additional immunizations required are the following:

- Pneumococcal vaccine at 2 years of age with a booster at 4 to 5 years
- Influenza vaccine

Analgesics are used to control pain during a crisis period. The only cure is thought to be a bone marrow transplant, which also involves risks. This may be a promising treatment modality in the near future.

INFECTIOUS DISEASES

Various types of infectious agents have effects on different body systems in newborns and children, which can cause infectious diseases. Discussion of the many infectious diseases that exist is beyond the scope of this text, but the following are a few examples that are seen more often in children.

Diarrhea

Diarrhea is one of the most common problems encountered by pediatricians. Diarrhea is defined as an increase in the frequency, fluidity, and volume of feces. During the first 3 years of life it is estimated that a child will experience an acute, severe episode of diarrhea one to three times. It may be caused by a variety of infectious agents such as bacteria, viruses, protozoans, and parasites. Hospitalization is usually necessary for severe diarrhea because of the possibility of bacterial disease, which should be treated there, and because hydration often requires fluid therapy.

Treatment for Diarrhea

Treatment for diarrhea is symptomatic. Antipyretic drugs are recommended for fever. Codeine, morphine, and the phenothiazine derivatives, often used for pain and vomiting but rarely needed for children, should be avoided because they may induce misleading signs and symptoms.

Bacteremia and Septicemia

The terms bacteremia and septicemia indicate the presence of bacteria in the blood. In **bacteremia**, bacteria are recovered from blood cultures of a patient and may or may not be associated with a disease. **Septicemia** is bacteremia associated with active disease, whether localized or systemic. In some patients, bacteremia or septicemia may be associated with focal infection (e.g., pneumonia, osteomyelitis, endocarditis, or meningitis). Primary bacteremia, however, also occurs in normal infants and children.

Treatment for Bacteremia and Septicemia

Treatment may be initiated with ampicillin and a semisynthetic penicillinase-resistant penicillin (methicillin, oxacillin, or nafcillin) administered intravenously. In some patients, the use of chloramphenicol may also be indicated.

Acute Bacterial Meningitis

The incidence of bacterial meningitis (especially that caused by *Haemophilus influenzae* type B and group B β-hemolytic streptococci) is increasing. Mortality and morbidity are significant, but the reported number of deaths has decreased over time. Acute bacterial meningitis may be caused by several types of bacteria, depending on the age group of the child. Table 31-4 shows the most common infectious agents that cause meningitis in different age groups.

Treatment for Meningitis

Initial therapy includes immediate administration of multiple antibiotics including a third-generation cephalosporin (such as ceftriaxone or cefotaxime), after an intravenous line has been placed and blood has been drawn for cultures. Vancomycin, with or without rifampin, is usually added, as is ampicillin or gentamycin. Heparin therapy should be considered for patients with the syndrome of disseminated intravascular coagulation. Corticosteroids have been suggested as a therapeutic adjunct that may reduce cerebral edema and inflammation.

Streptococcal Infections

Streptococci are among the most common causes of bacterial infections in infancy and childhood. Group A streptococci are the most common bacteria causing acute pharyngitis.

Treatment for Streptococcal Infections

Penicillin is the drug of choice for the treatment of streptococcal infections. The goal of therapy is to maintain, for at least 10 days, blood and tissue levels of penicillin sufficient to kill streptococci. Various subjects related to antimicrobial infections and the agents used to treat them are covered in Chapter 20.

Human Immunodeficiency Virus and Acquired Immunodeficiency Syndrome

The cause of acquired immunodeficiency syndrome (AIDS) is the human immunodeficiency virus (HIV). This virus attaches to lymphocytes and other immunological cells, which results in a gradual destruction of T-helper lymphocytes. Therefore, HIV is able to reduce and damage immune functions of the body. The virus is transmitted only through direct contact with infected blood or blood products and body fluids, through intravenous drug use, sexual contact, perinatal transmission from mother to infant, and breast-feeding. There is no evidence that HIV infection is acquired through casual contact. Zidovudine is given to pregnant HIV-infected women, which significantly reduces transmission from mother to child. Infants infected through perinatal transmission from infected mothers account for more than 85% of children with AIDS who are younger than 13 years. Infants who have been breast-fed (primarily in developing countries) and children who have received blood products (especially children with hemophilia) account for the remaining 15% of children with AIDS.

Treatment for AIDS

There is currently no cure for HIV infection and AIDS. Management begins with a staging evaluation to determine disease progression and the appropriate course of treatment. Zidovudine (AZT, ZDV), didanosine (DDI), zalcitabine (DDC), and lamivudine (3TC) slow down multiplication of the virus. Combination drug treatment is used, and many children are enrolled in research drug protocols. Trimethoprim-sulfamethoxazole (Septra®, Bactrim®) and pentamidine are used for treatment and prophylaxis of *Pneumocystis carinii* pneumonia. Monthly administration of intravenous immunoglobulin has been useful in prevention of serious bacterial infections in children, as well as hypogammaglobulinemia. Immunizations are recommended for children with HIV infection, but instead of the oral poliovirus vaccine, the inactivated poliovirus vaccine is given. See Chapter 28 for further discussion on immunological agents and related subjects.

TABLE 31-4. Most Common Infectious Agents Causing Meningitis in Different Age Groups	
AGE GROUP	**INFECTIVE CAUSES**
Neonates	Group B streptococci, *Escherichia coli*
Infants	*Haemophilus influenzae* type b, *Streptococcus pneumoniae*
Young children	*Streptococcus pneumoniae* or *Neisseria meningitidis*

SUMMARY

The administration of drugs to a growing and developing infant or child may present a unique problem for the physician, who must be constantly aware of the changes in drug dosages that are determined by alterations in processes of disposition at different ages. Underlying this approach is the concept that there are complex changes in the anatomy, physiology, biochemistry, and behavior from one stage of development to another over the time frame of growth from conception to adulthood. Drugs are double-edged swords. Although they can save lives, they can also endanger life. Effective and safe drug therapy in neonates, infants, and children requires an understanding of the differences in drug action, metabolism, and disposition that are apparent during growth and development. Virtually all pharmacokinetic parameters change with age. Therefore, pediatric drug dosage regimens must be adjusted for age, disease state, sex, and individual needs. Failure to make such adjustments may lead to ineffective treatment or even to toxicity. Pharmacy technicians must be educated so that they have the required knowledge about and pay proper attention to this important matter. It is impossible to cover each topic or aspect of pediatric diseases, conditions, and pharmacology in this chapter. Therefore, special considerations for selected diseases and their therapies were chosen for discussion.

<table>
<tr><td>■</td><td>**CRITICAL THINKING**</td></tr>
</table>

1. What characteristics that make children unique complicate drug administration?
2. Research a common disease or disorder affecting children. What types of therapies are available other than just drug therapies? What additional patient education is necessary when dealing with a child who has this disease/disorder and his or her parents?
3. What can pharmaceutical companies and the government do to make pediatric doses more accurate?

REVIEW QUESTIONS

1. Which of the following factors may cause slower drug excretion and increase the risk of drug toxicity in an infant?
   A. Kidney stones
   B. Pyelonephritis
   C. Urethritis
   D. Renal immaturity

2. Complications of apnea include which of the following?
   A. Sudden infant death syndrome
   B. Hypertension
   C. Asthma
   D. Congestive heart failure

3. Palivizumab (Synagis®) is used for the immunoprophylaxis against which of the following infections?
   A. Epiglottitis
   B. Pneumonia
   C. Respiratory syncytial virus
   D. Asthma

4. Which of the following years of age exhibits the peak onset for croup?
   A. 1
   B. 2
   C. 4
   D. 6

5. Which of the following is the most commonly encountered diagnosis of respiratory disorders in office visits for children younger than the age of 15 in the United States?
   A. Pneumonia
   B. Flu
   C. Epiglottitis
   D. Otitis media

6. Patent ductus arteriosus is one of the most common congenital cardiovascular anomalies associated with which of the following maternal infections?
   A. Hepatitis B
   B. Rubella
   C. AIDS
   D. Pneumonia

7. Ninety percent of infants with congenital heart defects develop which of the following complications within the first year of life?
   A. Iron deficiency anemia
   B. Cystic fibrosis
   C. Sickle cell anemia
   D. Congestive heart failure

8. The most common cause of death in children between 1 to 3 years, who are suffering from sickle cell anemia, is
   A. thrombosis of major organs.
   B. encephalitis.
   C. kidney failure.
   D. meningitis.

9. The first-line antibiotic medication most often prescribed for otitis media is
   A. tetracycline.
   B. Augmentin®.
   C. Septra®.
   D. amoxicillin.

10. Which of the following infectious diseases may be related to bacteremia?
    A. Hepatitis B
    B. Cystitis
    C. Osteomyelitis
    D. Epiglottitis

Continues

11. The goal of therapy for treatment of streptococcal infections is to
    A. maintain blood and tissue levels of penicillin sufficient to kill streptococci for at least 10 days.
    B. prevent myocarditis by using corticosteroids.
    C. maintain blood and tissue levels of corticosteroids to deal with stress for at least 3 days.
    D. prevent nephritic syndrome by using antineoplastic agents.

12. Which of the following infectious diseases probably requires monthly administration of intravenous immunoglobulin to prevent serious bacterial infections in children?
    A. Epiglottitis
    B. Croup
    C. Asthma
    D. AIDS

13. Which of the following types of insulin is classified as intermediate action?
    A. NPH
    B. Regular
    C. Ultralente
    D. Protamine zinc

14. The drug of choice for epilepsy is based on which of the following factors?
    A. Types of seizure
    B. Pregnancy
    C. Maturation of patients
    D. Race and age of patients

15. Treatment for patent ductus arteriosus includes which of the following agents?
    A. Oxygen
    B. Morphine
    C. Indomethacin
    D. Acetaminophen

32

Drug Therapy for Aging Patients

OUTLINE

OBJECTIVES

Upon completion of this chapter, the reader should be able to

1. Identify the most popular types of drugs that elderly patients need.
2. Discuss clinical concerns of drug therapy and the way elderly patients react to certain drugs differently from younger patients.
3. Compare the way aging affects drug interaction, absorption, and distribution.
4. Understand how drug metabolism changes with age.
5. Discuss renal function differences in elderly patients.
6. List some of the adverse effects that certain drugs have upon older patients.
7. Review some of the ways aging can be slowed with a healthy diet and exercise.
8. Identify age-related changes to the integumentary system.
9. Discuss common disorders in elderly patients.

GLOSSARY

alimentary canal The digestive tract.
collagen A strong fibrous protein found in connective tissue.
dermis A thick layer of loose connective tissue that is well-supplied with blood vessels, lymphatic vessels, nerves, and accessory organs.
elastin An extracellular connective tissue protein.
endocrine glands The structures that secrete hormones.
lower respiratory tract Consists of the bronchi, bronchioles, lower trachea, alveoli, and lungs.

pharmacodynamic interactions Differences in effects produced by a given plasma level of a drug.
pharmacokinetic interactions Differences in the plasma levels of a drug achieved with a given dose of that drug.
upper respiratory tract Consists of the nose and nasal cavities, pharynx, larynx, and upper trachea.

OVERVIEW

The phenomenon of aging is unavoidable because aging is a universal process. The difference between aging and disease is that the aging process is intrinsic and depends on genetic factors, whereas disease is intrinsic and extrinsic, depending on both genetic and environmental factors. Aging is always progressive, whereas disease may be discontinuous and may progress, regress, or be arrested entirely. Aging is irreversible, whereas disease may be treatable and often has a known cause. The average life expectancy in the United States, according to the Centers for Disease Control and Prevention, has risen from about 45 years in 1900 to 77 years in 2001. This increase is largely attributed to improvements in sanitation, food, and water supplies and to the advent of antibiotics and vaccinations. Most age-related biological functions peak before age 30; some show a subsequent gradual linear decline, having no practical implications for daily activity, but becoming critical in periods of great stress. Thus, disease, rather than normal aging, is the prime determinant of functional loss in old age.

AGING PATIENTS

The impact of age on medical care is substantial, and, thus, a significantly altered approach to treatment is needed for the older patient. As individuals age, they are more likely to be affected by many chronic disorders and disabilities. Consequently, they use more drugs than any other age group. Combined with a decrease in physiological reserve, these added burdens (if present) make the older person more vulnerable to environmental, pathological, or pharmacological illnesses. Understanding these facts is essential for optimal care of older patients. Aging alters pharmacodynamics and pharmacokinetics, affecting the choice, dose, and rate of administration of many drugs. In addition, pharmacotherapy may be complicated by an elderly patient's inability to purchase or obtain drugs or to comply with drug regimens.

In the United States about two thirds of persons older than 65 years of age take prescription and nonprescription (over-the-counter) drugs. Women take more drugs than men because they are, on average, older and because they use more psychoactive and antiarthritic drugs. The type of drug used most often by elderly persons varies with the setting. Community dwellers use analgesics, diuretics, cardiovascular drugs, and sedatives most often; nursing home residents use antipsychotics and sedative-hypnotics most commonly, followed by diuretics, antihypertensives, analgesics, cardiac drugs, and antibiotics.

Many drugs benefit elderly persons. Some can save lives, such as antibiotics and thrombolytic therapy in acute illness. Oral hypoglycemic drugs can improve independence and quality of life, while controlling chronic disease. Antihypertensive drugs and influenza vaccines can help prevent or decrease morbidity. Analgesics and antidepressants can control debilitating symptoms. Therefore, the appropriateness of the potential benefits in outweighing the potential risks should guide therapy. The health problems and medical management of elderly patients differs from those of younger ones in important ways, which explains the development of training in geriatrics as a medical specialty. Prescribing medications for elderly patients is always a challenge for physicians. Body functions decline dramatically in elderly patients. Safe, effective pharmacotherapy remains one of the greatest challenges in the practice of clinical geriatrics. Therefore, the normal aging process can lead to altered drug effects and the need for altered doses.

Physiological Aging

Not all functions in the human body show age-related changes. For example, the hematocrit value does not change with age. For some substances a balanced decline in both production and breakdown is seen; this seems to be true for testosterone and perhaps also for cortisol, thyroxine, aldosterone, and insulin. Age-related changes vary greatly, and a severe change in one organ does not mean severe changes in other organs.

It is extremely difficult to differentiate among primary age changes (physiological), secondary age changes (pathophysiological), and tertiary age changes (sociogenic and behavioral). Age-related changes may be responsible for the atypical presentation of diseases in elderly persons, which can be observed in hyperthyroidism, depression, uncontrolled diabetes mellitus, and rheumatoid arthritis. Although aging changes may lessen the severity of some diseases, they may also be responsible for more severe presentations. For example, normal human aging is associated with a progressive reduction in dopamine concentrations in the brain, which may influence the onset or severity of Parkinson's disease. Menopause clearly is related to an increase in osteoporosis and atherosclerosis. Arteriosclerosis accounts for the age-related increase in diastolic blood pressure, a major risk factor for cerebrovascular disease (stroke).

The Physiopathology of Aging

Many of the physiological changes associated with aging can be slowed to some extent with a healthy diet and a consistent regimen of moderate exercise. Many of the chronic diseases prevalent in elderly persons are either preventable or modifiable with healthy lifestyle habits. Reduction of dietary fat (especially saturated fats and cholesterol) lowers the risk of coronary artery disease and stroke as well as breast and colon cancer. It is clear that our health and well-being depend on the degree to which our organ systems can successfully work together to maintain homeostasis (internal stability) in the body. Diminished function in one organ system is lessened by appropriate compensatory mechanisms in other systems. The aging process affects all body systems physiologically.

The Immune System

The immune system includes all of the structures and processes that mount a defense against foreign agents such as microorganisms, pollens, toxins, and cancer cells. The immune system produces immunity, which involves many cells (see Table 32-1). Most cell-mediated and humoral immune responses decline with age. Aging has a pronounced effect on the thymus gland (located in the chest; it is one of the central pacemakers of the immune system). Over a person's life span, the weight of the thymus decreases. By age 50, the first functional impairments of thymic involution can be detected. The thymus is a very important site for the differentiation of stem cells into T lymphocytes, which mediate cellular immunity. As the thymic output of T cells diminishes, the differentiation of T cells occurs increasingly in the peripheral lymphoid structures, notably the spleen and the lymph nodes.

With humoral immunity, the B lymphocytes first recognize a foreign substance and then differentiate into plasma cells. Although no age-related change in the number of circulating B cells has been documented, they no longer function and respond normally in elderly persons. See Chapter 28 for more information on the immune system.

The Cardiovascular System

The cardiovascular system consists of the heart and blood vessels (arteries, veins, and capillaries). With advancing age, heart weight increases significantly. In the myocardium (the heart muscle), fat, **collagen**, and **elastin** increase. Arterial compliance in the internal and external carotid pathways

TABLE 32-1. White Blood Cells Involved in Immunity	
CELL TYPE	**FUNCTION**
Neutrophils	Phagocytosis
Basophils	Secrete histamine and heparin
Eosinophils	Destroy parasites
Monocytes	Phagocytosis; enter tissue and are transformed into macrophages
Lymphocytes	
1. B cells	Antibody-mediated immunity (30% of blood lymphocytes)
Plasma cells	Secrete antibodies
Memory B cells	Remember the antigens
2. T cells	Cell-mediated immunity (accounts for 70% of blood lymphocytes)
Killer T cells	Kill cells
Helper T cells	Secrete substances (lymphokines which activate B cells)
Suppressor T cells	Inhibit B cell and T cell activity (help control immune response)
Memory T cells	Remember the antigens
3. Natural killer cells	Kill cells

significantly decreases between the ages of 5 and 50 years, but the decreases then reach a plateau. Fibrous plaques are present in 30% of hearts at age 15 to 24 years; within another decade of life, 85% of hearts have these plaques. More than 60% of hearts at ages 55 to 64 years show vascular calcification. Narrowing heart vessels are also more prevalent with age. By ages 55 to 64, half of all hearts have greater than 50% occlusion in at least one of the three major coronary arteries. See Chapter 24 for more information on the cardiovascular system.

The Urinary System

The urinary system produces urine, temporarily stores it, and finally eliminates it from the body. The major organs of the urinary system include two kidneys, two ureters, one urinary bladder, and one urethra. Age-associated kidney changes can be categorized as anatomic or functional. Anatomic changes include loss of glomeruli, decreased kidney size, renal tubular changes, and renal vascular changes. Anatomic changes involving the lower urinary tract make men more susceptible to prostatic hypertrophy. Women become prone to pelvic relaxation, urinary incontinence, urinary tract infections, and the development of uterine and cervical cancers. Renal function declines progressively starting in the fifth decade, so that by age 70 normal renal function may be 40% less than that at age 30. Glomerular filtration rate declines by about 1 mL/min per year. Even in the absence of cardiovascular, renal, or acute illness, the decline is more rapid in men than in women. Renal blood flow and plasma flow also decrease with age. See Chapter 24 for more information on the urinary system.

The Endocrine System

The endocrine system is composed of endocrine glands, which are widely distributed throughout the body. **Endocrine glands** secrete chemical substances called hormones.

Specific age-related disturbances in extrahepatic hormonal regulatory mechanisms have been proposed. The reduced availability of hormones results in diminished endocrine regulatory mechanisms, deficiencies in hormonal feedback mechanisms, and decreased binding affinities and receptors. Altered pancreatic and adrenal hormone concentrations decrease glucose tolerance with age. Insulin release is impaired in some older individuals, whereas others have fewer insulin receptors or exhibit postreceptor abnormalities. The peripheral glucose disposal rate is significantly lower in older than in younger persons. Production of sex hormones also decreases with age. In postmenopausal women, reduced estrogen concentrations have been linked to increased incidence of osteoporosis and cardiovascular disease. See Chapter 26 for more information on the endocrine system.

The Respiratory System

The respiratory system contains the upper and lower respiratory tracts. The **upper respiratory tract** contains the respiratory organs located outside the chest cavity: the nose and nasal cavities, pharynx, and upper trachea. The **lower respiratory tract** consists of organs located in the chest cavity: larynx, the lower trachea, bronchi, bronchioles, alveoli, and lungs. The lower parts of the bronchi, bronchioles, and alveoli are located in the lungs. The pleural membranes and the muscles that form the chest cavity are also part of the lower respiratory tract.

Changes in the respiratory system with age have been reviewed. The diameters of the trachea and central airways increase, enlarging anatomic dead space. The volume of the alveolar ducts increases, whereas the membranous bronchioles narrow. Lung weight loss exceeds 20%, and chest wall compliance also decreases. These and other changes result in less elastic recoil in the lungs, increased closing volume, and decreased maximal expiratory flow.

Thus, elderly persons have an increased risk for respiratory failure. Aspiration or inhalation of foreign material into the tracheobronchial tree can produce major respiratory illness, which is more likely to occur in older than in younger people. Finally, asthma in elderly persons must be differentiated from other causes of airflow obstruction, such as acute bronchitis or congestive heart failure. See Chapter 22 for more information on the respiratory system.

The Gastrointestinal System

The digestive tract and the accessory organs of digestion make up the digestive system. The digestive tract is a hollow tube extending from the mouth to the anus. It is also called the **alimentary canal**. The structures of the digestive tract include the mouth, pharynx, esophagus, stomach, small intestine, large intestine, rectum, and anus.

Accessory organs include the salivary glands, teeth, liver, gallbladder, and pancreas. The secretions from the salivary glands empty into the mouth, whereas secretions from the liver, gallbladder, and pancreas empty into the small intestine.

Age-associated changes in the gastrointestinal system have been reviewed. The gastrointestinal system starts with the oral cavity, where age-related changes reflect perturbations in oral health resulting from poor hygiene, disease, or disease treatment, rather than from dysfunction directly related to age. Nevertheless, oral disorders are common among elderly persons. As many as 50% of older people experience traumatic lesions of the oral cavity, which may be ulcerative, atrophic, or hyperplastic. These changes make the oral mucosa more susceptible to disease, a problem that can be exacerbated by corticosteroids, antibiotics, cytotoxic agents, and immunosuppressive therapy. Elderly persons may have an increased risk of local adverse drug reactions such as fixed eruptions (round or oval patches of reddened blisters on the skin), swelling, glossitis (inflammation of the tongue), and stomatitis (inflammation of the mouth). About

80% of people older than 50 years of age have gastric muscular atrophy and thinning of the gastric mucosa.

Gastric secretion declines with age. Gastric cell function decreases and gastric pH rises. Gastric emptying is about 2.5 times faster in younger than in older persons, perhaps because it is under the control of the central nervous system, which may lose efficiency with advancing age. Slowing of gastric emptying also follows a reduction in gastric acid secretion. Gastric emptying is reduced by stress, lack of ambulation, gastric ulcer, intestinal obstruction, myocardial infarction, and diabetes mellitus. Emptying is delayed by fatty meals in elderly persons more so than in younger people. Bleeding is a fairly common complication of ulcers in elderly persons. The normal aging process leads to a reduction in vitamin D absorption and a profound decline in the intestinal absorption of calcium. There is little existing evidence that the motility of the small intestine is altered by the aging process. Constipation is common because of alterations of motility in the large intestine.

The liver is the organ least affected by primary age changes. It continues to function in those persons not affected by disease. In general, just a small part can perform the tasks of the entire liver. Liver weight correlates with body weight, and both decrease starting in the fifth or sixth decade.

Primary aging may be responsible for decreased hepatic blood flow, which is equal to approximately 25% of the cardiac output or 30% of the total circulating blood. Decreased hepatic blood flow probably affects the metabolic clearance of certain drugs. These functional changes are thought to be most relevant with drugs that have a high first-pass extraction ratio. Clearance is limited by the capacity of the organ, and hepatic clearance cannot exceed hepatic blood flow, which is approximately 1.5 L/min. Thus, reduced blood flow can alter drug action in elderly patients. For at least some drugs, hepatic metabolism in elderly persons apparently is altered. See Chapter 25 for more information on the gastrointestinal system.

The Nervous System

The structures of the nervous system are divided into two parts: the central nervous system and the peripheral nervous system. The central nervous system (CNS) includes the brain and the spinal cord. The CNS is located in the dorsal cavity. The brain is located in the cranium; the spinal cord is enclosed in the spinal cavity. The peripheral nervous system is located outside the CNS and consists of the nerves that connect the CNS with the rest of the body.

With age, cellular brain mass and cerebral blood flow decrease. Sensory conduction takes longer, and the blood-brain barrier may become more permeable. These changes may decrease coordination, prolong reaction time, and impair short-term memory. Manifestations include more falls (particularly among elderly women), urinary incontinence, and confusion. The homeostatic response (balance of the internal body systems) also declines.

In short, the brain shrinks with advancing age and loses nerve cells. The brain weighs 10% less at 70 years of age and older than it weighs at age 30. Various areas of the brain lose 10% to 50% of their nerve cells, although the nerve cells that control eye movement are not affected. The greatest loss of cells appears to take place in the temporal area, but the functional effect is surprisingly small. Cerebral blood flow is controlled by autoregulation, metabolic regulation, and chemical factors. Its regulation is influenced by the disease processes prevailing in old age, such as dementia, atherosclerosis, diabetes mellitus, stroke, and hypertension.

Short-term memory is significantly affected by aging, a loss that can be minimized by teaching methods of memorization to older adults. The declines in both learning facility and information retrieval and perhaps also the loss in processing speed appear to contribute to failing short-term memory.

Serotonin (a neurotransmitter) is widely distributed throughout the CNS. It is implicated in a variety of neural functions, such as pain, feeding, sleep, sexual behavior, cardiac regulation, and cognition. Changes in the serotonin system occur in association with healthy aging. See Chapter 23 for more information on the nervous system.

The Integumentary System

The integumentary system consists of three major layers (epidermis, dermis, and subcutaneous) and accessory structures such as hair, nails, sebaceous (oil) glands, and sweat glands. Cells in the epidermis, which contain melanocytes (that produce the melanin pigment), must be continuously replaced with new cells that divide, by mitosis, in the lower layers. The rate of production of these new cells decreases by 30% to 50% between ages 20 and 70. It is clear that during long periods of time, individual epidermal cells are exposed to carcinogens (cancer-causing agents), such as ultraviolet light, from the sun. Furthermore, the number of melanocytes and the amount of protective melanin pigment decrease with age, making ultraviolet light more dangerous.

The **dermis** is a thick layer of loose connective tissue that is well supplied with blood vessels, lymphatic vessels, nerves, and accessory organs. The predominant cells found in the dermis are fibroblasts, mast cells, and macrophages. Fibroblasts produce and release collagen and elastin into the extracellular matrix, which give skin its strength and elasticity, respectively.

The amount of collagen and elastin in the dermis decreases as people age, accounting for the thinning and wrinkling of the skin in elderly persons. Loss of collagen makes the skin more susceptible to wear and tear, whereas loss of elastin causes skin to lose its resiliency over time.

Perhaps the most striking age-related changes in the integumentary system are the graying, thinning, and loss of hair. Hair color depends on varying amounts of melanin pigment within specialized cells. Physiological changes may affect many organs or systems such as the nervous system, body composition (decrease of lean body mass, skeletal mass, and total body water), ears (loss of high-frequency hearing), endocrine system (menopause and decrease of testosterone), growth hormone secretion, increased incidence of diabetes, bone mineral loss, and increase secretion of antidiuretic hormone in response to osmolar stimuli. The physiological changes can also affect the eyes, gastrointestinal tract, heart, immune system, joints, sense of smell, and kidneys. Many of the physiological changes in body systems are summarized in Table 32-2.

PRINCIPLES OF DRUG THERAPY IN ELDERLY PATIENTS

The principal clinical concerns of drug therapy include efficacy and safety, dosage, complexity of regimen, number of drugs, cost, and patient compliance. There are several reasons for the greater incidence of adverse reactions to drugs in the elderly population. Drug metabolism is often impaired in this group because of a decrease in the glomerular filtration rate and reduced hepatic clearance. The reduction in hepatic clearance is due to decreased activity of microsomal enzymes and reduced hepatic perfusion with aging. The distribution of drugs is also affected. Because elderly persons have a decrease in total body water content and a relative increase in body fat, water-soluble drugs become more concentrated and fat-soluble drugs have longer half-lives. In addition, serum albumin levels decrease, especially in sick patients, so that protein binding of some drugs (e.g., warfarin and phenytoin) is reduced, leaving more free (active) drugs available. In addition, older individuals often have altered responses to a given serum drug level. Thus, they are more sensitive to some drugs (e.g., opioids), and less sensitive to others (e.g., β-blocking agents). Finally, the older patient with multiple chronic conditions is likely to be receiving many drugs, including nonprescribed agents. Thus, adverse drug reactions and dosage errors are more likely to occur, especially if the patient has visual, hearing, or memory deficits. Drug doses in elderly patients must often be reduced, although dose requirements may vary considerably from person to person. In general, starting doses of about one third to one half the usual adult dose are indicated for drugs with a low therapeutic index.

COMMON DISORDERS IN THE ELDERLY

Some disorders occur almost exclusively in elderly persons, and some occur in persons of all ages, but are far more common in elderly persons than in other age groups. For example, multiple disorders, accidental hypothermia, and urinary incontinence are almost exclusively found in elderly persons. Some other examples include lymphoma, chronic

TABLE 32-2.   Summary of Age-Related Decline of Body Systems

BODY SYSTEM	AGE-RELATED EFFECTS	BODY SYSTEM	AGE-RELATED EFFECTS
Immune System		**Respiratory System**	
Thymus gland	Decreases in weight	Trachea	Increases in size allowing more dead space
	Diminished output of T cells	Alveolar ducts	Increase in volume
B cells	No longer respond optimally	Bronchioles	Narrow
		Lungs	Decrease in weight
The Cardiovascular System			Chest compliance decreases
Heart	Weight increases		Less elastic recoil
	Fat, collagen, and elastin in the myocardium increase		Increase in closing volume
Arteries	Build up of plaques cause narrowing and calcification		Decreased maximal expiratory flow
		Gastrointestinal System	
The Urinary System		Oral cavity	Tooth decay
Kidneys	Loss of glomeruli		Oral lesions
	Decreased size	Stomach	Thinning of gastric mucosa
	Renal tubular changes		Decreased gastric secretions
	Renal vascular changes		Increased pH
	Decline in renal function		Slower gastric emptying
	Decline in glomerular filtration		Declined absorption of some vitamins and minerals
Bladder	Prostatic hypertrophy in men	Large intestine	Alterations in motility
	Urinary incontinence in women	**Nervous System**	
Urethra	Urinary tract infections in women	Brain	Cerebral mass decreases
	Uterine and cervical cancers in women		Cerebral blood flow decreases
			Sensory conduction takes longer
Endocrine System			Blood-brain barrier becomes more permeable
Hormones	Diminished endocrine regulatory mechanisms		Declines in short term memory
	Deficiencies in hormone feedback mechanisms	**Integumentary System**	Decreased production of new skin cells
	Decreased binding affinities and receptors		Prolonged exposure to carcinogens increases cancer risk
	Decreased glucose tolerance		Decrease in the amount of collagen and elastin in the dermis
	Decrease in production of sex hormones		Graying, thinning, and loss of hair

lymphocytic leukemia, prostate cancer, degenerative osteoarthritis, dementia, falls, hip fracture, osteoporosis, parkinsonism, hypertension, heart failure, stroke, and herpes zoster. These disorders are available for study and review in many medical textbooks. In this chapter, the most common disorders in elderly persons will be discussed selectively.

Multiple Disorders

Normal and abnormal effects of the aging process on different systems of the body in elderly persons may cause multiple disorders after middle age. A patient may suffer from several disorders, such as peptic ulcer, hypertension, and diabetes mellitus. Therefore, some patients are receiving several different medications that may cause drug interactions and side effects.

Cardiovascular Disorders

The incidence and prevalence of most cardiovascular disorders increase markedly with advancing age. Significant fat accumulations and calcifications in the blood vessels of the heart (coronary arteries), brain, or peripheral arterial system are found in the majority of men and women older than 70 years of age. The combined effects of the pathological and physiological changes contribute to a high prevalence of problems, such as heart failure and cardiac arrhythmias in elderly patients. Often, the prognosis for elderly patients is worse than that for their younger counterparts. For example, early mortality rates after acute myocardial infarction are more than four times greater in the older than 70 age group than in the younger than 60 age group. However, this situation can create a greater opportunity to use specific drugs for their beneficial effects. Furthermore, there is good evidence that risk factors such as hypertension and hyperlipidemia can be successfully modified in older people, reducing the risk of ischemic vascular events. Multiple disorders are common in old age and coexistent diseases often can influence the choice of drugs for a cardiovascular condition. In addition, both pharmacokinetic and pharmacodynamic drug profiles may be altered in older subjects. These can influence both choice of drug and dosing regimen.

Ischemic Heart Disease

Aging is associated with a progressive increase in morbidity and mortality due to ischemic heart disease, which is the most common cause of death in elderly people in the United States. The three main groups of drugs used to treat angina pectoris are β-adrenergic receptor blocking agents, calcium channel blockers, and nitrates, which are discussed in Chapter 24.

Acute Myocardial Infarction

Acute myocardial infarction (AMI) is painless in approximately 50% of persons older than 70 years of age. The mortality from AMI is greater in older subjects than in young and middle-aged subjects. This is due to a number of factors including increased severity of underlying coronary artery disease, a greater prevalence of previous myocardial infarction, and an associated increase in the incidence of cardiac failure. The aims of treatment are to relieve symptoms, reduce mortality, and prevent late cardiovascular disability. Pain relief is usually attempted by the use of intravenous opiates such as diamorphine. Intravenous nitrates are sometimes used to reduce opiate requirements and may also be helpful in the treatment of associated cardiac failure; however, adverse effects including hypotension and bradycardia are more common in elderly subjects. When used in elderly persons, the dosage should be reduced.

Aspirin has been shown to significantly reduce mortality, reinfarction, and stroke rate after AMI in older patients. Treatment with the combination of thrombolytic agents and oral aspirin confers additional benefits.

Cardiac Failure

The incidence and prevalence of cardiac failure increase sharply with increasing age. At post mortem examination of elderly persons, the most common underlying pathologic conditions are ischemia and hypertensive heart disease. The appropriate treatment of cardiac failure depends on accurate diagnosis including the underlying cardiac pathological conditions. Treatments for cardiac failure are discussed in Chapter 24.

Hypertension

The major causes of death and morbidity associated with hypertension are myocardial infarction and stroke. In addition, congestive heart failure is more common in elderly hypertensive patients than in their younger counterparts. Blood pressure rises with age up to about 75 years. Hypertension is perhaps best defined as the blood pressure level at which treatment is likely to confer benefits.

The best choice of antihypertensive treatment for elderly patients remains highly controversial. Drugs that are effective in younger patients also will lower blood pressure in elderly patients. In the absence of specific contraindications, different agents seem to be tolerated equally well in elderly patients; approximately 10% to 15% develop adverse reactions requiring a change of drug. Treatment of hypertension is discussed in Chapter 24.

Cerebrovascular Disease

Stroke continues to be a significant public health problem in the United States. It is estimated that every minute, one person in the United States suffers a stroke, making it the third leading cause of death, and the major cause of long-term disability in adults. Because two thirds of all patients affected by stroke are older than age 65, this disease mostly affects the elderly population.

The most significant unmodifiable risk factor for stroke is advanced age. The risk for stroke in African-Americans is greater than 60% higher than that in whites, even after controlling for the effects of age, hypertension, and diabetes. Cigarette smoking and excessive alcohol consumption are important independent risk factors for stroke. Hypertension is by far the most important modifiable risk factor. It is a contributing factor in more than 70% of strokes, and lowering diastolic blood pressure by 6 mm Hg reduces stroke risk by 40%.

General therapeutic measures for stroke patients include maintaining an open airway, hydration with intravenous fluids, and judicious treatment of hypertension and hypoglycemia.

Cancer

The management of cancer with aging is an increasingly common problem as the number of elderly patients with cancer grows. Elderly persons comprise approximately 12% of the U.S. population, and the number of elderly people (those aged 65 years or older) is projected to reach almost 40 million by 2010. After heart disease, cancer is the second leading cause of death in the United States.

Malignant tumor incidence increases progressively with age, although the increase is not uniform for each type of cancer. The reason for the increased incidence of cancer with age is not fully understood. The duration of carcinogenesis (agents that cause cancers), and the prolonged exposure to chemical, physical, or biological carcinogens may explain the association.

Cancer in older persons should be considered differently because of the physiological effects of aging. There are two important pharmacokinetic factors that occur with aging: a change in the volume of distribution and a decrease in the concentration of serum albumin. Treatment of different types of cancers is discussed in Chapter 21.

Arthritis

Arthritis is the most common chronic ailment in elderly persons. More than 50% of persons aged 70 years or older report having arthritis. Physical limitations resulting from arthritis occur in approximately 12% of elderly people. After age 65, the prevalence is approximately 50%, and it increases every decade thereafter.

The two most common forms of arthritis in elderly persons are rheumatoid arthritis (RA) and osteoarthritis (OA).

Rheumatoid Arthritis

The clinical manifestations of RA in elderly people may differ from those in the typical younger adult patient with this disease. The abrupt appearance of symptoms is more common in elderly-onset disease, whereas bone erosions and nodules are less common. A multidisciplinary treatment approach is required for elderly patients with RA. It includes physical therapy, occupational therapy, pharmacotherapy, and, occasionally, surgical intervention. The goals of therapy for elderly patients are the same as those for younger patients: to relieve symptoms, reduce inflammation, avoid joint destruction, prevent deformities, maintain functional capacity, and preserve quality of life. The pharmacotherapy of RA is similar in young and old patients. Age alone does not contraindicate the use of the first- or second-line antirheumatic drugs (see Chapter 27). The adverse effects of some drugs are more pronounced in elderly patients. Nonsteroidal anti-inflammatory drugs (NSAIDs), including aspirin and nonacetylated salicylates, are useful in treating arthritic symptoms in elderly subjects. Drug therapy must be monitored vigilantly in elderly patients because of the increased risk of complications. Anti-inflammatory complications of NSAIDs in elderly patients include cardiovascular (congestive heart failure and hypertension), central nervous system (confusion, dizziness, headaches, and hearing loss), gastrointestinal (gastritis, ulcers, and epigastric pain), and renal (electrolyte imbalances, fluid retention, and renal insufficiency).

Osteoarthritis

The other common type of arthritis is OA, which is characterized by degeneration of cartilage, bone remodeling, and overgrowth of bone. This form of arthritis, also referred to as degenerative joint disease, is the most common form in elderly people. Approximately 10% of the population older than age 60 have symptoms related to OA. Radiographic evidence of OA is present in approximately 80% of those older than age 65, yet many are asymptomatic. Pain is the primary complaint of patients with OA. Pain can be absent despite severe joint damage. Joint stiffness, pain at night, pain at rest, and crepitus (a feeling of crackling as the joint is moved) also are common symptoms. Commonly affected joints include the interphalangeal joints of the hands, knees, and hips, the first metatarsophalangeal joint, and the lumbar and cervical spine.

The primary goals in treatment of OA are to minimize joint pain, maintain functional mobility, and allow use of the affected joints. A combination of pharmacotherapy and non-pharmacological therapeutic interventions is often necessary. Resting the joints sometimes relieves pain. Joint replacement may be the treatment of choice in patients with severe OA that cannot be adequately managed with other modalities. For more information on pharmacotherapy, refer to Chapter 27.

Osteoporosis

Osteoporosis is a metabolic bone disorder in which the rate of bone reabsorption accelerates while the rate of bone formation slows down, causing a loss of bone mass. Bones affected by this disease lose calcium and phosphate salts and thus become porous, brittle, and abnormally vulnerable to fractures. Osteoporosis may be primary or secondary to an underlying disease. Primary osteoporosis is often called postmenopausal osteoporosis because it develops more commonly in postmenopausal women. Osteoporosis is usually discovered when an elderly person bends to lift something, hears a snapping sound, then feels a sudden pain in the lower back. Osteoporosis can develop insidiously with increasing deformity, kyphosis, and loss of height. As bones weaken, spontaneous wedge fractures, pathological fractures of the neck or femur and hip, become increasingly common. Osteoporosis, often affecting older people, is a major risk factor for vertebral compression fractures and hip fractures.

The aims of treatment are to prevent additional fractures and control pain. A physical therapy program, emphasizing gentle exercise and activity, is an important part of the treatment. Hormone replacement therapy (HRT) with estrogen and progesterone may retard bone loss and prevent the occurrence of fractures. HRT decreases bone reabsorption and increases bone mass. Other medications may include alendronate (Fosamax®) and calcitonin; however, adequate calcium and vitamin D intakes are needed for maximum effect. Drug therapy merely arrests osteoporosis; it does not cure it. Surgery can correct pathological fractures.

Ophthalmic Disorders

One of the consequences of aging is a gradual impairment of vision. Like other tissues and organs in the body, the eye is constantly undergoing change, both physical and functional. Changes may be a consequence of the aging process, diet, environment, or disease. Conditions that are commonly associated with age-related deterioration of ocular function include a reduction in precorneal tear production, changes affecting the clarity and flexibility of the crystalline lens, an elevation in intraocular pressure, and changes in vessels supplying blood to regions in the eye.

Dry Eye Syndrome

Dry eye syndrome (xerosis) in elderly persons may be caused by a number of conditions, including trachoma, vitamin A deficiency, chemical burn, radiation, and chemotherapy. Dry eye is a common disorder affecting the elderly population, especially individuals older than 40 years of age. In elderly persons, a thinned conjunctiva and diminished corneal sensation add to the problem of dry eyes.

The primary treatment for dry eyes is replacement of deficient tear production with artificial tear preparations. Sterile isotonic saline preparations have been used to replace aqueous tear deficiencies, but the duration of relief is extremely short, requiring frequent dosing. Relief can be prolonged by the addition of water-soluble polymers, which increase the viscosity of the solution and provide an aqueous film over the corneal surface for an extended period.

The Crystalline Lens

As one ages, the crystalline lens progressively loses elasticity, and its ability to change its curvature and modify its focal length decrease, thus reducing its capacity to accommodate close vision. In addition, the transparency of the lens decreases with development of opacities that reduce light transmission and clarity of visual images.

Presbyopia

In the normal resting state, the eye can focus on an image of a distant object. However, to focus on a near object, the refractive power of the lens must increase. This is accomplished by contraction of the ciliary muscles, which causes the lens to become more spherical. This process is referred to as *accommodation*. The closest distance that the eye is able to accommodate (near point) is extremely short in infancy, and it progressively increases with age. When a person reaches the mid-40s, presbyopia, a condition in which the near point of accommodation moves beyond a comfortable reading distance, gradually develops. Presbyopia is presently treated using corrective eyeglasses. Bifocal or trifocal contact lenses are also available, but they have had limited acceptance.

Cataract

A cataract is defined as any opacity or loss in transparency in the crystalline lens of the eye. When a cataract interferes with transmission of light to the retina, some loss in visual acuity and possibly complete loss of vision may result. Cataracts are a leading cause of blindness and visual impairment worldwide.

Cataracts may be congenital or acquired (secondary). Most cataracts have no known etiology, and they usually occur in individuals younger than 50 years of age. There is significant correlation between age and the occurrence of lens opacities, which are found to some degree in more than 80% of persons older than 60.

At present, no medical treatment will restore an opaque lens to its transparent state. Surgery remains the only effective method of treatment.

Glaucoma

Glaucoma includes a group of ocular diseases that are characterized by increased intraocular pressure, which may produce compression of the optic disk, resulting in damage to the optic nerve that leads to loss of the peripheral visual field and visual acuity.

Glaucoma is the second leading cause of blindness in the world. It is estimated that 67 million people worldwide have primary glaucoma. It is also a common cause of blindness in the United States.

The treatment of glaucoma centers on reduction of elevated intraocular pressure. Currently, this is accomplished with medical, laser, or surgical treatment.

■ DRUG INTERACTIONS

A drug interaction occurs whenever the pharmacological action of a drug is altered by a second substance. This change may be related to **pharmacokinetic interactions** (differences in the plasma levels of a drug achieved with a given dose of that drug) and **pharmacodynamic interactions** (differences in effects produced by a given plasma level of a drug). The duration and intensity of the action of a drug are a function of the plasma level of the drug, which is related directly to the absorption, distribution, metabolism, and excretion of that drug. These rates may be altered by previous drug therapy, dietary factors, and exposure to environmental chemicals (chemicals not used for therapeutic purposes). Physical factors such as ambient temperature and effects of disease (e.g., fever) may also have an impact.

Pharmacodynamics

Drug action is defined as physiological changes in the body caused by a drug or responses to the pharmacological effects of a drug. Pharmacodynamics refers to the chemical reaction of drugs in the body. This can be different in elderly persons because of physiological changes that occur with aging. Drugs can modify the way the body acts, but they do not give body organs and tissues a new function. They usually either slow down or speed up ordinary cell processes.

The most common way in which drugs display their action is by forming a chemical bond with specific receptors within the body. This binding may occur if the drug and its receptors have a compatible chemical shape. Figure 32-1 illustrates a drug-receptor interaction.

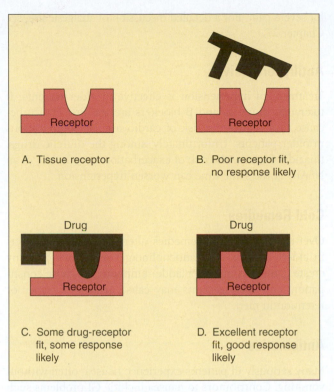

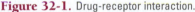

Figure 32-1. Drug-receptor interaction.

The effects of similar concentrations of drugs at the site of action may be greater or lesser in elderly than in younger persons. The difference may be due to changes in drug-receptor interactions. The increased sensitivity that occurs with aging must be considered when drugs that can have serious adverse effects are used. These drugs include morphine, pentazocine, warfarin, angiotensin-converting enzyme inhibitors, diazepam (especially when given parenterally), and levodopa. Some drugs whose effects are reduced with aging (e.g., tolbutamide, glyburide, and β-blockers) should also be used with caution because serious dose-related toxicity can still occur, and signs of toxicity may be delayed.

Drug Absorption

Physiological changes with aging, such as changes in gastric pH, slowed gastric emptying rate, reduced cardiac output (blood flow), reductions of absorptive surfaces, and slowed gastrointestinal (GI) tract motility, are factors that affect not only drug absorption but also drug distribution and metabolism. Different diseases and conditions of the GI tract are also obvious factors that affect drug absorption. Examples are peptic ulcer, diarrhea, constipation, and others.

Drug Distribution

Alterations in drug distribution in elderly patients depend on many factors, such as a reduction in total body water content, decreased plasma albumin concentration, reduced lean body mass, and increased body fat. Many drugs, especially acidic ones, bind to plasma proteins. Drugs can compete for plasma protein-binding sites. Plasma protein-binding sites are especially significant when a high percentage of the drug (more than 90%) is normally protein bound, as with coumarin anticoagulants, sulfonamides, salicylates, indomethacin, and most other nonsteroidal anti-inflammatory agents. Lipid-soluble drugs such as lidocaine and diazepam have a large volume of distribution in elderly persons, whereas water-soluble drugs such as ethanol and acetaminophen have a smaller volume of distribution. Digoxin also has a lower volume of distribution in elderly persons, and, therefore, doses must be reduced.

Drug Metabolism

The most common and most important cause for differences in plasma levels of a drug is a change in the rate of biotransformation of the drug. Variations in a person's plasma drug levels are more common with drugs that undergo extensive GI metabolism or first-pass hepatic metabolism. The total liver blood flow declines 40% to 45% with aging because of a reduction in cardiac output. Therefore, if severe and progressive liver damage is present in an elderly person, drug metabolism would be affected. Otherwise, the decline in the ability of elderly persons to metabolize most drugs is relatively small and difficult to predict. In older persons, presystemic (first-pass) metabolism of some drugs given orally is decreased and their serum concentration and bioavailability are increased. Examples of these drugs include labetalol, propranolol, and verapamil. Consequently, initial doses of these drugs should be reduced by about 30%. However, presystemic metabolism of other metabolized drugs such as imipramine, amitriptyline, morphine, and meperidine is not decreased. The effects of cigarette smoking, diet, and alcohol consumption may be more important than the physiological changes in the liver.

Drug Elimination

Drugs may be eliminated from the body by many routes, including urine, feces (e.g., unabsorbed drugs or those secreted in bile), saliva, sweat, tears, breast milk, and lungs (e.g., alcohols and anesthetics). Any route may be important for a given drug, but the kidney is the most important route for the elimination of the majority of drugs. Some drugs are excreted unchanged in the urine, whereas other drugs are so extensively metabolized that only a small fraction of the original chemical substance is excreted unchanged. Different responses to drug therapy may be seen in elderly individuals because of a decline in hepatic and renal function, which is often accompanied by a concurrent disease process. The rate of elimination of any drug by the kidney is reduced in elderly persons. Renal blood flow, mainly in the renal cortex, decreases significantly with aging. This physiological change causes a decrease in renal drug elimination.

Because renal function is dynamic, maintenance doses of drugs should be adjusted when a patient becomes acutely ill or dehydrated or has recently recovered from dehydration. In addition, because renal function continues to decline, the dose of drugs given long-term should be reviewed periodically. Examples of these drugs are aminoglycosides, chlorpropamide, digoxin, and lithium carbonate. To prevent drug toxicity, renal function must be estimated, and the dosage of the drug should be adjusted. Most elderly patients do not have normal renal function, and the majority require adjustments in the dosages of drugs that are eliminated primarily by the kidneys. See Chapter 24 for more information on drug elimination and the renal system.

SPECIFIC DRUG CONSIDERATIONS FOR ELDERLY PATIENTS

Several classes of drugs that are commonly prescribed for elderly persons should be given specific consideration. These include anticoagulants, glaucoma medications, analgesics, antihypertensives, cold remedies, antiemetics, and benzodiazepines.

Anticoagulants

Many elderly patients with atrial fibrillation are not given anticoagulants because physicians fear injuries and secondary bleeding due to falls. Head injuries from falling are usually of greatest concern. Given that anticoagulation can result in an annual absolute reduction in the risk of stroke, the benefits of anticoagulation outweigh the risks of falling in most instances (see Chapter 24).

Glaucoma Medications

Topical β-blockers can cause systemic side effects (bradycardia, asthma, and heart failure) as can oral carbonic anhydrase inhibitors. The latter may produce malaise, anorexia, and weight loss (see Chapter 24).

Analgesics

About one half of patients with cancer who are dying have severe pain. Patients perceive pain differently, depending on factors such as fatigue, insomnia, anxiety, depression, and nausea. Addressing these factors together with a supportive environment can help control pain.

The choice of analgesic depends largely on pain intensity, which can be determined only by talking with and observing the patient. All pain can be relieved by an appropriately potent drug at the right dosage, which may also produce sedation or confusion. Commonly used drugs are aspirin, acetaminophen, or NSAIDs for mild pain; codeine or oxycodone for moderate pain; and hydromorphone or morphine for severe pain. For a detailed discussion of analgesic use, see Chapter 27.

Antihypertensives

Treatment of hypertension is effective in older patients. If tolerated, diuretics and β-blockers are the first choice because they reduce the risk of cardiovascular complications in older patients. Unfortunately, among the diuretic drugs, thiazides increase the risk of exacerbation of gout. Use of an NSAID at the same time can worsen hypertension.

Cold Remedies

Over-the-counter cold remedies often cause adverse effects in elderly people. The anticholinergic properties of many create confusion, impair bladder emptying, or cause constipation, and decongestants may cause urinary hesitance or retention in men.

Antiemetics

Many seriously ill patients experience nausea, often without vomiting. Contributors to nausea include GI problems such as constipation and gastritis, metabolic abnormalities such as hypercalcemia and uremia (elevation of urea in blood), drug side effects, and increased intracranial pressure due to brain cancer. Treatment should be guided by the probable etiology, such as discontinuation of NSAIDs and administration of H_2 blockers such as ranitidine (Zantac®), famotidine (Pepcid®), or cimetidine (Tagamet®) in a patient with gastritis. In contrast, a patient with known or suspected brain metastasis may have nausea due to increased intracranial pressure and would best be treated with a course of corticosteroids. Metoclopramide, orally or by injection, is useful for nausea caused by gastric distension. If a reason for mild nausea is not identifiable, nonspecific treatment with phenothiazines such as promethazine or prochlorperazine before meals may be given. Anticholinergic drugs such as scopolamine and the antihistamine meclizine prevent recurrent nausea in many patients. Second-line drugs for intractable nausea include haloperidol and granisetron.

Treatment of Constipation

Constipation is common in elderly people because of inactivity, use of opioid and anticholinergic drugs, and decreased fluid and dietary fiber intake. Laxatives help prevent fecal impaction, especially for those receiving opioids. Laxative drugs are discussed in Chapter 25.

Benzodiazepines

Different benzodiazepines appear to be equally effective in relieving symptoms of anxiety. Selection depends on the drug's pharmacokinetics and pharmacodynamics. Longer-acting benzodiazepines should be avoided because the risk of accumulation and of toxicity is increased, leading to drowsiness, memory impairment, and impaired balance with falls and fractures. Treatment of anxiety or insomnia with these agents should be limited (see Chapter 23).

SUMMARY

Throughout the aging process, individuals are more likely to be affected by many chronic disorders and disabilities. Consequently, elderly persons use more drugs than any other age group. The normal function of each system and organ of the body changes during the aging process.

However, some functions in the human body do not show age-related changes. There are three factors that are associated with the aging process: physiological, pathophysiological, and sociogenic or behavioral. The principles of drug therapy in elderly patients are based on efficacy and safety, dosage, complexity of regimen, number of drugs, cost, and patient compliance. Many disorders and conditions are more common in elderly men or women or both. The most common diseases seen in elderly persons in the United States have been selectively discussed. Several classes of drugs that are commonly prescribed for elderly patients should be given special consideration because of their side effects, drug interactions, and dosages. They include anticoagulants, glaucoma medications, analgesics, antihypertensives, cold remedies, antiemetics, and benzodiazepines.

REVIEW QUESTIONS

1. Which of the following disorders is the most common cause of death in the United States?
   A. Cancer
   B. AIDS
   C. Rheumatoid arthritis
   D. Myocardial infarction

2. The goal of treatment for osteoporosis includes
   A. stopping the aging process.
   B. preventing additional fractures and controlling pain.
   C. preventing surgery for pathologic fractures and controlling pain.
   D. stopping the use of hormone replacement.

3. In postmenopausal women, reduced estrogen blood levels have been linked to increased incidence of which of the following conditions or diseases?
   A. Upper respiratory tract infections
   B. Rheumatoid arthritis
   C. Breast cancer
   D. Cardiovascular disease

4. Which of the following drugs requires a lower dosage in elderly persons because of reduction of renal function?
   A. Warfarin
   B. Gentamicin
   C. Digoxin
   D. Zantac

5. Which of the following medications in elderly patients may cause falls and hip fractures?
   A. Thiazides
   B. Diazepam
   C. Vitamin B_{12}
   D. Cimetidine

6. Physiological changes with aging may alter all of the following, except
   A. reduction of cardiac output.
   B. reduction of absorptive surfaces.
   C. increased gastric emptying rate.
   D. changes in gastric pH.

7. All of the following are reasons for the greater incidence of adverse reactions of drugs in elderly individuals, except
   A. increased total body fluid.
   B. impaired drug metabolism.
   C. decreased serum albumin levels.
   D. medication errors are more likely to occur.

8. Which of the following drugs has a large volume of distribution?
   A. Diazepam
   B. Acetaminophen
   C. Digoxin
   D. Ethanol

9. Which of the following body systems is the most important for elimination of the majority of drugs?
   A. Digestive
   B. Respiratory
   C. Reproductive
   D. Urinary

10. Which of the following agents can cause systemic side effects such as bradycardia, asthma, and heart failure?
    A. Diazepam
    B. Diphenhydramine
    C. β-blockers
    D. Bethanechol

Continues

11. The number of melanocytes and the amount of protective melanin _____ in elderly people.
    A. increases
    B. decreases
    C. does not change
    D. depends on what types of medication are being taken

12. The most important route for the elimination of the majority of drugs includes which of the following?
    A. Sweat
    B. Saliva
    C. Lungs
    D. Kidneys

13. The effects of similar drug concentrations at the site of action are called
    A. pharmacology.
    B. pharmacokinetic.
    C. pharmacodynamic.
    D. pharmacogenetic.

14. In the United States, about _____ of persons older than 65 years of age take prescription and nonprescription (over-the-counter) drugs.
    A. one half
    B. one fourth
    C. two thirds
    D. three fifths

15. Primary age changes are also known as _____ age changes.
    A. physiological
    B. pathophysiological
    C. sociogenic
    D. tertiary

The Most Commonly Prescribed Drugs in 2005

GENERIC NAME	BRAND NAME	GENERIC NAME	BRAND NAME
hydrocodone w/APAP	Hydrocodone w/APAP	propoxyphene N/APAP	Darvon-N
atorvastatin	Lipitor	alendronate sodium	Fosamax
atenolol	Tenormin	metformin hydrochloride	Glucophage, Fortamet
levothyroxine	Synthroid	ranitidine hydrochloride	Zantac
conjugated estrogens	Premarin	amitriptyline hydrochloride	Elavil
azithromycin	Zithromax	sildenafil citrate	Viagra
furosemide	Lasix	conjugated estrog ens/medroxyprogesterone	Prempro
amoxicillin	Amoxil		
amlodipine	Norvasc	amoxicillin	Trimox
hydrochlorothiazide	Ezide, Hydro-Diuril, Esidrex	gabapentin	Neurontin
		bupropion HCL	Wellbutrin SR
alprazolam	Xanax	pravastatin sodium	Pravachol
albuterol	Proventil, Ventolin	amoxicillin/clavulanate	Augmentin
sertraline hydrochloride	Zoloft	esomeprazole	Nexium
paroxetine hydrochloride	Paxil	quinapril hydrochloride	Accupril
simvastatin	Zocor	lisinopril	Prinivil, Zestrile
lansoprazole	Prevacid	venlafaxine	Effexor XR
ibuprofen	Motrin, Advil, Nuprin	Montelukast sodium	Singulair
triamterene	Dyrenium	lisinopril	Zestril
metoprolol succinate	Toprol-XL	potassium chloride	Potassium chloride, (K-Lease), Klorvess
cephalexin monohydrate	Keflex		
celecoxib	Celebrex	clonazepam	Klonopin
cetirizine hydrochloride	Zyrtec	naproxen	Naprosyn
levothyroxine sodium	Levoxyl	warfarin sodium	Coumadin
fexofenadine hydrochloride	Allegra	trazodone hydrochloride	Desgrel
norgestimate/ethinyl estradiol	Ortho Evra	ciprofloxacin hydrochloride	Cipro
citalopram hydrobromide	Celexa	fluticasone propionate	Flonase
prednisone	Deltasone	cyclobenzaprine hydrochloride	Flexeril
omeprazole	Prilosec	verapamil	Calan, Isoptin
loratidine	Claritin	enalapril moneate	Vasotec
fluoxetine hydrochloride	Prozac	isosorbide mononitrate	Ismo, Imdur
acetaminophen	Tylenol	levofloxacin	Levaquin
zolpidem tartrate	Ambien	diazepam	Valium
metoprolol tartrate	Lopressor	glipizide	Glucotrol XL
lorazepam	Ativan	warfarin	Coumadin

The Most Commonly Prescribed Drugs in 2005

GENERIC NAME	BRAND NAME	GENERIC NAME	BRAND NAME
clopidogrel bisulfate	Plavix	loratadine	Claritin
fluconazole	Diflucan	glimepiride	Amaryl
salmeterol/xinafoate	Serevent Diskus	spironolactone	Aldactrone
pantoprazole sodium	Protonix	fenofibrate	Tricor
amlodipine	Norvase	norethindrone/ethinyl estradiol	Ortho-Novum
valsartan	Diovan	hydroxyzine hydrochloride	Atarax, Vistaril
glyburide	Gen-Glybe, Micronase	fosinopril sodium	Monopril
ramipril	Altace	ipratropium/albuterol	Combivent
allopurinol	Allopurinol Zyloprim	meclizine hydrochloride	Antivert
estradiol	Estrogel	triamcinolone acetonide	Kenalog, Aristocart
rosiglitazone maleate	Avandia	metoclopramide	Reglan, Maxdon
pioglitazone hydrochloride	Actos	bisoprolol fumorate	Zebeta
benazepril hydrochloride	Lotensin	propranolol hydrochloride	Inderal
desloratadine	Clarinex	propoxyphene hydrochloride	Darvon
medroxyprogesterone acetate	Depo-Provera C-150, Provero	valacyclovir hydrochloride	Valtrex
		mirtazapine	Remeron
oxycodone hydrochloride	Roxicodone	famotidine	Pepcid
doxycycline hylate	Vibramycin	metronidazole	Flagyl
digoxin	Lanoxin	irbesartan	Avapro
losartan potassium	Cozaar	glipizide	Glucotrol
mometasone furoate monohydrate	Nasonex	buspirone hydrochloride	BuSpar
diltiazem hydrochloride	Cardizem	nystatin	Mycostatin, Nilstat, Nystex
clonidine hydrochloride	Catapres	phenytoin	Dilantin
digoxin	Digitek	ethinyl estradiol/norethindrone	Necon
methylprednisolone	Medrol	captopril	Capoten
raloxifene hydrochloride	Evista	clindamycin hydrochloride	Cleacin hydrochloride
folic acid	Folvite	aspirin	Aspirin
metformin hydrochloride	Glucophage XR	quetiapine fumarate	Seroquel
penicillin V Potassium	Penicillin VK	acyclovir	Zovirax
risperidone	Risperdal	amoxicillin potassium clavulanate	Augmentin
trimethoprim sulfamethoxazole	Cotrim, Sactrim, Septra	amphetamine mixed salts	Adderall XR
valsartan	Diovan	clarithromycin	Biaxin
rabeprazole sodium	Aciphex	levonorgestrel/ethinyl estradiol	Trivora-28
olanzapine	Zyprexa	norgestimate/ethinyl estradiol	Ortho-Cyclen
levothyroxine sodium	Levothroid	cefprozil	Cefzil
doxazosin mesylate	Cardura	isophanc insulin suspension	Humulin 70/30
latanoprost	Xalatan	tolterodine tetrate	Detrol LA
gemfibrozil	Lopid	carvedilol	Coreg
tamsulosin hydrochloride	Flomax	diltiazem hydrochloride	Tiazac
temazepam	Restoril	tramadol hydrochloride	Ultram
tramadol hydrochloride	Ultram	insulin lispro	Humalog
isophane insulin suspension	Humulin N	oxycodone/APAP	Endocet
divalproex sodium	Depakote	mupirocin	Bactroban
methylphenidate hydrochloride	Concerta	penicillin V potassium	Veetids
glyburide	Micronase	timolol maleate	Blacadren, Timoptic, Betimol
sumatriptan succinate	Imitrex		
terazosin	Hytrin	budesonide	Rhinocort

The Most Commonly Prescribed Drugs in 2005

GENERIC NAME	BRAND NAME	GENERIC NAME	BRAND NAME
nortriptyline hydrochloride	Aventyl	nifedipine	Adalat, Procardic
levonorgestrel/ethinyl estradiol	Aviane	tetracycline hydrochloride	Actisite, Sumycin
risedronate sodium	Actonel	desogestrel/ethinyl estradiol	Apri
topiramate	Topamax	diclofenac sodium	Voltaren
norethindrone/ethinyl estradiol	Microgestin Fe	carbidopa/levodopa	Sinemet
tamoxifen	Nolvadex	astelin	Dapac
desogestrel/ethinyl estradiol	Mircette		

abbreviations Shortened forms of words.

absorption The movement of a drug from its site of administration into the bloodstream.

accessory Any individual who helps a person to violate the law either directly or indirectly.

acetylcholine (ACh) A neurotransmitter that stimulates nerve endings.

acromegaly An overdevelopment of the bones of the hands, face, and feet as a result of excess growth hormone secreted as an adult.

active acquired immunity Immunity resulting from the development of antibodies within a person's body that renders the person immune; it may occur from exposure through a disease process or from immunizations.

administrative law Regulations set forth by governmental agencies, such as the Internal Revenue Service (IRS) and the Social Security Administration (SSA).

β-adrenergic agents Drugs that work as both cardiac and respiratory agonists.

β-adrenergic blockers Drugs used to reverse sympathetic heart action caused by exercise, stress, or physical exertion.

adrenogenital syndrome A disorder resulting from excess secretion of androgens.

agent An entity capable of causing disease.

agonist The drug that produces a functional change in a cell.

air-borne transmission Contaminated droplets or dust particles suspended in the air are transferred to a susceptible host.

alimentary canal The digestive tract.

alkylating agent An antineoplastic agent that affects cell growth.

allergic rhinitis Inflammation of the nasal mucosa that is due to the sensitivity of the nasal tissue to an allergen.

allergy A state of hypersensitivity induced by exposure to a particular antigen.

alveolar sacs Air cells found in the lung; also known as alveoli.

alveoli Air sacs found in the lung; also known as alveolar sacs.

Alzheimer's disease An illness characterized by progressive memory failure, impaired thinking, confusion, disorientation, personality changes, restlessness, speech disturbances, and inability to perform routine tasks.

American Association of Colleges of Pharmacy (AACP) A national organization that includes all 89 pharmacy colleges and schools in the United States, representing the interests of pharmaceutical education and educators; http://www.aacp.org.

American Association of Pharmaceutical Scientists (AAPS) An organization that represents pharmaceutical scientists employed in academia, industry, government, and other research institutions; http://www.aaps.org.

American Association of Pharmacy Technicians (AAPT) An organization that represents pharmacy technicians and promotes certification of technicians; http://www.pharmacytechnician.com.

American College of Clinical Pharmacy (ACCP) A professional and scientific society that provides leadership, education, advocacy, and resources for clinical pharmacists; http://www.accp.com.

American Council on Pharmaceutical Education (ACPE) A national accrediting agency for pharmacy education programs.

American Pharmacists Association (APhA) The largest of the national pharmacy organizations, consisting of three academies: the Academy of Pharmacy Practice and Management (APhA-APPM), the Academy of Pharmaceutical Research and Science (APhA-APRS), and the Academy of Students of Pharmacy (APhA-APS); http://www.aphanet.org.

American Society of Health-System Pharmacists (ASHP) A large organization that represents pharmacists who practice in hospitals, health maintenance organizations (HMOs), long-term care facilities, home care agencies, and other institutions; http://www.ashp.org.

amide A chemical compound formed from an organic acid by the substitution of an amino (NR2) group for the hydroxyl of a carboxyl (COOH) group.

ampule A sealed glass container that usually contains a single dose of medicine. The top of the ampule must be broken off to open the container.

analgesics Pain-relieving drugs.

anaphylactic shock A severe and sometimes fatal allergic reaction.

anesthetics Agents that act on nervous tissue to produce a loss of sensation or unconsciousness.

angina pectoris An episodic, reversible oxygen insufficiency.

angiotensin II receptor antagonists Drugs that block the binding of angiotensin II to the angiotensin II type 1 receptor.

angiotensin-converting enzyme inhibitors Drugs that competitively inhibit conversion of angiotensin I to angiotensin II, a potent vasoconstrictor, through the angiotensin-converting enzyme activity, with resultant lower levels of angiotensin II.

antacid mixtures Drugs used to treat pain related to peptic ulcer disorders; provide even more sustained action than single antacids and permit lower dosage.

antagonism When two drugs act to decrease the effects of each other.

anthrax A zoonotic disease caused by the anthrax bacillus that can infect humans in a number of ways and can be fatal.

antibiotics Substances that have the ability to destroy or interfere with the development of a living organism.

antibodies Proteins that develop in response to the presence of antigen in the body and react with the antigen on the next exposure. Antibodies may be formed from infections, immunization, transfer from mother to child, or unknown antigen stimulation.

anticoagulants Agents that prevent clot formation.

antigens A substance that is introduced into the body and induces the formation of antibodies.

antihistamines Drugs that counteract the action of histamine.

antimetabolite A substance that prevents cancer growth by affecting DNA production.

antineoplastic agents Drugs used to treat cancers and malignant neoplasms.

antiplatelet agents Drugs used to suppress aggregation (clumping) of platelets.

antitoxin Antibodies that neutralize toxins.

antitussives Agents that relieve or prevent coughing.

anxiety A persistent and irrational fear of a specific object, activity, or situation.

apathy A lack of feeling, emotion, interest, or concern.

apnea The cessation of respiration for more than 20 seconds with or without cyanosis, hypotonia, or bradycardia.

apothecary system An old English system of measurement.

Arabic numbers Standard numerical numbers.

aromatic water A mixture of distilled water with an aromatic volatile water.

arrhythmias Deviations from the normal pattern of the heartbeat.

arthritis Disease of the joints.

ascorbic acid A water-soluble vitamin that is essential for the formation of collagen and fibroid tissue for teeth, bones, cartilage, connective tissue, and skin. It also aids in fighting bacterial infections, bleeding gums, the tendency to bruise, nosebleeds, and anemia.

assay and control A group with the responsibility for auditing the control system and evaluating product quality.

assignment of benefits An authorization to an insurance company to make payment directly to the pharmacy or physician.

asthma A chronic inflammatory disorder of the airways of the respiratory system.

attenuation The process of weakening pathogens.

aura A sensation that may precede an attack of an epileptic seizure.

autoclave A sterilizing machine. An autoclave uses a combination of heat, steam, and pressure to sterilize equipment.

automated touch-tone response system A system in which the patient can call in an order or refill and the system routes the refill orders to the proper pharmacy and assigns each order a place in the order fulfillment sequence.

autonomy The right of an individual to make informed decisions for his or her own good.

aversive agent A nontoxic substance that is added to poisonous substances to cause the taste or smell of the poisonous substance to be offensive.

avoirdupois An old English system of weights.

bacteremia A condition in which bacteria are recovered from blood cultures of a patient and may or may not be associated with the disease.

bar coding Placing a code on packaging to help standardize and regulate inventory control.

batch repackaging The reassembling of a specific dosage and dosage form of medication at a given time.

beneficiary An individual entitled to receive insurance policy or government program health care benefits.

benign Nonprogressive.

bioavailability Measurement of the rate of absorption and total amount of drug that reach the systemic circulation.

bioethics A discipline dealing with the ethical and moral implications of biological research and applications.

biohazard symbol An image or object that serves as an alert that there is a risk to organisms, such as ionizing radiation or harmful bacteria or viruses.

biological agents Living organisms that invade the host.

biotin A water-soluble B complex vitamin that acts as a coenzyme in fatty acid production and in the oxidation of fatty acids and carbohydrates.

biotransformation The conversion of a drug within the body; also known as metabolism.

B lymphocytes Cells of the adaptive immune system that express cell surface immunoglobulins specific for an epitope on an antigen.

brand name A word, symbol, or device assigned to a product by its manufacturer, registered or not registered, as a trademark of its identity.

broad-spectrum antibiotic Antibiotics that are used for the treatment of diseases caused by multiple organisms.

broad-spectrum penicillins Drugs that have a wider antibacterial spectrum.

bronchodilators Agents that relax the smooth muscle of the bronchial tubes.

buccal Pertaining to the inside of the cheek.

buffered tablet A tablet that prevents ulceration or irritation of the stomach wall.

bulimia An eating disorder characterized by binge eating followed by purging.

bulk-forming laxatives Natural or synthetic polysaccharide derivatives that absorb water to soften the stool and increase bulk to stimulate peristalsis.

bursa A closed sac with a synovial membrane lining.

calciferol A fat-soluble vitamin chemically related to the steroids and essential for the normal formation of bones and teeth. It is important for the absorption of calcium and phosphorus from the gastrointestinal tract.

calcium An alkaline earth metal element. The body requires calcium ions for the transmission of nerve impulses, muscle contraction, blood coagulation, cardiac functions, and other processes.

calcium carbonate A substance that causes acid rebound, which may delay ulcer-related pain relief and ulcer healing.

calcium channel blockers Drugs used to treat stable angina.

caplet A tablet shaped like a capsule.

capsule A solid dosage form in which the drug is enclosed in either a hard or soft shell of soluble material.

carbohydrates Nutrients providing the main energy source in the average diet.

carcinogenic A substance that causes cancer.

cardiac toxicity Adverse effects on the heart by drugs or chemical substances.

case law Law established by judicial decision in legal cases and used as legal precedent.

caustic A substance that eats away at something.

Centers for Medicare & Medicaid (CMS) An organization that inspects and approves institutions to provide Medicaid and Medicare services.

central processing unit (CPU) The part of the computer that actually does the computations.

CHAMPVA Civilian Health and Medical Program of the Veterans Administration; a program to cover medical expenses of the dependent spouse and children of veterans with total, permanent service-connected disabilities.

channels Spoken words, written messages, and body language.

chemical agents Substances that can interact with the body.

chemical digestion Alteration of food into different forms through chemicals and enzymes.

chemical name Drug name derived from the chemical composition of the drug.

chemical sterilization A method of cleaning equipment used for instruments that cannot be exposed to the high temperatures of steam sterilization.

chloride An anion of chlorine. The most common form is sodium chloride (table salt).

cholesterol A waxy lipid found only in animal tissues. A member of a group of lipids called sterols, it is widely distributed in the body.

civil law Rules and regulations that govern the relationship between individuals within society.

class A prescription balance A two-pan device that may be used for weighing small amounts of drugs (not more than 120 g).

coinsurance An arrangement in which the insured must pay a percentage of the cost of medical services covered by the insurer.

collagen A strong fibrous protein found in connective tissue.

combining form A root with an added vowel (known as a combining vowel) that connects the root with the suffix or the root to another root.

common fraction Equal parts of a whole.

common law Derives authority from ancient usages and customs affirmed by court judgments and decrees.

communication The sharing of information, ideas, thoughts, and feelings.

compensation An unconscious mechanism by which an individual tries to make up for fancied or real deficiencies.

complex fraction The numerator or the denominator or both as a whole number, proper fraction, or mixed number. The value may be less than, greater than, or equal to 1.

compounding slab A plate made of ground glass with a hard, flat, and nonabsorbent surface for mixing compounds.

compromised host A person whose normal defense mechanisms are impaired and is therefore more susceptible to a disease.

computer A piece of programmable equipment that stores, retrieves, and processes data.

computerized physician order entry system (CPOE) A computerized system in which the physician inputs the medication order directly for electronic receipt in the pharmacy.

congestive heart failure A disorder in which the heart cannot pump the blood returning to the right side of the heart or provide adequate circulation to meet the needs of organs and tissues in the body.

conical graduates Devices used for measuring liquids that have wide tops and wide bases and taper from the top to the bottom.

conjugation The biosynthetic process of combining a chemical compound with a highly polar and water-soluble natural substance to yield a water-soluble, usually inactive, product.

Conn's syndrome A disorder resulting from excess secretion of aldosterone.

constitutional law Deals with interpretation and implementation of the United States Constitution.

consumer The person coming to you for the filling of prescriptions or the purchase of over-the-counter remedies for a wide variety of situations.

contact transmission The physical transfer of an agent from an infected person to an uninfected person.

contract An insurance policy; this is a legally enforceable agreement.

contraindication A condition that increases the chance of a serious adverse reaction.

controlled substance medication order An order for medication (generally narcotics) that requires monitored documentation of procurement, dispensing, and administration.

conversion factor Used to determine equivalents of specific units of measure.

convulsion Abnormal motor movements.

coordination of benefits The prevention of duplicate payment for the same service.

co-payment A patient's payment of a portion of the cost at the time the service is rendered.

copper A metallic element that is a component of several important enzymes in the body and is essential to good health.

corticosteroids The most potent and consistently effective antiinflammatory agents that are currently available for relief of respiratory conditions.

cost analysis All information regarding the disbursements of an activity, department, program, or agency.

cost-benefit analysis The procedure of evaluating costs and benefits of only those programs whose benefits are found to supersede the costs.

cost control The implementation of managerial efforts to achieve cost objectives.

counter balance A device capable of weighing much larger quantities, up to about 5 kg. It is a double-pan balance.

cream A semisolid emulsion of either the oil-in-water or the water-in-oil type, ordinarily intended for topical use.

crime A violation of the law.

criminal An individual who violates the law.

criminal law Rules and regulations that govern the relationship of the individual to society as a whole.

cross-dependence The ability of one drug to substitute for another drug in the same drug class to maintain a dependent state or prevent withdrawal.

cross-tolerance Tolerance to one drug conferring tolerance to other drugs in the same drug class.

croup A viral infection that affects the larynx and the trachea.

Cushing's syndrome A disorder resulting from an excess of glucocorticoid hormones, which raises the blood glucose level.

cyanocobalamin A water-soluble substance that is the common pharmaceutical form of vitamin B_{12}. It is involved in the metabolism of protein, fats, and carbohydrates. Vitamin B_{12} is also involved in normal blood formation and neural function.

cylindrical graduates Devices used for measuring liquids that have narrow diameters that are the same from top to base.

cytochrome P-450 A system of enzymes that contribute to drug interactions.

data The raw facts the computer can manipulate.

decimal A numerator that is expressed in numerals with a decimal point placed so that it designates the value of the denominator, and the denominator, which is understood to be 10 or some power of 10; also called decimal fraction.

decimal fraction A numerator that is expressed in numerals, with a decimal point placed so that it designates the value of the denominator, and the denominator, which is understood to be 10 or some power of 10; also called decimal.

decode Translation of a message by the receiver into what is perceived to be said.

decongestant A drug that causes vasoconstriction of nasal mucosa and reduces congestion or swelling.

deductible A specific amount of money that must be paid each year before the policy benefits begin (e.g., $50, $100, $300, or $500).

defense mechanisms Tools an individual uses when required to deal with uncomfortable or threatening situations.

demand/stat medication order An order for medication to be given in rapid response to a specific medication condition.

denial A psychological defense mechanism in which confrontation with a personal problem or with reality is avoided by denying the existence of the problem or reality.

denominator The number the whole is divided into.

Department of Health (DPH) An organization that oversees hospitals, including the pharmacy department.

dependence The psychological, physiological, or biochemical need to continue to take a drug.

dependents The insured's spouse and children under the terms of the policy.

depot-medroxyprogesterone (Depo-Provera®) A long-acting progestin.

derivatives Substances that are made from another substance.

dermis A thick layer of loose connective tissue that is well-supplied with blood vessels, lymphatic vessels, nerves, and accessory organs.

diffusion Particles in a fluid move from an area of higher concentration to an area of lower concentration, resulting in an even distribution of the particles in the fluid.

diphtheria An acute, toxin-mediated disease caused by *Corynebacterium diphtheriae*.

direct costs Costs caused directly by or resulting from providing the service.

disinfection Destruction of pathogens by physical or chemical means.

displacement The transfer of impulses from one expression to another, such as from fighting to talking.

distribution The process by which blood leaves the bloodstream and enters the tissues of the body.

diuretics Drugs that increase sodium excretion and lower blood volume.

divisor The number performing the division.

dosage form The make up of a particular type of drug; the form in which it is given.

dosage strength The amount of medication per unit of measure.

dram A unit of weight in the apothecary system; 1 dram equals 60 grains.

drive through An external site at a pharmacy that can be accessed by driving up in the car.

drop rate The number of drops an intravenous infusion is administered at over a specific period of time.

drug abuse Nonmedical use of a drug that is deemed unacceptable by society.

drug control A method used to eliminate or reduce the potential harm of the drug distributed.

drug interaction An interference of a drug with the effect of another drug, nutrient, or laboratory test.

drug label factor The form of the drug dose with its equivalent in unit.

dry heat sterilization A method of sterilization that uses heated dry air at a temperature of 320 to 356°F (160 to 180°C) for 90 minutes to 3 hours.

dry powder inhaler (DPI) A device used to deliver medication in the form of micronized powder into the lungs.

dwarfism Reduction in growth of long bones as a result of too little growth hormone secretion during childhood.

elastin An extracellular connective tissue protein.

electrolytes Compounds that dissociate into ions when dissolved in water.

electronic balance A two-pan device that may be used for weighing small amounts of drugs (not more than 120 g).

eligibility The specific terms of coverage under a policy.

elixir A clear, sweetened, hydroalcoholic liquid intended for oral use.

emergency medication order An order for a medication to be given in response to a medical emergency.

emollient laxatives Substances that act as surfactants by allowing absorption of water into the stool.

emulsion A system containing two liquids that cannot be mixed together in which one is dispersed, in the form of very small globules, throughout the other.

endocrine glands The structures that secrete hormones.

endogenous depression Feelings of intense sadness, helplessness, and worthlessness that have no external cause and may be the result of genetic factors or biochemical changes in the brain.

enteral nutrition (EN) Feeding by tube directly into the patient's digestive tract.

enteric-coated tablet A tablet covered in a special coating to protect it from stomach acid, allowing the drug to dissolve in the intestines.

epiglottitis An acute bacterial infection of the epiglottis (an appendage which closes the glottis while food or drink is passing through the pharynx), and the surrounding areas that cause airway obstruction.

epilepsy A disorder characterized by recurrent, unprovoked seizures, in which seizures are of primary cerebral origin, indicating underlying brain dysfunction.

ester A class of chemical compounds formed by the bonding of an alcohol and one or more organic acids. Fats are esters produced by the bonding of fatty acids with the alcohol glycerol.

ethics The branch of philosophy that deals with the distinction between right and wrong and with the moral consequences of human actions.

ethinyl estradiol A chemical derivative of natural estrogens.

exogenous depression Feelings of intense sadness, helplessness, and worthlessness that occur in response to a loss, disappointment, or illness.

expectorants Agents that promote the removal of mucous secretions from the lung, bronchi, and trachea, usually by coughing.

exposure control plan A written procedure for the treatment of persons exposed to biohazardous or similar chemically harmful materials.

expressive aphasia Inability of an individual to form language and express his or her thoughts accurately even though thought processes are intact.

extemporaneous compounding The preparation, mixing, assembling, packaging, and labeling of a drug product based on a prescription order from a licensed practitioner for the individual patient.

external noise Physical noise such as typing or traffic that interferes with hearing a message.

extravasation Leakage of fluid from vessels into surrounding tissues.

extremes The two outside terms in a ratio.

fats Substances composed of lipids or fatty acids and occurring in various forms.

fatty acids Any of several organic acids produced by the hydrolysis of neutral fats.

felony A serious crime, such as murder, kidnapping, assault, or rape, that is punishable by imprisonment for more than 1 year.

file A set of data or a program that has been given a name.

filtration The movement of water and dissolved substances from the glomerulus to the Bowman's capsule.

fire safety plan A written procedure that includes fire extinguisher locations, fire alarm pull-box locations, sprinkler system location, exit signs, and clear directions to the quickest and safest exit of a building during an emergency.

first-pass effect The drug reaches the liver where it is partially metabolized before being sent to the body.

floor stock system A system of drug distribution in which drugs are issued in bulk form and stored in medication rooms on patient care units.

fluidextract A pharmacopeial liquid preparation of vegetable drugs, made by filtration, containing alcohol as a solvent or as a preservative or both.

fluoride A substance that prevents tooth decay and protects against osteoporosis and gum disease.

folacin A water-soluble vitamin essential for cell growth and the reproduction of red blood cells.

folic acid A water-soluble vitamin essential for cell growth and the reproduction of red blood cells.

fomites Objects contaminated with an infectious agent but are symptom free.

food additive Any substance that becomes part of a food product.

form The structure and composition of a drug.

formulary A document that specifies particular drug forms and compositions.

fraction An expression of division with a number that is the portion or part of a whole.

fungi Microorganisms that grow in single cells or in colonies.

gas sterilization The use of a gas such as ethylene oxide to sterilize medical equipment.

gavage Feeding with a stomach tube.

gel A jelly or the solid or semisolid phase of a colloidal solution.

gelcap An oil-based medication that is enclosed in a soft gelatin capsule.

generic name The name the manufacturer uses for a drug.

geometric dilution When mixing agents, the medicament is first mixed with an equal weight of diluent. A further quantity of diluent equal in weight to the mixture is then incorporated. This process is repeated until all of the diluent has been mixed in.

giantism A disorder resulting from excess growth hormone secreted before puberty.

glomerular filtration rate (GFR) The rate of filtration in the kidney.

glucagon A hormone that works antagonistically with insulin and is released when blood glucose levels fall below normal.

grain The basic unit of weight in the apothecary system.

gram The basic unit for weight in the metric system.

gram-negative Microorganisms that stain red or pink with Gram stain.

gram-positive Microorganisms that stain blue or purple with Gram stain.

Gram stain A sequential procedure involving crystal violet and iodine solutions followed by alcohol that allows rapid identification of organisms as gram-positive or gram-negative types.

granule A very small pill, usually gelatin- or sugar-coated, containing a drug to be given in a small dose.

group purchasing Procurement contracts are negotiated on behalf of the members of a group (e.g., hospitals, nursing home pharmacies, and home infusion pharmacies). The group purchasing organization uses the collective buying power of its members to negotiate discounts from manufacturers, wholesalers, and other suppliers.

Haemophilus influenzae A gram-negative bacterium that commonly causes otitis media or bacterial meningitis in children.

half-life The time it takes for the plasma concentration to be reduced by 50%.

haloperidol An antipsychotic drug.

hardware The parts of the computer that you can touch.

hazard communication plan Application of warning labels for all hazardous chemicals.

health insurance A contract between a policyholder and an insurance carrier or government program to reimburse the policyholder for all or a portion of the cost of medical care rendered by health care professionals.

hepatitis Inflammation of the liver caused by microorganisms, especially viruses, or drugs such as alcohol and other poisons.

high-density lipoproteins (HDLs) Lipoproteins that carry cholesterol from cells to the liver for eventual excretion.

hirsutism Excessive hair growth.

histamine A chemical substance found in all the body tissues that protects the body from factors in the environment that produce allergic and inflammatory reactions.

hormonal agents Substances consisting of a heterogeneous compound that either blocks hormone production or blocks hormone action.

hormone A natural chemical secreted into the bloodstream from the endocrine glands to regulate and control the activity of an organ or tissues in another part of the body.

hospice Originally a facility, usually within a hospital, intended to care for the terminally ill, in particular, by providing physical comfort to the patient and emotional support and counseling to the patient and the family.

hospital pharmacy The provision of pharmaceutical care within an institutional or hospital setting.

household system System of measurement used in most homes; this is not an accurate system of measurement for medications.

hydrolysis The process of adding a water molecule to split a molecule into smaller portions.

hydrophobia A fear of water; a symptom caused by rabies as the disease progresses.

hyperactive Secretion of an excessive amount of a substance.

hyperalimentation The administration of a nutritionally adequate hypertonic solution consisting of glucose, protein, minerals, and vitamins through an indwelling catheter into the superior vena cava.

hypercalcemia A disorder resulting from an overactive parathyroid gland.

hyperlipidemia An increase in triglycerides.

hyperpituitarism A disorder resulting from overactivity of the pituitary gland.

hypertension An abnormal increase in arterial blood pressure.

hypervitaminosis An abnormal condition resulting from excessive intake of toxic amounts of one or more vitamins, especially over a long period.

hypnosis An increased tendency to sleep.

hypnotics Drugs that depress the central nervous system by inhibiting transmission of nerve impulses.

hypoactive Secretion of an inadequate amount of a substance.

hypovitaminosis A condition related to the deficiency of one or more vitamins.

idiosyncratic reaction Experience of a unique, strange, or unpredicted reaction to a drug.

immunity An immunologic reaction that destroys or resists antigens.

immunogen An antigen.

immunoglobulins Blood products that contain disease-specific antibodies for passive immunity.

immunology The study of immune responses.

improper fraction The numerator is greater than or equal to the denominator.

inactivated vaccines Vaccines in which the infectious components have been destroyed by chemical or physical treatments.

independent practice association (IPA) A type of health maintenance organization (HMO) in which the HMO contracts directly with physicians, who continue in their existing practices.

independent purchasing The director of the pharmacy or buyer directly contacts and negotiates pricing with pharmaceutical manufacturers.

indirect costs Costs not caused directly by or that do not result from providing the service.

induration An excessive hardening or firmness of any body site. It is one of the signs of inflammation.

influenza A A virus causing moderate to severe illness, affecting all age groups.

influenza B A virus causing a mild illness; usually only affects children.

influenza C A viral infection of the upper respiratory tract.

input devices Any piece of equipment that allows data to be entered into the computer system.

inscription Medication prescribed.

insulin A hormone synthesized and secreted by the pancreas.

insulin-dependent diabetes mellitus A disorder caused by complete lack of insulin secretion of the pancreas.

internal noise An individual's beliefs or prejudices that interfere with decoding a message.

international law Law based on treaties and other agreements between two or more countries.

international units A standardized amount of medication required to produce a certain effect.

intradermal injection Between the layers of the skin. A dose of an agent administered between the layers of the skin.

intramuscular injection Inside a muscle. Normally used in the context of an injection given into a muscle.

intravenous injection Into a vein. Most commonly used in the context of an injection given directly into a vein.

inventory The stock of medications a pharmacy keeps immediately on hand.

inventory control Controlling the amount of product on hand to maximize the return on investment.

inventory turnover rate A mathematical calculation used to determine the number of times the average inventory is replaced over a period of time, usually annually.

investigational medication order An order for a medication given under direction of research protocols that also require strict documentation of procurement, dispensing, and administration.

invoice A form describing a purchase and the amount due.

iodine An essential micronutrient of the thyroid hormone (thyroxine).

iron A common metallic element essential for the synthesis of hemoglobin.

iron deficiency anemia A microcytic hypochromic anemia caused by inadequate supplies of iron needed to synthesize hemoglobin.

ischemic heart disease A condition in which there is an insufficient supply of oxygen to the myocardium (cardiac muscle).

Joint Commission on Accreditation of Healthcare Organizations (JCAHO) An organization that surveys and accredits health care organizations.

judicial law Rules and regulations resulting from court decisions.

just in time (JIT) system An inventory control system in which stock arrives just before it is needed.

killer cells Large, granular lymphocytes that appear to have the ability to destroy tumor cells.

kwashiorkor A deficiency disease caused by extreme lack of protein.

laminar airflow hood A system of circulating filtered air in parallel-flowing planes in hospitals or other health care facilities. The system reduces the risk of airborne contamination and exposure to chemical pollutants in surgical theaters, food preparation areas, hospital pharmacies, and laboratories.

law A principle or rule that is advisable or obligatory to observe.

legend drug A medication that may be dispensed only with a prescription; also know as prescription drug.

leukotrines Substances that contribute to the inflammation associated with asthma.

levigate To grind into a smooth substance with moisture.

levonorgestrel A contraceptive implant; also known as the Norplant® system.

liniment A liquid preparation for external use, usually applied by friction to the skin.

lipids Fats.

liquid antacid Drug used to treat pain related to peptic ulcer disorders; has a greater buffering capacity than tablets.

liter The basic unit for volume in the metric system.

live attenuated vaccines Vaccines containing living organisms or intact viruses that have undergone radiation or temperature conditioning to produce safe vaccinations which will help the patient become immune to a specific disease.

long-term care A wide range of health and health-related support services.

long-term care pharmacy organization An organization involving a licensed professional pharmacy or practice that provides medications and clinical services to long-term care facilities and their residents.

low-density lipoproteins (LDLs) Lipoproteins that carry blood cholesterol from all cells.

lower respiratory tract Consists of the bronchi, bronchioles, lower trachea, alveoli, and lungs.

lozenge A small, disk-shaped tablet composed of solidifying paste containing an astringent, an antiseptic, or an oil-based drug used for local treatment of the mouth or throat. It is held in the mouth until dissolved. Also known as a troche.

lubricant laxative A substance such as mineral oil that works by increasing water retention in the stool to soften it.

Lugol's solution A popular strong iodide solution containing 5% iodine and 10% potassium iodide and saturated solution of potassium iodide.

magnesium A silver-white mineral element. It is the second most abundant cation of the intracellular fluids in the body and is essential for many enzyme activities.

mail-order pharmacy A licensed pharmacy that uses the mail or other carriers (e.g., overnight carriers or parcel services) to deliver prescriptions to patients.

malignant Spreading.

malnutrition Ingestion of nutrients inadequate to maintain health and well-being.

Mantoux test An intradermal screening for tuberculin hypersensitivity. A red, firm patch of skin at the injection site greater than 10 mm in diameter after 48 hours is a positive result that indicates current or prior exposure to tubercle bacilli.

marasmus Severe wasting caused by lack of protein and all nutrients or faulty absorption.

markup method A pricing mechanism in which the price charged to the patient is calculated by adding a percentage markup, in addition to a dispensing fee, to the acquisition cost of the drug.

material safety data sheet (MSDS) Written or printed material concerning a hazardous chemical that includes information on the chemical's identity and physical and chemical characteristics.

means The two inside terms in a ratio.

measles An acute viral infectious disease.

mechanical digestion The breakdown of large food particles into smaller pieces by physical means.

Medicaid A federal/state medical assistance program to provide health insurance for specific populations.

medical asepsis Complete destruction of organisms after they leave the body.

Medicare A federal health insurance program created as part of the Social Security Act.

medication order The written order for particular medications and services to be provided to a patient within an institutional setting; medication orders are written by physicians, nurse practitioners, or physician's assistants.

memory The ability of the computer to store data and retrieve data.

menadione A water-soluble injectable form of the product of vitamin K_3.

meningitis An inflammation of the meninges (membranes) that surround and protect the brain. It is often caused by bacteria.

meniscus Meaning "moon-shaped body"; indicates that the level of the liquid will be slightly higher at the edges.

mestranol A chemical derivative of natural estrogens.

metabolism The conversion of a drug within the body; also known as biotransformation.

metastasis Uncontrollable growth characteristic of cancer cells.

meter The basic unit for length in the metric system.

metered dose inhaler (MDI) A hand-held pressurized device used to deliver medications for inhalation.

metric system Worldwide standard system of measurement.

migraine headache A disorder characterized by unilateral throbbing or nonthrobbing pain that is often accompanied by nausea, vomiting, and sensitivity to noise and light.

milliequivalent A unit of measure based upon the chemical combining power of a substance.

milliunit One thousandth of a unit.

minerals Inorganic substances occurring naturally in the earth's crust, having a characteristic chemical composition.

minim The basic unit of volume in the apothecary system.

misdemeanor A less serious crime, punishable by a fine or imprisonment for less than 1 year.

mixed fraction A whole number and a proper fraction that are combined. The value of the mixed number is always greater than 1.

mixture A mutual incorporation of two or more substances, without chemical union, in which the physical characteristics of each of the components are retained.

mode of transmission The process that bridges the gap between the portal of exit of the infectious agent and the portal of entry of the susceptible host.

modem A device used to transfer information from one computer to another.

mortar A cup-shaped vessel in which materials are ground or crushed.

mucolytic Destroying or dissolving the active agents that make up mucus.

multiplicand The number to be multiplied by another.

multiplier A number by which another is multiplied.

mumps An acute viral illness.

mutagen A substance that is capable of making changes at the cellular level.

myocardial infarction An area of dead cardiac muscle tissue, with or without hemorrhage.

myocarditis Inflammation of the heart.

narrow-spectrum antibiotics Antibiotics that are effective against only a few organisms.

National Drug Code (NDC) A unique and permanent product code assigned to each new drug as it becomes available in the marketplace; it identifies the manufacturer or distributor, the drug formulation, and the size and type of its packaging.

National Formulary (NF) A database of officially recognized drug names.

natural active acquired immunity Resistance to the causative pathogen in individuals who have had a specific infection because of the presence of antibodies and stimulated lymphocytes.

neonatal period The time from birth to approximately 28 days of age.

neoplasm A tumor.

neurohormones Neurotransmitters.

neurohypophysis The posterior pituitary gland.

neuron The basic structure of a nerve consisting of dendrites, cell body, and axon.

neurosis A disease of the nerves or a mental disorder.

neutral fats Fats consisting of about 95% triglycerides or triacylglycerols.

niacin A part of two enzymes that regulate energy metabolism.

nitrates Drugs used for the treatment of angina.

nitrosoureas Newer forms of alkylating agent that are lipid soluble.

nomogram A quick reference for calculating pediatric doses.

nonsteroidal anti-inflammatory drugs (NSAIDs) Drugs that inhibit the synthesis of the prostaglandin responsible for causing pain and inflammation.

Norplant® system A contraceptive implant; also known as levonorgestrel.

nuclear pharmacy A pharmacy that is specially licensed to work with radioactive materials. Previously called radiopharmacy.

numerator The portion of the whole being considered.

nutrient A chemical substance found in food that is necessary for good health.

nutrition The sum of the processes involved in the taking in of nutrients and their assimilation and use for proper body functioning and maintenance of health.

ointment A semisolid preparation that usually contains medicinal substances and is intended for external application.

oral Pertaining to the mouth. Medication given by mouth.

orphan drug A drug that is developed for small populations of people in need of the drug.

osteoporosis A disease characterized by a reduction in bone mass.

otitis media An inflammation of the middle ear.

ounce A unit of weight in the apothecary system; 1 ounce equals 8 drams.

output devices Any piece of equipment that allows data to exit the computer system.

overpayment Payment by the insurer or by the patient of more than the amount due.

over-the-counter (OTC) A medication that may be purchased without a prescription directly from the pharmacy.

oxidation The process by which oxygen combines with another chemical; the removal of hydrogen or the loss of electrons.

pantothenic acid A member of the vitamin B complex. It is widely distributed in plant and animal tissues and may be an important element in human nutrition.

parenteral Administration by some means other than through the gastrointestinal tract; referring particularly to introduction of substances into an organism by intravenous, subcutaneous, intramuscular, or intramedullary injection.

parenteral nutrition A combination of amino acids, dextrose, fats, vitamins, minerals, electrolytes, and water administered intravenously. Parenteral nutrition is capable of providing all the nutrients needed to sustain life.

Parkinson's disease A disorder characterized by resting tremor, rigidity or resistance to passive movement, akinesia, and loss of postural reflexes.

parotitis Inflammation of the salivary glands.

passive acquired immunity Immunity acquired from the injection or passage of antibodies from an immune person or animal to another for short-term immunity or immunity passed from mother to child.

patent ductus arteriosus A disorder in which the ductus remains patent when pulmonary vascular resistance falls, resulting in aortic blood being shunted into the pulmonary artery.

patient prescription system A system of drug distribution in which a nurse supplies the pharmacy with a transcribed medication order for a particular patient and the pharmacy prepares a 3-day supply of the medication.

pediatric period The period from birth to approximately age 18.

percent A fraction whose numerator is expressed and whose denominator is understood to be 100.

perpetual inventory system An inventory control system that allows review of drug use monthly.

personal digital assistant (PDA) A hand-held device that runs on its own battery power so that it may be used anywhere.

pertussis An acute infectious disease caused by the bacterium *Bordetella pertussis;* also known as whooping cough.

pestle A solid device that is used to crush or grind materials in a mortar.

pharma food A system of nourishing through breathing.

pharmaceutical care Term used to describe the care provided to a patient by the pharmacy, which encompasses all aspects of drug therapy from dispensing to drug monitoring.

pharmacodynamic interactions Differences in effects produced by a given plasma level of a drug.

pharmacodynamics The study of the biochemical and physiological effects of drugs.

pharmacokinetic interactions Differences in the plasma levels of a drug achieved with a given dose of that drug.

pharmacokinetics The study of the absorption, distribution, metabolism, and excretion of drugs.

pharmacy The art and science of dispensing and preparing medication and providing of drug-related information to the public.

pharmacy compounding The preparation, mixing, assembling, packaging, or labeling of a drug or device.

pharmacy shop Term used to describe the first stand-alone pharmacies.

Pharmacy Technician Certification Board (PTCB) An organization that prepares and administers the standard national exam for certification as a pharmacy technician; http://www.ptcb.org.

Pharmacy Technician Certification Exam (PTCE) A standardized national exam for certification to become a pharmacy technician.

Pharmacy Technician Educators Council (PTEC) An association of educators who prepare people for careers as pharmacy technicians; http://www.rxptec.org.

phospholipid A phosphorus-containing lipid.

phosphorus A nonmetallic chemical element occurring extensively in nature as a component of phosphate rock. Phosphorus is essential for the metabolism of protein, calcium, and glucose.

physical agent Factors in the environment that interact with the body.

physical dependence The necessity to continue drug use to avoid a withdrawal syndrome.

pill A small, globular mass of soluble material containing a medicinal substance to be swallowed.

pipette A long, thin, calibrated hollow tube, which is made of glass used for measuring liquids.

placebo Sugar pill.

plasma cells Differentiated B cells that secrete antibodies.

plaster A solid preparation that can be spread when heated and that becomes adhesive at the temperature of the body.

pneumonia An acute inflammation of the lungs, often caused by inhaled *Streptococcus pneumoniae.*

point of sale (POS) master An inventory control system that allows inventory to be tracked as it is used.

poison Any substance that causes injury, illness, or death of a living organism.

poisoning The development of dose-related adverse effects after exposure to chemicals, drugs, or other substances foreign to the body.

policy Statement of the definite course or method of action selected to support goals of the overall organization.

policy and procedure manual A formal document specifying guidelines for operations of an institution.

policy limitation Policies that exclude certain types of coverage.

poliomyelitis Inflammation of the spinal cord that leads to paralysis.

portal of entry The route by which an infectious agent enters the host.

portal of exit The route by which an infectious agent leaves the reservoir to be transferred to a susceptible host.

potassium An alkali metal element. Potassium salts are necessary to the life of all plants and animals. Potassium in the body helps to regulate neuromuscular excitability and muscle contraction.

potentiation One drug prolongs the effects of another drug.

powder A dry mass of minute separate particles of any substance.

preauthorization The requirement of notification and permission to receive additional types of services before one obtains those services.

precaution Specific warning to consider when medications are prescribed or administered.

preferred provider organization (PPO) A managed care organization that contracts with a group of providers, who are called *preferred providers,* to offer services to the managed care organization's members.

prefix A part of a word structure that occurs before or in front of the word and modifies the meaning of the root.

prejudice A preformed and unsubstantiated judgment or opinion about an individual or a group, either favorable or unfavorable.

premium The cost of the coverage that the insurance policy contains; this may vary greatly depending on the age and health of the individual and the type of insurance protection.

prime supplier Establishment of a relationship with a single supplier to obtain lower prices.

PRN (as needed) medication order An order for medication to be given in response to a specific defined parameter or condition.

procedure Statement of a series of steps to implement the policies of the department of organization.

product The number resulting from the multiplication of two or more quantities together.

profession A group that requires specialized education and intellectual knowledge.

professional fee method A set dollar amount added to the ingredient cost to determine prescription price.

professionalism The following of a profession as an occupation. A person who conforms to the rules and standard of their chosen profession.

programs A set of electronic instructions that tell the computer what to do.

projection A defense mechanism by which a repressed complex in the individual is denied and conceived as belonging to another person, such as when faults that the person tends to commit are perceived in or attributed to others.

proper fraction The numerator is smaller than the denominator and designates less than one whole unit.

proportion The relationship between two equal ratios.

propoxyphene An analgesic.

protein The only one of six essential nutrients containing nitrogen.

psychological dependence The overwhelming need to take a drug to maintain a sense of well-being.

psychosis A mental illness accompanied by bizarre behavior and altered personality with failure to perceive reality.

pulmonary toxicity Adverse effects on the lungs by drugs or chemical substances.

pyridoxine A water-soluble vitamin that is part of the B complex. It acts as a coenzyme essential for the synthesis and breakdown of amino acids.

quality control An organized effort of all individuals directly or indirectly involved in the production, packaging, and distribution of quality medications, which are safe, effective, and acceptable.

quality control unit A group with the responsibility for auditing the control system and evaluating product quality.

quotient The answer to a division problem.

rabies The only rhabdovirus that infects humans; it is a zoonotic disease characterized by fatal meningoencephalitis.

radiopharmaceutical A drug that is or has been made to be radioactive. Although a few radiopharmaceuticals are used to treat diseases (e.g., radioactive iodine), most are used as diagnostic agents.

ratio A mathematical expression that compares two numbers by division.

rationalization A psychoanalytic defense mechanism through which irrational behavior, motives, or feelings are made to appear reasonable.

reabsorption The movement of water and selected substances from the tubules to the peritubular capillaries.

reagent kit Vials containing particular compounds, usually in freeze-dried form used in nuclear pharmacy.

receptive aphasia A physical limitation after certain neurological injuries, which leaves the person incapable of understanding all that is said.

receptor The cell that a drug has an affinity to.

regression An unconscious defense mechanism involving a return to earlier patterns of adaptation.

regulatory law Regulations set forth by governmental agencies. It is also called administrative law.

repression A defense mechanism of keeping out and ejecting or banishing from consciousness an unacceptable idea or impulse.

reservoir The place where an agent can survive.

respiratory distress syndrome (RDS) The result of the absence, deficiency, or alteration of the components of pulmonary surfactant.

respiratory syncytial virus (RSV) The major cause of bronchiolitis and pneumonia in infants younger than 1 year of age; caused by a virus and exhibits mild cold-like symptoms.

retinol A fat-soluble vitamin essential for skeletal growth, maintenance of normal mucosal epithelium, reproduction, and visual acuity.

Reye syndrome A complication that occurs almost exclusively in children taking aspirin, primarily in association with influenza B or varicella zoster, and presents with severe vomiting and confusion, which may progress to coma, due to swelling of the brain.

riboflavin One of the heat-stable components of the B complex. It is involved as a coenzyme in the oxidative processes of carbohydrates, fats, and proteins.

root The main part of a word that gives the word its central meaning.

rubella A mild, highly infectious viral disease common in childhood.

salicylism Salicylate intoxication.

saline laxatives Substances that create an osmotic effect to increase water content and volume of stool.

sanitization A process of cleansing to remove undesirable debris.

sarcasm Hostile and cruel language intended to hurt someone.

scheduled intravenous (IV)/total parenteral nutrition (TPN) solution order An order for medication given via an injection; these medications are to be prepared in a controlled (sterile) environment.

scheduled medication order An order for medication that is to be given on a continuous schedule.

sedation A state of consciousness characterized by decreased anxiety, motor activity, and mental acuity.

sedatives Drugs that depress the central nervous system by inhibiting transmission of nerve impulses.

seizure A sudden, transient alteration in brain function as a result of abnormal neuronal activity and excessive cerebral electric discharge.

sepsis A syndrome involving multiple organ systems that is the result of microorganisms or their toxins in the blood.

septicemia A systemic infection caused by multiplication of microorganisms in the blood circulation.

sexual harassment Intentional, clearly understood statements or intentional, clearly understood action that causes another to feel that his or her job is at risk if the sexual advances are rejected.

sickle cell anemia An inherited disorder characterized by the presence of abnormal hemoglobin; hemoglobin contains hemoglobin S (HbS).

signa Directions for patient.

sliding scale method Variable markup percentages or professional fees that are used to calculate prescription prices.

smallpox Acute viral disease that was essentially eradicated in 1979. It causes a disfiguring rash, headache, vomiting, and fever.

sodium One of the most important elements in the body. Sodium ions are involved in acid-base balance, water balance, transmission of nerve impulses, and contraction of muscles.

software A set of electronic instructions that tell the computer what to do.

solution A liquid dosage form in which active ingredients are dissolved in a liquid vehicle.

solvent The liquid substance in which another substance is being dissolved.

spasticity A form of muscular contraction.

specific affinity The attraction a drug has for particular cells.

spirits An alcoholic or hydroalcoholic solution of volatile substances.

spores A resistant stage of bacteria that can withstand an unfavorable environment.

standard code sets Under HIPAA, "codes used to encode data elements, tables of terms, medical concepts, diagnostic codes, or medical procedure." A code set includes the codes and descriptors of the codes.

standard precautions A set of guidelines for infection control.

standards Established by authority, custom, or general consent as a model or example; something set up and established by authority as a rule for the measure of quantity, weight, extent, value, or quality.

starter kit A group of medications provided to a hospice patient by the hospice pharmacy to provide a "start" in treatment for the majority of urgent problems that can develop during the last days or weeks of life.

State Board of Pharmacy (BOP) An agency that registers pharmacists and pharmacy technicians.

statins A class of drugs that inhibits the activity of an enzyme that forms cholesterol in the body. Statins are named as such because all of their generic names end with "-statin" (e.g., lovastatin).

statutes Rules and regulations resulting from decisions by legislatures.

statutory law The body of laws enacted by a legislative body with the power to make law.

sterile product A substance that contains no living microorganisms.

sterilization Complete destruction of all forms of microbial life.

stimulant laxatives Substances that stimulate bowel mobility and increase secretion of fluids in the bowel.

stool softeners Substances that decrease the consistency of stool by reducing surface tension.

subcutaneous injection The administration of medication by means of a needle and syringe into the layer of fat and blood vessels beneath the skin.

sublimation An unconscious defense mechanism in which unacceptable instinctual drives and wishes are modified into more personally and socially acceptable channels.

sublingual Pertaining to the area under the tongue.

subscriber The individual or organization protected in case of loss under the terms of an insurance policy.

subscription Dispensing directions to pharmacist.

succinylcholine A depolarizing, noncompetitive, neuromuscular blocking agent.

suffix A word ending that modifies the meaning of the root.

superscription Rx symbol.

supply dosage Refers to both the dosage strength and the form of the drug: the number of measured units per tablet of the concentration of a drug.

suppository A small, solid body shaped for ready introduction into one of the orifices of the body other than the oral cavity (e.g., rectum, urethra, or vagina), made of a substance, usually medicated, that is solid at ordinary temperature but melts at body temperature.

surgical asepsis The complete destruction of organisms before they enter the body.

susceptible host A person who lacks resistance to an agent and is vulnerable to contracting a disease.

suspension A liquid dosage form that contains solid drug particles floating in a liquid medium.

sustained release (SR) A capsule with a controlled release of the dosage over a special period of time.

sympatholytic drugs A group of drugs that blocks or inhibits the effects of epinephrine or norepinephrine on the cells that normally react to them.

synergism The cooperative effect of two or more drugs given together to produce a stronger effect than that of the either drug given alone.

syrup A liquid preparation in a concentrated aqueous solution of a sugar used for medicinal purposes or to add flavor to a substance.

tablet A solid dosage form containing medicinal substances with or without suitable diluents.

tablet triturate Solid, small, and usually cylindrically molded or compressed tablets.

tardive dyskinesia An abnormal condition characterized by involuntary repetitious movements of the muscles of the face, limbs, and trunk.

tare The weight of an empty capsule used to compare with the full capsule.

teratogen A substance that is capable of affecting the fetus.

teratogenic A substance that causes developmental malformation.

tetanus An acute, often fatal disease caused by an exotoxin produced by *Clostridium tetani*.

thiamin A water-soluble, crystalline compound of the B complex, essential for normal metabolism and health of the cardiovascular and nervous systems.

third-party payer The fee for services provided is paid by an insurance company and not by the patient.

time limit The amount of time from the date of service to the date (deadline) the claim can be filed with the insurance company.

time purchase The time that the purchase order was made.

tincture An alcoholic solution prepared from vegetable materials or from chemical substances.

tine test In this test, the tuberculin antigen is injected just under the skin with a multipronged instrument. The antigen is located on the spikes (tines) that penetrate the skin. If results are positive, the skin around the injection site will be red and swollen like a mosquito bite 48 to 72 hours after the injection. It is not as accurate as the Mantoux test.

T lymphocytes Lymphocytes that exhibit cell surface receptors that recognize specific antigenic peptide—major histocompatibility complexes.

tocopherol A fat-soluble vitamin essential for normal reproduction, muscle development, resistance of erythrocytes to hemolysis, and various other biochemical functions.

tolerance A reduced drug effect with repeated use of a drug and a need for higher doses to produce the same effect.

topical Pertaining to a drug that is applied to the surface of the body.

tort A civil wrong committed against person or property.

total parenteral nutrition (TPN) An intravenous feeding that supplies all of the nutrients necessary for life.

total volume The quantity contained in a package.

touch screen A monitor with a touch-sensitive surface, on which the touch of a finger makes a selection as a mouse pointer does.

toxicity The degree to which something is poisonous.

toxoid A toxin that has been treated with chemicals or heat to decrease its toxic effect but retain its antigenic powers.

trade name A drug name, followed by the symbol ®, which indicates that the name is registered to a specific manufacturer or owner and that no one else can use it.

tremors Shakiness of the hands.

TRICARE A federally funded comprehensive health benefits program for dependents of personnel serving in the uniformed services.

triglycerides Simple fat compounds consisting of three molecules of fatty acid and glycerol. Triglycerides make up most animal and vegetable fats and are the principal lipids in the blood, where they circulate within lipoproteins.

triturate To reduce a fine powder by friction.

troche A small, disk-shaped tablet composed of solidifying paste containing an astringent, antiseptic, or oil-based drug used for local treatment of the mouth or throat. It is held in the mouth until dissolved. Also known as a lozenge.

tuberculosis A chronic granulomatous infection caused by *Mycobacterium tuberculosis*. It is generally transmitted by the inhalation or ingestion of infected droplets and usually affects the lungs.

tubular secretion The active secretion of substances such as potassium from the peritubular capillaries into the tubules.

unit The amount of medication required to produce a certain effect.

unit-dose drug distribution system A system for distributing medication in which the pharmacy prepares single doses of medications for a patient for a 24-hour period.

United States Pharmacopeia (USP) A nonprofit organization that sets standards for the identity, strength, quality, purity, packaging, and labeling of drug products.

unit-of-use packaging The packaging from bulk containers into patient-specific containers.

upper respiratory tract Consists of the nose and nasal cavities, pharynx, larynx, and upper trachea.

users The individuals who work with computers on a regular basis.

vaccination The process of immunization for prevention of diseases.

vasoconstrictors Drugs used mostly to prolong the duration of action of local anesthetics or to help control bleeding.

vasodilators Drugs used to relax or dilate vessels throughout the body.

vector-borne transmission An agent is transferred to a susceptible host by animate means.

vehicle transmission An inanimate material (solid object, liquid, or air) that serves as a transmission agent for pathogens.

very low-density lipoproteins (VLDLs) Lipoproteins made by the liver to transport lipids throughout the body.

vial A small glass or plastic bottle intended to hold medicine.

vitamin A A fat-soluble vitamin essential for skeletal growth, maintenance of normal mucosal epithelium, reproduction, and visual acuity. This vitamin is also called retinol.

vitamin B complex A group of water-soluble compound vitamins.

vitamin B$_1$ A water-soluble, crystalline compound of the B complex, essential for normal metabolism and health of the cardiovascular and nervous systems. This vitamin is also called thiamin.

vitamin B$_2$ One of the heat-stable components of the B complex. It is involved as a coenzyme in the oxidative processes of carbohydrates, fats, and proteins. This vitamin is also called riboflavin.

vitamin B$_3$ A part of two enzymes that regulate energy metabolism. This vitamin is also called niacin.

vitamin B$_6$ A water-soluble vitamin that is part of the B complex. It acts as a coenzyme essential for the synthesis and breakdown of amino acids. This vitamin is also called pyridoxine.

vitamin B$_7$ A water-soluble B complex vitamin that acts as a coenzyme in fatty acid production, in the oxidation of fatty acids, and carbohydrates. This vitamin is also called biotin.

vitamin B$_9$ A water-soluble vitamin essential for cell growth and the reproduction of red blood cells. This vitamin is also called folic acid or folacin.

vitamin B$_{12}$ A water-soluble substance that is the common pharmaceutical form of vitamin B$_{12}$. It is involved in the metabolism of protein, fats, and carbohydrates. Vitamin B$_{12}$ is also involved in normal blood formation and neural function. This vitamin is called cyanocobalamin.

vitamin C A water-soluble vitamin that is essential for the formation of collagen and fibroid tissue for teeth, bones, cartilage, connective tissue, and skin. It also aids in fighting bacterial infections, bleeding gums, tendency to bruise, nosebleeds, and anemia. This vitamin is also called ascorbic acid.

vitamin D A fat-soluble vitamin chemically related to the steroids and essential for the normal formation of bones and teeth. It is important for the absorption of calcium and phosphorus from the gastrointestinal (GI) tract. This vitamin is also called calciferol.

vitamin E A fat-soluble vitamin essential for normal reproduction, muscle development, resistance of erythrocytes to hemolysis, and various other biochemical functions. This vitamin is also called tocopherol.

vitamin K A group of fat-soluble vitamins that are essential for the synthesis of prothrombin in the liver and are involved in the clotting of blood. These vitamins are also called quinones.

vitamins Organic substances necessary for life although they do not, independently, provide energy.

waiting period The period of time that an individual must wait to become eligible for insurance coverage (e.g., 30 days) before coverage commences or for a specific benefit.

want book A list of drugs and devices that routinely need to be reordered.

wheal An intensely itchy skin eruption larger than a hive.

xanthine derivatives A substance that is effective for relief of bronchospasm in asthma, chronic bronchitis, and emphysema.

zinc A metallic element that is an essential nutrient in the body and is used in numerous pharmaceuticals such as zinc acetate and zinc oxide.

Z-track method A method of intramuscular injection of medication in which the skin must be pulled to one side before the tissue is grasped for the injection of such medication. It is used when a drug is highly irritating to subcutaneous tissues or has the ability to permanently stain the skin.

Answer Key

CHAPTER 1

Multiple Choice

1.	C	5.	A	9.	C
2.	D	6.	C	10.	D
3.	C	7.	C		
4.	B	8.	A		

Critical Thinking
Answers may vary.

CHAPTER 2

Multiple Choice

1.	C	5.	B	9.	C
2.	C	6.	D	10.	C
3.	A	7.	C		
4.	B	8.	B		

Critical Thinking
Answers may vary.

CHAPTER 3

Multiple Choice

1.	B	6.	C	11.	D
2.	A	7.	A	12.	A
3.	D	8.	C	13.	C
4.	B	9.	D	14.	C
5.	B	10.	A	15.	B

Critical Thinking
Answers may vary.

CHAPTER 4

Multiple Choice

1.	D	6.	A	11.	C
2.	B	7.	B	12.	A
3.	D	8.	A	13.	C
4.	C	9.	C	14.	D
5.	C	10.	D	15.	C

Critical Thinking
Answers may vary.

CHAPTER 5

Multiple Choice

1.	B	5.	C	9.	C	13.	D
2.	D	6.	C	10.	B	14.	A
3.	B	7.	B	11.	B	15.	C
4.	A	8.	A	12.	D		

Critical Thinking
Answers may vary.

CHAPTER 6

Multiple Choice

1.	B	6.	C	11.	A
2.	A	7.	B	12.	D
3.	D	8.	B	13.	B
4.	D	9.	D	14.	C
5.	A	10.	A		

Critical Thinking
Answers may vary.

CHAPTER 7

Multiple Choice

1. A	6. A	11. B
2. C	7. B	12. C
3. A	8. B	13. B
4. A	9. B	14. C
5. B	10. A	15. B

Critical Thinking
Answers may vary.

CHAPTER 8

Multiple Choice

1. D	8. C	15. A
2. B	9. C	16. D
3. C	10. D	17. B
4. A	11. A	18. A
5. A	12. B	19. B
6. B	13. D	20. C
7. A	14. D	

Critical Thinking
Answers may vary.

CHAPTER 9

Multiple Choice

1. A	6. B	11. D
2. D	7. D	12. D
3. C	8. C	13. D
4. B	9. B	14. C
5. D	10. A	15. B

Critical Thinking
Answers may vary.

CHAPTER 10

Multiple Choice

1. A	4. D	7. C
2. B	5. D	8. B
3. A	6. D	9. D

Critical Thinking
Answers may vary.

CHAPTER 11

1. A	6. D	11. C
2. D	7. B	12. A
3. B	8. C	13. B
4. C	9. A	14. D
5. A	10. D	15. B

Critical Thinking
Answers may vary.

CHAPTER 12

Multiple Choice

1. B	6. B	11. A
2. D	7. C	12. C
3. C	8. B	13. B
4. A	9. B	14. D
5. D	10. C	15. A

Critical Thinking
Answers may vary.

CHAPTER 13

Multiple Choice

1. C	6. D	11. C
2. D	7. B	12. D
3. B	8. C	13. B
4. A	9. C	14. B
5. C	10. A	15. A

Critical Thinking
Answers may vary.

CHAPTER 14

Multiple Choice

1. C	6. A	11. D
2. A	7. C	12. C
3. C	8. B	13. D
4. C	9. D	14. B
5. A	10. C	15. D

Critical Thinking
Answers may vary.

CHAPTER 15

Multiple Choice

1. B	6. B	11. B
2. D	7. B	12. A
3. D	8. C	13. A
4. B	9. D	14. C
5. A	10. C	15. D

Critical Thinking
Answers may vary.

CHAPTER 16

Multiple Choice

1. B	5. D	9. A
2. D	6. A	10. A
3. A	7. C	
4. B	8. B	

Calculations
11. 1,038
12. 2,258
13. 657, 292
14. 276.5 after rounding up
15. 3,000
16. 57
17. $\frac{1}{3} = \frac{8}{24}$
18. $\frac{1}{51}$
19. $4\frac{11}{15}$
20. 1:8
21. $1\frac{5}{18}$
22. $140\frac{1}{2}$
23. $\frac{7}{18}$
24. $\frac{71}{8} = 8\frac{7}{8}$
25. $\frac{71}{72}$
26. $\frac{779}{17} = 45\frac{14}{17}$
27. $\frac{7}{8}, \frac{3}{4}, \frac{1}{2}, \frac{2}{16}$
28. $\frac{15776}{45} = 350\frac{26}{45}$
29. $\frac{1}{25}$
30. $\frac{22}{5} = 4\frac{2}{5}$
31. $\frac{12}{65}$
32. $\frac{31}{3}$
33. $3\frac{1}{2}$
34. 21
35. 4.72
36. 0.4, 0.044, 0.04, 0.0040
37. 111.1298
38. 0.063

CHAPTER 17

Calculations
1. weight
2. 1000
3. 1,000,000
4. 1
5. volume
6. 1000
7. 100
8. linear measurement or length
9. 10,000
10. 0.001
11. 0.002
12. 3000
13. 11,000
14. 5000
15. 0.009
16. 0.76
17. $2\frac{1}{2}$
18. 8500
19. 36,000
20. 3500
21. 20
22. 12
23. 12

39. 3020.6317
40. 76.58
41. 3.06
42. 23,850
43. 0.103
44. $100\frac{23}{50}$
45. 0.17
46. 40
47. 7.5
48. 1.5 tablets
49. 3
50. 125
51. 640
52. 0.445
53. 7.6%
54. 5%
55. 105
56. $75.96 is the amount of the discount. $113.94 is the discounted sale price
57. 20%
58. 11.1%
59. 6.4%
60. 75%
61. 67%

Critical Thinking
Answers may vary.

24. 180
25. $3\frac{2}{3}$
26. $2\frac{1}{3}$
27. $2\frac{1}{2}$
28. 8
29. 15
30. 20
31. 90
32. $3\frac{1}{3}$
33. $3\frac{1}{2}$
34. $1\frac{2}{3}$
35. $2\frac{3}{4}$
36. 4
37. $7\frac{1}{3}$
38. 48
39. 12
40. 24
41. 180
42. 64
43. 40
44. 10
45. $5\frac{5}{8}$
46. $\frac{3}{8}$
47. 8
48. 48

49. $5\frac{2}{3}$
50. 0.5
51. 7.5
52. 8
53. .226795
54. 0.28125
55. $1\frac{1}{2}$
56. $\frac{1}{4}$
57. 320
58. $2\frac{3}{4}$
59. 24
60. 1
61. 1
62. 0.026
63. 19,500
64. 300
65. 70
66. 0.14
67. 0.25
68. 600
69. 36,000
70. 7.5
71. 12,500
72. 2400
73. 12,760
74. 235
75. 8
76. 1
77. 125
78. 125
79. 45.25
80. 0.001
81. 5.524
82. 125
83. 90
84. 100
85. 8.5
86. 750
87. 0.0546
88. 14,000
89. 0.00001
90. 15
91. 0.000008 mg
92. 0.25 m
93. 65,000 cc
94. $\frac{1}{2}$
95. $1\frac{1}{4}$
96. 10
97. 225
98. $\frac{1}{200}$
99. 90
100. 1000, 1
101. 225, 15
102. 15, 15,000
103. 30, .03
104. 240, .24
105. 15
106. 4

107. 2496
108. 5
109. 75
110. 4
111. 30
112. 62.5
113. 2240
114. 7
115. 480
116. $\frac{1}{200}$
117. 300
118. 0.4
119. 480
120. 1400
121. 25
122. x
123. 75
124. 4
125. 900
126. 4480
127. $\frac{1}{600}$
128. $4\frac{2}{3}$
129. 320
130. 24
131. 880
132. 3 tablets
133. 3 tablets
134. 0.5 mL
135. 0.5 mL
136. 6 tablets
137. 40 mL
138. $1\frac{2}{3}$ caplets
139. 4 tablets
140. $1\frac{1}{2}$ tablets
141. 2 tablets
142. 2.5 tablets
143. 2 caplets
144. 2.5 tablets
145. $\frac{1}{2}$ tablet
146. 4 tablets
147. 5
148. $\frac{1}{200}$
149. 25 mL
150. 8 mL, 3 ii
151. 20 mL
152. 2.5 tablets
153. 2 tablets
154. 160
155. 7870
156. 2/9
157. 500
158. $\frac{1}{50}$
159. 10.3
160. 3.128

Critical Thinking
Answers may vary.

CHAPTER 18

Multiple Choice

1. A	21. C	41. B
2. C	22. C	42. C
3. C	23. D	43. B
4. D	24. B	44. A
5. D	25. C	45. C
6. A	26. B	46. C
7. B	27. D	47. B
8. A	28. C	48. C
9. C	29. B	49. A
10. D	30. B	50. C
11. C	31. A	51. D
12. C	32. B	52. C
13. B	33. B	53. B
14. B	34. A	54. C
15. C	35. C	55. C
16. D	36. D	56. D
17. D	37. B	57. C
18. C	38. A	58. D
19. C	39. B	59. B
20. B	40. A	60. D

Critical Thinking
Answers may vary.

CHAPTER 19

Multiple Choice

1. C	6. D	11. C
2. B	7. D	12. D
3. C	8. A	13. A
4. A	9. C	14. C
5. B	10. B	15. B

Critical Thinking
Answers may vary.

CHAPTER 20

Multiple Choice

1. D	6. C	11. B
2. B	7. D	12. A
3. D	8. A	13. D
4. A	9. B	14. B
5. C	10. D	15. C

Critical Thinking
Answers may vary.

CHAPTER 21

Multiple Choice

1. A	6. A	11. C
2. B	7. C	12. B
3. C	8. B	13. C
4. D	9. D	14. D
5. C	10. A	15. C

Critical Thinking
Answers may vary.

CHAPTER 22

Multiple Choice

1. D	6. B	11. A
2. A	7. D	12. C
3. C	8. B	13. B
4. B	9. D	14. A
5. A	10. B	15. C

CHAPTER 23

Multiple Choice

1. D	6. B	11. D
2. B	7. C	12. B
3. C	8. D	13. A
4. A	9. A	14. C
5. D	10. C	15. B

Critical Thinking
Answers may vary.

CHAPTER 24

Multiple Choice

1. D	6. B	11. B
2. B	7. A	12. D
3. A	8. C	13. A
4. C	9. B	14. C
5. B	10. D	15. B

Critical Thinking
Answers may vary.

CHAPTER 25

Multiple Choice

1. A	6. B	11. D
2. C	7. A	12. B
3. D	8. B	13. C
4. D	9. D	14. D
5. B	10. B	

Critical Thinking
Answers may vary.

CHAPTER 26

Multiple Choice

1. C	6. C	11. B
2. D	7. D	12. B
3. B	8. B	13. C
4. C	9. A	14. A
5. A	10. B	15. D

Critical Thinking
Answers may vary.

CHAPTER 27

Multiple Choice

1. B	6. B	11. B
2. C	7. C	12. D
3. A	8. B	13. A
4. A	9. C	14. C
5. C	10. B	15. D

Critical Thinking
Answers may vary.

CHAPTER 28

Multiple Choice

1. B	6. C	11. C
2. D	7. C	12. A
3. C	8. D	13. A
4. A	9. B	14. C
5. A	10. A	15. D

Critical Thinking
Answers may vary.

CHAPTER 29

Multiple Choice

1. B	6. A	11. C
2. B	7. C	12. D
3. B	8. B	13. C
4. B	9. D	14. A
5. D	10. B	15. B

Critical Thinking
Answers may vary.

CHAPTER 30

Multiple Choice

1. C	6. C	11. D
2. A	7. B	12. B
3. D	8. C	13. C
4. A	9. B	14. C
5. B	10. B	15. A

Critical Thinking
Answers may vary.

CHAPTER 31

Multiple Choice

1. D	6. B	11. A
2. A	7. D	12. D
3. C	8. A	13. A
4. B	9. D	14. A
5. D	10. C	15. C

Critical Thinking
Answers may vary.

CHAPTER 32

Multiple Choice

1. D	6. C	11. B
2. B	7. A	12. D
3. D	8. A	13. C
4. C	9. D	14. C
5. B	10. D	15. A

Index